Diagnostic Radiology
Paediatric Imaging

PIONEERS OF AIIMS-MAMC-PGI IMAGING COURSE SERIES

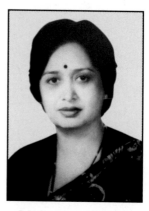

Manorama Berry

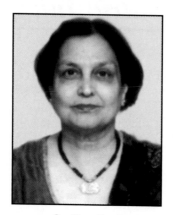

Sudha Suri

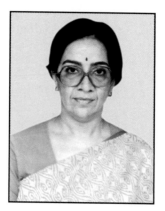

Veena Chowdhury

PAST EDITORS

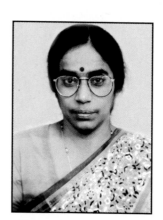

Sima Mukhopadhyay

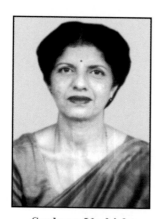

Sushma Vashisht

Diagnostic Radiology
Paediatric Imaging

THIRD EDITION

Editors

Arun Kumar Gupta MD MAMS
Professor and Head
Department of Radiodiagnosis
All India Institute of Medical Sciences
Ansari Nagar, New Delhi, India

Veena Chowdhury MD
Director Professor and Head
Department of Radiodiagnosis
Maulana Azad Medical College
New Delhi, India

Niranjan Khandelwal MD DNB FICR
Professor and Head
Department of Radiodiagnosis
PGIMER, Chandigarh, India

Associate Editors

Ashu Seith Bhalla MD
Associate Professor
Department of Radiodiagnosis
All India Institute of Medical Sciences
Ansari Nagar, New Delhi, India

Sanjay Thulkar MD
Associate Professor
Department of Radiodiagnosis (IRCH)
All India Institute of Medical Sciences
Ansari Nagar, New Delhi, India

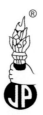

JAYPEE BROTHERS MEDICAL PUBLISHERS (P) LTD

New Delhi • St Louis • Panama City • London

Published by

Jaypee Brothers Medical Publishers (P) Ltd

Corporate Office

4838/24, Ansari Road, Daryaganj, **New Delhi** 110 002, India
Phone: +91-11-43574357, Fax: +91-11-43574314

Offices in India

- **Ahmedabad**, e-mail: ahmedabad@jaypeebrothers.com
- **Bengaluru**, e-mail: bangalore@jaypeebrothers.com
- **Chennai**, e-mail: chennai@jaypeebrothers.com
- **Delhi**, e-mail: jaypee@jaypeebrothers.com
- **Hyderabad**, e-mail: hyderabad@jaypeebrothers.com
- **Kochi**, e-mail: kochi@jaypeebrothers.com
- **Kolkata**, e-mail: kolkata@jaypeebrothers.com
- **Lucknow**, e-mail: lucknow@jaypeebrothers.com
- **Mumbai**, e-mail: mumbai@jaypeebrothers.com
- **Nagpur**, e-mail: nagpur@jaypeebrothers.com

Overseas Offices

- **North America Office, USA**, Ph: 001-636-6279734
  e-mail: jaypee@jaypeebrothers.com, anjulav@jaypeebrothers.com
- **Central America Office, Panama City, Panama**, Ph: 001-507-317-0160
  e-mail: cservice@jphmedical.com, Website: www.jphmedical.com
- **Europe Office, UK**, Ph: +44 (0) 2031708910
  e-mail: info@jpmedpub.com

Diagnostic Radiology: Paediatric Imaging

© 2011, Jaypee Brothers Medical Publishers

First Edition: 1997
Second Edition: 2004
Third Edition: **2011**

ISBN 978-93-5025-205-5

Typeset at JPBMP typesetting unit

Printed at Ajanta Offset & Packagings Ltd

CONTRIBUTORS

Ajay Garg MD
Assistant Professor
Department of Neuroradiology
All India Institute of Medical Sciences
Ansari Nagar
New Delhi, India

Akshay Kumar Saxena MD
Associate Professor
Department of Radiodiagnosis
PGIMER, Chandigarh, India

Alpana Manchanda MD
Professor
Department of Radiodiagnosis
Maulana Azad Medical College
New Delhi, India

Amar Mukund MD
Pool Officer
Department of Radiodiagnosis
All India Institute of Medical Sciences
Ansari Nagar, New Delhi, India

Anjali Prakash DMRD DNB MNAMS
Professor
Department of Radiodiagnosis
Maulana Azad Medical College
New Delhi, India

Anju Garg MD
Director Professor
Department of Radiodiagnosis
Maulana Azad Medical College
New Delhi, India

Ankur Gadodia MD DNB FRCR
Senior Resident
Department of Radiodiagnosis
All India Institute of Medical Sciences
Ansari Nagar, New Delhi, India

Arun Kumar Gupta MD MNAMS
Professor and Head
Department of Radiodiagnosis
All India Institute of Medical Sciences
Ansari Nagar, New Delhi, India

Ashu Seith Bhalla MD
Associate Professor
Department of Radiodiagnosis
All India Institute of Medical Sciences
Ansari Nagar
New Delhi, India

Atin Kumar MD MNAMS DNB
Assistant Professor
Department of Radiodiagnosis
Trauma Centre
All India Institute of Medical Sciences
Ansari Nagar, New Delhi, India

Deep N Srivastava
MD MNAMS MBA
Professor
Department of Radiodiagnosis
All India Institute of Medical Sciences
Ansari Nagar, New Delhi, India

Gaurav S Pradhan DMRD DNB
Professor
Department of Radiodiagnosis
Maulana Azad Medical College
New Delhi, India

Gurpreet Singh Gulati MD
Assistant Professor
Department of Cardiac Radiology
Cardio-Thoracic Centre
All India Institute of Medical Sciences
Ansari Nagar, New Delhi, India

Jyoti Kumar MD
Associate Professor
Department of Radiodiagnosis
Maulana Azad Medical College
New Delhi, India

Kushaljit Singh Sodhi
Assistant Professor
Department of Radiodiagnosis
PGIMER, Chandigarh, India

Mahesh Prakash
Assistant Professor

Department of Radiodiagnosis
PGIMER, Chandigarh, India

Manisha Jana MD DNB FRCR
Senior Resident
Department of Radiodiagnosis
All India Institute of Medical Sciences
Ansari Nagar, New Delhi, India

Naveen Kalra MD
Associate Professor
Department of Radiodiagnosis
PGIMER, Chandigarh, India

Niranjan Khandelwal MD DNB FICR
Professor and Head
Department of Radiodiagnosis
PGIMER, Chandigarh, India

P Singh
Additional Professor
Department of Radiodiagnosis
PGIMER, Chandigarh, India

Raju Sharma MD MNAMS
Additional Professor
Department of Radiodiagnosis
All India Institute of Medical Sciences
Ansari Nagar, New Delhi, India

Rashmi Dixit MD
Professor
Department of Radiodiagnosis
Maulana Azad Medical College
New Delhi, India

Sanjay Sharma MD FRCR DNB
Associate Professor
Department of Radiodiagnosis
All India Institute of Medical Sciences
Ansari Nagar, New Delhi, India

Sanjay Thulkar MD
Associate Professor
Department of Radiodiagnosis (IRCH)
All India Institute of Medical Sciences
Ansari Nagar, New Delhi, India

Sanjiv Sharma MD
Professor and Head
Department of Cardiac Radiology
Cardio-Thoracic Centre
All India Institute of Medical Sciences
Ansari Nagar, New Delhi, India

Sapna Singh MD DNB MNAS
Associate Professor
Department of Radiodiagnosis
Maulana Azad Medical College
New Delhi, India

Shailesh B Gaikwad MD
Additional Professor
Department of Neuroradiology

All India Institute of Medical Sciences
Ansari Nagar
New Delhi, India

Shivanand Gamanagatti MD MNAMS
Assistant Professor
Department of Radiodiagnosis
Trauma Centre
All India Institute of Medical Sciences
Ansari Nagar, New Delhi, India

Smriti Hari MD
Assistant Professor
Department of Radiodiagnosis
All India Institute of Medical Sciences
Ansari Nagar, New Delhi, India

Sumedha Pawa MD
Director Professor
Department of Radiodiagnosis
Maulana Azad Medical College
New Delhi, India

Veena Chowdhury MD
Director Professor and Head
Department of Radiodiagnosis
Maulana Azad Medical College
New Delhi, India

Vivek Gupta MD
Assistant Professor
Department of Radiodiagnosis
PGIMER, Chandigarh, India

PREFACE TO THE THIRD EDITION

The first edition of diagnostic radiology on Paediatric Imaging was published in 1997, while the second edition followed in 2004. The ever-evolving field of radiology and our commitment to our readers has motivated us to publish the third edition now.

Rapid advances are taking place in the field of imaging. This results in the need for re-evaluating and redefining the role of a modality in different clinical scenarios. Coupled to this, particularly in paediatric radiology is the need for ensuring patient safety. The industry has made significant attempts to minimize radiation exposures in imaging and this is pre-requisite that cannot be over-emphasized in children. Paediatric radiology is already a well-established subspecialty in the West, but in the developing world due to the paucity of trained radiologists in proportion to our population, every practicing radiologist needs to be aware of the special needs and disease entities in children.

The third edition of the book has been designed to include current recommendations, guidelines and existing knowledge on the subject. The content of all chapters has been updated, while some have been significantly restructured. New chapters have also been added. It is our earnest hope that our readers will find this text informative and that it will aid in their learning process and daily practice.

We wish to thank all the contributors from the institutions, i.e. All India Institute of Medical Sciences, New Delhi; Maulana Azad Medical College, New Delhi and Postgraduate Institute of Medical Education and Research, Chandigarh for their efforts in updating this edition. We would also like to express our sincere appreciation to Shri Jitendar P Vij, Chairman and Managing Director, Mr Tarun Duneja (Director-Publishing), Mr Subrato Adhikary (Author Co-ordinator), Mrs Samina Khan (PA to Director-Publishing) and other staff of M/s Jaypee Brothers Medical Publishers (P) Ltd, for their professionalism and dedication towards publication of this edition.

Arun Kumar Gupta
Veena Chowdhury
Niranjan Khandelwal

PREFACE TO THE FIRST EDITION

If we are to reach real peace in this world and we are to carry on real war against war; we shall have to begin with children

MK Gandhi

Just as paediatrics is now justifiably recognized as a specialized area of medical practice, so has paediatric radiology, in recent years gained recognition as a specialized branch of general radiology requiring specific knowledge of the diseases of the young.

Children are not merely "little people" or "young adults", nor are the disorders to which they are particularly susceptible, merely variants of the diseases of adult life. The paediatric radiologist therefore must deal with many disorders, some of which are encountered only in the young and others only in the newborn. This book although not a complete text on paediatric radiology, is aimed at touching upon some aspects of basic and up-to-date paediatric radiology. It covers both conventional radiology and advances in imaging. This incorporates a collaborative effort of many distinguished teachers who have contributed in their own ways giving us a unique opportunity to share the art and science of radiology.

However, reader must remember the words of Dr John Caffey, the father of Paediatric Radiology "A diagnosis is not made from a single type of examination such as a radiograph, but rather from a cluster of findings derived from history, physical examination and laboratory studies including a radiograph". Reader must therefore always remember the basic rule to interpret radiological features in the background knowledge of clinical and biochemical information. Our goal in this book has been to be concise, relevant and reader-friendly. We hope the readers will find it useful.

We wish to take this opportunity to thank Prof K Subbarao, Dr Ashok Khurana and our faculty colleagues from AIIMS, MAMC and PGIMER, for their active support, coordination and timely submission of the manuscripts. We also express our sincere thanks to the publishers M/s Jaypee Brothers Medical Publishers (P) Ltd for timely publication of this volume in the series of AIIMS-MAMC-PGI Imaging Courses in Diagnostic Radiology.

Manorama Berry
Sudha Suri
Veena Chowdhury
Arun Kumar Gupta
Sudha Katariya

CONTENTS

SECTION 2—CHEST

SECTION 3—GASTROINTESTINAL AND BILIARY TRACT, LIVER AND PANCREAS

SECTION 4—GENITOURINARY

SECTION 5—MUSCULOSKELETAL

SECTION 6—CENTRAL NERVOUS SYSTEM

PLATE 1

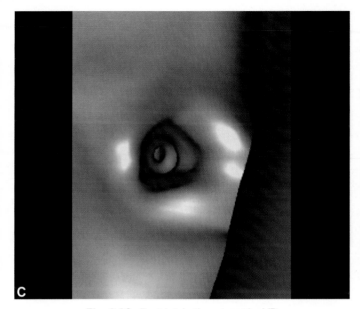

Fig. 8.6C: Post-intubation stenosis: VB

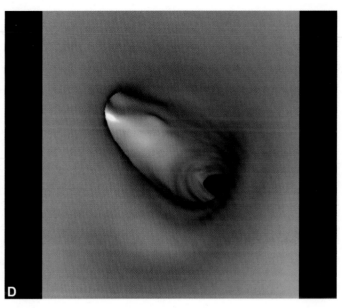

Fig. 8.17D: Inflammatory stricture: Confirm the main bronchus stricture with non-visualization of the distal airway

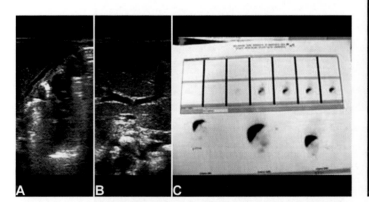

Figs 13.3A to C: Sonography reveals an atretic gallbladder. The length of the gallbladder is less than 19 mm with an irregular wall and an indistinct mucosal lining (A) Bile duct is not identified anterior to the portal vein (B) HIDA scan reveals no bowel opacification (C) Biliary atresia.

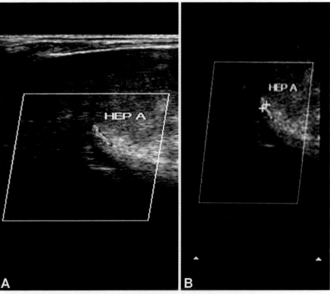

Figs 13.6A and B: Color Doppler showing color fill in of the hepatic artery which is enlarged. The diameter of the artery >1.5 mm – Biliary atresia.

PLATE 2

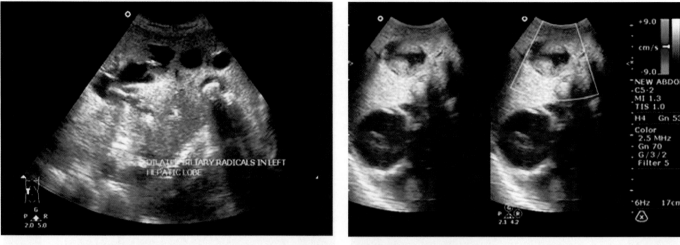

Fig. 13.21: Ultrasound images in an adolescent male showing multiple saccular areas of biliary dilatation within the liver parenchyma. Echogenic foci with distal acoustic shadowing seen in one of the cysts s/o intraductal calculi. One of the larger cysts shows presence of soft tissue along the walls

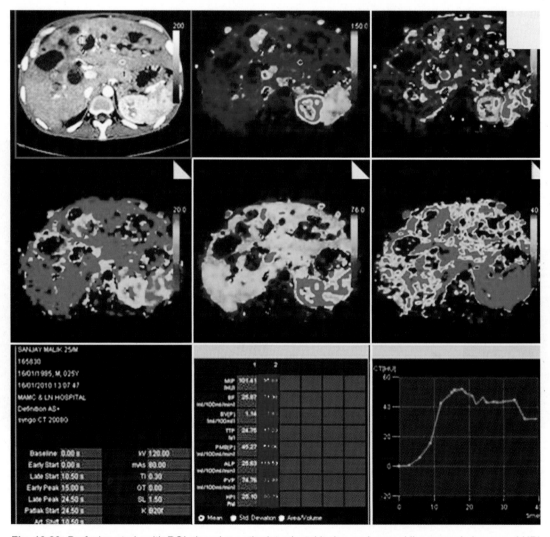

Fig. 13.23: Perfusion study with ROI placed over the intraductal lesion and normal liver reveals increased HPI values 80.79% for the lesion. Higher BF BV PMB HPI are observed. Biopsy revealed it to be a intraductal cholangiocarcinoma

PLATE 3

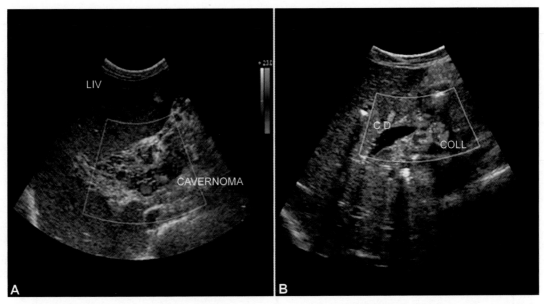

Figs 13.30A and B: Doppler images revealing multiple anechoic tubular structures replacing the portal vein with color fill in s/o portal cavernoma formation.There is extrinsic compression with resultant dilatation of the common bile duct – portal hypertensive biliopathy

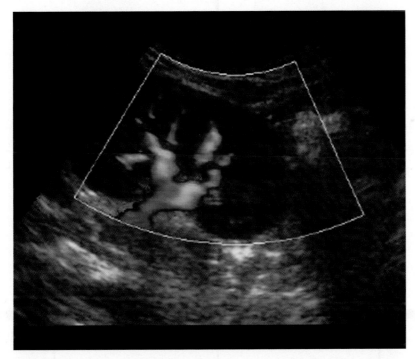

Fig. 15.1: Power Doppler ultrasound of kidney reveals a well defined area of altered echogenicity at lower pole, which demonstrates decreased flow and perfusion, corresponding to acute pyelonephritis

PLATE 4

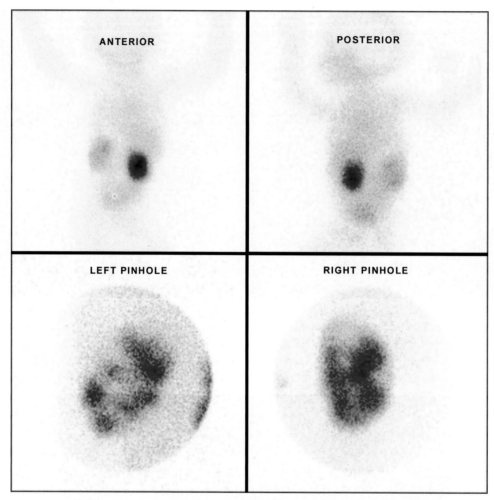

Fig. 15.2: ^{99m}Tc DMSA scan showing multiple photopenic areas in both kidneys, suggestive of pyelonephritis

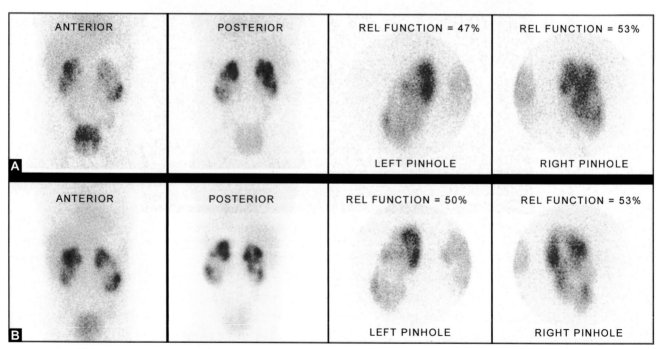

Figs 15.3A and B: Consecutive ^{99m}Tc DMSA scans in 2008 (A) and 2010 (B) showing persistent photopenic defects
in both kidney cortices, indicative of renal scarring

PLATE 5

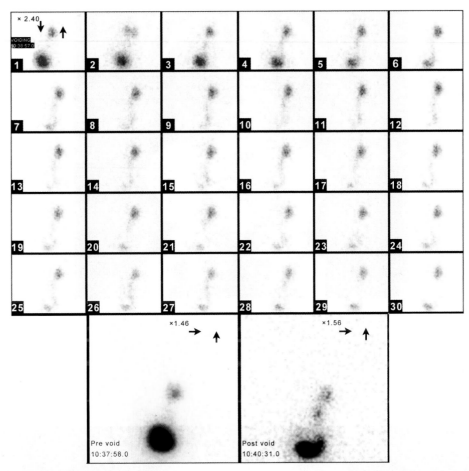

Fig. 15.7: ^{99m}Tc sulphur colloid DRCG: Retrograde movement of tracer is seen from the right kidney into the upper ureter, indicative of high grade right sided VU reflux

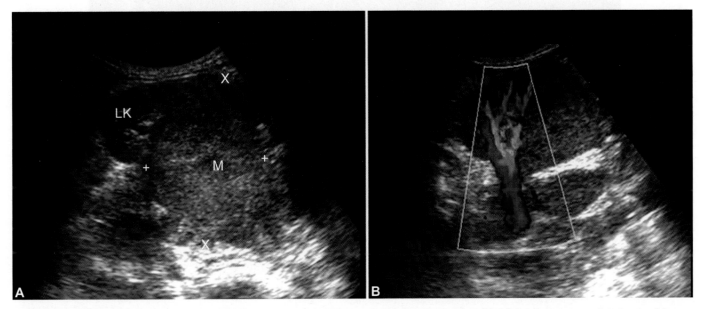

Figs 16.3A to E: Wilms' tumor in a 4-year-old girl – US, CT and MRI. (A) Longitudinal US through the left flank shows a well defined solid mass arising from the lower pole of the left kidney. A hypoechoic rim (pseudocapsule) can be seen separating it from the normal renal parenchyma. (B) Color Doppler image shows the normal intrarenal vasculature along with the patent left renal vein (C) Axial postcontrast CT scan shows the tumor as a hypodense, minimally enhancing mass with small low attenuation areas of necrosis. (D and E) Axial and coronal T2-weighted MR images show a well defined iso- to hypointense mass, with small focal hyperintense areas of necrosis and a hypointense pseudocapsule separating it from the normal renal parenchyma (displaced anterolaterally) exhibiting the positive 'beak" sign. Multiple retroperitoneal nodes are seen on both CT and MRI

PLATE 6

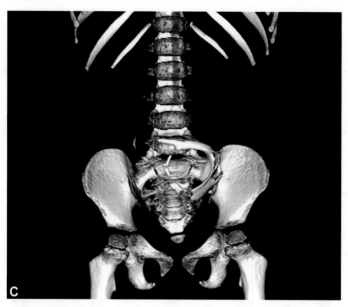

Fig. 17.4C: CT abdomen (A to C) demonstrates a pelvic cystic tumor with bony elements in axial (A), coronal (B) and volume rendered images (C) in a case of mature teratoma in a 3-year-old girl

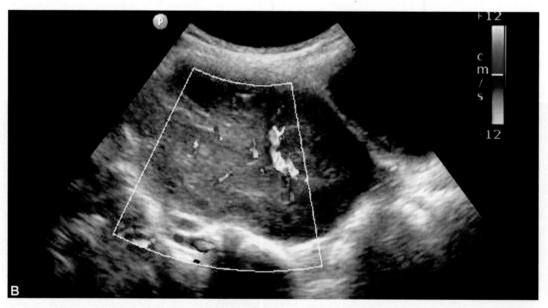

Fig. 17.8B: Dysgerminoma right ovary. Ultrasound pelvis reveals a solid pelvic mass in the right adnexa (A), which on color Doppler (B) demonstrates mild increased central vascularity

PLATE 7

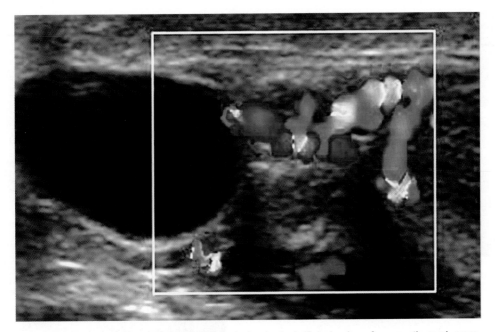

Fig. 17.9: Color Doppler ultrasound demonstrates typical dilated veins of spermatic cord, seen in child with varicocele along with encysted cord hydrocele

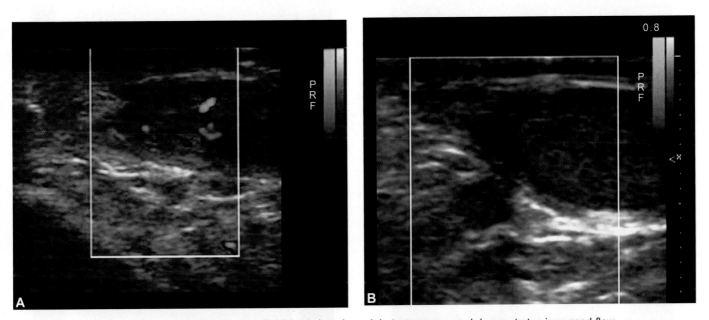

Figs 17.12A and B: Epididymitis. Epididymis is enlarged, heterogeneous and demonstrates increased flow on color Doppler (A). Normal opposite epididymis is shown for comparison (B)

PLATE 8

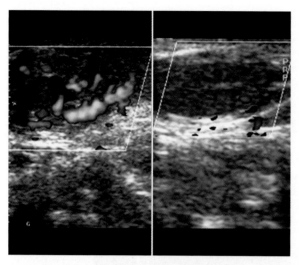

Fig. 17.13: Epididymo-orchitis in a 9-year-old boy. Ultrasound revealed enlarged epididymal head with heterogeneous echotexture of epididymus and testes, which demonstrated increased vascularity on power Doppler. Oppisite normal left testis is shown for comparison

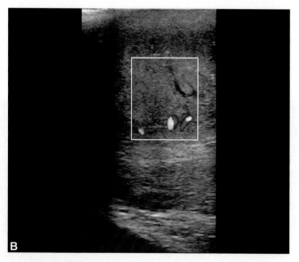

Fig. 17.17B: Ultrasound reveals diffuse leukemic infiltration of testes in a child with lymphoblastic leukemia

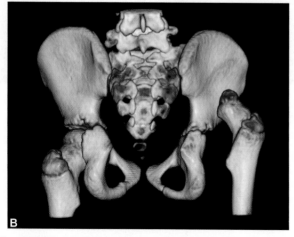

Fig. 22.25B: CT-VRT shows right femoral epiphysis dislocated superiorly and posteriorly

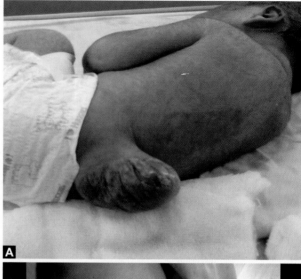

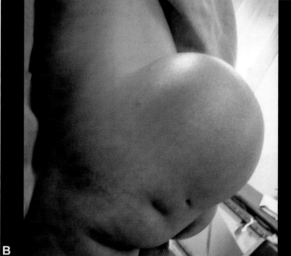

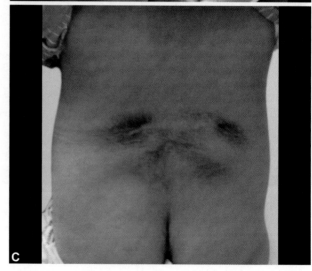

Figs 21.2A to C: Clinical photographs (A) One-day-old male child with meningomyelocele (Open spinal dysraphism). (B) Six-month old child with skin covered mass in lumbo sacral region showing associated abnormal skin dimples. Findings are suggestive of lipomyelomeningocele (CSD with subcutaneous mass). (C) Five-year-old child with split cord malformation showing tuft of hair at high lumbar region (CSD without subcutaneous mass)

PLATE 9

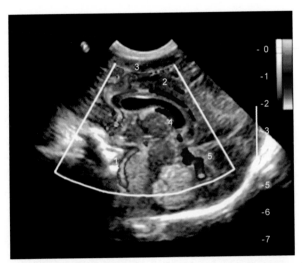

Fig. 27.3: Midline sagittal color Doppler scan showing internal cerebral artery (1), pericallosal artery (2) callosomarginal artery (3) internal cerebral vein (4) straight sinus (5)

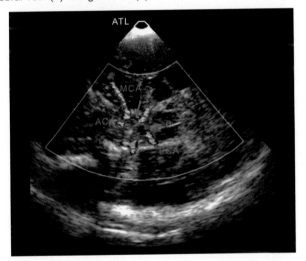

Fig. 27.4: Axial section through the squamous temporal bone showing the vessels of the circle of Willis. Arrow points to the posterior communicating artery

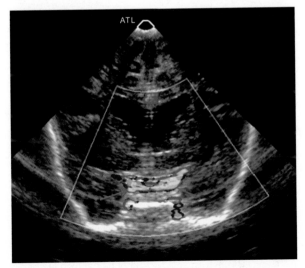

Fig. 27.5: Coronal CDFI scan showing ICA on both sides, arrow points to their bifurcation on both sides

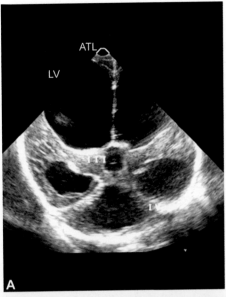

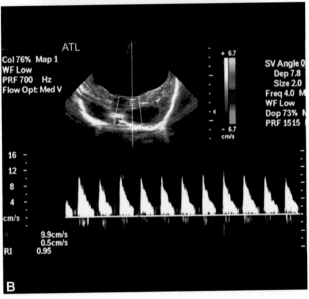

Figs 27.16A and B: (A) Coronal sonogram showing generalized dilatation of the ventricular system. (B) CDFI of the same patient showing markedly elevated RI in the MCA s/o increased ICP

CHAPTER **1**

Technical Considerations in Pediatric Imaging

Ashu Seith Bhalla, Arun Kumar Gupta, Amar Mukund

Technical factors such as the ability to position the patient and expose the radiograph with the patient immobile, which are often taken for granted in adult radiography, may appear as crippling problems in pediatric radiography. For this reason and because of the importance of minimizing radiation to the child, special attention must be paid to certain technical points. These will be discussed under the following five broad groups:

   I. Minimizing heat loss
  II. Immobilization
 III. Sedation
 IV. Reduction of radiation dosage
  V. Use of contrast media

MINIMIZING HEAT LOSS

Neonates and infants lose body heat rapidly, the risk of hypothermia being greatest in the premature baby with little subcutaneous fat. Local warmth may be obtained by special table-top heating cradles, but the most convenient way of avoiding heat loss is to maintain a room temperature of about 27°C in room. A room thermometer is an important piece of equipment. Enhanced humidity is not normally required for the duration of an X-ray examination.[1]

IMMOBILIZATION

Atraumatic immobilization is essential in order to ensure proper positioning and to minimize patient motion. Newborn babies and small infants need only soft sandbags and adhesive tape to stop movement. Towels and sheets can also be used to tightly wrap babies. Older, stronger children require wrapping on immobilization boards in addition to tape and sandbags. Special X-ray equipment is available which is designed specifically for the examination of infants and children. The essential factors for an immobilization device are (1) absence of artifacts, (2) safety, (3) no disturbance of the patient's sedation, and (4) ease of handling. It is not always possible to accommodate older children on such apparatus. Cradle holding devices are provided which enable the infant to be rotated in relation to the tabletop. When this type of equipment is not available, views such as the prone shoot through swallow for tracheoesophageal fistula may be obtained by using a device such as the Charteris baby holder inverted on the step of an up-right adult screening table.[1-3]

SEDATION

One fundamental technical component for imaging is the need for the child to remain motionless during the duration of imaging. Babies and infants under 6 months of age will often sleep after a feed and may not need sedation unless they are known to be restless, or the procedure is painful. Adjunctive measures such as sleep deprivation can also be useful. In older children verbal reassurance may be sufficient. Venous access produces less disturbance if a cannula is put in place after the area has been treated with a topical gel. Two possible area can be prepared about 30 mins before injection. Small gage needles are used, often 22 to 25 gage. Warming of contrast medium makes injection through fine needles easier and less painful.[1,4,5]

Sedation, however, is often necessary, especially for procedures like MRI due to its long duration, and for interventions due to the pain involved. Once it is deemed that both the procedure and sedation are necessary, every effort must be made to provide safety for the child. Even if the radiologist is not directly responsible for the sedation procedure, he or she must expedite the procedure in order to minimize the length of sedation. The timing of sedation and of the procedure need careful coordination.[1,5]

Monitoring the patient in the radiology suite is not an easy task for the clinicians. Observing children from the CT or MRI control room through a glass window is much more difficult for the clinician than direct observation at the bedside and increases their reliance on monitoring devices. Hence, adequate monitoring devices should be available. Pulse oximetry is commonly used during sedation. Monitoring is further complicated during MRI because the scanner generates strong static, radio-frequency and time varied magnetic fields which interfere with the monitoring devices. New nonferromagnetic monitors and cables have been deviced which are safe and reliable within the scanning suite. Standard ferromagnetic monitors if used need to be placed outside the magnetic field or carefully shielded.[4,5]

The radiology suite is a less than ideal environment for dealing with respiratory arrest or cardiovascular collapse. Hence, the most important prerequisite to sedation is the availability of adequate equipment for resuscitation and personnel experienced in managing sedation complications. If the radiology suite is not equipped with wall outlets for oxygen and suction, portable oxygen cylinders and suction apparatus should be available. Also, a cart with resuscitation drugs, defibrillator, and age and size appropriate equipment for different age groups and body sizes for purpose of oxygen administration and intubation are absolutely essential.[4,5]

Risk factors must be taken into consideration before planning sedation. If the child's condition is tenuous enough for sedation to be a significant risk, precautionary measures like securing the airway should be taken before the child arrives in the radiology department. Knowledge of both the past and the present medical history is equally important.

NIL PER ORALLY (NPO) STATUS

Aspiration is a significant concern in sedated children and NPO guidelines should be as stringent as those in children undergoing general anaesthesia. Guidelines recommended by American Academy of Pediatrics Committee on Drugs (AAPCOD) are as follows: clear liquids are allowable up to 2 hours before the procedure for any age; semisolid liquid (including breast milk) and solid foods are acceptable for up to 4 hours for children less than 6 months, 6 hours for children 6 to 36 months old and 8 hours for older children. Whenever possible these recommendations must be followed. Bowel obstruction or ileus are other factors that increase the risk of aspiration because they delay gastric emptying. In these patients, nasogastric suction of gastric contents should be performed and agents given that promote gastric emptying, such as metoclopramide. The actual risk of aspiration in children undergoing diagnostic imaging, is unknown, but it is probably quite low. In one recent report, aspiration of gastric contrast was present in no more than 4 percent of children undergoing CT scan examination in a setting of trauma.[4,6]

The practice of administering oral contrast material in children before sedation for abdominal CT is controversial. At some institutions, the practice of administering an enteric contrast material before sedation is being discouraged because it violates the "nothing by mouth" status that is otherwise strictly enforced before sedation. However, recent studies have indicated that oral contrast appears to be safe when using the sedation drugs like chloral hydrate and propofol. Further study of the safety of this practice is required.[7]

Pharmacological Agents

Several different agents have been successfully used for sedation of children for imaging studies. The choice of the agent depends on availability, local expertise and patient risk factors. The route of administration could be oral or parenteral. Intravenous route has the advantage of faster onset and reliable titration of dose. Other non-parenteral routes include the intranasal or rectal route.

The most commonly used sedative agents belong to one of the three classes of drugs:
1. Barbiturates,
2. Benzodiazepines, or
3. Narcotics.

The most often used *barbiturate* is pentobarbital. Others being methohexital and thiopental sodium. Pentobarbital and Quinalbarbitone are safe, effective oral agents in children under the age of 5 years. The *benzodiazepines* include diazepam and midazolam. Diazepam is not used routinely as a sedative for diagnostic imaging in children. Respiratory depression is the most important concern with barbiturates while vomiting is often seen with midazolam. *Narcotics* are commonly used as an adjunct to other sedative agents in situations where pain control is desirable in addition to sedation.[4,5]

Besides these three groups of drugs, other commonly used agents include triclofos, chloral hydrate, propofol, ketamine and a combination of meperidine (Demerol), chlorpromazine (Phenargan) and promethazine (Thorazine) {also known as DPT, or the "lytic" cocktail}, injected intramuscularly. Triclofos (pedicloryl) is a good sedative agent which can be used orally to sedate infants and children <5 year undergoing procedure or imaging. Maximum dose of 70-100 mg/kg body weight may be given.[8] Years of experience, ease of administration, and an excellent safety record have made chloral hydrate the most widely used sedative for children undergoing radiologic imaging. It is most effective in children under 2 years of age. Use of propofol by radiologists is not widespread due to its anaesthetic properties. Ketamine is a safe and effective agent for pediatric outpatient sedation and analgesia. Ketamine can be given by multiple routes and is one of only a few agents that are extremely predictable when administered intramuscularly. Furthermore, unlike benzodiazepines, barbiturates, and sedative/hypnotic agents; ketamine seldom causes respiratory depression. Ketamine, however, may cause raised intracranial pressure and should not be used when this is an issue. DPT has been popular as an analgesic and sedative to facilitate a variety of painful or anxiety-provoking procedures in children, but prolonged sedation times and the possibility of respiratory depression argue against the use of DPT in any setting. Table 1.1 enlists the routes and doses of frequently used sedatives.[4,9]

REDUCTION OF RADIATION DOSAGE

It is essential to limit the dose of ionizing radiation to children as much as possible. Based on information concerning the effects of low-dose radiation to atomic bomb survivors who were irradiated as children with doses that are comparable to those received by children in helical CT, it is now known that there is a statistically significant, albeit, small individual risk for excess cancer in patients with doses used in CT. Children are more sensitive than adults by a factor of 10 because firstly, they have more time to express cancers than do adults and also because they have more dividing cells. Also, girls are more sensitive than boys. Hence, applying the ALARA principle in imaging becomes especially important in children. Gonad protection especially is essential.[10-12] Reduction of dose during an examination can be done at several levels, i.e. rational use of referral criteria, modification of equipment and technique. The most important prerequisite is the evaluation of need for an examination and the choice of most suitable modality accordingly. Specific pediatric adaptation of equipment such as restriction devices, tubes for immobilization and a removable grid are very useful for dose saving. Besides modification of equipment, operator dependent factors, i.e. the technique is equally

Table 1.1: Sedative agents and antagonists for pediatric imaging[4,8]				
Agent	Class and Route *	Effect and Onset	Dose	Duration
Chloral hydrate	PO (PR)	Sedative	50-100 mg/kg; up to 120 mg/kg. reported. Maximum single dose 2 g	30-90 min
Pentobarbital sodium	Barbiturate IV (PO, IM)	Sedative 5-10 min	2-3 mg/kg dose titrated over 5-7 min until sedated, maximum cumulative dose of 8 mg/kg or 150-200 mg	40-60 min
Fentanyl citrate	Narcotic IV	Analgesic with sedative properties 1-2 min	1 mg/kg slowly IV over 5 min; adult-size paitents 25-50 mg/dose; maximum cumulative dose 4 mg/kg	30-60 min
Midazolam	Benzodiazepine IV (PO)	Sedative, anxiolytic, amnestic 1-5 min (IV)	0.02-0.05 mg/kg; titrate using half of original dose (over 2-4 min) based on effect and oxygen saturation; maximum of 1 mg	20-30 min

IV—Intravenous, IM—Intramuscular, PO—Per os, PR—Per rectum. Preferred route listed first with alternate routes in brackets

important.[12,13] Two major areas where reduction of radiation dose are critical are:
1. Radiography and fluoroscopy
2. Computed tomography

Radiography and Fluoroscopy

In procedures involving radiography and fluoroscopy, radiation dose reduction can be achieved at two broad levels:
A. Radiographic equipment factors
B. Operator dependent techniques

Radiographic Equipment Factors

- Use of increased film-screen sensitivity
- Use of digital radiography
- Addition of filtration
- Use of carbon fiber materials
- In fluoroscopy
  - Modern image intensifiers
  - Pulsed fluoroscopy
  - Last image hold up system
  - Dynamic recording on videotape for screening procedures.

Potential reduction using these changes have been studied by many investigators like Gozalez *et al* (1995), Martin *et al* (1994), Mooney *et al* (1998), etc. who found dose reduction ranging from 30 to 85 percent.[14-16]

Screen-Film Combinations

The choice of the optimal screen-film combination has the greatest impact on dose reduction. The higher the sensitivity of the screen-film combination, the lower the patient dose. A dose reduction by a factor of 8 to 10 in comparison to universal screens is possible when rare earth screens with a high speed are used. Generally speaking, for routine examinations (with the exception of some bone disease like osteomyelitis, battered child), screens with a speed of at least 400 should be used. Some authors recommend systems with a speed of 600 because the radiation doses are minimum and their use permits very short exposure times, which

also prevents motion blurring artifacts. These advantages outweigh the slightly lower resolution.[12,17]

Digital Radiography

Phosphor plates are now frequently used for intensive care radiography and even portable DR systems are available. Most modern CR and DR systems now effectively offer substantial patient dose reduction compared to screen-film radiography, however in pediatric radiography this may not be true due to lack of standardization in exposure factors due to lack of understanding of fundamentals of CR and DR technology.[18,19] Moreover, other advantages of digital radiography are the fact that images can be stored and transferred electronically. Repeated exposures are no longer necessary because the contrast resolution is sufficient over a wider range than with conventional screen-film combinations; in particular, fine catheters and tubes are clearly seen. Also modern equipment have integrated 'diagnostic reference dose levels'. This is defined as dose levels for typical examinations for groups of standard sized patients. Using these presets, exposure can be adjusted as per the patient's size and hence dose may be reduced. Despite these advantages, these may be counterbalanced by dose increases due to the radiographer's unawareness of possible overexposure, since the visible film blackening is standardized by the reading mechanism of the laser imaging device. So, in order to reduce the radiation dose all guidelines implemented for conventional radiography, including appropriate collimation, appropriate source-to-image distance (SID), focal spot size, and patient positioning should be practiced in digital techniques as well.[18,19] It should be emphasized that while doing various portable examinations and pediatric applications requiring manual tube settings, special care should be taken as there may be unnoticed increase in exposure.

Additional Filtration

Additional filtration can reduce the entrance surface dose considerably up to about 50 percent, depending on the material used. Its use has the disadvantage that the image contrast is deteriorated and the tube load is increased. Adjustable additional filtration should be available for all X-ray tubes, which are used for pediatric exposures (Bucky tables, fluoroscopic equipment and mobile X-ray units). The recommended materials for additional filtration are 1.0 mm aluminum and 0.1-0.2 mm copper. Steel filtration (0.7 mm) can also be used.[12,20,21]

Use of Carbon Materials

The use of carbon materials for patient support, in anti-scatter grids and for the radiographic cassette face, allows transmission of a larger portion of the X-ray beam. The overall reduction in the absorbed dose due to this measure is in the range of about 30 percent to more than 50 percent.[13]

Fluoroscopy

Image intensifiers: Direct dark room fluoroscopy delivers higher radiation dose to the patient than fluoroscopy with image intensification, and produces images of lower quality. The use of direct fluoroscopy should hence be discontinued.

Also, the size of the image intensifier determines the receptor dose rate. The rule is that because of the need for constancy of brightness at the image intensifier input, smaller sizes of the image intensifier require higher dose rates. A similar increase in dose occurs if electronic magnification is used. Two different dose rates should be available in order to select the lower dose for simple follow-through contrast studies, such as the barium enema, and to switch to the higher dose rate if a high contrast examine is needed, such as the tracheoesophageal fistula. Electronic magnification during fluoroscopy should be restricted to rare cases.[12,13]

Pulsed fluoroscopy: Pulsed fluoroscopy with and without grid controlled tubes reduces the effective screening time and hence, the dose can be dramatically reduced.[12,13]

Last image hold up system, Dynamic recording on videotape for screening procedures: Use of these techniques essentially contributes to a decrease in screening time by the operator and thus the dose.[12,13]

Flat panel detector units: Recently flat panel detector units have been introduced for fluoroscopic and angiographic use. These units offer high quality images. However the available studies do not show these units to be superior to conventional units with image intensifiers in reducing the radiation dose.[22,23] Hence, the guidelines implemented for conventional fluoroscopy should be followed to reduce patients dose.

Operator Dependent Techniques

- Field size
- Focus film distance
- Use of high voltage
- Shielding of sensitive organs
- Beam direction
- Avoid use of anti-scatter grid
- Minimizing fluoroscopic time
- Decrease in number of films

Studies in the previous decade have shown that operator dependent changes could lead to dose reductions of about 30-50 percent with no increase in the cost.

Field Size

This is the most important and most variable factor in the amount of radiation dose imparted to the patient and hence accurate field collimation should be meticulously followed. This is especially important in children because an increase in the field size in pediatric patients will cause a proportionally greater increase in individual exposure as compared to adults. This relatively higher increase is due to the smaller anatomical size of young patients. Compared to adults a similar edge length increase in pediatric patients will lead to a larger percentage of the body surface area being irradiated. Also because, upto 35 percent of the red bone marrow of infants is in the long bones of the arms and the legs, correct patient positioning and collimation in the transverse axis is also important when chest and/or abdominal films are taken.[12,13]

The actual field size also depends on a correctly functioning collimating system. In most machines, an automatic setting prevents collimation of radiographic exposure even if fluoroscopic field is collimated. This can be identified and switched off[12,24] (Figs 1.1A and B).

Five frequent reasons for bad collimation in daily practice, and consequently for oversized field areas, are:
- Lack of knowledge of age dependent anatomy
- No information on pathology
- Difficulty in patient positioning
- Difficulty in patient immobilization
- Difficulty in handling of the X-ray equipment

Permanent training and supervision of the technicians and young radiologists is needed to optimize collimation, especially in neonates. In a European survey on neonatal chest radiography only 15 percent of the films had an acceptable field size.[25] In chest X-ray inadvertent exposure of both the skull and the abdomen, and in abdominal films of both the chest and the legs is too high, thereby increasing the red bone marrow dose. Up to 40 percent of the red bone marrow of infants and toddlers is in the skull, and 25 percent in the femora of premature babies.[12]

Focus Film Distance

The radiographer should always try to select the largest possible focus-patient distance during radiography. For example the longest distances are used for the upright anteroposterior spine for scoliosis (up to 300 cm). On the other hand, the focus-film distances (FFD) for X-rays performed with mobile units in neonatal wards (mainly chest and abdominal films) are often too short (less than 80 cm, sometimes even less than 60 cm). Ideally, the focus-film distance should be at least 100 cm. Incorrect and varying focus-film distances are the most important factor responsible for over-exposure of patients in the intensive care units.[12,13]

Use of High Voltage

In terms of radiation protection, there is an important relationship between the absorbed dose and the voltage used. A reduction in the kV causes a steep increase in the relative dose. A basic rule of radiation protection is that voltage values below 60 kV should not be used for X-rays of the body, trunk and head. The highest possible kV should be used. An increase in the voltage up to

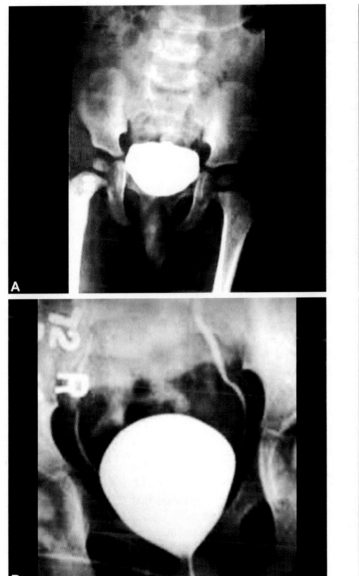

Figs 1.1A and B: MCU, AP view bladder area (A) without automatic setting switched off showing unsatisfactory collimation, (B) With the setting is switched off, desired collimation is achieved

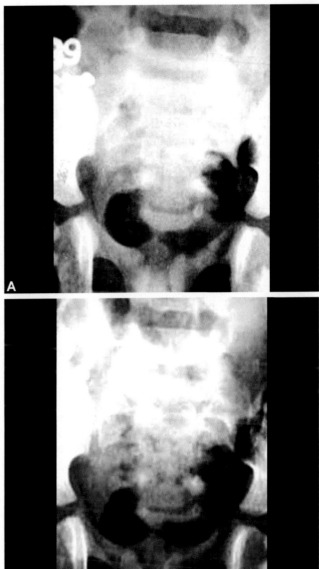

Figs 1.2A and B: Pelvis AP view: (A) Taken at 48 kV and 8 mA, (B) Taken at 58.5 kV and 3.6 mA. No significant difference in image quality, dose reduction by 28 percent in high kV technique

120 kV can diminish the dose slightly further, but is not at all useful in infants and young children because the image contrast is significantly degraded. Many generators cannot cope with the short switching times needed for high kV exposures. When voltage settings above 50 kV are used for small patients, one should use additional filtration to counterbalance the very small mAs-product, and thus allow for longer switching times.[12,13,24]

An increase in patient thickness causes an enormous increase in the required dose. The anteroposterior diameter in children up to one year of age is only 10-12 cm and is about 15 cm in older children up to five. In patients with a body diameter above 15 cm the dose increase is very steep. In order to deal with these relatively higher doses in school children, one should at first increase the kV-setting to avoid an undesirable concomitant increase in exposure time. This simple relationship is also important for fluoroscopy

when lateral views have to be performed during voiding cystoure-thrography. Increasing the kV not only reduces the dose but also shortens the exposure time and thereby reduces motion blurring artifacts. However, the scatter will be increased with the use of higher kV. Scattered radiation can be diminished if the irradiated volume can be kept small by good collimation.[12]

In a study in our department at AIIMS, the use of high kV and low mA in radiographic exposures was studied during micturating cystourethrograms, under fluoroscopic guidance. The kV used was about 25 percent higher and mA about 50 percent lower than the routinely used parameters. It was found that the resultant dose area product (DAP) value per radiograph during an exposure was 25-28 percent lower than the DAP value per radiograph at the routinely used parameters when the same degree of collimation was used, and comparable image quality was obtained[23] (Figs 1.2A and B).

Low kV settings for the bones are only rarely needed for special indications, i.e. mostly for special skeletal disorders (osteogenesis imperfecta, etc).[12]

Shielding of Sensitive Organs

The best gonadal protection is tight collimation to exclude the gonads from direct exposure. If this is not possible, gonadal shielding should be used. It is recommended that the gonads should be shielded when they are directly in the X-ray beam or within 5 cms of it, unless such shielding excludes or degrades important diagnostic information. Various gonadal shields are available. Every pediatric radiology department must have different size shields for the various age groups. Contrary to general opinion, it has been shown that shields like lead capsules, can be used in over 90 percent of cases for a voiding micturition cystourethrography without overshadowing the urethra, and even for pelvic examinations.

Effective protection of the ovaries is more difficult because these generally lie within the pelvis.[13] Ovarial masks (fixation of the shadowing material at the collimator) should be preferred over contact shielding which can be easily displaced during the examination, thereby possibly shadowing the hip joints causing a need for retakes.[3,25,26,27]

Beam Direction

Another important aspect for patient exposure is the beam direction {anteroposterior (AP)/posteroanterior (PA)}. The standard AP projection can be replaced by prone positions for a large number of examinations (Table 1.2). For example, the gonadal and breast tissue dose in gastrointestinal or urographic examinations can greatly be decreased using PA instead of AP projection. In addition patient thickness is decreased by compression of the belly in prone positioning, thereby decreasing the scattered dose.[12]

Anti-scatter Grid

Scattered radiation plays no major role in pediatric patients. Use of anti-scatter grid increases patient dose by a factor of 3 to 5. No grid is needed if the object thickness is less than 12 cm. No anti-scatter grid is needed for chest X-ray in patients upto 8 years of age, for the infant hip, for abdominal films in infants or for most of the fluoroscopic examinations (with the exception of double-contrast examinations of the gastrointestinal tract studies in older children). However, a grid is needed for imaging of fat patients (diameter over 15 cm) and for high kV exposures (over 90 kV). A grid ratio of 8:1 is sufficient for all pediatric examinations.[12,13,29]

In nearly all pediatric fluoroscopic examinations, grids are not needed, because no significant scatter is produced, especially when collimation is good. A removable grid is essential for pediatric fluoroscopy equipment. Gridless screening may reduce the radiation dose by as much as 50 percent. Infants under 1 year of age are always examined with the explorator grid removed since there is little scatter and no appreciable loss of detail. When fine detail such as mucosal pattern is not required, gridless screening may be used in children upto 5 years of age.[1,12,13,29]

Table 1.2: The possible use of posterior-anterior beam projection for radiographic examinations in pediatric patients[11]

Radiographic Examinations	Clinical Setting	Critical Organ
Skull	Trauma, ventriculoperitoneal shunt	Lens
Chest in lateral decubitus	Foreign body aspiration, empyema	Breast
Abdomen in lateral decubitus	Bowel perforation, ileus	Breast
Spine	Scoliosis	Breast, gonads
Abdomen post-contrast films	Intravenous urography	Breast
Abdomen	Enteroclysis	Breast

Minimizing Fluoroscopic Time

The most important factor for dose reduction in fluoroscopy is the limitation of screening time. This depends mostly on the clear definition of the clinical questions, on the patient's disease and on the radiologist's experience. Reduction of fluoroscopic time can be achieved by modifying some practices as a habit. Techniques like collimating fluoroscopic field before placing the child on the table and use of fluoroscopy only after satisfactory positioning of the child and the explorator are useful.[1,13,24]

Decrease in Number of Films

Tailoring an examination based on clinical problem and minimizing the number of films can significantly reduce the radiation dose.[13,24]

Computed Tomography (CT)

Various studies have established that CT scans performed in children result in a significantly increased life time radiation risk over adult CT, both because of the increased dose per milliampere second as well as the increased life time unit dose. This underlines the importance of dose reduction in pediatric CT examinations. In older helical CT scanners parameters were not adjusted on the basis of examination type or age of the child so that most pediatric CT scans were performed using the same parameters as for adult CT. Donnelly et al suggested a number of techniques for minimizing radiation dose in pediatric helical CT. Most important of these include reduction in mA and increase in pitch.[30,31]

Dose is directly proportional to the product of scan time and tube current. Hence, keeping other parameters constant, absorbed dose shows a linear relationship with mA. This has been shown by numerous investigators including Fearon et al and Donnelly et al in phantom studies.[30,31] Selection of most appropriate mA is a compromise between image quality and radiation dose. Phantom experiments have shown that an increase in mAs will always result in a decrease in image noise and thus an improvement in image quality. But at high tube current settings the gain in image quality will not be significant. Tube current should be adjusted to provide the lowest dose consistent with adequate diagnostic quality. A technique chart that relates current to patient's weight is appropriate. Scan time can be shortened by more rapid gantry rotation or by decreasing beam rotation to less than a full 360°. In general, the fastest scan time that uses full rotation should be used.[31,33]

Similarly it has been seen that radiation dose in helical CT is inversely proportional to the pitch used. When pitch is doubled, radiation dose gets halved.[31]

The dose increase caused by increasing kilovoltage is not linear, and is greater than often appreciated. An increase from 120 to 140 kilovoltage peak increase dose by approximately 40 percent. Pediatric patients are rarely large enough to warrant the use of increased kilovoltage peak.[33]

Newer multidetector CT scanners are equipped with automatic exposure control system (AEC) under different names (Care dose 4D, Dose right, AutomA etc.). These dose modulation systems work in various ways, so as to adjust the radiation dose according to the patient's body size and attenuation. AEC reduces the patient's dose without compromising image quality.[34,35] The radiation dose is essentially reduced by controlling the tube current which is performed by three methods. These methods are based on (a) patient size , (b) z axis and (c) angular or rotational AEC. Most of the scanners use combination of all these methods.[35] The scanner uses the projection radiograph data (topogram/scanogram) to assess size and attenuation of patient and accordingly dose is modulated using patient size and z axis. In angular AEC, the dose is modulated so as to equalize the photon flux to the detector while the tube is rotating. This is needed because the human body is non circular and hence the attenuation of the beam varies at different projections. Generally lateral projections are more attenuating than antero-posterior projections. By using AEC there is considerable reduction in the magnitude exposure dose, in the range of 35-60%.[36] AEC thus is helpful in reducing the patient's dose, especially in pediatric cases.

Despite these developments following facts should always be taken into account while performing a CT in pediatric cases. In a neonate approximately 30 percent of the marrow is contained in the skull and the marrow absorbed dose for a CT brain examination in a 6 years old patient phantom has been reported to be even higher than that for a CT chest or abdomen examination. Therefore, high priority should be given to dose reduction measures for head scans in children. Results of a study in our department at AIIMS also showed that a reduction of mAs from 115 or 141 mAs to 77 or 94 mA, which represents a 53-65 percent reduction in dose did not result in any significant difference in diagnostic accuracy although there was a slight reduction in image quality which was also not statistically significant,[37] (Figs 1.3A and B). Chest is a naturally high contrast area because of large attenuation differences that result from the presence of air in lungs and fat in mediastinum. Scans of objects with large differences in attenuation values such as lungs are less likely to be sensitive to image noise as image noise mainly affects low-contrast resolution. So, low doses may be used. Low radiation dose technique was used by Rogalla et al in their study of chest CT. Rogalla et al had found that although there is no consensus regarding which mA setting may be regarded as ideal low dose technique for spiral CT scanning of pediatric chest, 25-75 mAs is sufficient for lung

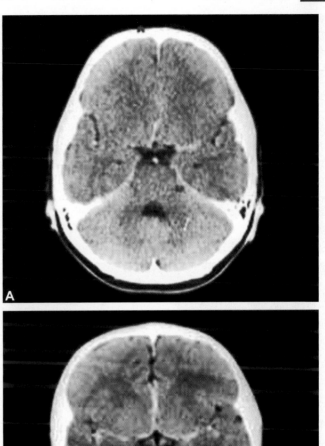

Figs 1.3A and B: CT head at 94 mA (A) and at 206 mA (B). No significant difference in overall image quality. Radiation dose in A is 50 percent of B

window and 50-75 mAs for mediastinal window. A mA of 77 (57.5 mAs) time represents a nearly 67 percent reduction in dose as compared to mA of 240 (180 mAs) with no significant loss of diagnostic information.[38] Our departmental study also showed similar results[37] (Figs 1.4A and B). Now-a-days most of the modern scanners provide CT dose index (CTDI) which is the most commonly used dose indicator. It does not provide the precise dose, rather it is an index of dose measured using a phantom. However, CTDI may greatly help in comparing radiation dose at different scanning parameters.[35]

Various manufacturers provide multiple protocols for different examination and as per the age of patient. Hence when imaging for children, pediatric protocols should be followed. Ideally, all institutions must set their own scanning protocol, involving various

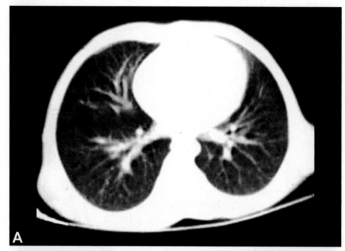

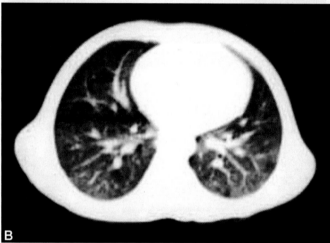

Figs 1.4A and B: Chest CT at 240 mA (A) and at 77 mA (B). Image quality is comparable while radiation dose in B is less than one-third of that in A

Weight	mA	
kg	Chest	Abdomen or pelvis
4.5-8.9	40	60
9.0-17.9	50	70
18.0-26.9	60	80
27.0-35.9	70	100
36.0-45.0	80	120
45.1-70.0	100-120	140-150
> 70	≥ 140	≥ 170

Table 1.3: Suggested tube current (mA) by weight of paediatric patients for single-detector Helical CT[38]

parameters (tube voltage, tube current, slice thickness, collimation and pitch) optimized as per the use. The important point to remember is that different manufacturers use different techniques for dose modulation so the user should know about the system's characteristics before trying to attempt any change in scanning parameters.[39] Any changes should be performed using appropriate (weight range) phantoms.

Recently dual energy CT scanners have been introduced which are faster and have ability to provide greater information about tissue composition than obtained by single energy scanners. Although not much is known about its use in pediatric cases, however with dual energy scanners non contrast CT scans are not needed as contrast media can be subtracted, and the patient is spared the radiation dose of a second scan.

USE OF CONTRAST MEDIA

Contrast media available for intravenous (IV) use in radiography are categorized as high-osmolality contrast media (HOCM), low-osmolality contrast media (LOCM) and isosmolar contrast media (IOCM). Considerations in choice amongst these are the concentra-

tion of iodine achieved within plasma and urine, economic factors, and safety factors.

High Osmolality Contrast Media

HOCM have an iodine content ranging from 280 to 480 mg/mL and an osmolality range from 1400 to 2500 mOsm/kg. Dosage of contrast material is based upon grams of iodine administered in relation to body mass. It is appropriate to use a dosage of approximately 300 mg of iodine per kilogram. This represents approximately 1.0 mL/kg in the most commonly used forms of diatrizoate or iothalamate. The total dose for excretory urography or for CT is usually 2.0 mL/kg in children or 3.0 mL/kg in the newborn.

Speed of injection is important for the resultant plasma concentration of contrast material. After rapid injection there is an increase in serum osmolality within 3 minutes, a decrease in serum sodium concentration, and an increase in heart rate. The osmotic effect is particularly significant in young infants. A mean increase of 3 percent in serum osmolality is observed in adults. Excretion occurs rapidly by renal glomerular filtration. Because of a high osmotic load, these contrast media also produce diuresis, opposing tubular resorption.[38]

Low Osmolality Contrast Agents

LOCM have an iodine content ranging from 128 to 320 mg/mL and an osmolality range from 290 to 702 mOsm/kg. Agents with low iodine content are most suitable for intra-arterial digital subtraction arteriography. Those with iodine content of 240 to 300 mg/mL are used for excretory urography, venography, venous injection digital subtraction arteriography, and bolus IV enhancement for CT scans. The contrast media with high iodine content, 320 to 370 mg/mL, are used for aortography and selective arteriography.

Iso Osmolar Contrast Agents

IOCM have an iodine content ranging from 270 to 320 mg/mL and an osmolality of 290 mOsm/kg.

Initial reports showed that the IOCM reduces the risk of contrast induced nephropathy (CIN) in patients with deranged renal parameters. However recently various meta-analysis of randomized control trials have shown that there is no statistically significant reduction in CIN associated with iodixanol as compared to LOCM.[39,40] Hence with this equivocal kind of reports IOCM offers no significant advantage over LOCM.

Unlike HOCM, LOCM and IOCM have little or no effect on serum osmolality, serum sodium, vasodilation, haemodilution, red blood cell morphology, or vascular permeability. There is little or no effect on the blood-brain barrier, fewer electrocardiographic changes, and fewer alterations in myocardial contractility, cardiac output, and left ventricular, pulmonary artery, and aortic pressures. There is less endothelial damage, and lower release or activation of vasoactive substances including complement activation, histamine release, and acetylcholinesterase inhibition. Diminished effects on coagulation pathways have been demonstrated. These effects are attributed to the lower osmolality and the reduced chemotactic effect of the molecules. Of importance is reduction in the nephrotoxic effect noted with HOCM. Hence, there are definite advantages to adoption of LOCM. A major consideration is degradation of the resulting examination resulting from pain, heat or vomiting with HOCM.[38]

Performing a multiphasic CT scans in neonate and infants may be challenging, as the IV cannula is of smaller gage limiting the injection rate of power injector, moreover only small amount of IV contrast can be used depending on the weight of the child. These situations may be handled by (i) using bolus tracking and saline chasing technique and (ii) large bore cannula.[41,42] An injection rate of 2-3 ml/sec is safe and provides good results.[40] Although there is no consensus, but contrast may be administered using central venous line with a maximum injection rate of 2 ml/sec.[41]

MR Contrast Agents

The most commonly used contrast agents are paramagnetic substances and amongst these Gadolinium diethylenetriamine penta-acetic acid (Gd DTPA) dimeglumine is most frequently used. Gd DTPA is excreted by glomerular filtration with 90 percent excreted within 24 hours. Rapid renal clearance, and low toxicity are important features of this contrast material. The clinical dose of Gd DTPA is 0.1 mmol/kg. It has an osmolality of 1,900 mOsm/kg. However, the high osmolality is of little importance because of the small volume administered.[38,43]

Although gadolinium-enhanced MR imaging was once considered one of the safer imaging procedures, but recently there has been a significant concern regarding nephrogenic systemic fibrosis (NSF) associated with gadolinium based contrast agents. The identified risk factors associated with development of NSF include - administration of a high dose of gadolinium-based contrast agent, acute or chronic renal failure, venous thrombosis and coagulopathy and vascular surgery.[44,45]

Some additional guiding principles for use of contrast in the neonates are:

1. Use warm contrast for maintenance of body temperature.
2. Use iso-osmolar+ve, non-ionic contrast in most instances.
3. When giving oral or rectal contrast, use low-osmolar, non-ionic agents instead of barium to avoid barium contamination of the peritoneal cavity.

4. Do not give contrast blindly; oral contrast may be aspirated, and rectal contrast may get into peritoneal cavity via a perforation. Even in the intact bowel, the contrast may not progress distally as quickly as predicted and therefore may lead to unnecessary radiographs.
5. Be judicious in the volume of contrast administered. Renal function in neonates is less than in babies over one month and age, therefore excretion of contrast may be delayed.
6. Gadolinium is the preferred contrast agent for magnetic resonance imaging. However, it should be used with a caution.[43,44,45]

In conclusion the aim of all departments and radiologists dealing with pediatric imaging should be to achieve a diagnostically adequate radiograph or examination, with minimum radiation exposure and discomfort to the child. This goal can only be achieved if the radiologists and technicians in charge are committed to quality control programs, and are aware of the necessity for radiation protection in children.

REFERENCES

1. Levick RK, Spriqq A. In Whitehouse GH, Worthington BS (Eds): Pediatric Radiology in Techniques in Diagnostic Imaging (3rd edn) 1996; 389-404.
2. Tani S, Mizuno N, Abe S. Availability and improvement of a vacuum-type immobilization device in pediatric CT. Abstract in English on pubmed. Nippon Hoshasen Gijutsu Gakkai Zasshi 2002; 58(8):1073-79.
3. Bontrages KL. Pediatric Radiography in Textbook of Radiographic Positioning and Related Anatomy (5th edn). St Louis: Mosby 2001; 629-64.
4. Frush DP, Bisset GS. Sedation of children for emergency imaging. RCNA 1997; 35(4):789-97.
5. Chudnofsky C, Krauss B, Brustowic Z (Eds): Sedation for Radiologic Imaging in Pediatric Procedural Sedation and Analgesia Maryland, USA: Lippincott Williams and Wilkins 2001; 169-78.
6. Lim-Dunham JE, Narra J, Benya EC, et al. Aspiration following oral contrast administration for pediatric trauma CT scans [abstract 46]. In 82nd Scientific Assembly and Annual Meeting, Radiological Society of North America. Chicago, Radiological Society of North America 1996; 137.
7. Ziegler MA, Fricke BL, Donnelly LF. Is administration of enteric contrast matrial safe before abdominal CT in children who require sedation? Experience with chloral hydrate and pentobarbital. AJR 2003; 180(1):13-15.
8. Iwata S, Okumura A, Kato T, Itomi K, Kuno K. Efficacy and adverse effects of rectal thiamylal with oral triclofos for children undergoing magnetic resonance imaging. Brain Dev. 2006; 28(3):175-7.
9. Frush DP, Bisset GS 3rd, Hal SC. Pediatric sedation in radiology: The practice of safe sleep. AJR Am J Roentgenol 1996; 167:1381.
10. Pierce DA, Preston DL. Radiation related cancer risks at low doses among atomic bomb survivors: Radiat Res 2000; 154:178-86.
11. Slovis TL. Executive summary, ALARA Conference: Pediatric Radiology 2002; 32:221.
12. Schneider K. Radiation Protection in pediatric radiology: How important is what? In syllabus of 20th Postgraduate Course European Society of Pediatric Radiology 1997; 95-101.

13. Protection of the patient in diagnostic radiology: Summary of the current ICRP principles, by Atomic Energy Regulatory Board: Mumbai 1987; 3-16.

14. Gonzalez L, Vano E, Ruiz MJ. Radiation dose to pediatric patients undergoing micturating cystourethography examinations and potential reduction by radiation protection optimization. Br J Radiol 1993; 68:291-95.

15. Martin CJ, Darragh CL, Mc Kenzie GA, et al. Implementation of a program for reduction of radiographic doses and result achieved through increase in tube potential. Br J Radiol 1993; 66:228-33.

16. Mooney, et al. Dose reduction in a pediatric X-ray department following optimization of radiographic technique. Br J Radiol 1998; 71:852-60.

17. Kohn MM, et al. Guidelines on Quality Criteria for Diagnostic Radiographic Images in Pediatrics. CEC Directorate General XII/D/3, Brussels, 1996.

18. Uffmann M, Schaefer-Prokop C. Digital radiography: The balance between image quality and required radiation dose. Eur J Radiol 2009; 72(2):202-8.

19. Willis CE. Optimizing digital radiography of children. Eur J Radiol 2009; 72(2):266-73.

20. Fearon T, Vucich J. Normalized pediatric organ absorbed doses from CT examinations. AJR 1987; 148:171-74.

21. Nicholson RA, Thornton A, Akpan M. Radiation dose reduction in pediatric fluoroscopy using added filtration. Br J Radiol 1995; 68(807):296-300.

22. Bogaert E, Bacher K, Lapere R, Thierens H. Does digital flat detector technology tip the scale towards better image quality or reduced patient dose in interventional cardiology? Eur J Radiol 2009; 72(2):348-53.

23. Chida K, Inaba Y, Saito H, Ishibashi T, Takahashi S, Kohzuki M, Zuguchi M. Radiation dose of interventional radiology system using a flat-panel detector. AJR Am J Roentgenol 2009; 193(6):1680-5.

24. Shah R, Gupta AK, Rehani M. Evaluation of radiation dose to children undergoing radiological examinations and reduction of dose by protective methods. (Unpublished data) Deptt. of Radiodiagnosis, AIIMS, 2002.

25. Schneider K. Evolution of Quality assurance in pediatric radiology. Radiation Protection Dosimetry 1995; 57:119-23.

26. Fendel H, Schineider K, Bakowski C, et al. Specific principles for optimization of image quality and patient exposure in pediatric diagnostic imaging. BJR 1990; 20:91-110.

27. Fendel H. Die zehn Gebote des Strahlenshutzes bei der Rontgendiagnostikim Kindesalter. Pediatric Prax 1976; 17:339-46.

28. Fendel H, Schneider K, Schofer H, et al. Optimization in pediatric radiology: Are there specific problems for quality – assurance in pediatric radiology. Brit J Radiol 1985; 18:159-65.

29. Drury P, Robinson A. Fluoroscopy without the grid: A method of reducing the radiation dose. Br J Radiol 1980; 53(626):93-99.

30. Brenner DJ, Ellison CD. Estimated risks of radiation induced fatal cancer from pediatric CT. AJR 2001; 176:289-96.

31. Frush DP, Donnelly LF. Helical CT in children technical considerations and body applications: Radiology 1998; 209:37-48.

32. Fearon T, Vucich J. Normalized pediatric organ absorbed doses from CT examinations. AJR 1987; 148:171-74.

33. Kuhn JP, Brody AS. High resolution of CT pediatric lung disease. RCNA 2002; 40(1):89-110.

34. McCollough CH, Bruesewitz MR, Kofler JM Jr. CT dose reduction and dose management tools: Overview of available options. Radiographics 2006; 26(2):503-12.

35. Lee CH, Goo JM, Ye HJ, Ye SJ, Park CM, Chun EJ, Im JG. Radiation dose modulation techniques in the multidetector CT era: From basics to practice. Radiographics 2008; 28(5):1451-9.

36. Söderberg M, Gunnarsson M. Automatic exposure control in computed tomography – an evaluation of systems from different manufacturers. Acta Radiol 2010; 51(6):625-34.

37. Shah R, Gupta AK, Rehani M M, Pandey AK, Mukhopadhyay S. Effect of reduction in tube current on reader confidence in pediatric computed tomography. Clinical Radiology 2005; 60(2):224-31.

38. Rogalla et al. Low dose spiral CT applicability to pediatric chest imaging: Pediatr Radiol 1999; 29:565-69.

39. Gudjónsdóttir J, Ween B, Olsen DR. Optimal use of AEC in CT: A literature review. Radiol Technol 2010; 81(4):309-17.

40. Currarino G, Wood B, Mayd: In Silverman FN, Kuhn JP (Eds). Diagnostic Procedures: The Genitourinary Tract and Retroperitoneum in Caffey's Pediatric X-Ray Diagnosis (9th edn). 1148-71, St Louis: Mosby, 1993.

41. From AM, Al Badarin FJ, McDonald FS, Bartholmai BJ, Cha SS, Rihal CS. Iodixanol Versus Low-Osmolar Contrast Media for Prevention of Contrast Induced Nephropathy: Meta-analysis of Randomized, Controlled Trials. Circ Cardiovasc Interv 2010; 3(4):351-8.

42. Heinrich MC, Häberle L, Müller V, Bautz W, Uder M. Nephrotoxicity of iso-osmolar iodixanol compared with nonionic low-osmolar contrast media: Meta-analysis of randomized controlled trials. Radiology 2009; 250(1):68-86.

43. Nievelstein RA, van Dam IM, van der Molen AJ. Multidetector CT in children: current concepts and dose reduction strategies. Pediatr Radiol. 2010 Aug;40(8):1324-44. Epub 2010 Jun 10.

44. Fleishmann D, Kamaya A. Optimal vascular and parenchymal contrast enhancement: The current state of the art. Radiol Clin North Am 2009; 47:13-26

45. Slovin TL: In Kuhn JP, Slovin TL, Halles JO (Eds). Neonatal Imaging: Overview in Caffey's Paediatric Diagnostic Imaging (10th edn). Penn Sylvania: Mosby 2004; 15-18.

46. Prince MR, Zhang HL, Prowda JC, Grossman ME, Silvers DN. Nephrogenic systemic fibrosis and its impact on abdominal imaging. Radiographics 2009; 29(6):1565-74.

47. Juluru K, Vogel-Claussen J, Macura KJ, Kamel IR, Steever A, Bluemke DA. MR imaging in patients at risk for developing nephrogenic systemic fibrosis: Protocols, practices, and imaging techniques to maximize patient safety. Radiographics 2009; 29(1):9-22.

CHAPTER 2

Recent Advances in Pediatric Radiology

Akshay Kumar Saxena, Kushaljit Singh Sodhi

The articles dwelling upon pediatric radiology are published not only in the radiology journals but also in journals in the fields of allied specialties like pediatrics and pediatric surgery. There is no strict definition of recent advances. For an avid reader, recent advances mean the literature published in last few months (say one year); for a research worker dedicated to a particular topic, only the articles published in that context would constitute recent advances while for a general radiologist, changing trends over last few years would qualify for recent advances. Given the vast plethora of articles available in medical literature and differing needs of radiologists, it is impossible to cater to the need of all. This chapter dwells upon some of the recent trends in speciality of pediatric radiology as applicable to Indian scenario. Readers are encouraged to update their knowledge by reading the recent journals.

RADIATION PROTECTION

The children are known to be at high risk for developing radiation induced malignancies. This is because the growing tissues are more radio sensitive. In addition, children have long life span available to manifest the ill effects of radiation. Hence, there is a need to keep the radiation dose to the minimum possible level in children. An Alliance for Radiation Safety in Pediatric Imaging (Image Gently campaign)[1] has recently taken shape with the objective increasing awareness in the imaging community of the need to adjust radiation dose when imaging children. It started as a committee within the Society for Pediatric Radiology in late 2006 and currently encompasses 56 professional associations globally. The ultimate goal of this alliance is to change practice. The initial focus of the alliance has been CT scan as there has been dramatic global increase in number of CT scans being performed for children. The alliance website (www.imagegently.org) provides information for radiologists, parents, pediatricians, medical physicists and radiology technologists. The alliance has evoked widespread interest. Already, the website has been visited over 300,000 times, the CT protocol has been downloaded over 20,000 times and 4528 medical professionals have taken the pledge. Recently, the alliance has started targeting radiation safety pediatric interventional radiology. It has been labeled "Image Gently, Step Lightly". It encourages the radiologists to "Step Lightly" on the fluoroscopy pedal during the pediatric interventional procedures. It also encourages the radiologists to use ultrasound or MRI for guidance during interventional procedures. The image gently campaign has been named to the 2009 Associations Advance America Honor Roll. This award is sponsored by the American Society of Association Executives to recognize the ways non-profit associations improve the quality of life in America. Detailed guidelines are now available for reducing radiation dose during fluoroscopy, CT scan and interventional procedures in children.[2-4]

NEURORADIOLOGY

CT scan of head is commonly performed for head trauma in children. However, very few of these patients show CT evidence of intracranial injury. Since CT scan imparts high radiation dose, it is desirable to minimize number of children who do not require CT scan after head trauma. Palchak and colleagues[5] conducted a prospective observational study to derive a decision rule for identifying children at low risk for traumatic brain injuries. They enrolled 2043 children and evaluated clinical predictors of traumatic brain injury on CT scan and traumatic brain injury requiring acute intervention, defined by (i) a neurosurgical procedure (ii) antiepileptic medications for more than 1 week (iii) persistent neurologic deficits or (iv) hospitalization for at least 2 nights. CT scan was performed in 1,271 (62%) patients of which 98 (7.7%) had traumatic brain injuries on CT scan. 105 (5.1% of 2043 enrolled patients) had traumatic brain injuries requiring acute intervention. Abnormal mental status, clinical signs of skull fracture, history of vomiting, scalp hematoma (in children ≤ 2 years of age), or headache identified 97/98 (99%) of those with traumatic brain injuries on CT scan and 105/105 (100%) of those with traumatic brain injuries requiring acute intervention. Amongst the 304 (24%) children undergoing CT with none of these predictors, only 1 (0.3%) patient had traumatic brain injury on CT. This patient was discharged from the emergency department without complications. The authors concluded that absence of abnormal mental status, clinical signs of skull fracture, history of vomiting, scalp hematoma (in children ≤ 2 years of age), and headache were important factors for identifying children at low risk for traumatic brain injuries after blunt head trauma.

Magnetic resonance imaging (MRI), diffusion tensor imaging (DTI) and MR spectroscopy are important constituents of evaluation of neonatal encephalopathy. Barkovich[6] and colleagues performed serial MRI in 10 neonates to describe the time course of changes in different brain regions during the first 2 weeks of life. In most of the patients DTI and MR spectroscopy revealed a characteristic evolution pattern during the first 2 weeks after birth. Although, the anatomic images were normal or nearly normal on the first 2 days after birth in most patients, abnormalities were detected on DTI and spectroscopy. The parameters tended to worsen until about day 5 and then normalize, though in several patients abnormal metabolite ratios on spectroscopy persisted. During the serial scans, the areas of reduced diffusion pseudonormalized in some parts while new abnormal areas developed in other parts. Thus, the pattern of injury looked very different on serial scans.

Liauw and colleagues[7] evaluated the predictive value of DWI and apparent diffusion coefficient (ADC) measurements for outcome in children with perinatal asphyxia. MRI was performed in term neonates with in ten days of life because of birth asphyxia. In survivors, developmental outcome until early school age was graded as: 1) normal, 2) mildly abnormal, and 3) definitely abnormal. For analysis, category 3 and death (category 4) were labeled "adverse," 1 and 2 were "favorable," and 2-3 and death were "abnormal" outcome. The study demonstrated that ADC values in normal-appearing basal ganglia and brain stem correlated with outcome independent of all MR imaging findings. However, ADC values in visibly abnormal brain tissue on DWI did not show a predictive value for outcome. Another study (by Vermeulen and colleagues) which evaluated diffusion-weighted and conventional MR imaging in neonatal hypoxic ischemia reported DW imaging to be a useful additional MR tool to predict the motor outcome at 2 years. In this study, local ADC values had a limited value. Recognition of the patterns of brain damage with DW and conventional MR imaging appeared useful as a diagnostic tool.

Although, ultrasound and MRI are frequently utilized for evaluation of neonatal hypoxic ischemic injury, there is striking paucity of prospective studies comparing these two modalities. Epelman and colleagues[8] prospective performed ultrasound and MRI of 76 neonates and young infants (age range 1-44 days; means age 9.8 days). Both the studies were done within two hours of each other. The diagnostic accuracy of ultrasound was found to be 95.7%. The authors recommended the use of ultrasound as screening modality with emphasis on correct technique. They also recommended early MRI for mapping delineating entent of injury.

Tovar-Moll F[9] and colleagues utilized magnetic resonance diffusion tensor imaging and tractography in patients of callosal dysgenesis to reveal the aberrant circuit. The study group consisted of eleven patients nine of which belonged to pediatric age group. Four main findings were reported:

1. In the presence of a callosal remnant or a hypoplastic corpus callosum, fibers therein largely connect the expected neocortical regions
2. Callosal remnants and hypoplastic corpus callosum display a fiber topography similar to normal

3. At least 2 long abnormal tracts are formed in patients with defective CC: Probst bundle and a sigmoid, asymmetrical aberrant bundle connecting the frontal lobe with the contralateral occipito parietal cortex
4. Whereas the PB is topographically organized and has an ipsilateral U-connectivity, the sigmoid bundle is a long, heterotopic commissural tract.

These observations suggested that when the process of corpus callosum fibers to cross the midline is hampered, some properties of the miswired fibers are maintained (such as side-by-side topography), whereas others are dramatically changed, leading to the formation of grossly abnormal white matter tracts.

MRI is considered inferior to CT scan in detecting calcification. However, susceptibility weighted imaging (SWI) technique can identify calcification by using phase images. Using this technique Wu and colleagues[10] were able to detect a partially calcified oligodendroglioma, multiple calcified cysticercosis lesions, and multiple physiologic calcifications in a single patient. The authors concluded that SWI filtered phase images can identify calcifications as well as CT scan.

Wang[11] and colleagues evaluated serial MRI changes compared to clinical outcome and evaluated their impact on clinical outcome in the follow-up of pyogenic spinal infection in children. In this study, 17 patients (age 2 months-16 years) underwent 51 follow-up MRI scans done 2 weeks-4.75 years after baseline scan. Follow-up scans done at short-term revealed epidural and/or paraspinal soft tissue changes which co-related with the clinical status and laboratory findings in all patients. However, in some cases progression of bone and disk abnormalities was noted in spite of clinical improvement. Long-term follow-up scans revealed soft tissue, bone and disk changes 1-3 years after initial scan in spite of these children being symptom free. The authors concluded that management should be based on the clinical response and that long-term or serial routine follow-ups are not necessary.

THORACIC IMAGING

Lung pathologies have traditionally been evaluated using radiography and CT scan. A few recent studies have explored utility of ultrasound and magnetic resonance imaging (MRI) in lung pathologies. Bober and Swietliñski[12] investigated the possible role of chest ultrasound in the diagnosis of the respiratory distress syndrome in newborn. Using transabdominal approach, they performed ultrasound examination in 131 consecutive newborns (admitted to the neonatal intensive care unit) in their first day of life with symptoms of respiratory failure. Retrohepatic or retrosplenic hyperechogenicity was shown in 109/131 newborns examined and the diagnosis of respiratory distress syndrome was confirmed by radiography in 101 cases. Respiratory distress syndrome was diagnosed in any patient without retrohepatic or retrosplenic hyperechogenicity. In eight patients with positive ultrasound images unconfirmed by chest X-ray (i.e. false positive sonographic examination), congenital pneumonia was diagnosed in four cases and pneumothorax in one case while in three cases no pathology was found. The authors reported 100% sensitivity and 92% specificity of ultrasound in diagnosis of respiratory distress syndrome.

Copetti and Cattarossi[13] evaluated sonographic appearance of transient tachypnea of newborn and its clinical relevance. They performed sonographic examination of 32 neonates with clinical suspicion of transient tachypnea of newborn (TTN) and compared the findings with 60 normal infants, 29 with respiratory distress syndrome, 6 with pneumonia and 5 each with pulmonary hemorrhage and atelectasis. They noted that in TTN the echogenecity of upper lung fields was different from lower lung fields. Specifically, the lower lung fields showed very compact comet tail artefacts while these were rare in superior lung fields. The authors labeled this as "double lung point" which had 100% sensitivity and specificity for diagnosis of TTN.

In another study, Copetti and colleagues[14] attempted to define the sonographic appearance of neonatal respiratory distress syndrome and evaluate its clinical relevance. They enrolled 40 neonates with respiratory distress syndrome and performed transthoracic ultrasound. In all the patients, sonography revealed echographic "white lung", pleural line abnormalities (small subpleural consolidations, thickening, irregularity and coarse appearance) and an absence of areas with a normal pattern (i.e. spared areas). When presented simultaneously, these signs had 100% sensitivity and specificity for diagnosis of respiratory distress syndrome.

Kurian and colleagues[15] compared the findngs of sonography and computed tomography in pediatric patients suffering from pneumonia complicated by parapneumonic effusion. In this retrospective study of 19 patients (age range 8 months-17 years), images were evaluated for effusion, loculation, fibrin strands, parenchymal consolidation, necrosis, and abscess. In this study CT of the thorax did not provide any additional clinically useful information that was not available on chest ultrasound. The authors suggested that the imaging workup of complicated pediatric pneumonia be done with chest radiography and chest ultrasound and CT be reserved for cases where the chest ultrasound is technically limited or discrepant with the clinical findings.

Montella and colleagues[16] compared the efficacy of high-field MRI and high resolution CT (HRCT) in children and adults with non cystic fibrosis chronic lung disease with the aims of assessing whether chest high-field MRI is as effective as chest HRCT in identifying pulmonary abnormalities; and to investigate the relationships between the severity and extent of lung disease, and functional data in patients with non-CF chronic lung disease. There were 30 children and 11 adults in this study (age range 5.9-29.3 years; median age 13.8 years. 14 patients each had primary ciliary dyskinesia and primary immunodeficiency while another 13 had recurrent pneumonia. All the patients underwent pulmonary function tests, chest HRCT (120 kV, dose-modulated mAs) and high-field 3.0-T MRI (HASTE; transversal orientation; repetition time/echo time/flip angle/acquisition time, infinite/92 milliseconds/ 150 degrees/approximately 90 seconds). The images of both HRCT and MRI were scored in consensus by 2 observers using a modified version of the Helbich scoring system. The maximal score was 25. HRCT and high-field MRI total scores were 11 (range: 1-20) and 11 (range: 1-17), respectively. There was good agreement between the 2 techniques for all scores (r > 0.8). HRCT and MRI total

scores, and extent of bronchiectasis scores were significantly related to pulmonary function tests (r = -0.4, P < 0.05). The MRI mucus plugging score was also significantly related to pulmonary function tests (r = -0.4, P < 0.05). The authors concluded that high-field 3.0-T MRI of chest appears to be as effective as HRCT in assessing the extent and severity of lung abnormalities in non-CF chronic lung diseases, and it might be a reliable radiation-free option to HRCT.

Bannier and colleagues[17] evaluated the sensitivity of hyperpolarized helium (3He) MRI for the detection of peripheral airway obstruction in younger cystic fibrosis (CF) patients showing normal spirometric results and the immediate effects of a single chest physical therapy (CPT) session. The study involved ten children of 8-16 years of age. Spirometry followed by proton and hyperpolarized 3He three-dimensional lung imaging were performed on a 1.5-Tesla MR unit before and after 20 minutes of CPT. The number of ventilation defects per image (VDI) and the ventilated lung fraction (VF) were quantified. Despite spirometery being normal in all the patients, ventilation defects were found in all patients (mean VDI, 5.1 ± 1.9; mean global VF, 78.5% ± 12.3; and mean peripheral VF, 75.5% ± 17.1). This was well above the VDI in healthy subjects (1.6) as reported in literature. After CPT, although disparate changes in the distribution of ventilation defects were observed, the average VDI and VF did not change significantly.

Tracheomalacia is characterized by excessive collapsibility of trachea in expiration. Lee and colleagues[18] evaluated air trapping in pediatric patients with and without tracheomalacia. In this retrospective study, the study group and comparison group had 15 patients each. Tracheomalacia was diagnosed if the cross sectional luminal area of trachea decreased by ≥ 50% during expiration as seen on CT scan and confirmed by bronchoscopy. The authors graded the severity of air trapping visually on a 5 point score. All the patients with tracheomalacia and 10/15 children without tracheomalacia showed air trapping. The median air trapping score was significantly higher (p = 0.002) in the study group. However, the patterns of air trapping were not significantly different. These findings have potential implications for diagnosis and management of children with tracheomalacia.

Chest radiography, catheter angiography and echocardiography have remained the mainstay of evaluation of patients with heart disease. With the recent availability of advanced multidetector scanners, it has now become possible to evaluate congenital heart diseases using CT scan. Cheng and colleagues[19] evaluated the clinical value of low-dose prospective ECG-triggered dual source CT angiography (DSCT) in infants and children with complex congenital cardiac diseases. They compared DSCT findings with transthoracic echocardiography (TTE). The study include 35 patients with the age range of 2 months-6 years. They demonstrated high sensitivity (97.3%) and specificity (99.8%) with mean effective dose of 0.38 ± 0.09 mSv. In this study, the subjective mean image quality score was 4.3 ± 0.7 using a five point scale. Another study evaluated[20] step-and-shoot DSCT for evaluation of heart coronary artery and other thoracic structures in young children (age <6 years) with congenital heart disease. They utilized prospective gating with end systolic reconstruction. The image quality was evaluated using a five point scoring system. They reported mean image quality score of 4.7 ± 0.6 and mean effective radiation dose of 0.26 ± 1.6 mSv.

GASTROINTESTINAL IMAGING

Necrotizing enterocolitis (NEC) refers almost exclusively to an idiopathic, often severe, enterocolitis that occurs in neonates with premature babies being more at risk.[21] The radiological evaluation is traditionally dependent upon radiography. Although there are sporadic reports of use of ultrasound in NEC, the first comprehensive evaluation of NEC with abdominal sonography was reported by Faingold and colleagues.[22] They enrolled 30 control and 32 neonated of proven or suspected NEC. They performed color Doppler of the bowel wall and described the normal and abnormal flow patterns. In this study, the sensitivity of absent flow in bowel wall on color Doppler, as marker for severe NEC, was 100% . This was significantly superior to 40% sensitivity of abdominal radiography which relied upon free air as sign of severe NEC.

A recent study[23] reported the findings of ultrasonography in early NEC. The authors evaluated 40 neonates with clinically diagnosed NEC and 10 controls. They evaluated the echogenicity of the bowel wall, involved region, ascites, and portal venous gas at initial and follow-up examinations. Echogenic dots were seen in bowel wall in 16 patients (40%) and dense granular echogenicities in 24 patients (60%). Portal venous gas was not visualized in any of the patients. None of the neonates in control group had echogenic foci in bowel wall. Follow-up examinations revealed decrease in the echogenicity of the bowel wall and ascites in 37 patients (93%).

Silva and colleague,[24] in a retrospective study (Ref), correlated the sonographic findings with clinical outcome in 40 neonates. They divided the patients into two groups based on outcome— group A included neonates who were treated medically and who recovered fully while the group B included neonates who required surgery for perforation in the acute setting (laparotomy or placement of a peritoneal drain), surgery for late strictures or those who died as a result of NEC. They calculated the risk ratios and 95% confidence intervals (CI) for those features for different sonographic patterns. They reported that an adverse outcome was associated with the sonographic findings of free gas, focal fluid collections or three or more of the following: increased bowel wall echogenicity, absent bowel perfusion, portal venous gas, bowel wall thinning, bowel wall thickening, free fluid with echoes and intramural gas. Interestingly, in this study, two babies in group A revealed absent flow in bowel wall suggesting that absent flow in bowel wall need not always be associated with adverse outcome.

Dilli and colleagues[25] also reported sonographic findings in NEC. They stated that sonography had high specificity but low sensitivity for detection of portal venous gas. In addition, sonography provided valuable information regarding intra-abdominal collections.

Bora and colleagues[26] evaluated the role of post natal superior mesenteric artery (SMA) flow in predicting feed intolerance and NEC in the babies of mothers showing absent end diastolic flow in umbilical arteries during antenatal sonography. There were three groups in this study: group 1 (n = 23) was small for gestational age with mothers having absent end diastolic flow; group 2 was small for gestational age (n = 20) while the group 3 was appropriate for gestational age (n = 19). Antenatal color Doppler revealed normal umbilical artery blood flow in group 2 and 3. In all the patients, postnatal superior mesenteric artery color Doppler was performed before test feed (0.5 ml) and repeated every 15 minutes till one hour after administration of test feed. The study revealed higher incidence of NEC and feed intolerance in group 1. The study also suggested that serial SMA flow evaluation, especially the 60 minutes post feed study may help in identifying babies likely to develop feed intolerance.

Extrahepatic biliary atresia (EHBA) and neonatal hepatitis are two important causes of neonatal conjugated hyperbilirubinemia. Together, they account for 60 - 90 percent of patients.[27,28] It is essential to differentiate between these two entities as the treatment is completely different. Some of the recent articles have utilized ultrasound and/or color Doppler for evaluation of babies suspected of having EHBA. Humphrey and Stringer[29] performed sonographic evaluation of 90 infants with conjugated hyperbilirubinemia for gallbladder morphology, triangular cord sign, presence of a common bile duct, liver size and echotexture, splenic appearance, and vascular anatomy. Using all of the above mentioned features, they were able to correctly classify 88/90 infants as having or not having EHBA (98% accuracy). The features with the greatest individual sensitivity and specificity, respectively, in the diagnosis of BA were triangular cord sign had sensitivity of 73% and specificity of 100% for diagnosis of EHBA. Corresponding figures were 91 percent and 95 percent for abnormal gallbladder wall; 70% and 100% for gallbladder shape, and 93% and 92% for absent common bile duct. The hepatic artery had statistically significant ($p < 0.001$) larger diameter in infants with EHBA than in those without EHBA. However, portal vein diameters were not significantly different between the two groups.

Kim and colleagues[30] prospectively evaluated prospectively evaluate the accuracy of hepatic artery diameter and hepatic artery diameter-to-portal vein diameter ratio for ultrasonographic diagnosis of biliary atresia. The diameter of right hepatic artery and the ratio of hepatic artery diameter-to-portal vein diameter were larger in the EHBA group. The authors suggested right hepatic arterial diameter of 1.5 mm and hepatic artery diameter-to-portal vein diameter ratio of 0.45 as optimal cut off values for diagnosis of EHBA.

Lee and colleagues[31] described the color Doppler ultrasonographic findings in livers of neonates with EHBA and compared them with US findings in livers of neonates with non-BA and control subjects. The study included 64 patients of neonatal cholestasis of which 29 had EHBA. In additional, they enrolled 19 control subjects. The authors evaluated the triangular cord sign and hepatic subcapsular flow. The images were interpreted by three pediatric radiologists independently and discrepancies were resolved by consensus. The triangular cord sign had sensitivity of 62% and specificity of 100% for diagnosis of EHBA.

Hepatic subcapsular flow on color Doppler had sensitivity and specificity of 100% and 86% respectively for diagnosis EHBA on the basis of consensus reading.

The gold standard for diagnosis of EHBA is intraoperative cholangiogram.[32] Unfortunately, some infants are found not to have EHBA on per-operative cholangiogram. In a retrospective study, Nwomeh and colleagues[33] evaluated the contribution of percutaneous cholecysto-cholangiography in preventing unnecessary laparotomy in infants with cholestatic jaundice. The study included 35 infants of which 9 had sonographically visible gallbladder. In these patients ultrasound guided percutaneous cholecysto-cholangiography was performed and diagnosis of EHBA excluded. This obviated the need of laparotomy in these patients.

Rectal bleeding is commonly evaluated using CT colonoscopy (CTC) in adult population. However, this modality has not been extensively used in pediatric population. Anupindi and colleagues[34] evaluated eight (3-17 years of age) children with non contrast CTC and reported it to be a well tolerated, safe and useful investigation. The estimated mean effective dose in this study for CTC was 2.17 mSv as compared to 5-6 mSv for a standard air contrast barium enema in a small child. Capuñay and colleagues[35] performed 100 CTC studies in children with rectal bleeding. No complications were encountered. They reported sensitivity and specificity of 89% and 80% of CTC in diagnosis of elevated colonic lesions. The authors concluded that virtual colonoscopy is an alternative method for the evaluation of children with elevated lesions. It is fast, has no complications, and uses a low radiation dose. The postulated advantages of using CTC included diagnosis of the exact location of the polyp, faster and easier polypectomy by conventional colonoscopist, reduction in the time of anesthesia and less complications related to conventional colonoscopy procedure.

Sugiyama et al[36] evaluated the feasibility of single scan CTC using polyethylene glycol electrolytes solution with contrast medium (PEG-C) bowel preparation in children. Seven patients suspected of colorectal elevated lesions were subjected to CTC. All patients underwent bowel preparation using PEG at a dose of 32 ± 3 ml/kgBW during the evening before the day of CTC. The water-soluble contrast agent (Gastrografin, Nihon Schering, Osaka, Japan) was given to the patients orally or through a nasogastric tube at a dose of 0.6 ± 0.1 ml/kgBW, the next morning. The water-soluble contrast agent was diluted 1:9 with PEG. The contrast agent was used for residual fluid tagging. Air was insufflated into the colon in the left decubitus position. The patient was scanned axially with a single run from the colonic flexures to the pelvis in the supine position. CTC were negative for polyps in two patients and positive in five patients. The endoscopic findings were similar to the CTC images. In two cases which did not reveal polyps on CTC, no symptoms were seen on follow-up over a period of 6 months. The authors concluded that the single scan CTC using polyethylene glycol with contrast medium (PEG-C) preparation was safe and less invasive compared to conventional colonoscopy due to the shorter examination time and lower radiation dose. Radiation exposure in this study was between 6.5 and 15.0 mGy (mean dose, 9.1 mGy).

Intussusception is a common emergency in infants and young children. Ultrasound or fluoroscopy guide reduction is frequently attempted to avoid surgery. However, many a times the reduction is incomplete. Curtis and colleagues[37] retrospectively reviewed whether a failed reduction of ileocolic intussusception at a referring hospital is predictor of failure of repeat attempt at a children's hospital. The children with pathological lead point, thise with age >10 years, those having successful reduction at referring hospital and those who did not undergo an enema reduction at the authors' institute were excluded. 152 patients met the enrollment criteria. The authors did not find any significant difference in the rate of successful reduction for the patients who initially presented to author's institute (60.5% as compared to those who had failed reduction at a referring hospital 60.7%). They concluded that children referred to a children's hospital after failed enema reduction at a referring hospital should undergo repeat enema reduction provided there are no other contraindications.

In another retrospective study, Pazo and Losek[38] evaluated the demographic and clinical characteristics of children with intussusception and failed initial air enema reduction who were managed by delayed repeat enema attempts. They attempted to identify predictors associated with successful reduction. In this study, there were 21 intussusception events in 20 patients which were managed by delayed repeat air enemas. 9/21 repeat enemas were successful. 4 of the patients who had unsuccessful reduction at first repeat enema underwent a second repeat enema with successful reduction in 3 patients. Thus, 12/25 (48%) repeat enemas were successful. The success rate of delayed repeat enemas was found to be greatest when the intussusception was initially reduced to the ileocecal valve. Demographic characteristics, clinical characteristics, or time from initial enema to first repeat enema were not significant determinant of success at repeat enema.

Cystic fibrosis frequently involves liver early in evolution. Liver Steatosis is the most common manifestation while focal biliary cirrhosis is the pathognomonic manifestation. Menten and colleagues[39] evaluated the role of transient elastography of liver in patients of cystic fibrosis. In this prospective study, the authors evaluated 134 patients of cystic fibrosis of which 75 were children. In addition, 31 children without cystic fibrosis were enrolled as controls. Liver morphology was classified on a scale of 1-5 representing increasingly severe liver disease. Ten measurements were recorded for tissue elastography for each subject and median value was considered the elastic modulus of liver. The authors found elasticity values of controls, pancreatic sufficient cystic fibrosis and pancreatic insufficient cystic fibrosis patients with ultrasound score < 3 to be comparable and significantly lower than compared to cystic fibrosis patients with ultrasound score of ≥3. In addition, male patients with cystic fibrosis had significantly higher median elasticity (4.7 kilopascals) as compared to female patients with cystic fibrosis (3.9 kilopascals). This preliminary study suggests that transient elastography may be an attractive non-invasive technique to assess and follow-up hepatic disease in cystic fibrosis patients.

URORADIOLOGY

Intravenous urography and micturating cystourethrography are important radiological investigations in pediatric uroradiology. However, both of these investigations impart ionizing radiation to the children. Magnetic resonance urography (MRU) and voiding ultrasonography are being evaluated as radiation free alternatives.

Hydronephrosis is common urological problem in pediatric population which is evaluated using a combination of several modalities. Perez-Brayfield[40] and colleagues conducted a prospective study to compare comparing ultrasound, nuclear scintigraphy and dynamic contrast enhanced magnetic resonance imaging in the evaluation of hydronephrosis. 96 children with mean age of 4 years (range 1 month to 17 years) were enrolled in the study. Patient sedation, an important issue in pediatric MRI, was administered without complications. The split renal function as calculated by nuclear and MRI scans were comparable in 71 cases (r = 0.93) evaluated. In 50/64 (78%) cases, the final diagnosis at MR urography was similar to that on a combination of ultrasound and nuclear scintigraphy. The authors concluded that dynamic contrast enhanced MRI provided equivalent information about renal function but superior information regarding morphology in a single study without ionizing radiation.

Akgun[41] and colleagues conducted a retrospective study to assess whether diuretic agent administration in MR urography has an effect on renal length and to determine whether the increase in length can be used to assess renal function. The study group consisted of 20 children of age group 10 months to 13 years. All these children had ureteropelvic junction stenosis. All had 99mTc-mercaptoacetyltriglicine (MAG-3) and 99mTc-diethylenetriamine-pentaacetic acid (DTPA) diuretic renography performed within 1 month of MR urography. The authors reported that the mean renal lengths measured before and after diuretic administration were 79.02 ± 16.84 mm and 85.61 ± 18.49 mm, respectively. This increase in renal length after diuretic administration was found to be statistically significant (p < 0.001; t = 8.082). In addition, a positive co-relation was observed between the increase in renal length after diuretic injection and functional status of kidneys (p < 0.001; r = 0.547). The better functioning kidneys had higher increase in renal length after diuretic administration.

Availability of sonographic contrast agents and harmonic imaging has contributed significantly to the sonographic evaluation of vesicoureteric reflux. In a recent study, Papadopoulou[42] and colleagues prospectively evaluated sensitivity of harmonic voiding urosonography (VUS HI) using a second-generation contrast agent (sulfur-hexafluoride gas microbubbles, SonoVue, Bracco, Italy) for the diagnosis of vesicoureteral reflux. The study group included 228 children with 463 kidney-ureter units (KUUs). The patients underwent two cycles of VUS HI and two cycles of VCUG at the same session. The findings of two modalities were compared. Vesicoureteric reflux was demonstrated in 161/463 (34.7%) KUUs, 57 by both methods, 90 only by VUS HI, and 14 only by micturating cystourethrogram. There was (77.5%) (k = 0.40) concordance (359/463 KUUs) in findings regarding the presence or absence of vesicoureteric reflux. The difference in the detection rate of reflux between the two methods was significant (P < 0.01). Apart from

showing inferior sensitivity, micturating cystourethrography also missed reflux of higher grade (2 grade I, 65 grade II, 19 grade III, 4 grade IV) as compared to VUS HI (8 grade I, 5 grade II, 1 grade III). The authors suggested that VUS HI and a second-generation contrast agent can be used as an alternative radiationfree imaging method for evaluation of vesicoureteric reflux.

Another radiation free approach to evaluation of vesicoureteric reflux involves utilization of MR fluoroscopy. Vasanwala and colleagues[43] have attempted to develop an MRI voiding cystography protocol with continuous real time MR fluoroscopy and validate it against micturating cystouretrography. In this study, eight follow-up patients of vesicouretric reflux were evaluated in a specially designed machine capable of performing MRI as well as fluoroscopic voiding cystourethrography. In this study, MRI had sensitivity of 88% when the grade of reflux differed by less than 1 on two modalities. MRI detected reflux in one patient which was not detected by fluoroscopic voiding cystourethrography.

MUSCULOSKELTAL IMAGING

Magni-Manzoni and colleagues[44] conducted a study to compare clinical evaluation and ultrasound in the assessment of joint synovitis in children with juvenile idiopathic arthritis. 52 joints in 32 children were evaluated by two pediatric rheumatologists for swelling, tenderness/pain on motion, and restricted motion. The same joints were evaluated by an experienced sonographer for synovial hyperplasia, joint effusion, and power Doppler signal. Overall, 1,664 joints were assessed both clinically and sonographically. On clinical examination joint swelling, tenderness and restricted motion were noticed in 98 (5.9%), 59 (3.5%) and 40 (2.4%) of joints respectively. Sonographic evaluation revealed synovial hyperplasia in 125 (7.5%), joint effusion in 153 (9.2%) and power Doppler signal in 53 (3.2%) joints. A total of 104 (6.3%) and 167 (10%) joints had clinical and sonographic evidence of synovitis, respectively. 86 (5.5%) of the clinically "normal" joints had sonographic features of synovitis. 5 patients were classified as having polyarthritis who were classified as having oligoarthritis or no synovitis on clinical evaluation. In this study, sonographic features moderately correlated with clinical measures of joint swelling, but poorly correlated with those of joint tenderness/pain on motion and restricted motion. The authors concluded that subclinical synovitis is common in juvenile idiopathic arthritis which may have important implications for patient classification and may affect the therapeutic strategy in individual patients.

Rooney, McAllister and Burns[45] prevalence of synovitis and tenosynovitis in children with juvenile idiopathic arthritis who were felt clinically to have active inflammatory disease of the ankle. Forty nine clinically swollen ankle joints in thirty four patients were included in this study. There were 19 patients with polyarticular disease and 13 with oligoarticular disease. One patient had systemic juvenile idiopathic arthritis. The authors found that 71% of ankles had tenosynovitis and 39% had tenosynovitis alone. Only 29% of clinically swollen ankles had tibiotalar joint effusion alone while 33% had both tenosynovitis and tibiotalar joint effusion. There was statistically significant difference between different subgroups for the frequency of occurrence of medial ankle tenosynovitis (p = 0.048) and lateral ankle tenosynovitis (p = 0.001).

SUMMARY

Several good articles have been published in recent years contributing to improved patient care. The current trends stress on the need of keeping the radiation dose to the minimum possible level when investigating the pediatric patients. Readers are encouraged to stay in touch with recent developments. Use of electronic resources is recommended as quick and inexpensive means for maintaining up to date knowledge.

REFERENCES

1. www.imagegently.org last accessed on 05.10.2010.
2. Strauss KJ, Kaste SC. The ALARA concept in pediatric interventional and fluoroscopic imaging: Striving to keep radiation doses as low as possible during fluoroscopy of pediatric patients—a white paper executive summary. AJR 2006; 187:818-9.
3. Strauss KJ, Goske MJ, Kaste SC, et al. Ten steps you can take to optimize image quality and lower CT dose for pediatric patients. AJR Am J Roentgenol. 2010; 194:868-73.
4. Sidhu M, Strauss KJ, Connolly B, et al. Radiation safety in pediatric interventional radiology. Tech Vasc Interv Radiol. 2010; 13:158-66.
5. Palchak MJ, Holmes JF, Vance CW, et al. A decision rule for identifying children at low risk for brain injuries after blunt head trauma. Ann Emerg Med. 2003; 42:492-506.
6. Barkovich AJ, Miller SP, Bartha A, et al. MR imaging, MR spectroscopy, and diffusion tensor imaging of sequential studies in neonates with encephalopathy. AJNR 2006; 27:533-47.
7. Liauw L, van Wezel-Meijler G, Veen S, van Buchem MA, van der Grond J. Do apparent diffusion coefficient measurements predict outcome in children with neonatal hypoxic-ischemic encephalopathy? AJNR 2009; 30:264-70.
8. Epelman M, Daneman A, Kellenberger CJ, et al. Neonatal encephalopathy: A prospective comparison of head US and MRI. Pediatr Radiol. 2010; 40:1640-50.
9. Tovar-Moll F, Moll J, de Oliveira-Souza R, Bramati I, Andreiuolo PA, Lent R. Neuroplasticity in human callosal dysgenesis: A diffusion tensor imaging study. Cereb Cortex. 2007; 17:531-41.
10. Wu Z, Mittal S, Kish K, Yu Y, Hu J, Haacke EM. Identification of calcification with MRI using susceptibility-weighted imaging: A case study. J Magn Reson Imaging. 2009; 29:177-82.
11. Wang Q, Babyn P, Branson H, Tran D, Davila J, Mueller EL. Utility of MRI in the follow-up of pyogenic spinal infection in children. Pediatr Radiol. 2010; 40:118-30.
12. Bober K, Swietliński J. Diagnostic utility of ultrasonography for respiratory distress syndrome in neonates. Med Sci Monit. 2006; 12:CR440-6.
13. Copetti R, Cattarossi L. The 'double lung point': An ultrasound sign diagnostic of transient tachypnea of the newborn. Neonatology. 2007; 91:203-9.
14. Copetti R, Cattarossi L, Macagno F, Violino M, Furlan R. Lung ultrasound in respiratory distress syndrome: a useful tool for early diagnosis. Neonatology. 2008; 94:52-9.
15. Kurian J, Levin TL, Han BK, Taragin BH, Weinstein S. Comparison of ultrasound and CT in the evaluation of pneumonia complicated by parapneumonic effusion in children. AJR 2009; 193:1648-54.
16. Montella S, Santamaria F, Salvatore M, et al. Assessment of chest high-field magnetic resonance imaging in children and young adults with non cystic fibrosis chronic lung disease: comparison to high-resolution computed tomography and correlation with pulmonary function. Invest Radiol. 2009; 44:532-8.
17. Bannier E, Cieslar K, Mosbah K, et al. Hyperpolarized 3He MR for sensitive imaging of ventilation function and treatment efficiency in young cystic fibrosis patients with normal lung function. Radiology. 2010; 255:225-32.
18. Lee EY, Tracy DA, Bastos M, Casey AM, Zurakowski D, Boiselle PM. Expiratory volumetric MDCT evaluation of air trapping in pediatric patients with and without tracheomalacia. AJR 2010; 194:1210-5.
19. Cheng Z, Wang X, Duan Y, Wu L, Wu D, Chao B, Liu C, Xu Z, Li H, Liang F, Xu J, Chen J. Low-dose prospective ECG-triggering dual-source CT angiography in infants and children with complex congenital heart disease: First experience. Eur Radiol. 2010; 20: 2503-11.
20. Paul JF, Rohnean A, Elfassy E, Sigal-Cinqualbre A. Radiation dose for thoracic and coronary step-and-shoot CT using a 128-slice dual-source machine in infants and small children with congenital heart disease. Pediatr Radiol. 2010 Sep 4. [Epub ahead of print].
21. Buonomo C. The radiology of necrotizing enterocolitis. Radiol Clin North Am 1999; 37:1187-98.
22. Faingold R, Daneman A, Tomlinson G, et al. Necrotizing enterocolitis: Assessment of bowel viability with color doppler US. Radiology 2005; 235:587-94.
23. Kim WY, Kim WS, Kim IO, et al. Sonographic evaluation of neonates with early-stage necrotizing enterocolitis. Pediatr Radiol 2005; 35:1056-61.
24. Silva CT, Daneman A, Navarro OM, et al. Correlation of sonographic findings and outcome in necrotizing enterocolitis. Pediatr Radiol 2007; 37:274-82.
25. Dilli D, Oguz SS, Ulu HO, Dumanli H, Dilmen U. Sonographic findings in premature infants with necrotising enterocolitis. Arch Dis Child Fetal Neonatal Ed. 2009; 94:F232-3.
26. Bora R, Mukhopadhyay K, Saxena AK, Jain V, Narang A. Prediction of feed intolerance and necrotizing enterocolitis in neonates with absent end diastolic flow in umbilical artery and the correlation of feed intolerance with postnatal superior mesenteric artery flow. J Matern Fetal Neonatal Med. 2009; 22:1092-6.
27. Jonas MM, Perez-Atayde AR. Liver disease in infancy and childhood. In: Schiff ER, Sorell MF, Maddrey WC, editors. Schiff's diseases of liver. USA. 10th edn. Lippincott Williams and Wilkins 2007; p. 1307, 1331.
28. Nicotra JJ, Kramer SS, Bellah RD, Redd DC. Congenital and acquired biliary disorders in children. Semin Roentgenol 1997; 32: 215-27.
29. Humphrey TM, Stringer MD. Biliary atresia: US diagnosis. Radiology 2007; 244:845-51.
30. Kim WS, Cheon JE, Youn BJ, et al. Hepatic arterial diameter measured with US: Adjunct for US diagnosis of biliary atresia. Radiology 2007; 245:549-55.
31. Lee MS, Kim MJ, Lee MJ, et al. Biliary atresia: Color Doppler US findings in neonates and infants. Radiology. 2009; 252:282-9.
32. de Carvalho E, Ivantes CA, Bezerra JA. Extrahepatic biliary atresia: Current concepts and future directions. *J Pediatr* 2007;83:105-20.
33. Nwomeh BC, Caniano DA, Hogan M. Definitive exclusion of biliary atresia in infants with cholestatic jaundice: The role of percutaneous cholecysto-cholangiography. Pediatr Surg Int. 2007; 23:845-9.

34. Anupindi S, Perumpillichira J, Jaramillo D, Zalis ME, Israel EJ. Low-dose CT colonography in children: Initial experience, technical feasibility, and utility. Pediatr Radiol 2005; 35:518-24.

35. Capuñay CM, Carrascosa PM, Bou-Khair A, Castagnino N, Ninomiya I, Carrascosa JM. Low radiation dose multislice CT colonography in children: Experience after 100 studies. Eur J Radiol 2005; 56:398-402.

36. Sugiyama A, Ohashi Y, Gomi A, Moriya K, Sanada Y, Yatsuzuka M et al. Colorectal screening with single scan CT colonography in children. Pediatr Sur Int 2007; 23:987-90.

37. Curtis JL, Gutierrez IM, Kirk SR, Gollin G. Failure of enema reduction for ileocolic intussusception at a referring hospital does not preclude repeat attempts at a children's hospital. J Pediatr Surg. 2010; 45:1178-81.

38. Pazo A, Hill J, Losek JD. Delayed repeat enema in the management of intussusception. Pediatr Emerg Care. 2010; 26:640-5.

39. Menten R, Leonard A, Clapuyt P, Vincke P, Nicolae AC, Lebecque P. Transient elastography in patients with cystic fibrosis. Pediatr Radiol. 2010; 40:1231-5.

40. Perez-Brayfield MR, Kirsch AJ, Jones RA, Grattan-Smith JD. A prospective study comparing ultrasound, nuclear scintigraphy and dynamic contrast enhanced magnetic resonance imaging in the evaluation of hydronephrosis. J Urol. 2003; 170:1330-4.

41. Akgun V, Kocaoglu M, Ilgan S, Dayanc M, Gok F, Bulakbasi N. Diuretic-induced renal length changes in the estimation of renal function with MR urography. AJR 2010; 194:W218-20.

42. Papadopoulou F, Anthopoulou A, Siomou E, Efremidis S, Tsamboulas C, Darge K. Harmonic voiding urosonography with a second-generation contrast agent for the diagnosis of vesicoureteral reflux. Pediatr Radiol. 2009; 39:239-44.

43. Vasanawala SS, Kennedy WA, Ganguly A, et al. MR voiding cystography for evaluation of vesicoureteral reflux. AJR 2009; 192:W206-11

44. Magni-Manzoni S, Epis O, Ravelli A, et al. Comparison of clinical versus ultrasound-determined synovitis in juvenile idiopathic arthritis. Arthritis Rheum. 2009; 61:1497-504.

45. Rooney ME, McAllister C, Burns JF. Ankle disease in juvenile idiopathic arthritis: Ultrasound findings in clinically swollen ankles. J Rheumatol. 2009; 36:1725-9.

CHAPTER 3

Interventions in Children

PART A—Vascular Interventions

Gurpreet Singh Gulati, Sanjiv Sharma

INTRODUCTION

Interventional procedures in the pediatric age group have a long history. Probably the first intervention performed in a pediatric patient was the reduction of intussusception. The earliest cardiovascular intervention in children performed with angiographic guidance was balloon atrial septostomy. Over the years, although vascular interventional techniques as applied to the adult population have undergone dramatic and continuous innovation, their application to pediatric patients has been delayed, due to a conservative attitude of pediatric medicine practitioners, lack of adequately trained physicians and staff in this subspecialty, and need for special equipment appropriate for pediatric use.

Children are not merely "little adults", nor are the diseases to which they are particularly susceptible, variants of diseases in adult life. Excessive crying, unwillingness for examination, and their inability to describe complaints make a child the most difficult patient. However, it is a challenge to the pediatric interventionist to master the art of 'talking' and achieve a successful examination. A friendly environment, affectionate attitude of the medical staff, and a carefully and rapidly performed study, go a long way in conducting a successful procedure.

Special Considerations for the Pediatric Patient

A discussion between the interventional radiologist and referring physician ensures that the appropriate procedure is performed, the risks for the particular patient are appreciated, and the likely benefit to accrue to the patient is understood. It is particularly imperative to pay special attention to the following details while conducting a pediatric angiography or intervention. These are:
1. Choice of sedation or anesthesia
2. Maintenance of temperature control
3. Fluid balance
4. Radiation safety
5. Equipment selection

A dedicated team consisting of the operating radiologist, the radiation and hemodynamic technologists, and the nursing attendant are needed to prepare the catheterization laboratory, prepare and handle the patient, and assist during the procedure. A high-resolution digital angiography system is required to obtain reliable diagnostic images quickly and to monitor the interventional procedure.

Patient Preparation

History and Physical Examination

A detailed discussion on the patient's history taking and examination relevant to general as well as specific angiographic interventional procedures is outside the scope of this chapter. Table 3.1 lists the several components that need to be assessed while evaluating the patient.

Informed Consent

The parent or guardian of a minor child, and when possible, the patient himself, should understand the reasons for undergoing the procedure, the risks and benefits, the consequences of refusing the procedure, and the alternative therapies available. He or she should then give consent for the procedure.

Coagulation

Whenever there is a bleeding diathesis, risk of hemorrhage, or a plan to perform systemic thrombolysis, coagulation studies are obtained. Blood is sent for grouping and cross-matching whenever there is ongoing or expected blood loss. Heparin is

Table 3.1: Pre-procedure clinical evaluation of the patient
1. History of the current problem
2. Pertinent medical and surgical history
3. Review of the organ systems
• Cardiac
• Pulmonary
• Renal
• Hepatic
• Hematologic (e.g. coagulopathy, hyper-coagulable state)
• Endocrine (diabetes)
4. History of allergies
5. Current medications
6. Directed physical examination

administered for arterial catheterization procedures in a dose of 50 units/kg for diagnostic and 100 units/kg for revascularization procedures.

Anesthesia

Most diagnostic studies are carried out with intravenous sedation. Difficult interventions such as device implantation or particularly painful procedures are conducted under general anesthesia.

In most children, conscious sedation is used, in which the child is conscious, drowsy, and may even close his eyes, but is responsive to verbal commands and able to protect his reflexes and airway. *Midazolam* is a commonly used, short-acting benzodiazepine that is metabolised by the liver. Its dose is 0.2-1 mg/KBW I.V. The onset of action is 3-5 minutes and the duration of action is 60 minutes. The major side effects are respiratory depression and apnea. A combination of 3 drugs namely, *demerol* (50 mg), *promethazine* (12.5 mg) and *triclofos* (12.5 mg), known as *DPT,* is the other agent used for conscious sedation. A mixture of the 3 is made into a 2 ml solution, to be given in a dose of 0.06–0.1 ml/KBW I.M. For deeper sedation, a combination of *diazepam* (0.1 mg/KBW) and *morphine* (0.1 mg/KBW) may be given I.V. Respiratory depression may occur with higher doses.

Patient Immobilization

Smaller children are immobilized on a restraining board. Older children will have hand and leg restraints but, if uncooperative, will need to be anesthetized.

Temperature Control

Neonates and especially premature babies may become hypothermic if a warm operating environment is not maintained. The room temperature should be increased, radiation heaters are required, and the child should be covered quickly while preparing the groin and draping.

Diet and Medications

Small children need not be kept fasting for more than 3-4 hours prior to the procedure. Routine antibiotics are not prescribed except for high-risk procedures, e.g. splenic embolization.

Dose of Radiation and Fluids

Isky Gordon et al[1] calculated and published the ratio of radiation dose to the skin (in rads) for various procedures as follows:

Age (years)	1	5	10	15
Angiography – 20 films	1.4	3.0	4.8	7.5
Fluoroscopy – 4 minutes	3.2	4.8	6.8	8.8

One must try and minimize the radiation exposure to children who are believed to be more sensitive to the effects of radiation and likely to live for many years with these effects. Digital systems probably do not reduce radiation exposure. However, several precautions may be taken by the operator to reduce the dose. Fluoroscopy at the lowest dose possible (reduce the mAS), pulsed fluoroscopy, removing the scatter grids, and addition of rare earth filters in the X-ray tubes help to reduce radiation doses to the patient.

All fluids and medication must be scaled to the patient size. One may easily administer excessive amounts of fluids and contrast without realizing it. Digital systems (more so with bi-plane angiography systems) help to bring down the volume of contrast material and speeding up procedures. Most infants can tolerate 4 ml/kg of contrast, whereas children over 6 months can tolerate 6 ml/kg, if it is delivered as several injections spread over a period of time. It is important to maintain patient hydration if such large doses are employed.

TECHNIQUES

Vascular procedures in pediatric patients require a substantially different approach than that used in the adult population. Many considerations must be taken into account when treating the pediatric population, including the small caliber vessel size, anticipation of spasm, the risk for infection, the propensity for children to rapidly form collateral circulation, the inevitability of growth, and the strong tendency for restenosis and growth arrest to occur.

Access

Introducer sheaths should be used to preserve vascular access, since multiple catheter/guide wire insertions or exchanges may be needed. Special pediatric access sheaths are available in 4-6 F sizes. These are usually introduced by using a cannula (18-21 G) and an 0.021" guide wire. The angle of entry of the needle should be less perpendicular to the skin, and a small nick in the skin with the blade should be given before introducing the sheath, to prevent pain and a possible vasovagal reaction. Care should be taken to prevent an inadvertent incision in the anterior vessel wall while using the blade.

PROCEDURES

The major vascular interventional procedures performed in children can be grouped into:
A. Embolization
B. Angioplasty
C. Thrombolysis
D. Foreign body removal

Embolization

Percutaneous transcatheter embolization has replaced surgery for many pediatric vascular problems, and is a treatment alternative in patients where surgery has little to offer. Microcatheter systems, which were initially developed for adult neurovascular interventions, are ideal for pediatric applications. They permit access to small vessels and territories that were previously inaccessible. Hydrophilic coated steerable guidewires permit negotiation of complex vascular loops without provoking spasm or causing dissection.

Embolization procedures should only be performed by experienced physicians familiar with the equipment and technical aspects of the procedure. Discussion with the pediatric physicians or surgeons, their support and backup is essential for a safe and successful procedure.

The various pediatric vascular conditions treated by using embolotherapy can be grouped as follows:

1. Vascular anomalies, e.g. arteriovenous malformation (AVM), arteriovenous fistula (AVF), venous malformation (VM), lymphatic malformation (LM), and hemangioma.
2. Hemorrhage from bleeding vessels (due to pseudoaneurysms or vascular involvement in trauma, tumor or inflammation) in various organ systems.
3. Other conditions, e.g. tumors and organ ablation.

Goals of embolotherapy include: (i) an adjunctive goal, e.g. preoperative, adjunct to chemotherapy or radiation therapy; (ii) a curative goal, e.g. definitive treatment such as that performed in cases of aneurysms, AVFs, AVMs, and traumatic bleeding; and (iii) a palliative goal, e.g. relieving symptoms, such as of a large AVM, which cannot be cured by using embolotherapy alone.

EMBOLIZATION MATERIALS AND SUBSTANCES

Materials used in embolization include coils, ethanol, sodium tetradecyl sulfate, n-butyl cyanoacrylate (NBCA) glue, polyvinyl alcohol (PVA) particles, microspheres, and gelatin sponge (Gelfoam).

Vascular Anomalies

Vascular anomalies are grouped into 2 categories: hemangiomas and vascular malformations. Vascular malformations are categorised further as high-flow lesions (AVM, AVF), low-flow lesions (capillary malformation, VM, LM), or combined vascular malformations. Embolotherapy with a variety of embolic materials is commonly used in the treatment of vascular anomalies

Hemangioma

Hemangiomas are benign tumors that require no treatment in most patients. In rare cases, embolization may be necessary (particularly in patients in whom therapy is needed urgently) because of spontaneous hemorrhage or functional abnormality caused by the extreme size of the lesion or the particular anatomic location or because of significant congestive heart failure.[2] In addition, embolotherapy is considered useful prior to surgical resection in select patients, and in patients in whom a hemangio-endothelioma causes Kasabach-Merritt phenomenon (platelet trapping).[2] Embolotherapy of a hemangioma or hemangioendothelioma can be performed with the use of PVA particles. Coils are infrequently used since they cause more proximal occlusion with potential for recruitment of supply from other arteries and they block future access to the lesion if needed.

The goal of embolotherapy is to block a large percentage of the tumoral vessels, thereby preventing further trapping and destruction of the platelets and hastening involution of the lesion. Some tumors may require several sessions of embolotherapy because of revascularization of the tumor or to prevent exceeding the limits of radiation and contrast burden in one session. Infantile hepatic hemangioendotheliomas, a variant of infantile hemangioma, usually are multiple and frequently are complicated by congestive heart failure. In the clinical setting, the goal of embolotherapy is to reduce hepatic arterial flow, which

sufficiently relieves high-output cardiac failure. A variety of embolic materials have been used. In some patients, embolization of other nearby arteries (e.g. intercostals) may also be necessary.[3] Arterial portography should be performed to exclude the possibility of feeders from the portal system.

A rare entity called noninvoluting hemangioma, which is found in the adult population, may also respond to transcatheter embolization (usually with particles such as PVA or microspheres). This procedure is usually performed to improve the cosmetic appearance.

AVM

AVMs are typically characterized by a nidus of abnormal vessels in which shunting of arterial blood to veins occurs. These vascular anomalies are usually present during childhood but often demonstrate a sudden increase in size in response to trauma, hormones, or other stimuli. Although a clinical grading system has been used among surgeons, no grading system has been developed for imaging. Most AVMs can be managed by transcatheter embolization and/or sclerotherapy. Some focal AVMs can be treated by surgical excision. Proximal embolization or ligation of the feeding arteries usually worsens matters because of subsequent recruitment of collaterals, and transluminal embolization of the nidus cannot be performed afterwards. The collaterals that develop are more problematic in terms of transcatheter treatment; however, proximal embolization of the feeding arteries may be performed if indicated prior to surgical excision.

Whenever possible during primary embolotherapy, the nidus should be embolized.[2] Absolute alcohol is the most effective agent in the treatment of AVMs. If the nidus cannot be reached through the feeding arteries, direct percutaneous cannulation of the nidus can be attempted. In selected patients with AVMs, another therapeutic approach is embolic occlusion of the venous outflow.

Cervicofacial AVMs

For dental arcade AVMs, spontaneous or catastrophic hemorrhage during tooth extraction is a common presentation. Embolization of an AVM in this region requires superselective catheterization of the involved branches of external carotid artery and other regional arterial branches (e.g. thyrocervical trunk) using microcatheters and the coaxial technique.[4]

Embolotherapy can be performed with NBCA, alcohol, particles, and/or microcoils, depending on the nature and extent of the malformation. Gelfoam can also be used for preoperative embolization. Patients with dental AVMs associated with acute bleeding and loose teeth should undergo embolization immediately prior to tooth extraction. Possible complications of embolotherapy of cervicofacial AVMs include stroke, nerve paralysis, skin necrosis, infection, blindness, and pulmonary embolism.

Extremity AVMs

In the extremities, AVMs can be diffuse and may involve the entire extremity (Parkes-Weber syndrome). Extremity AVMs typically

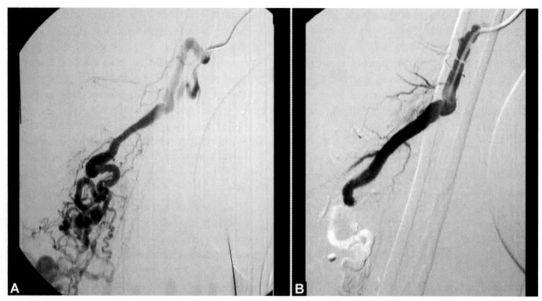

Figs 3.1A and B: An arteriovenous malformation of the right arm, with feeders from the profunda brachii artery. Pre (A)- and post (B) – embolization (polyvinyl alcohol particles) angiograms

present with extremity-length discrepancy, high cardiac output, pain, and ulceration. Extremity lesions can be treated with multiple embolizations[5] and/or surgical resections or amputation of the extremity (Figs 3.1A and B).

A detailed pre-embolization angiographic examination is important for mapping the feeders and draining veins. During the injection of contrast material, the injection rate and duration should be adjusted so that arteriovenous connections can be identified accurately. A high injection rate in a short period is appropriate for AVMs.

Selective catheterization with microcatheters is required to reach the nidus of the AVM. Significant complications of embolotherapy possibly include skin necrosis (blisters), nontarget embolization (which also includes pulmonary emboli), and systemic sclerosant toxicity if a liquid agent (e.g., alcohol) is used.

Pulmonary AVMs

Pulmonary AVMs are also called pulmonary AVFs. They have a high association with Osler-Weber-Rendu syndrome (also called hereditary hemorrhagic telangiectasia syndrome). Symptoms may include dyspnea, cyanosis, and clubbing. Paradoxical embolization may cause stroke or brain abscess. This anomaly can be classified as simple or complex on the basis of the number of feeders and draining veins. In simple lesions, a single artery and vein are involved; in complex lesions, 2 or more supplying arteries and 1 or more draining veins are involved.

Most pulmonary AVMs (80%) are simple. Although a surgical approach (thoracotomy and resection) is the traditional mode of therapy, transcatheter embolization is currently a preferred alternative.[6] Transcatheter embolization offers significantly reduced morbidity and mortality rates, particularly in hereditary hemorrhagic telangiectasia syndrome.

Embolotherapy for AVMs can be performed with coils, vascular plugs or detachable balloons. Possible complications of

embolotherapy include non-target embolization in the systemic circulation (through the AVM shunt) or in other noninvolved pulmonary arteries. Therefore, properly sizing the coil to the feeding (afferent) artery is essential. A preliminary detailed angiography is essential for mapping the feeders and draining veins, paying particular attention to the size of the feeders. Basically, a successful embolization is accomplished by nesting 1 or more coils in the feeding artery, which occludes flow through the AVM shunt (Figs 3.2A and B).

Generally, feeding arteries larger than 3 mm should be embolized. Feeders smaller than 3 mm have low risk of paradoxic embolization and should be left alone unless they are simple and straightforward technically. A coil that is 2 to 3 mm larger than the feeding artery is usually selected. For vascular plug, a 30-50 percent oversizing is recommended. If the feeding artery is large in caliber (>12 mm), a balloon occlusion of the proximal artery via a second groin puncture can be used for a more controlled coil deployment. Postembolization syndrome can occur and is characterized by pleuritic chest pain, pleural fluid, atelectasis, fever, and leukocytosis.

AVF

AVFs are relatively large arteriovenous connections and may be congenital or secondary to trauma, surgery, or underlying vascular abnormality (e.g. neurofibromatosis). AVFs may be seen in any part of the body. A patient may present with cardiac failure, localized growth disturbances, neurologic deficits, and ischemic changes. Unlike AVMs, AVFs can be cured with embolotherapy. The embolotherapy technique used depends on the size, location, and hemodynamics of individual lesions. The goal of embolotherapy is to occlude the fistula and the immediate draining vein.

Embolization can be achieved by using detachable coils or balloons, or tissue adhesives (glue or onyx). Gelfoam or particles are not appropriate for use in AVF embolization. Detachable coils[7]

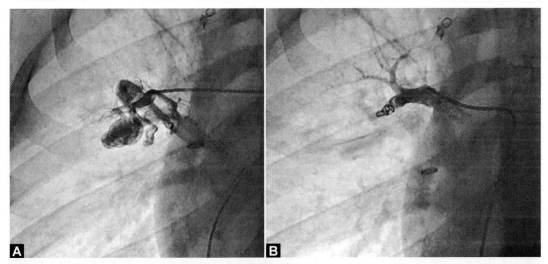

Figs 3.2A and B: Right upper lobe pulmonary arteriovenous malformation. Pre (A)- and post (B)-embolization (fibered platinum coils) angiograms. Coils elsewhere are from embolization carried out for other PAVMs in the right lung

or balloons are ideal because these embolic materials can be positioned optimally before they are detached. Balloons also have the advantage of conforming to the size and shape of the abnormal vessels. Microcoils can be dislodged; however, this complication can be minimized by performing flow-control techniques (e.g. balloon occlusion, tourniquet, or blood pressure cuff control). The other disadvantage of coil embolization is that the clot that forms around the coil may dissolve, resulting in recanalization. Appropriate nesting of several coils (packing) can minimize recanalization. Also, thrombosis can be augmented by soaking the coils in thrombin before deployment or by injecting sclerosants around the coils. If adequate coil packing cannot be accomplished, tissue adhesive can be effectively used in combination with coils. Covered stents can also be particularly useful for acquired AVFs (single communications). They have the advantage of maintaining patency of the parent artery. Often, a combined strategy using different techniques is necessary.

VM

VMs are the most common type of vascular malformations and can vary significantly in size and clinical presentation. These lesions (usually distinguished by a bluish discoloration with swelling and pain) may also be associated with systemic syndromes such as blue rubber-bleb nevus syndrome or Maffucci syndrome. Sinus pericranii (communication between intracranial and extracranial venous drainage) is also commonly associated with craniofacial VMs. These lesions can be treated with embolotherapy (sclerotherapy) and/or surgical excision.[8,9] The type of treatment used depends on the morphology, size, and location of the malformation.

A preliminary venogram is usually obtained to evaluate the deep venous system and to determine if any communication exists between the VM and the extremity veins. In particular, a venogram is performed on extremity VMs. The lesion is localized by using ultrasonography, and the largest-appearing cystic portion of the lesion is selected. Then, the lesion is accessed by using real-time ultrasonographic guidance and a small Angiocath needle (typically, 20-22 gauge). The lesion is studied with contrast agent injections under fluoroscopy as well as digital subtraction angiography. Subsequently, sclerotherapy is performed by using ethanol (absolute alcohol) or sodium tetradecyl sulfate mixed with a contrast medium (Ethiodol or iodinated contrast) under real-time fluoroscopic control (Figs 3.3A and B). Foam sclerotherapy is a technique where a mixture of room air and sclerosant is injected and potentially results in greater agent-malformation contact and lowers volume of sclerosant required.

If draining veins are present (as they commonly are), manual compression or a tourniquet should be used to reduce washout of the sclerosant material from the malformation. If large draining veins are present, these veins can be embolized with coils via a percutaneous approach before sclerotherapy. For large head and neck VMs, airway involvement can be a challenging component of the condition in terms of treating the patients. Because alcohol and sodium tetradecyl cause significant edema after sclerotherapy, airway patency should be carefully monitored during and after the sclerotherapy procedure. In patients with large head and neck VMs requiring surgical debulking, presurgical sclerotherapy with NBCA glue can be performed because NBCA causes no significant edema.

Two common problems associated with sclerotherapy include skin necrosis (blisters) and/or nerve damage or paralysis. Nerve damage or paralysis can result from the direct toxic effect of the sclerosant agent and/or compression of the nerve by focal compartmental tissue edema (compartment syndrome). In addition, hemoglobulinuria is a relatively common complication; this is treated by aggressive hydration and alkalinization. A less common but more severe complication is cardiac toxicity resulting from the systemic effect of absolute alcohol.

LM

LMs can be grouped as microcystic, macrocystic, and mixed. The mixed form of anomaly is probably the most common form of LM.

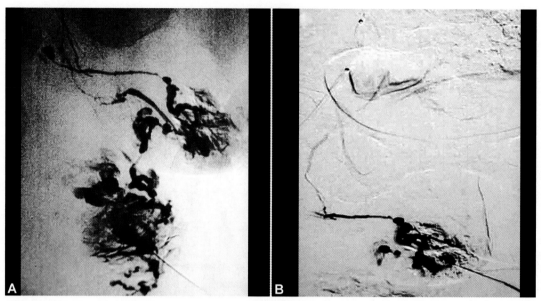

Figs 3.3A and B: A diffuse venous malformation in the right thigh. Direct puncture venogram showed minimal flow into deep veins (A). Sodium tetradecyl sulphate was slowly injected under fluoroscopic control. Successful occlusion of the malformation was achieved (B)

Lymphatic cysts contain lymphatic fluid. When a single cystic mass (previously termed cystic hygroma when found in the neck) or a conglomerate mass containing a few macrocysts is encountered, surgical excision is considered the most effective treatment. However, some lesions respond really well to sclerotherapy without any complications after 1 or several sclerotherapy sessions.

When a mixed form of LM is encountered, the best therapeutic approach may be sclerotherapy for cystic masses, followed by surgical debulking. The microcystic LM, or the microcystic component of the mixed form, does not contain cystic spaces on radiologic studies (including MRI). It demonstrates a characteristic contrast-enhanced pattern of rings and arcs. The sclerosant agents most commonly used are antibiotics (doxycycline), ethanol, sodium tetradecyl sulfate and, most recently, OK-432 (a derivative of group A streptococci). For patients older than 8 years, doxycycline is the most commonly used sclerosant agent. If the patient is younger than 8 years, the options are alcohol, sodium tetradecyl, or OK-432. The amount of alcohol used depends on the patient's weight, which is a limiting factor in most procedures involving alcohol.

The interventional therapeutic approach used for LMs is similar to the sclerotherapy technique used for VMs; however, an initial venogram is usually unnecessary.

Hemorrhage

Several types of hemorrhage can be treated with embolization. Examples include hemoptysis; epistaxis; and GI tract, post-traumatic, and iatrogenic hemorrhage (e.g. postbiopsy or nephrostomy tube insertion).

GI Hemorrhage

Major causes of upper GI tract hemorrhage are ulcer disease, gastritis and varices. The most common causes of a lower GI tract hemorrhage are vascular malformations and bleeding after endoscopic biopsy. If the bleeding source is identified on arterial angiogram, the patient is treated by using either intra-arterial vasopressin infusion (Pitressin) or embolization of the bleeding mesenteric artery. Embolization is usually the first line of treatment in patients with upper GI tract bleeding and is used as the second line of treatment in patients with lower GI tract bleeding (usually used if vasopressin treatment fails).[10]

Embolization in the arcades proximal to the bleeding vasa recta is recommended to minimize the risk of bowel necrosis. The most commonly used embolic agents are coils (macrocoils or microcoils) and Gelfoam pieces (torpedoes). Coil embolization is particularly helpful if the bleeding is caused by focal vascular abnormalities such as a false aneurysm. Some interventional radiologists have also used PVA, although the use of PVA or other particles should be avoided because of the risk of bowel infarction. After embolization, control angiography is performed to determine if bleeding (contrast material extra-vasation) continues via any collaterals. The primary advantage of embolotherapy is the immediate cessation of bleeding without need for prolonged catheterization (unlike vasopressin infusion therapy).

Pelvic Hemorrhage

Intractable pelvic hemorrhage, usually post-traumatic, should be approached in a similar interventional fashion. A surgical approach to control active bleeding in acute trauma setting is usually not favored. Detailed angiographic examination with superselective injections in the branches of the internal iliac artery is mandatory. Embolization can be performed by using an autologous blood clot, Gelfoam torpedoes, PVA particles, NBCA, coils, or detachable balloons.[11] At the capillary level, embolization with small particles or Gelfoam powder is contraindicated (because of the elimination of collateral flow, which results in massive tissue necrosis).

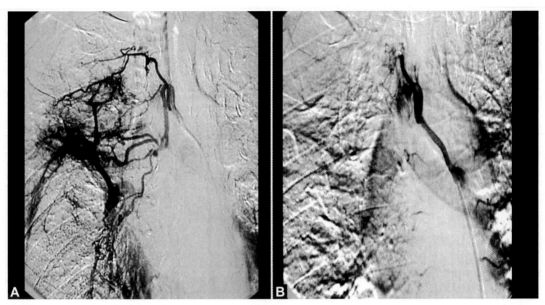

Figs 3.4A and B: A patient with hemoptysis due to bronchiectasis in the right upper and middle lobe. Selective injection of the hypertrophied right intercosto-bronchial trunk (A) revealed multiple feeders with parenchymal blush. After embolization with PVA particles and gelfoam, the culprit vessel is completely occluded (B)

A specific anatomic relationship between the fracture site and the affected vessel often allows embolization of the branch (frequently the obturator artery) even when no obvious bleeding site is detected.[12] In particular, liquid or particle embolization of the inferior gluteal branch of the anterior division should be avoided to minimize the possibility of sciatic nerve injury (this branch supplies muscles of the thigh and buttocks and the sciatic nerve). In addition, embolization of the posterior division of the internal iliac artery should be avoided because of the risk of gluteal necrosis.

Hemoptysis

Hemoptysis is considered massive when at least 300 ml of blood is lost in less than 24 hours, and it may be life-threatening. Common causes of massive hemoptysis are cystic fibrosis, bronchiectasis, tuberculosis, and aspergillosis. Malignancy is rarely a cause. Surgical intervention is usually not feasible because of severe pulmonary disease; therefore, embolization of the bleeding bronchial arteries can be life saving.[13]

Bronchial arteries are variable. They usually arise from the descending thoracic aorta between thoracic vertebre T4 and T7. The right bronchial artery arises from the intercostobronchial trunk in most patients (> 90%). The left bronchial artery usually arises directly from the aorta and is multiple in most patients. Occasionally, the right and left bronchial arteries arise from a common trunk.

Although some bronchial branches may supply the spinal cord, the most important of these branches is the artery of Adamkiewicz. This artery usually arises from an intercostal or lumbar artery on the left. Other spinal branches from the right intercostobronchial artery, thyrocervical, or costocervical arteries may be identified. A preliminary thoracic aortogram may be performed, which usually shows abnormal bronchial arteries. An aortogram helps in outlining the bronchial anatomy.

Because of potential source of collaterals, a subclavian arteriogram also is obtained, particularly if the upper lung field is involved. Then, the bronchial arteries are catheterized and studied with selective injections. The most common appearance of the abnormal bronchial artery (the bleeding source) is increased caliber of the bronchial artery with some hypervascularity over the lung field. Contrast agent extravasation, shunting from bronchial to pulmonary arteries, or aneurysmal changes in the involved bronchial artery rarely are identified.

Embolotherapy is usually performed with particles (PVA or embospheres) and Gelfoam pledgets (Figs 3.4A and B). When the decision is made to use particles, appropriately sized particles should be used. Sizes are usually 500-710 µm for PVA and 500-800 µm for embospheres. Use of coils is inappropriate, and absolute alcohol or cyanoacrylate is no longer used for bronchial artery embolization because of the risk of tissue necrosis (bronchial and/or esophageal).

Embolization is performed as selectively as possible (when necessary, by using a microcatheter and coaxial technique) to minimize tissue necrosis and nontarget embolization (e.g. spinal artery). Special care should be taken to prevent reflux by injecting the embolic material slowly under continuous fluoroscopic control. Gelfoam pledgets/torpedoes usually are used to occlude the abnormal artery more proximally after particle embolization.

Epistaxis

Intractable epistaxis is a nosebleed that does not respond to conservative treatment (nasal spraying of vasoconstrictors, nasal packing, blood transfusion). Etiologies include uncontrolled hypertension with or without superficial mucosal abnormality (e.g. Osler-Weber-Rendu syndrome).

Epistaxis can be treated by either surgical means (e.g. cautery, vascular ligation) or endovascular embolotherapy. Internal carotid

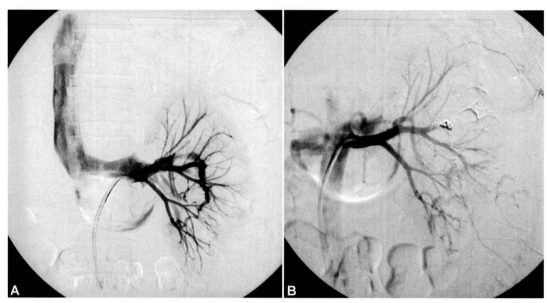

Figs 3.5A and B: A patient with postrenal biopsy hematuria. Selective left renal angiogram (A) shows an arteriovenous fistula from an interlobar artery in the midpole with early filling of the inferior vena cava. Complete occlusion of the branch was achieved with coils (B)

arteriograms are obtained to exclude aneurysms. Then, the external carotid artery is catheterized and control angiography is performed initially to map the vascular anatomy and to check for the presence of a collateral supply to the intracranial circulation.

During catheterization of the external carotid artery and its branches, vasospasm is a common problem. Nitroglycerin can be used to treat this. The target branch is usually the pterygopalatine division of the internal maxillary artery, which is distal to the origin of the meningeal and temporal arteries. By using a microcatheter, the pterygopalatine division is catheterized and embolized with particles (most commonly PVA). If bleeding is not caused by a neoplastic entity, embolotherapy can be performed in the 250 to 500 μm range. If a neoplastic entity is the cause, the capillary bed needs to be embolized. This embolization can be accomplished by using smaller particles (150-250 μm).

Although the procedure is considered safe if performed by an experienced physician, possible complications can occur. These include ischemia, pain, cranial nerve damage, blindness, and stroke.

Post-traumatic Hemorrhage

Post-traumatic hemorrhage can be due to either a blunt or penetrating injury to a vessel, typically arteries in the extremities with penetrating injuries or associated fractures or arteries to the organs (e.g. renal arteries, after blunt trauma). Some patients may present after an orthopedic procedure, such as total hip replacement. An angiographic study is mandatory, not only to aid selecting in the appropriate subsequent embolization procedure but also in planning for possible future surgical interventions.

Coil embolization is appropriate in extremity branch arteries responsible for the bleeding because it offers a fast and permanent occlusion of the vessel. The bleeding vessel should be embolized proximal and distal to the site of arterial injury. Avoid embolization

of arteries that endangers limb viability. Hemorrhage or AVF formation after organ biopsy (particularly renal biopsy), or iatrogenic traumatic hemorrhage, is a common complication (i.e. iatrogenic traumatic hemorrhage) that can be treated with embolization (Figs 3.5A and B).

Pseudoaneurysm

Pseudoaneurysms occur secondary to trauma or infection and consist of leakage of blood into the confined perivascular space at the site of a vessel wall disruption. Embolization is a good alternative to surgical repair, and is often the treatment of choice, especially when pseudoaneurysms are not accessible or when the patient is not a surgical candidate because of sepsis or other medical conditions.[14,15]

Embolic materials used for pseudoaneurysms include coils, detachable balloons, thrombin, gelfoam, and NBCA. In large-neck pseudo-aneurysms, a stent placement combined with coil embolization has been described. If the involved vessel cannot be catheterized or if a pseudoaneurysm is close to the skin surface (typically a pseudoaneurysm in the groin after cardiac catheterization), the pseudoaneurysm can be directly punctured with a fine needle (e.g. 22 gauge), and thrombin or NBCA can be injected (Figs 3.6A to D). When the involved artery is embolized with coils, the artery also should be embolized distal to the origin of the pseudoaneurysm so that collaterals do not fill the aneurysm

Malignant Tumors

Indications for embolotherapy in neoplastic conditions include preoperative embolization and palliative embolization. Embolization helps alleviate symptoms, reduces further dissemination, and increases the response to other treatment modalities (e.g. radiation therapy). Embolotherapy can be used for many types of malignant tumors.[16] Renal malignancy is the most common type of tumor treated with embolotherapy. In particular, tumors extending into

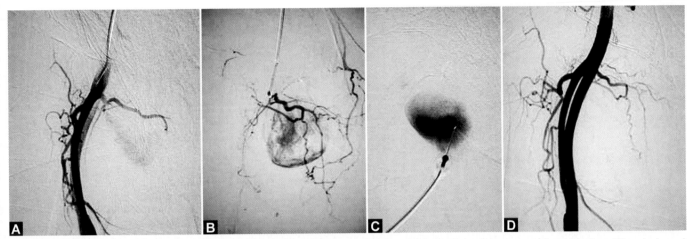

Figs 3.6A to D: A postcatheterization pseudoaneurysm in the right groin. Selective injections into the right common femoral artery (A) and a branch of the profunda femoris artery (B) shows the jet and the lesion. The lesion was percutaneously punctured and 800 U thrombin was injected (C). Though the pseudoaneurysm occluded immediately (D), it recanalized a few days later and needed surgical repair

the hilum or other adjacent structures for which surgical removal is difficult are treated by using embolotherapy. In these patients, prior embolization of the tumor shrinks the mass and minimizes blood loss during surgical removal.

Unresectable tumors can be made operable by means of embolotherapy. If the entity is in its end-stage (disseminated metastatic deposits), the technique can be used for palliation to control pain and hematuria. Other reported malignancies in which embolotherapy has been used include pelvic malignancies and bone tumors. Hemorrhage resulting from malignancy or radiotherapy (e.g. due to radiation cystitis) can be controlled by using embolotherapy.

Chemoembolization

Chemoembolization is commonly performed in hepatic malignancies.[17] The technique is used in patients with unresectable liver tumors and metastatic liver disease. An essential prerequisite for chemoinfusion/chemoembolization is the presence of a patent portal vein with hepatopetal flow. The bilirubin level should be less than 3 mg/dl to perform chemoinfusion/chemoembolization safely.

Vigorous intravenous hydration is required before the procedure for at least 24 hours. Initially, a superior mesenteric arteriogram is usually obtained to demonstrate a variant origin of hepatic artery (accessory or replaced, originating from the superior mesenteric artery) and to demonstrate patency of the portal vein. Then, the celiac trunk and, subsequently, the common hepatic artery are catheterized and studied to outline the vascular anatomy.

The involved lobar hepatic artery or, more commonly, the first- or second-order branches of this artery is subsequently catheterized by using a microcatheter and the chemoinfusion material is injected under fluoroscopic guidance. The tip of the catheter must be placed distal to the cystic and gastroduodenal arteries. The most commonly used chemoinfusion mixture consists of 10 ml of iopamidol (Isovue), 20 ml of Ethiodol, and

60 mg of doxorubicin. The chemoinfusion is usually followed by embolization with a slurry of gelatin sponge powder (Gelfoam).

Lidocaine is intra-arterially administered to reduce pain after the chemoinfusion/chemoembolization treatment.

Organ Ablation

Splenic embolization can be used as a preoperative therapy or as an alternative to surgical removal of the spleen. Indications include post-traumatic bleeding, variceal bleeding secondary to portal hypertension or splenic vein thrombosis, hypersplenism, thalassemia major, thrombocytopenia, idiopathic thrombocytopenic purpura, Gaucher's disease, and Hodgkin's disease. Embolotherapy is performed with superselective catheterization/embolization of the splenic artery by using embolic particles while the tip of the catheter is beyond the caudal pancreatic artery. Careful fluoroscopic control of the splenic area is required to limit the total infarction to approximately 60 percent of the spleen.

Renal embolization is an alternative to surgical removal of the kidney, and indications include end-stage renal disease or renovascular hypertension requiring unilateral or bilateral nephrectomy and renal transplant with native kidneys *in situ*. The procedure requires selective catheterization of the renal artery with further advancement of the catheter so that the catheter is wedged or with the use of a balloon occlusion catheter to minimise the possibility of embolic material spillage into the aorta. The preferred embolic agents are particles (e.g. PVA) and/or liquid agents such as ethanol or NBCA. Postinfarction syndrome is relatively common and characterized by pain, which can be managed with narcotics. This pain usually subsides within 48-72 hours.

ANGIOPLASTY

The techniques for balloon dilatation of vascular stenosis are the same for children as for adults. Balloon dilatation can be carried out safely even in small children and can permit access to peripheral stenoses. Small balloon catheters (2 mm) and small shaft

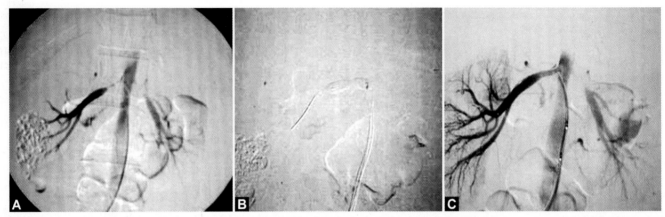

Figs 3.7A to C: A 12-year-old female with hypertension: Tight bilateral ostial renal artery stenosis (A) due to aortoarteritis. The right stenosis was treated with balloon angioplasty (B) with a mild residual waist. The lesion opened up well (C) with mild residual disease. The left stenosis was then subjected to angioplasty with a similar result

catheters (3.8 F) can be used with 4 F delivery systems. Small steerable guidewires (e.g. 0.018" or 0.014" PTCA wires) can be used to cross small distal stenosis. For the renal arteries, low profile balloons in diameters of 3-4 mm are employed. Larger balloons up to 20 mm in size are used to treat recurrent coarctation or peripheral pulmonary stenosis. High pressure balloons (up to 17 atm burst pressure) are available with smaller sizes for fibrous stenosis or restenotic lesions.

The major indications for angioplasty in children are:
1. Renal artery stenosis (RAS)
2. Aortic stenosis
3. Coarctation of aorta
4. Transplant renal artery stenosis
5. Peripheral pulmonary stenosis
6. Systemic-to-pulmonary artery shunt stenosis
7. Budd-Chiari syndrome due to hepatic vein/IVC stenosis

Percutaneous transluminal renal angioplasty (PTRA) is the treatment of choice for RAS. Nonspecific aortoarteritis (NSAA) is responsible for 61% of RAS in our country. Other causes include fibromuscular dysplasia (28%), atherosclerosis (8%), polyarteritis nodosa (2.5%) and renal artery aneurysm of indeterminate etiology (0.5%). NSAA is a chronic and progressive panarteritis of unknown cause that commonly affects the aorta, its major branches and the pulmonary arteries, and results in stenosis, occlusion, dilatation or formation of aneurysms in the involved blood vessels.[18,19] Stenosis or obstruction is the most common angiographic abnormality, frequently involving the aorta and the renal arteries, and resulting in systemic hypertension. The complexity of pathological changes in the wall of the aorta and widespread nature of involvement make surgical revascularization a very difficult option. There is also a high prevalence of graft occlusion. Due to these reasons, nonsurgical revascularization techniques have been increasingly used in the treatment of this group of patients.[20-22]

The goals of therapy in RVH include control of blood pressure (BP) and restoration of renal blood flow. We accept the patients for treatment by nonsurgical revascularization if they have hypertension uncontrolled by single-drug therapy, angiographic evidence of at least 70 percent stenosis in the renal artery or the aorta with a pressure gradient of more than 20 mm Hg and a normal ESR. Patients with an elevated ESR and/or a positive C-reactive protein test are considered to have an active arteritis and are not generally accepted for this treatment except in certain situations (uncontrolled hypertension, severe ventricular dysfunction, flash pulmonary edema and deteriorating renal function).

Anti-hypertensive medication is stopped 24 hr before angioplasty, except for sublingual administration of 5-10 mg nifedipine if the blood pressure is more than 170/110 mm Hg. The patients are treated with aspirin (175-330 mg) daily for 3 days before angioplasty, and this treatment is continued for 6 months after treatment. Heparin (100 IU/kg body weight) is given IV during the procedure and is not reversed afterwards. Blood pressure medication is withheld for 24 hr after the procedure, except for sublingual administration of nifedipine (5-10 mg) if the blood pressure is more than 160/100 mm Hg. If there is severe, uncontrolled hypertension before renal angioplasty, the BP is controlled with nitroprusside drip infusion.

For renal angioplasty (Figs 3.7A to C), a pigtail catheter is positioned in the abdominal aorta above the origin of renal arteries for continuous pressure measurement and diagnostic DSA. The diseased renal artery is selectively catheterized through another arterial sheath in the opposite groin and transstenotic pressure gradient is measured. The angiographic catheter is replaced by a commercially available, appropriate sized balloon catheter by using standard exchange technique. The diameter of the involved vessel is measured and a balloon catheter of same size is used for angioplasty. Three to five inflations, for up to 45 sec each, are performed until the balloon "waist" is no longer present or has decreased substantially. We do not use oversized balloon catheters in patients with mild residual stenosis or transstenotic pressure gradients in order to avoid the risk of arterial rupture. Immediately after the procedure, transstenotic pressure is measured and an angiogram is obtained to assess the adequacy of angioplasty.

Alternatively, the procedure can be completed through a single groin approach too. After crossing the stenosis with the angiographic catheter, an 0.014" or 0.018" exchange guidewire is placed in a distal intrarenal branch, and a 6F or 7F (depending upon the patient size) guiding (right coronary or renal double curve configuration) catheter is placed at the ostium of the diseased artery. The appropriately compatible balloon catheters (sometimes, PTCA balloons in monorail configuration may also be used) are then used to dilate the lesion. The advantage of this approach is the avoidance of a second puncture, although the cost of hardware increases.

If there is an obstructive dissection or a recurrent ostial stenosis, renal artery stent placement is considered. Pretreatment with ticlopidine (250 mg twice daily) beginning three days before angioplasty is then advisable. This should be continued for atleast six weeks after the procedure. A preshaped renal guiding catheter is positioned at the ostium of the diseased renal artery over an exchange guide wire positioned in a secure distal location in the artery. The selection of the diameter and length of the stent is based on the angiographic morphology of the involved artery. It is advisable to give sublingual nifedipine (5-10 mg) or an intraarterial bolus of trinitroglycerine (100-200 mg) in the renal artery before stent placement. The stent is positioned across the lesion and released by inflating the balloon at the desired inflation pressure for up to 30 sec. Various stent designs are available for use in this location. Balloon-mounted stents are generally preferred for an ostial stenosis. A check angiogram is obtained at the end of the procedure to assess the adequacy of stent release. Intravascular ultrasound is a useful technique to define the endpoint of intervention. Angioplasty or stent placement in the aorta is performed by a similar technique.

Angioplasty is considered technically successful if: (i) the aortic or renal artery lumen after angioplasty has less than 30 percent residual stenosis (ii) the arterial lumen is atleast 50 percent larger than its pretreatment diameter, and (iii) the pressure gradient is less than 20 mm Hg and has decreased at least 15 mmHg from the pretreatment gradient.

The clinical results of the angioplasty are judged as follows: (i) cure (normal BP after the procedure without antihypertensive drug therapy), (ii) improved (atleast 15 percent reduction in diastolic pressure or a diastolic pressure less than 90 mmHg with the patient taking less antihypertensive medication than before the procedure), and (iii) failed (no change in BP after the procedure).[27,28] All patients cured or improved are considered to have benefited from angioplasty. Follow-up is performed by BP and medication evaluation one day, one week, and four to six weeks after treatment and then at six-month intervals. Follow-up angiograms are performed in patients with recurrence of hypertension, in whom contralateral nephrectomy of poorly or nonfunctioning kidney for residual hypertension is planned and in those patients who consent for the procedure. Angioplasty is repeated if restenosis is detected.

PTA of the aortic stenosis in NSAA can also be carried out by a similar technique (Figs 3.8A and B). The angiographic features, including eccentricity of the stenosis and presence of

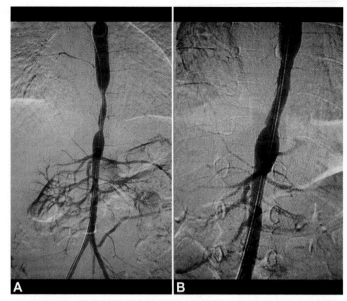

Figs 3.8A and B: Juxtadiaphgramatic aortic stenosis (due to aortoarteritis) in an 18-year-old girl with resistant hypertension. The stenosis responded well to balloon angioplasty alone with a small dissection flap (B). The systolic pressure gradient across the lesion was significantly reduced and the patient did well on clinical follow-up

diffuse adjacent disease, location of the stenosis in juxtadiaphragmatic segment of the aorta and presence of calcification adversely affect the outcome of PTA, most of whom develop large intimal flaps. Stents have been occasionally used as a "bail-out" measure in salvaging an obstructive dissection in such situations and rarely electively in the treatment of native stenosis. Stents provide an immediate relief of symptomatic obstructive dissection and are also useful in the treatment of recurrent stenosis after successful angioplasty. We do not advocate elective use of stents due to young age of the patients, the cost involved and lack of knowledge about the long-term behavior of stents in the aorta at a growing age. Until recently, it was felt that this diesease is characterized by skip areas of involvement. The findings of recent studies, using crosssectional imaging techniques, suggest that nonspecific aortitis involves a continuous length of the aorta, producing mural and luminal changes in some areas, and only mural changes in the intervening segments. This observation has therapeutic implications. The site of surgical reconstruction or balloon positioning in PTA is based on the demonstration of angiographically normal adjacent segments. The results of cross-sectional imaging suggest that there are extensive wall changes even in angiographically normal areas. The unpredictable outcome of PTA and surgical revascularization in nonspecific aortitis, in our opinion, is caused by the placement of a bypass graft or the balloon catheter within the diseased segments and not from normal to normal aortic segment. In this regard, intravascular ultrasound may be useful in guiding the interventional procedures. Overall, aortic PTA has specific technical problems but has a high technical and clinical success rate. The complication rate is low. Late remodeling occurs in most patients and is responsible for delayed clinical benefit despite poor technical success in some patients.

Arterial stenosis associated with renal transplantation can often be improved. These obstructions may be at or beyond the suture line. It is important to evaluate the hemodynamic significance of proximal stenosis because in some of these patients extensive peripheral disease due to rejection nullifies the benefit of dilating the proximal lesions.

Peripheral pulmonary artery stenosis can sometimes be treated effectively but at moderate risk. Because of the elasticity of pulmonary arteries, these lesions require large balloons for small increases in artery size. Arterial rupture can occur, resulting in death. Because there are no surgical options to treat these lesions, balloon dilatation is the procedure of choice when treatment is clinically indicated. Stenting is a safer and more effective approach to these lesions.

After the modified Blalock-Taussig (BT shunt) is placed, stenosis can develop in the subclavian artery, the proximal or distal anastomosis, the graft, or the pulmonary artery. All of these may be treated except the graft stenosis. The best results are obtained in those patients with a traditional BT shunt where the subclavian artery has been directly connected to the pulmonary artery, but this surgery is rarely performed nowadays. Most BT shunts are performed with Goretex grafts, which limit the amount of stretching of the stenosis. Narrowing within the graft is probably caused by kinking, thrombosis, or fibrointimal proliferation.

Complications of Angioplasty Procedures

Vascular spasm can occur, particularly in PTRA, and may in turn provoke thrombosis and segmental infarction. 100 Units/kg of heparin is usually given to prevent this, and more may be required for prolonged procedures. Monitoring of heparinisation with measurements of Activated Clotting Time (ACT) should be done. Spasm may be treated with direct intraarterial injection of nitroglycerin (0.25-1.00 µg/kg/min).

Thrombosis may occur at the PTA site or at the groin. If it does, then thrombolytic therapy is indicated. Intimal dissection is part of any PTA procedure, and usually does not cause flow obstruction. If an obstructive dissection develops, stents may be used. Vascular rupture is always a concern but can be avoided by appropriate balloon selection.

THROMBOLYSIS

Experience with thrombolysis in children is limited but has increased because of the need to treat complications of cardiac or peripheral angiography or intervention. Procedures requiring insertion of devices mounted on large shafts are more likely to result in femoral artery thrombosis. The other indications include thrombosis of BT shunts, dialysis fistula, pulmonary artery thrombosis, iliofemoral thrombophlebitis, aortic thrombosis in neonates, and brachial artery occlusion after supracondylar fracture. Contraindications for the procedure include recent surgery or trauma (within the past 6 weeks), any intracranial or gastrointestinal bleed within the past 3 months, renal failure,

gangrene or significant pregangrenous changes in the affected organ system or extremity.

Thrombolytic agents include streptokinase, urokinase, or r-tpa. Urokinase is the most commonly employed agent. Local lowdose therapy is unlikely to produce systemic changes in coagulation, whereas systemic therapy may cause undesirable bleeding. The dose of urokinase for local lowdose infusion is 300-500 IU/kg/hr. High dose, short duration treatment given locally often produces clearing of thrombus (Figs 3.9A to D). Treatment failures usually relate to delays in implementing therapy, resulting in maturation of thrombus. The fibrinogen level, thrombin time, prothrombin time, and activated partial thromboplastin time are monitored at regular intervals, and the children are observed in an intensive care unit or neonatal nursery.

Complications of intraarterial thrombolysis include systemic bleeding (<5% cases), compartment syndrome due to extremity edema, tissue breakdown products entering systemic circulation causing renal shut down, hyperkalemia causing cardiac arrhythmias, etc. Appropriate patient selection and preprocedure evaluation may help prevent these complications.

FOREIGN BODY REMOVAL

Intravascular foreign bodies may result from the complex interventional hardware, monitoring systems, and indweling catheters that are increasingly being used these days. These may be catheter fragments, pieces of guidewires, metallic coils, stents, electrodes, or ventriculoatrial shunt tubing. Large fragments are believed to pose a risk of thrombosis, spasm, hemorrhage, and arrhythmia. Snares, deflectable guidewires, wire baskets, and intravascular forceps (bioptomes) may be used to retrieve these objects.

CONCLUSION

The future is indeed bright for the practice and practitioners of pediatric vascular interventions. As more and more of the procedures that are currently being performed in adults get gradually adapted for use in the pediatric population, it may be possible to perform safe and successful interventions in many of the pediatric vascular lesions that are otherwise being referred for surgery. These include use of atherectomy devices or lasers that may be used for fibrointimal proliferation that develops in bypass grafts or stents, or in cases of coarctation and recoarctation of the aorta once the vessel wall structure is better understood. Endovascular stenting of the neonatal ductus may replace the surgical creation of aortopulmonary shunts. Percutaneous insertion of central lines and creation of portocaval anastomosis may increasingly get applied to the pediatric patients as well.

However, a note of caution may be made at this point. Risk of radiation damage and the long lasting impact of its after effects may be a serious problem in this age-group, particularly in interventional procedures that require increased fluoroscopic times or multiple sessions. Newer devices or materials or those with uncertain safety should be used with caution in children, and only in situations where other more suitable and safer alternatives do not exist.

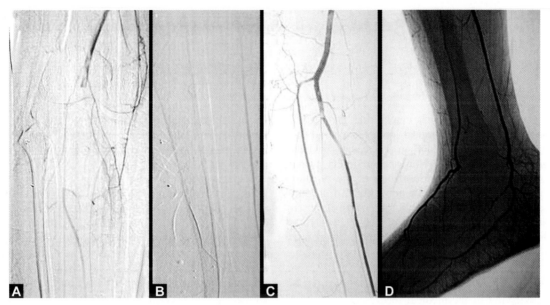

Figs 3.9A to D: Acute thrombotic occlusion of the right popliteal artery (A). The infrapopliteal arteries are not visualized (B). After intraarterial mechanical and pharmacological thrombolysis with urokinase (C and D), antegrade flow has been reestablished

REFERENCES

1. Gordon I, Evans K, Peters AM, Kelly J, et al. Diagnostic Imaging in Pediatrics 1987; 21:661-70.
2. Castaneda-Zuniga WR. Vascular embolotherapy. In Interventional Radiology. Lippincott William and Wilkins, 1997.
3. Tadavarthy SM, Knight L, Ovitt TW, et al. Therapeutic transcatheter arterial embolization. Radiology 1974; 112(1):13-16.
4. Yakes WF, Rossi P, Odink H. How I do it. Arteriovenous malformation management. Cardiovasc Intervent Radiol 1996; 19(2):65-71.
5. Yoshimoto T, Takahashi A, Kinouchi H, et al. Role of embolization in the management of arteriovenous malformations. Clin Neurosurg 1995; 42:313-27.
6. White RI Jr, Pollak JS, Wirth JA. Pulmonary arteriovenous malformations: Diagnosis and transcatheter embolotherapy. J Vasc Interv Radiol 1996; 7(6):787-804.
7. Kaufman SL, Martin LG, Zuckerman AM, et al. Peripheral transcatheter embolization with platinum microcoils. Radiology 1992; 184(2):369-72.
8. Berenguer B, Burrows PE, Zurakowski D, et al. Sclerotherapy of craniofacial venous malformations: Complications and results. Plast Reconstr Surg 1999; 104(1):1-11; discussion 12-5.
9. Dubois JM, Sebag GH, De Prost Y, et al. Soft-tissue venous malformations in children: Percutaneous sclerotherapy with Ethibloc. Radiology 1991; 180(1):195-8.
10. Goldman ML, LAND WC, Bradley EL, et al. Transcatheter therapeutic embolization in the management of massive upper gastrointestinal bleeding. Radiology 1976; 120(3):513-21.
11. Moore HM, List A, Holden A, et al. Therapeutic embolization for acute hemorrhage in the abdomen and pelvis. Australas Radiol 2000; 44(2):161-8.
12. Agolini SF, Shah K, Jaffe J, et al. Arterial embolization is a rapid and effective technique for controlling pelvic fracture hemorrhage. J Trauma 1997; 43(3):395-9.
13. Fellows KE, Khaw KT, Schuster S, et al. Bronchial artery embolization in cystic fibrosis; technique and long-term results. J Pediatr 1979; 95(6):959-63.
14. Mazer MJ, Baltaxe HA, Wolf GL. Therapeutic embolization of the renal artery with Gianturco coils: Limitations and technical pitfalls. Radiology 1981; 138(1):37-46.
15. Stambo GW, Hallisey MJ, Gallagher JJ Jr. Arteriographic embolization of visceral artery pseudoaneurysms. Ann Vasc Surg 1996; 10(5):476-80.
16. Chuang VP, Soo CS, Wallace S. Ivalon embolization in abdominal neoplasms. AJR Am J Roentgenol 1981; 136(4):729-33.
17. Gates J, Hartnell GG, Stuart KE, Clouse ME. Chemoembolization of hepatic neoplasms: Safety, complications, and when to worry. Radiographics 1999; 19(2):399-414.
18. Liu YQ. Radiology of aortoarteritis. Radiol Clin North Am 1985; 23:671-88.
19. Sharma S, Rajani M, Talwar KK. Angiographic morphology in nonspecific Aortoarteritis (Takayasu's arteritis): A study of 126 patients from North India. Cardiovasc Intervent Radiol 1992; 15:160-5.
20. Sharma S, Saxena A, Talwar KK, et al. Renal artery stenosis caused by nonspecific arteritis (Takayasu disease): Results of treatment with percutaneous transluminal angioplasty. AJR 1992; 157:417-22.
21. Sharma S, Bahl VK, Saxena A, et al. Stenosis in the aorta caused by nonspecific aortitis: Results of treatment by percutaneous stent placement. Clin Radiol 1999; 54:46-50.
22. Sharma S, Gupta H, Saxena A, et al. Results of renal angioplasty in nonspecific aortoarteritis (Takayasu's disease). JVIR 1998; 9:429-35.

PART B—Nonvascular Interventions

Amar Mukund, Ashu Seith Bhalla, Shivanand Gamanagatti

Pediatric interventional radiology has emerged as an essential adjunct to management of various surgical and medical conditions of children. The interventional procedure may be categorized into: (a) Vascular interventions and (b) Nonvascular interventions. Vascular interventions have been described in the previous section of this chapter, and in this section nonvascular procedures will be addressed. Prior to any intervention the most important step consists of patient evaluation and pre-procedure care. Every intervention should have a proper and valid referral. If necessary, a direct discussion with the referring physician is appropriate.

PATIENT EVALUATION

This includes reviewing of the medical records as well as the available imaging. Patient/guardian counseling with proper explanation about the procedure should be done and then an informed consent obtained. Other prerequisite prior to the procedure is evaluation of the various necessary laboratory reports. The coagulation parameters should be within normal limits or else these should be rectified prior to intervention. Renal function parameters should be evaluated prior to any intervention needing administration of intravenous (IV) contrast media; however IV contrast is seldom needed in nonvascular procedures.

SEDATION AND ANESTHESIA

Sedation is one the most important factors determining the technical success of a procedure and it also decrease the actual time of procedure. Children may be unable to cooperate for the procedure and crying and body movements can significantly impair the procedure. Hence, anesthetic agents are required to perform a successful intervention. Choice of anesthetic agent depends upon the estimated duration and the degree of pain associated with the procedure. Longer and painful procedure may need general anesthesia (GA) while shorter and less painful procedure may be performed under conscious sedation. Moreover, all procedures should be done in a room well equipped with pulse oximeter monitor, resuscitation devices and emergency drugs needed to handle any adverse situation.

BASIC PROCEDURES

Fine Needle Aspiration (FNA)/Biopsy

The most common image guided nonvascular procedures requested are fine needle aspiration (FNA) and biopsy. Common indications for these procedures are diagnosis of underlying inflammatory/malignant pathology, metastatic disease and tumor staging. The few contraindications, although relative, include – uncorrectable coagulation abnormalities and non availability of safe percutaneous pathway to reach the desired lesion. For abdominal biopsies ascites is also considered a contraindication.

The basic prerequisite for FNA and biopsies are the same as described earlier. Special care should be taken for correcting the coagulopathies, if any, prior to the procedure. A 22-23 gauge (G)

spinal (LP) needle is the most preferred needle for FNA. For deep seated lesions 22 G chiba needle may be needed. Most of the FNAs may be performed under sedation and local anesthesia (LA).

Image guided biopsies although, safe still carry a risk of bleeding and hence, should always be performed with all precautions. Nowadays most of the procedures are performed using either automated or semiautomated biopsy guns. In certain situations coaxial system may prove to be very helpful in cases where multiple passes are required like FNAs and biopsies from lung lesions. Generally, 18 - 20 G biopsy gun suffices for most of the true cut biopsies but the throw length of the cutting needle should be chosen depending upon the size of the lesion. US guidance is preferred over CT guidance for most of the pediatric FNAs and biopsies barring few procedures related to lung lesions, where CT may be needed.[1] Also US guidance prevents the child from unnecessary radiation.

Sampling Technique

Patient should be kept in a comfortable position preferably supine for most of the procedures, but other positions like prone, oblique and even sitting position may be opted for, if deemed necessary. For all FNAs and biopsies the shortest and safest path should be chosen and any vital structure lying in the path between the target and skin should be avoided (Fig. 3.10). Lesions situated on the surface of the liver should be approached by a path having a sizable amount of normal liver parenchyma between the lesion and site of capsular puncture to reduce hemorrhagic complications. FNAs and biopsies should not be attempted if the child is crying or restless as patient movement may cause inadvertent needle movement resulting in organ injury and bleeding. Also the needle tip should always be monitored throughout the procedure.

For FNA, once the needle tip reaches the target organ the stylet should be removed and small to and fro as well as rotating movement should be done with the tip placed in the lesion. Sample for FNA may be obtained using either slight suction technique with a 10 ml syringe or non suction technique to prevent contamination of sample by red blood cells.

Various needles and biopsy guns are commercially available, and prior to any biopsy proper knowledge of the device is mandatory. The performing radiologist should know about the functioning of device (automated or semiautomated gun) and throw length of the cutting needle. While performing biopsy special care is to be taken (more than FNA) to avoid any vital structure as slight negligence leading to vital structure injury may be catastrophic.

Abscess Drainage

Percutaneous drainage is the preferred treatment for various abdominal/pleural collections and abscesses. This may be performed using either of the two basic techniques. For large and superficial collections one step procedure (*Trochar technique*)

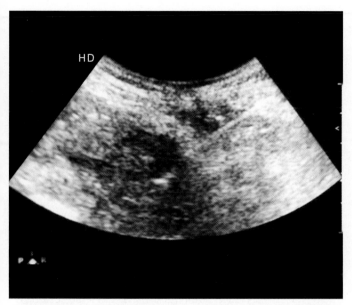

Fig. 3.10: USG image showing FNA being performed with needle tip in retroperitoneal lymph node

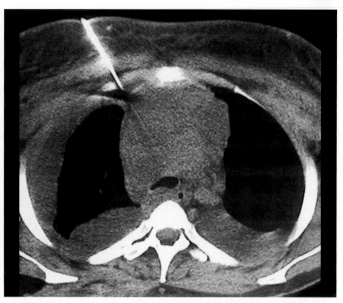

Fig. 3.11: Anterior mediastinal mass being sampled through right parasternal approach under CT guidance

may be used; whereas relatively small and deeper collections or collections adjoining vital structures are suitable for *Seldinger technique*. In trochar technique, the catheter is mounted over a stiff cannula with a stylet; and this assembly is directly inserted into the collection under image guidance as a one step procedure. In Seldinger technique 18/17.5 G needle is used for the initial puncture and a guidewire is introduced into the collection via this needle. Further serial dilatation of the track is done and then a catheter is placed. Choice of catheter depends upon the consistency of the collection. For thick collections wide bore catheters (10-14 F) with large holes like Malecot's may be required whereas for clear or less viscous collections 8-10 F pigtail catheter may suffice.

THORACIC INTERVENTIONS

Guided aspiration of pleural fluid is the most commonly requested nonvascular intervention of the thorax. Other interventions include guided insertion of percutaneous drainage catheters for large/thick/septated pleural/mediastinal collections and FNA/biopsy of lung/mediastinal lesions.

Pleural fluid aspiration may be requested either for diagnostic purpose or sometimes it may be a therapeutic tap. Single time aspiration using a small gauge needle is performed for small and clear pleural effusions, however thick/septated and non resolving effusions require continuous drainage via a percutaneous drainage catheter. For large collections *trochar technique* may be used but for smaller collections *Seldinger technique* is preferable. Special care should be taken to prevent pneumothorax while attempting these procedures, for instance in single time aspiration a three way stop cock along with tubing should be attached to the hub of the needle to prevent entry of air into the pleural cavity. Similarly, if a drainage catheter is placed it should be connected to an under water seal bag rather than a routine urobag. Fibrinolytic therapy may be needed for thick and septated collections and various agents like streptokinase, urokinase and tPA (tissue type plasminogen activator) are available. Studies have shown urokinase and tPA to be safer options.[2,3]

Thoracic lesions in contact with the chest wall and hence, visible on US should be sampled under US guidance; however, lung/mediastinal lesions not visible on US will require CT guidance (Fig. 3.11). The basic technique remains the same as described above except for few modifications and precautions. Multiple pleural punctures should be avoided to prevent pneumothorax and for this purpose coaxial devices are useful. Facility for oxygen administration, suction and chest tube insertion should be available.

GASTROINTESTINAL INTERVENTIONS

Salivary Gland Interventions

These include US guided injection of botulinum toxin in submandibular and sometimes parotid glands. Botulinum injection is performed for treatment of drooling in children with neurological impairment.[4] While injecting botulinum, care should be taken so as to provide uniform distribution of drug throughout the gland. This may be achieved by placing the needle at deeper level and withdrawing it while drug is being injected. FNAs and biopsy of salivary gland lesions may be safely done under US guidance; however the risk of needle track seeding exists in cases of epithelial malignancy.

Esophageal Interventions

One of the common childhood problems is *esophageal stricture*, which may be secondary to corrosive ingestion or anstomosis.[5,6] Balloon dilatation for esophageal strictures is a well recognized radiological treatment (Figs 3.12A to D).[5,6] It should be done under sedation/GA and fluoroscopic guidance. Curved/straight tip angiographic catheter with (0.035 in) hydrophilic, floppy J tip guidewire may be used to cross the stricture. Size of balloon depends upon the size of patient and ranges from 8-18 mm. A rough guide maybe obtained from the width of the thumb of the child, which should be the upper limit of the size of the balloon to be used.[5] Complete dilatation should be attempted progressively in two or more sessions.[7] There is no consensus

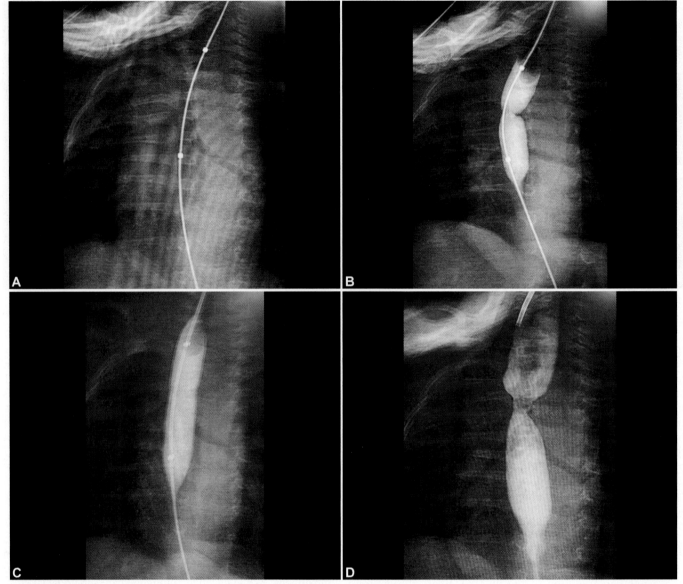

Figs 3.12A to D: (A) Image showing balloon catheter placed across the stricture (B) Balloon catheter being inflated with formation of waist at the site of stricture (C) The waist within the balloon was removed (D) Post dilatation contrast study showing free flow of contrast, however, residual stricture seen, which requires another session

regarding the time to keep balloon inflated, however authors have suggested balloon inflation for 10-30 seconds.[8]

Gastric Interventions

Percutaneous gastrostomy is one of the radiological interventions which may be requested in patients requiring long term (>6 weeks) nutritional supplementation such as patients having neurodisability, craniofacial anomalies, severe gastroesophageal reflux disease etc. This is done under fluoroscopic guidance and initially the stomach is distended with air and punctured by a thin gauge needle. An anchor device is then inserted and pulled to fix the anterior wall of stomach to the abdominal wall.[9] Thereafter, again the stomach is punctured and the tract is dilated in order to insert a pigtail catheter. This may be further converted to gastrojejunostomy by passing the guide wire into the jejunum

through the same track and inserting the catheter over it (Fig. 3.13). Care should be taken during the procedure to prevent colonic puncture/injury, which may lead to formation of gastro-colic fistula.

Hepatic Interventions

Common hepatic interventions requested in pediatric patients are percutaneous FNA, biopsy and drainage of liver abscess. The technique remains the same for FNA and biopsy as described previously. However, the coagulation profile should be within normal limits for any patient undergoing hepatic intervention, especially biopsy. Also the lesion should be approached via substantial normal liver parenchyma.

Percutaneous insertion of the drainage catheter may be required in selected cases of liver abscess.[10,11] Depending upon

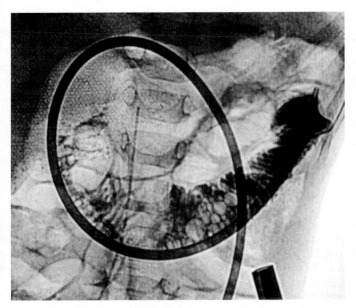

Fig. 3.13: Gastro-jejunostomy image with tip of malecots in proximal jejunum

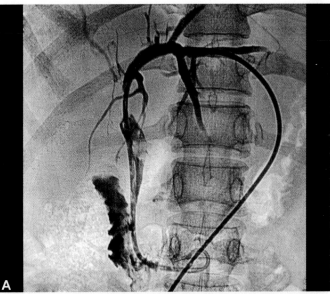

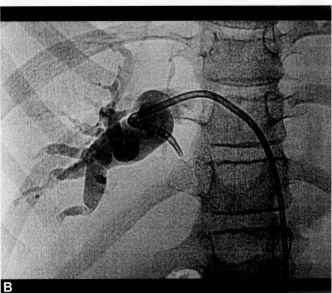

Figs 3.14A and B: (A) Image showing internal external drainage catheter (Ring biliary catheter) placed across the stricture with collapsed biliary system (B) Grossly dilated biliary system with external drainage catheter *in situ*

the size and location of the abscess either trochar or Seldinger technique may be used.

Biliary Intervention

Percutaneous biliary drainage may be required in children having malignant obstructive jaundice as in patients with metastatic lymph nodes encasing the common bile duct, primary pancreatic tumors or metastatic involvement of pancreas.[12] Prior to the procedure, status of biliary confluence (patent/blocked) should be ascertained and accordingly procedure should be performed. In case of a patent primary confluence the catheter may either be placed in the right or the left ductal system. Left sided drainage is generally better tolerated by the children because of less inconvenience caused; and also it is easy to perform under US guidance. In case of a blocked primary confluence the duct which is draining the maximum part of liver should be targeted and at least one third of liver should be drained.

Sedation is a must with coagulation profile under normal limits. For patients with a deranged prothrombin time FFP (fresh frozen plasma) may be required. Ideally, the puncture should be performed using a micropuncture set containing a 21G needle and 018' guidewire which can be further dilated to accommodate 035' guidewire. After initial puncture performed under US guidance the procedure should be carried under fluoroscopic guidance and efforts should be made to cross the strictured segment and place an internal-external drainage catheter across the stricture reaching upto the duodenum (Fig. 3.14A). However at times, it may not be possible to negotiate the stricture in the first attempt when the system is grossly dilated. In these cases patient may be scheduled for a second session to attempt internalization while the external drain is left in place (Fig. 3.14B). Once the system collapses the internalization of the biliary drainage becomes easier. If internalization fails and the patient is on an external drainage then adequate care should be taken to maintain hydration and electrolyte balance caused by bile loss.

Pancreatic Interventions

Pancreatic interventions include FNA/biopsy of pancreatic mass and drainage of peripancreatic collections. While attempting pancreatic FNA/biopsy, care should be taken to avoid traversing through spleen, colon and normal pancreatic parenchyma.

Pancreatitis is relatively rare in children and is generally seen secondary to trauma. Sometimes, a pseudocyst may form and drainage may be required. While planning drainage the smallest and safest pathway without any intervening abdominal viscera should be chosen for catheter placement, however, if no safe pathway is available transgastric approach may be taken.[13] US guidance is preferred for drainage of various abdominal collections, however if proper acoustic window is not available then the drainage should be performed under CT guidance.

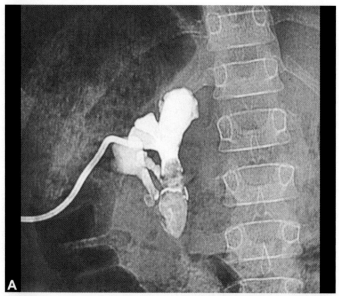

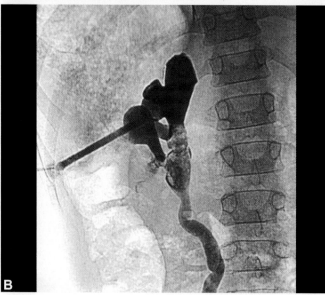

Figs 3.15A and B: (A) PCN (Pigtail drainage catheter) through upper pole calyx, as patient planned for PCNL (B) Pigtail catheter replaced with a 12F sheath in upper pole calyx for PCNL

GENITOURINARY INTERVENTIONS

Common interventions of genitourinary system include renal biopsies, drainage procedures, percutaneous nephrostomy and ureteric dilatation and stenting.

Renal Biopsy

Renal biopsy is required for the diagnosis of renal parenchymal disease or renal masses for tissue diagnosis. Being a painful procedure sedation/GA may be needed for a successful biopsy. All renal biopsies are done under US guidance and retroperitoneal approach is preferred especially in cases with renal masses to prevent intraperitoneal seeding. While sampling renal masses a coaxial technique is preferred.[14] Sampling of renal capsule should be avoided as it may increase the chances of bleeding/hematoma. Post biopsy hematuria though common is

minimal and self limiting. In cases of continuous significant hematuria, patient should be worked up to rule out pseudoaneurysm/arteriovenous fistula, which if present, may need angiographic embolization for treatment.

Percutaneous Nephrostomy (PCN)

Common indications for PCN are obstructive renal disease, urinary diversion, for removal of renal stones or placement of antegrade ureteric stent. In cases of obstructive disease or when simply urinary diversion is needed lower polar calyx puncture is preferred. However, if PCN is performed as an initial step for ureteric stenting or percutaneous nephrolithotomy then upper/interpolar calyx should be punctured (Figs 3.15A and B). Intercostal approach may be needed to access the upper pole calyx.[15]

Commonly, the patient is placed in a prone or semiprone position. The initial puncture of selected calyx (upper or lower) is done under USG guidance. It is preferable to puncture the selected calyx via an oblique posterolateral approach (at 25° from the median plane, with the hub towards patient's flank) to avoid renal hilar vessels.[16] Once the needle tip is inside the calyceal system, urine is seen coming out of the needle as soon as the stylet is removed. At this point, a small amount of diluted contrast may be injected to map the anatomy of pelvicalyceal system and ureter. Further, a floppy tip wire is inserted and directed towards the ureter and using Seldinger technique drainage catheter is positioned in the renal pelvis. The catheter should be properly secured by using various commercially available devices or may be sutured to the skin and dressing should be applied.

Ureteric Dilatation and Stenting

Common indication of ureteric dilatation and stenting in pediatric patients is post transplant ureteral stricture. Upper pole calyx or interpolar calyx puncture is required for all ureteric interventions (Fig. 3.16A). Dilatation and stenting may be done via a pre-existing PCN catheter or through a new antegrade puncture. Initially, a 0.035' hydrophilic floppy J tip guide wire is placed in the ureter (Fig. 3.16B). Then an angled 5F angiographic catheter is advanced over it to reach the stricture site and using the combination of guide wire and catheter the stricture is negotiated (Fig. 3.16C). Sometimes, floppy straight tip guide wire may be needed to cross the stricture. After crossing the stricture hydrophilic floppy guide wire is exchanged for a stiff metallic (0.035' Amplatz extra stiff) guide wire, over which the balloon dilatation of stricture is done. Thereafter, a double J ureteric stent is inserted over the same guide wire using the stent pusher (Fig. 3.16D). The proximal end of the stent may be secured using a suture anchored in one of the side hole so as to position the proximal end of the stent in the renal pelvis while the wire is being withdrawn. A PCN tube should also be placed in the renal pelvis with external end capped for next 24 hours so as to perform antegrade nephrostogram to ensure proper functioning of the stent. Later these stents are removed cystoscopically.

CONCLUSION

Barring a few, most interventions performed in children are similar to adults; but interventions in children are more challenging due to their small size and uncooperative nature due to the associated pain. It is thus essential to have an experienced team consisting of interventional radiologists, anesthetists and nurses for successful pediatric interventions. Also critical is the availability

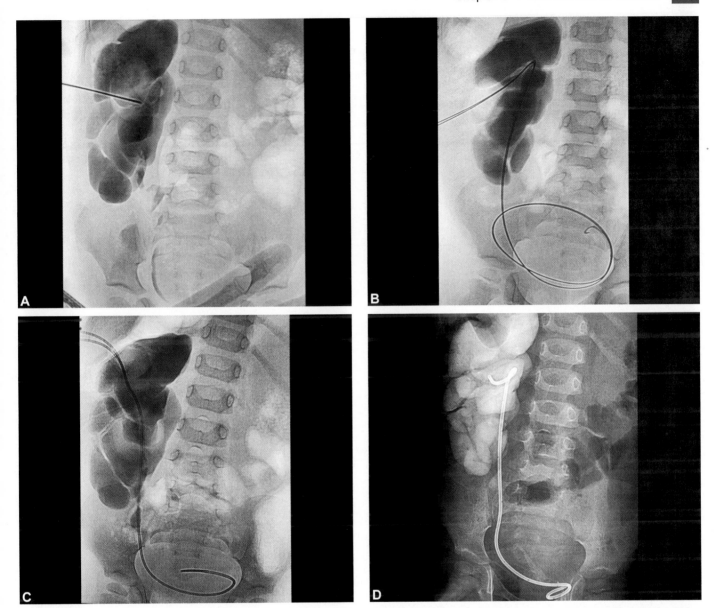

Figs 3.16A to D: (A) Contrast study following interpolar calyx puncture (B) Guide wire was negotiated across the stricture with tip lying within the urinary bladder lumen (C) Further catheter was advanced into the bladder (D) Double J stent was placed over the stiff metallic guide wire

of size appropriate hardware. Concern regarding radiation may be addressed by performing most of the interventions under US guidance, with judicious use of fluoroscopy/CT.

REFERENCES

1. Roebuck DJ. Pediatric interventional radiology. Imaging 2001; 13:302-20.
2. Haaga JR, Nakamoto D, Stellato T, Novak RD, Gavant ML, Silverman SG, Bellmore M. Intracavitary urokinase for enhancement of percutaneous abscess drainage: Phase II trial. AJR Am J Roentgenol 2000; 174(6):1681-5.
3. Beland MD, Gervais DA, Levis DA, Hahn PF, Arellano RS, Mueller PR. Complex abdominal and pelvic abscesses: Efficacy of adjunctive tissue-type plasminogen activator for drainage. Radiology 2008; 247(2):567-73.
4. Pena AH, Cahill AM, Gonzalez L, et al. Botulinum toxin A injection of salivary glands in children with drooling and chronic aspiration. J Vasc Interv Radiol 2009; 20:368-73.
5. Hamza AF, Abdelhay S, Sherif H, et al. Caustic esophageal strictures in children: 30 years' experience. J Pediatr Surg 2003; 38:828–33.
6. Ko HK, Shin JH, Song HY, et al. Balloon dilation of anastomotic strictures secondary to surgical repair of esophageal atresia in a pediatric population: Long-term results. J Vasc Interv Radiol 2006; 17:1327-33.
7. Gercek A, Ay B, Dogan V, et al. Esophageal balloon dilation in children: Prospective analysis of hemodynamic changes and complications during general anesthesia. J Clin Anesth 2007; 19:286-9.
8. Roebuck DJ, McLaren CA. Gastrointestinal intervention in children. Pediatr Radiol 2010; 29.

9. Amaral J, Connolly B. Pediatric interventional radiology. In: Geary DF, Schefer F (Eds) Comprehensive pediatric nephrology. Elsevier, Philadelphia 2008; 1053-78.

10. Simeunovic E, Arnold M, Sidler D, et al. Liver abscess in neonates. Pediatr Surg Int 2009; 25:153-6.

11. Lee SH, Tomlinson C, Temple M, et al. Imaging-guided percutaneous needle aspiration or catheter drainage of neonatal liver abscesses: 14-year experience. AJR 2008; 190:616-22.

12. Roebuck DJ, Stanley P. External and internal-external biliary drainage in children with malignant obstructive jaundice. Pediatr Radiol 2000; 30:659-64.

13. Curry L, Sookur P, Low D, et al. Percutaneous cystgastrostomy as a single-step procedure. Cardiovasc Intervent Radiol 2009; 32:289-95.

14. Roebuck D, Michalski AJ. Core biopsy of renal tumors in childhood [abstract]. Med Pediatr Oncol 2003; 41:283.

15. El-Nahas AR, Shokeir AA, El-Kenawy MR, et al. Safety and efficacy of supracostal percutaneous nephrolithotomy in pediatric patients. J Urol 2008; 180:676-80.

16. Roebuck D. Pediatric interventional radiology: An overview. In: Spitz L, Coran A (Eds) Operative pediatric surgery. Hodder Arnold, London 2006; 1025-37.

CHAPTER 4

Imaging of Pediatric Trauma

Shivanand Gamanagatti, Atin Kumar

Nearly 50% of all deaths in children from 1 to 14 years are the result of trauma.[1] The estimates of mortality for children hospitalized after injury are uniformly low because most fatalities occur prior to arrival at a health care facility.[1,2]

The most common single organ system injury which is associated with highest mortality in pediatric age group is head trauma and nearly 80% of patients with head injuries have associated other organ injuries such as thoracoabdominal injuries. Children are not simple mini adults. Pediatric patients have major anatomic, physiologic, and psychological differences in comparison to adult patients, which play a significant role in the evaluation and management of pediatric trauma patient.

List of anatomic differences in adults and children: Implications for pediatric trauma management [3]

1. Pediatric body size allows a greater distribution of traumatic injuries, hence multiple injuries are common.
2. Relatively greater body surface area of children contributes to greater heat loss.
3. More anterior position of liver and spleen with less protective musculature and subcutaneous tissue mass, makes them more susceptible to injury.
4. Relatively large size of the kidneys compared to their body size, more mobility and less protection from rib cage makes them very susceptible to deceleration injury.
5. The child's growth plates are not yet closed, leading to Salter-type fractures with possible limb-length abnormalities following healing.
6. Children have larger head-to-body ratio and thinner cranial bones (< age of 4 years, the calvarium is unilaminar and lacks dipole) due to which injuries to the head are more serious.

Imaging differences in children from adults[3-5]

Imaging differences in children is based on following aspects:

- In children, periosteum is stronger, thicker, highly vascularized, loosely attached to the underlying bone, biologically more active, and often remains intact even in the presence of significant trauma. The bones have more elasticity and plasticity and therefore sometimes may lead to reversible deformities, without manifesting a typical fracture.
- Because of increased elasticity of the pediatric bones—we may come across significant organ injuries without any osseous injuries. The child's cortical bone is also relatively thicker.

- The growth zone, (consists of transition zone between the elastic metaphysis, with a thinner cortical layer and more spongiosa that is prone to bulge fractures, and the initially purely cartilaginous epiphysis) is the most vulnerable part of the growing bone.
- In children, the bones and also other injuries heal quicker. Growth potentially corrects axial deviations, hence an anatomically exact repositioning of a fracture may not always be necessary as in adults, and even severe parenchymal injuries may be completely compensated by organ growth. On the other hand, even slight injuries of the growth zone may cause severe growth retardation, osseous deformities and joint problems.
- Abdominal parenchymal organs are more mobile in childhood, and less protected by the osseous thoracic skeleton. This exposes them to a higher risk of injury.
- In children, circulation remains stable for very long time but can deteriorate dramatically at any point. Hence, reliable initial assessment as well as effective continuous monitoring and precautionary measures have to be taken to either preventively stabilize the patient or to ensure prompt treatment, particularly important in the era of conservative treatment approach.
- Children are smaller, have higher breathing and heart rates, and have less fatty tissue or not yet ossified skeletal parts, hence their imaging demands a higher spatial and temporal resolution. Some conditions can be assessed by ultrasound (US) in infants and children that in adults could only be reliably assessed by computed tomography (CT); e.g. injuries of abdominal parenchymal organs, neonatal cerebral hemorrhage.
- Children are more sensitive to radiation, and have a higher probability to develop radiation-induced cancer. Therefore, utmost radiation protection is compulsory, one should use dedicated imaging algorithms, alternative imaging modality, and radiation reduction imaging protocols (e.g. reduce X-rays, adapt CT protocols).
- Finally, non-accidental injuries comprise an important aspect of pediatric trauma imaging. It is the duty of any radiologist to pick up potential victims as early as possible to prevent future harm or even life-threatening events.

IMAGING METHODS[6]

The initial assessment of any child should focus on the following questions:

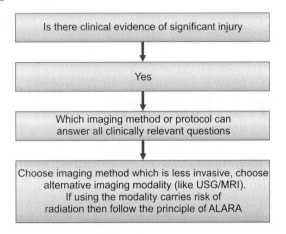

Radiographs: Radiographs are the first imaging method used following trauma. Radiographs will be obtained based on the physical examination. For patients sustaining minor trauma, radiographs may not be needed. Plain film radiography is the method most often relied upon in the assessment of suspected non-accidental injury of children. Children younger than 2 years of age with injuries consistent with child abuse will need a skeletal survey including skull, chest, abdomen, and long bone radiographs It is important that good quality radiographs are obtained in all circumstances and that quality should not be compromised just because of the age and lack of cooperation of the child. It is important that all individuals interpreting radiographs in the acute trauma situation should have an understanding of the normal anatomy and basic radiographic projections used. In majority of the cases, X-ray films are taken because of medicolegal considerations rather than clinical necessity.[7]

Ultrasound: High frequency transducers (7-5 MHz) and ultrasound machines with high spatial and temporal resolution having color Doppler ability are mandatory for a thorough investigation, particularly for imaging neonates and infants. However, in the emergency room just for checking free fluid can be performed using normal equipment using 3-5 MHz transducer. An important use of ultrasound in the acutely traumatized pediatric patient is the 'Focused Abdominal Sonography for Trauma (FAST)' exam. When used by a trained radiologist, the FAST evaluation has the potential to provide sensitive and specific identification of intraperitoneal hemorrhage without invasive measures. The FAST examination does not have the ability to reliably detect specific organ injuries.

Potential Uses of the FAST Examination[8]

- Rapidly identify the source of hypotension in the hemodynamically unstable patient
- Assist in decision making in the child with head and abdominal trauma (head and abdominal CT versus laparotomy and/or craniotomy)
- Evaluate a stable and alert trauma patient with negative physical examination who otherwise would not routinely undergo radiology imaging
- Help prioritize imaging studies in the multiple-trauma patient
- Help avoid additional imaging in a child with an already low likelihood of intra-abdominal injury.

CT: CT is still and will remain (at least for the near future) the modality of choice for a quick, reliable and comprehensive assessment of any polytraumatized child. The current generation CT scanners are very fast, have extremely short rotation time, improved Z axis resolution and offer multiplanar reconstruction facilities. Contrast media is essential just as in adults, using weight adapted contrast media dose and age adapted delay. The modern CT scanners have automated radiation dose reduction techniques such as *automatic tube current modulation* that can substantially reduce patient dose. Currently There are two methods used in the CT systems: z-axis modulation and angular (x- and y-axis) modulation. The aim of this dose reduction or low dose CT strategy is to still achieve a diagnostically reliable image quality at lowest possible radiation dose, by accepting some noise and speckle with consecutive image degradation. In pediatric patients, however, a more critical approach should be adopted with the CT examination being tailored to the specific clinical question being asked, to avoid unnecessary radiation dose.[9]

The specific indications for chest CT in blunt trauma should be guided by the findings of the initial clinical examination and chest radiograph.

- A spinal fracture or fractures of the upper ribs, shoulder girdle, and sternum will often necessitate a contrast-enhanced CT to look for vascular injury
- If there is persistent hemorrhagic output from these tubes or progressive pneumomediastinum, to look for bronchial or vascular injury
- In the presence of an abnormal mediastinum on plain radiographs, to evaluate for thoracic aortic injury.

The most common indications for abdominal CT include lap-belt ecchymosis, gross hematuria, positive FAST scan, all patients with penetrating injury and signs of peritonitis to look for bowel injury.

There are three arguments against the routine use of total-body CT in pediatric trauma imaging[9]

1. An important issue of radiation dose in the pediatric age group
2. Consideration of cost effectiveness in the use of expensive imaging resources
3. There is the risk of the possible demonstration of pseudo-disease and clinically unimportant findings by over-interpretation of CT findings

Hence, there is a critical need for developing clinical appropriateness criteria for the application of CT in pediatric trauma patients.

Given these controversies, the initial imaging evaluation of pediatric trauma should consist of the conventional trauma series (lateral radiograph of the cervical spine, AP radiograph of the pelvis and chest radiograph), in conjunction with a careful and rapid triage by an experienced clinician after taking the mechanism and force of injury into account. This approach will determine the need for additional imaging with cross-sectional techniques, such as ultrasound and spiral or multidetector-row CT.

MRI: MRI is rarely used for the initial assessment of acute severe trauma except in some rare situations, most commonly related to the central nervous system and spinal cord. However, MRI is also widely used for assessment of traumatic musculoskeletal changes at multiple body areas, particularly the joints. Diagnostic MRI needs appropriate sequence selection and good quality images. Sequence selection is dependent on the clinical question being asked and the possible pathological processes that may be encountered. Image quality is dependent on the signal to noise ratio, spatial resolution, image contrast and any associated artifacts.[10]

Abdominal Trauma[11-13]

The management of pediatric blunt abdominal trauma has become increasingly nonoperative over the past several decades. Blunt trauma accounts for nearly 90% of injuries in children. Although skeletal, thoracic, and central nervous system injuries are often clinically evident but intra-abdominal injuries in children are difficult to detect on physical examination, especially in an unconscious child. Hence, imaging plays an important role in diagnosis and management.

Contrast-enhanced CT is the preferred imaging modality in the evaluation of intra-abdominal injury. The radiologist's job is not simply to recognize injuries but also to actively seek imaging signs that indicate the need for surgery. Imaging signs that indicate need of either surgical or endovascular intervention include presence of pneumoperitoneum, intraperitoneal bladder rupture, grade V renovascular injury and active contrast extravasation.[14]

Nonoperative management is typical for uncomplicated spleen and liver injuries and is gaining popularity for uncomplicated pancreatic and renal injuries. The injuries detected at CT help in determining the appropriate degree of patient monitoring in the hospital (i.e. intensive care unit versus regular ward), length of hospitalization, and amount of activity restriction after discharge. In children, following blunt abdominal trauma, solid-organ injuries predominate, with the spleen being the most commonly injured organ, followed by the liver and kidney.

Spleen and Liver

Injury to the liver and spleen occurs in 6 to 9% of pediatric patients after blunt abdominal trauma. Although these injuries occur with nearly equal frequency, mortality is greater in patients with hepatic injuries. Patterns of hepatic and splenic injury includes laceration, fracture, hematoma, and rupture (Figs 4.1 and 4.2A to D). Complications of splenic and liver injury include arterial pseudoaneurysm, active intra-abdominal hemorrhage, delayed hemorrhage, and biloma.

Pancreas

Pancreatic injuries occur in approximately 1 to 2% of children undergoing CT for blunt abdominal trauma. Bicycle handlebar injuries are the most common mechanism of pancreatic injury in children. Pediatric pancreatic injuries are most often isolated, whereas in adults they commonly accompany other abdominal injuries.

Direct signs of pancreatic injury include pancreatic laceration, transection, and comminution (Figs 4.3A to D). Peri-pancreatic fat stranding, hemorrhage, and fluid between the splenic vein and

pancreas are useful secondary signs of pancreatic injury. Presence of peri-pancreatic fluid in the absence of other abdominal visceral injury should strongly suggest pancreatic injury.

CT is useful in delineating the location of pancreatic injury in relation to superior mesenteric artery and vein, as well as the status of main pancreatic duct.

Common complications of pancreatic injury in children include pancreatitis and pseudocyst formation. In contrast to adults, trauma is the most common cause of pancreatitis in children.

Nonoperative management is preferred in children with blunt pancreatic trauma in contrast to adult patients who undergo surgery in most cases.

Kidney

Injury to kidney occurs in 4 to 14% of children presenting with blunt abdominal trauma. Children are more susceptible to renal injury after trauma than adults due to the relatively increased renal size and mobility, decreased amount of perinephric fat, and decreased chest wall protection. Presence of an underlying abnormality such as a mass, horseshoe kidney, hydronephrosis, or multiple cysts may increase that susceptibility by causing the kidney to become bulky and oversized. Most patients with significant renal injury present with hematuria. In some cases significant renal injuries are present in children with only microscopic hematuria or a normal urinalysis.

Majority (64-96%) of renal injuries is mild (grade 1-2) (Figs 4.4A to D). Just as with other solid organ injuries in children, nonoperative management is preferred in the management of renal trauma.

Complications of nonoperative management include delayed hemorrhage, renal pseudoaneurysm, delayed hematuria, renal scarring, renal cysts, hypertension, infections, and persistent urinoma.

Bowel and Mesentery

A specific history of lap-belt or handlebar injury should heighten suspicion for bowel injury. Bowel injury occurs in 1 to 8.5% of children after blunt abdominal trauma.

Although bowel perforation is one of the few indications for surgery after abdominal trauma, the diagnosis is difficult to establish at CT. Differentiating perforating from nonperforating bowel injury remains a challenge even for an experienced radiologist.

Most common CT findings in children with bowel rupture are free peritoneal fluid and bowel wall enhancement (Figs 4.5A and B). Other CT findings include extraluminal gas, bowel wall thickening, bowel dilation, bowel wall defect, mesenteric stranding, fluid at the mesenteric root, focal hematoma, active hemorrhage, and mesenteric pseudoaneurysm.

Unexplained peritoneal fluid (free fluid without any solid parenchymal injury, pelvic fracture, or hypoperfusion complex) is another useful indicator of bowel or mesenteric injury.

Duodenal injury is rare, occurring in less than 1% of children after blunt abdominal trauma. CT findings that are strongly suggestive of a nonperforating duodenal injury include a thickened

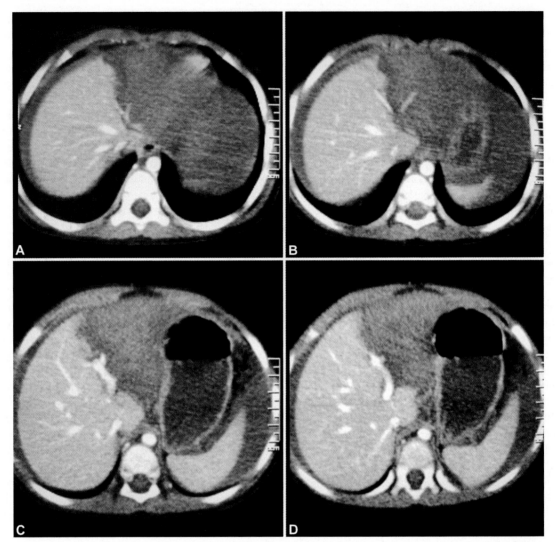

Fig. 4.1: Axial CT sections of liver showing large contusion involving lateral segment of left lobe of liver with hemoperitoneum

duodenum, mural hematoma, retroperitoneal fluid, and intraperitoneal fluid. Presence of retroperitoneal air has a strong association with duodenal perforation. The distinction is critical, as perforating injuries require surgery, while duodenal hematomas can be managed nonoperatively.

Complications of bowel injury include abscess, fistula formation, bowel obstruction, and wound infection.

One common mimicker of bowel injury at CT is overhydration, or increased central venous pressure that occurs during aggressive resuscitation. This can lead to bowel wall or mesenteric edema that can obscure or simulate bowel injury.

Chest Trauma

Blunt Trauma Chest [9]

Thoracic injury is a leading cause of death resulting from trauma in children, second only to head injury. Blunt chest injuries are more common than penetrating injury. Physical evaluation of chest is limited in children with polytrauma either because of loss of consciousness due to head injury, or because of lack of co-operation; imaging plays an important role in diagnosis.

The supine anteroposterior (AP) chest radiograph performed in emergency room may be limited because of technical factors and artifact from overlying immobilization hardware; however, it remains an important tool for the prompt diagnosis of life-threatening conditions such as a tension pneumothorax.

Focused sonography of the lower chest and pericardial space may be very helpful in identifying presence of significant hemo-thorax or hemopericardium, which may require urgent drainage.

Once a severely injured child is stabilized hemodynamically, further imaging tests need to be undertaken to identify internal injury such as contusion, laceration, pneumothorax, hemothorax, pericardial effusion or any vascular injury.

Currently, CT is the imaging modality of choice to evaluate chest injury in multitrauma patients, not only in adults, but increasingly in the pediatric population.

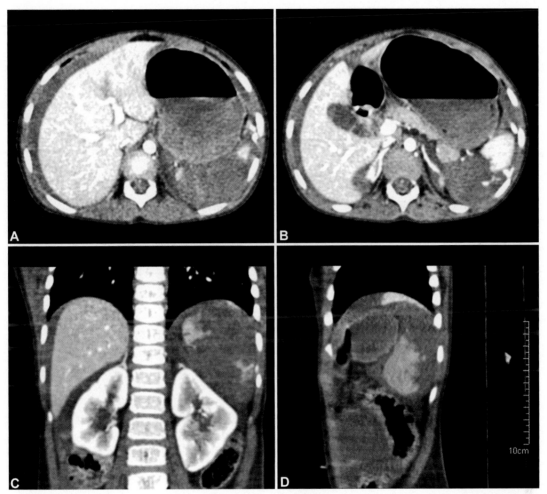

Figs 4.2A to D: Axial CT (A,B) and coronal (C) and sagittal MPR (D) images of upper abdomen showing large contusion involving more than 50% of splenic parenchyma suggesting Grade 3 lesion with hemoperitoneum

Chest wall injuries; Rib fractures are less common in children than in adults because of the compliance/elasticity of the anterior chest wall in children, hence, major internal injuries can occur without rib fractures. Dislocated rib fractures/ unstable flail chest are rarely seen in smaller children. Fractures of the upper ribs and clavicle are often combined with either vascular or esophago-tracheo-bronchial injuries.

Lower rib fractures are often combined with lacerations of the upper abdominal organs. The fractures of the upper ribs, clavicles, sternum, scapulae, and vertebral bodies or processes are all better assessed with CT than with plain films.

Fracture of the trachea or of a bronchus gives following radiological findings:

- Misplaced endotracheal tube, but a deformed bronchial contour can also be helpful in the diagnosis.
- In the most advanced cases fallen lung sign with collapse of the lung *not to* the hilum *but towards* the diaphragm can be seen.

Pleura

Pneumothorax can result from penetrating injury to the chest wall, from air leak into the pleural space from an injured lung (laceration),

or in association with central air leak from the tracheobronchial tree (pneumomediastinum).

Diagnosis of pneumothorax is straightforward on upright chest radiographs, with demonstration of the visceral pleural line outlined by free pleural air in the apex of the chest. Expiratory films may enhance the visibility of pneumothoraces. In the multitrauma situation, patient is typically in the supine position hence pneumothorax is more difficult to detect and often can be diagnosed only by indirect signs such as deep sulcus sign and double diaphragm sign.

CT is more sensitive than chest radiography for small pneumothoraces (Fig. 4.6A), but it is of no clinical significance unless the patient is receiving positive-pressure ventilation support.

Presence of a tension pneumothorax (Fig. 4.6B), as evidenced by midline shift on chest radiograph, requires urgent chest tube insertion and therefore this information should be communicated to the treatment team.

Hemothorax: Hemothorax is a result of venous or arterial bleeding into the pleural cavity.

On supine chest radiography, pleural effusions manifest as a veil-like increased density over the involved hemithorax with

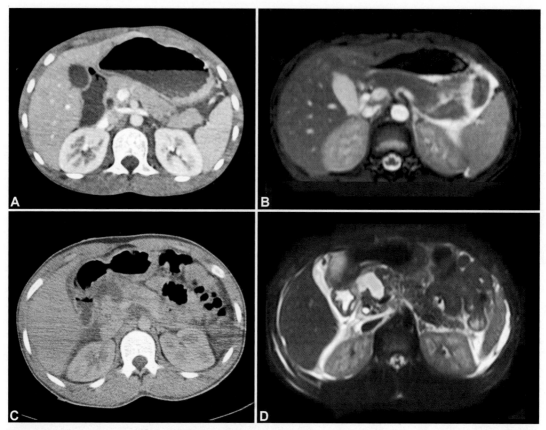

Figs 4.3A to D: Axial CT and TRUE FISP MR images showing linear complete laceration involving tail of pancreas with peripancreatic minimal free fluid collection (A, B). Axial CT and T2W-FS image showing complete laceration with fluid collection in the region of head of pancreas (C,D)

preserved visibility of pulmonary vascular markings and, in the case of larger amounts of fluid, thickening of the lateral pleural line. CT is more sensitive than radiography for demonstrating small effusions, and Hounsfield density measurements may help confirm their hemorrhagic nature (Figs 4.7A and B). CT is also superior for accurate assessment of chest tube placement and related complications.

Pulmonary parenchyma: The radiological findings in pulmonary contusion can vary considerably from patient to patient. There is no air bronchogram but the pattern and extent varies. There are many different radiological appearances. They can be patchy or extensive and confluent, they can be solitary or multifocal, and they can be unilateral or bilateral. Simultaneous aspiration can sometimes confuse the radiological assessment and complicate the outcome. Lung laceration initially may be indistinguishable from the surrounding contusion (Figs 4.8A to D). Because of the disruption of lung tissue, one or more air cavities develop over time and may contain a central density or fluid level because of intrapulmonary hematoma. In the case of large lacerations involving the pleural surface, a bronchopleural fistula may develop. Cavitation of contusions or hematomas, sometimes with air-blood levels on upright chest films or on CT occurs earlier

in time in children than in adults. They can be seen as residual infiltrates for months.

Mediastinum: The momentary chest compression and re-expansion of the chest at the time of incident may lead to mediastinal injury and a pneumomediastinum with air tracking and sometimes extending into the neck as subcutaneous emphysema. Pneumomediastinum is recognized by streaky air collections outlining mediastinal structures such as thymus. Another sign of pneumomediastinum is the so called 'continuous diaphragm sign' which is due to air beneath the heart.

Perforation/rupture of the esophagus may be caused by blunt trauma of chest or by penetrating injury. Unexplained pneumomediastinum and pleural effusions are the most important radiologic signs. If the injury is suspected, an esophagogram should be performed, initially with water-soluble contrast material, followed by dilute barium (Figs 4.9A and B).

Detection of a *mediastinal hematoma* is extremely important, because it may be a clue to an occult traumatic aortic injury (TAI), which is often clinically silent. Mediastinal measurement criteria published in the adult, i.e. mediastinal width greater than 8 cm, mediastinum-to-chest ratio greater than 0.25 have been proven to lack a sufficient predictive value for TAI and do not necessarily

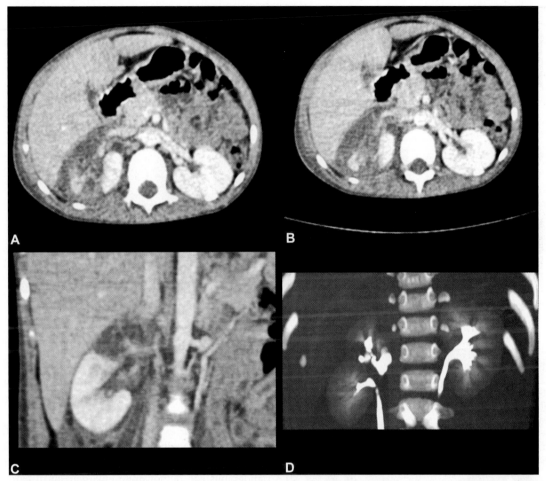

Figs 4.4A to D: Axial CT (A,B) and Coronal MPR (C) images of upper abdomen showing laceration involving upper pole of right kidney with perinephric hematoma and there is evidence of contrast leakage from the upper pole calyx in delayed scan (D)

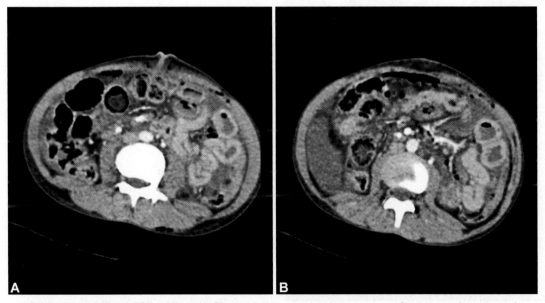

Figs 4.5A and B: Axial CT sections (A, B) of mid abdomen showing presence of pneumoperitoneum and abnormal enhancement of walls of small bowel loops with hemoperitoneum suggestive of bowel injury

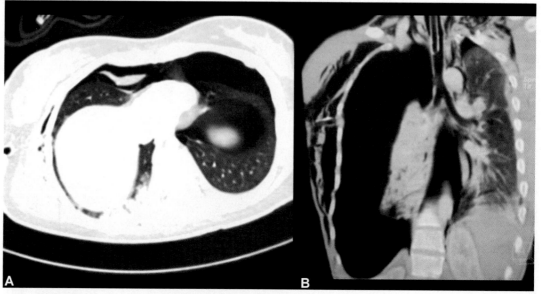

Figs 4.6A and B: Axial and coronal MPR images of lungs showing bilateral minimal pneumothorax (A) and tension pneumothorax on right side with collapse of underlying lung (B)

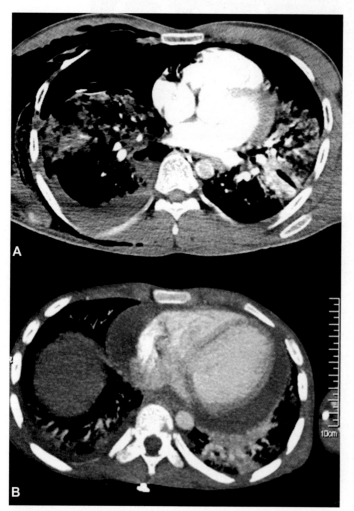

Figs 4.7A and B: Axial CT section of thorax showing right side hemothorax with contusion in bilateral lungs (A) and hemopericardium with minimal right side hemothorax (B)

apply to children. Multidetector-row CT angiography has emerged in recent years as a test that is helpful to rule out or demonstrate TAI in patients with an abnormal mediastinum on chest radiography.[9]

Cardiac injuries are rare but may include both myocardial laceration with ventricular shunting or pericardial hemorrhage (Figs 4.7A and B) and possibly a cardiac tamponade. Chest radiographs can demonstrate enlargement of cardiac silhouette, but they are generally more accurately assessed by CT.

Traumatic ruptures of the diaphragm are more common on the left side but are generally very rare.

Penetrating Chest Trauma

When they involve the lungs, heart or great vessels they produce similar findings to those that occur with blunt chest trauma. Gunshot wounds are relatively common and the pellet is most often accompanied by a pulmonary consolidation. Even if the pellet has passed through the body a circular tube-like consolidation around the track of the bullet can be seen. Specifically, penetrating pediatric chest trauma tends to produce air within the pleural space, heart, mediastinum or great vessels. Metallic and sometimes other foreign bodies may be seen.

Musculoskeletal Injuries[7,10]

Many unique features of the growing skeleton pose specific challenges in imaging skeletal trauma (Vide supra). Differences in the composition and development of the pediatric skeleton (as compared with adults) result in characteristic injuries and fractures. Imaging of these injuries typically begin with plain films, and in the majority no further radiologic evaluation is required. However, Computed tomography (CT) and magnetic resonance imaging (MRI) are used as supplementary imaging studies in pediatric patients with suspected skeletal trauma.

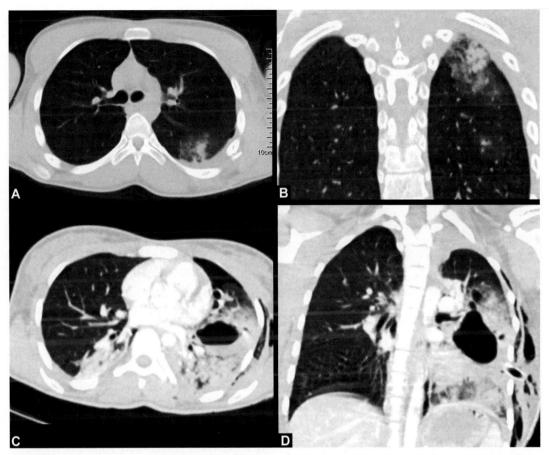

Figs 4.8A to D: Axial and coronal MIP images (A,B) of lung showing ground glass attenuation lesion in left upper lobe close to the chest wall suggestive of lung contusion. Axial and coronal MIP (C,D) images of lung showing large air filled cavity in left upper lobe with surrounding consolidation suggestive of laceration with surrounding contusion. Note; minimal pneumothorax on left side

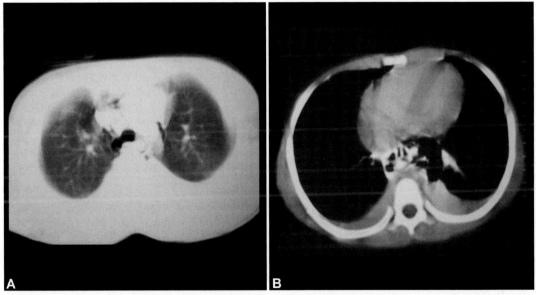

Figs 4.9A and B: Axial CT sections of thorax showing pneumomediastinum (A) and contrast leakage from the esophagus (B) given orally suggestive of esophageal rupture

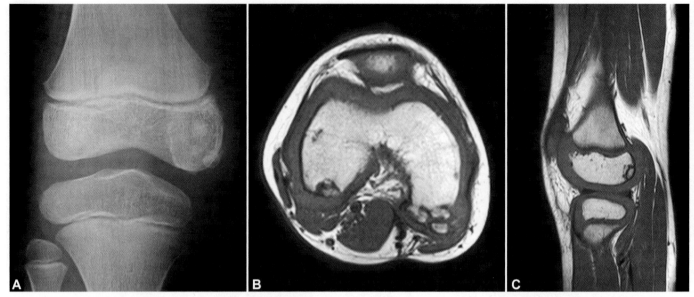

Figs 4.10A to C: AP radiograph of left knee (A) showing multiple loose bodies overlying the medial condyle of left femur. Axial and sagittal MR (B,C) images showing osteochondral lesions involving both condyles of left femur with multiple loose bodies in relation to medial condyle

Imaging [15]

Plain Radiographs

In most cases, imaging of pediatric skeletal trauma begins with radiographs, and very few patients require imaging beyond plain films, this is particularly true in cases of common fractures.

At least two perpendicular views should be performed. Occasionally, oblique or other views may be needed to diagnose a fracture.

CT Scan

Multidetector CT (MDCT) with multiplanar and 3-D reconstruction may help in the identification or exclusion of fractures in anatomically complex areas such as the pelvis, spine, elbow and ankle that are not definite on plain radiography. MDCT is also excellent for the evaluation of fracture healing and complications such as pseudoarthrosis formation, post-traumatic physeal closure and growth arrest.

MRI

With acute pediatric trauma, although plain radiography is still the primary imaging tool, MR imaging has evolved into an essential adjunct diagnostic tool for the prompt identification of occult musculoskeletal injuries. Growth plate injuries and their complications, osteochondritis dissecans (Figs 4.10A to D), avulsion, stress fractures, and soft tissue injuries can be diagnosed early and confidently with MR imaging when other imaging modalities are equivocal. MR imaging, therefore, offers invaluable aid in clinical decisions regarding the timely institution of necessary management to help alleviate symptoms, promote healing, and, more importantly, prevent further complications, such as fractures, degenerative changes, malunion, and growth arrest. MRI is able to accurately evaluate occult and physeal fractures. MRI has been shown to change the classification of physeal fractures significantly, thus affecting surgical management of these patients. Complications such as physeal growth arrest are also well demonstrated on MRI. In other circumstances it is of limited value, being relatively insensitive in detecting small ossific fragments within a joint and when there is a considerable amount of metallic hardware within the bone. While protocols are important, each examination should be tailored to the individual patient and address the specific area of clinical concern. Drawbacks of MRI include longer imaging times, dependence on patient cooperation, and frequent need for sedation.

Musculoskeletal injuries account for 12% of pediatric visits to the emergency department, with fractures making up a large proportion of these numbers. Pediatric bone is more elastic than adult bone and can bend without breaking. This results in unique childhood fractures such as the plastic deformation, torus and greenstick fractures.[7,10]

Fractures extending into the physeal plate may cause growth arrest, and angular deformity may result. Fractures involving the physis have been classified and described by Salter and Harris.

Types of Pediatric Fractures

- Plastic deformation of bone
- Torus
- Greenstick
- Complete diaphyseal fractures
  - Plastic deformation occurs as a result of longitudinal compression of a long bone. With increasing force, microfractures occur and the bone then loses its capacity to regain its original shape and remains bowed. This fracture occurs most commonly in the radius and ulna.
  - Torus fractures are also known as buckle fractures and are incomplete fractures occurring on the concave side of the bone with outward buckling of the cortical margin. These

fractures occur most commonly in the metaphyseal regions of long bones (Fig. 4.12).

– A greenstick fracture is an incomplete fracture occurring only on the convex side of the long bone (Figs 4.11A and B).

– A complete fracture occurs when the fracture line propagates completely through the bone and most commonly involve the diaphyseal region.

Physeal Fractures

The Salter-Harris classification of physeal fractures is the most widely accepted classification and it relates the radiological appearance of physeal fractures with treatment and morbidity.

Salter-Harris Classification

I : Transverse through physis.
II : Through physis but with a metaphyseal fragment.
III : Through physis and epiphysis and therefore intra-articular.
IV : Through epiphysis, across physis and through metaphysis (II and III).
V : Physeal crush injury (Figs 4.13A to C).

A useful rule of thumb is that the higher the grades of injuries, the greater likelihood that the growth plate will be damaged, which can result in long-term complications. Types I, II and III have a relatively good prognosis, whereas type V has a poorer prognosis due to damage to the growth plate. Complications of growth plate injuries include malunion, premature fusion resulting in growth impairment and avascular necrosis.

Head Trauma[16]

Pediatric head trauma is one of the primary causes of injury, mortality and morbidity in childhood. Imaging supports the diagnosis and treatment of intracranial injuries.

The mechanisms of injury in children vary depending on age. The younger the child, the higher the risk of injury, and the risk for asymptomatic intracranial injury is highest for infants younger than 6 months, because of their large heads, weak neck musculature, and relatively thin calvarium. As the child gets older, falls become a less frequent cause of accidental trauma, whereas bicycle injuries and motor vehicle accidents become more common.

Broad Classification

• *Primary lesions:* Are the direct result of trauma (Already occurred at the time of presentation)

• *Secondary lesions:* As complications of primary lesions (preventable)

 – *Acute and subacute:* Include cerebral edema, ischemia, and brain herniation.

 – *Chronic:* Hydrocephalus, the cerebrospinal fluid (CSF) leak, leptomeningeal cyst, and encephalomalacia.

According to Location of Lesions

• *Intra-axial:* Cortical contusions, intracerebral hematoma, axonal shearing injuries, gray matter injury, and vascular injury

• *Extra-axial:* Epidural, subdural, subarachnoid, and intraventricular hemorrhage.

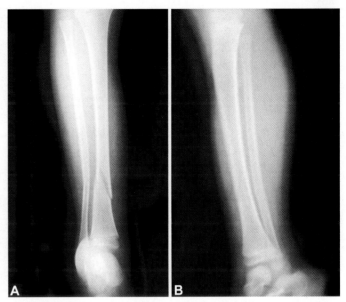

Figs 4.11A and B: AP (A) and lateral radiographs (B) of right leg showing a greenstick fracture of fibula and oblique fracture of tibia

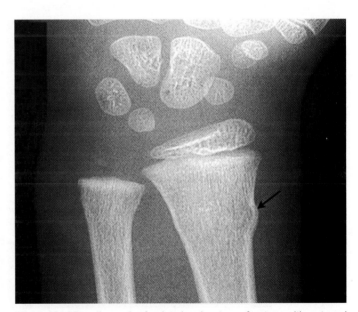

Fig. 4.12: AP radiograph of wrist showing torus fracture with outward buckling of the cortical margin of lower end of radius in the metaphyseal region (arrow)

Skull Fractures[17]

Skull fractures in neonates may be of the following types: linear, diastatic, depressed, compound or buckled. Skull fractures may be diagnosed by CT or plain radiography. Complications from depressed skull fractures include dural tear, cerebral contusion, retained osseous fragments, and cosmetic deformity.

Imaging findings of these abnormalities in children are similar to those in adults.

However, there are few differences as compared to adults [18]

• Skull fractures from minor trauma are more common in children than adults, especially in children younger than 2 years of age.

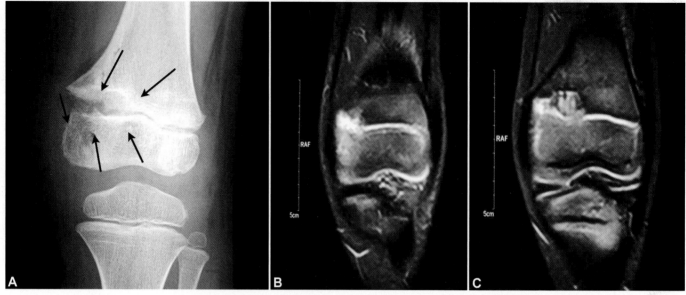

Figs 4.13A to C: AP radiograph (A) and coronal STIR MR images (B,C) of right knee showing type V fracture of Salter-Harris classification involving the medial aspect of growth plate

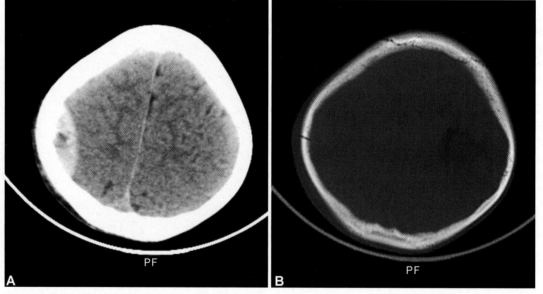

Figs 4.14A and B: Axial CT sections in brain window (A) and bone window (B) showing small biconvex epidural hematoma in parietal region with linear non-depressed fracture of overlying parietal bone

The calvarium in a child is softer and thinner than an adult' and is, therefore, susceptible to fracture.

- The calvarium is unilaminar without diploe till the age of 4 years. Therefore, skull offers less protection to the child's brain than it does in the adult, and children with skull fractures are at an increased risk of having intracranial injury.

Extra-axial Injury

1. Epidural hematoma (EDH) (Figs 4.14A and B)
2. Subdural hematoma (SDH) (Figs 4.15A and B)
3. Subarachnoid hemorrhage
4. Intraventricular hemorrhage

Imaging findings of these abnormalities in children are similar to those in adults.

However, there are few differences as compared to adults

- SDH are more common than EDH
- In children, the dura is more firmly adherent to the inner table of the skull and the groove for the middle meningeal artery is shallow, allowing for more mobility of the vessel. For these reasons EDH is less common, and when it does occur, is more often from venous bleeding than arterial.
- Skull fractures are less commonly associated with EDH in children because of the increased plasticity of the child' skull.

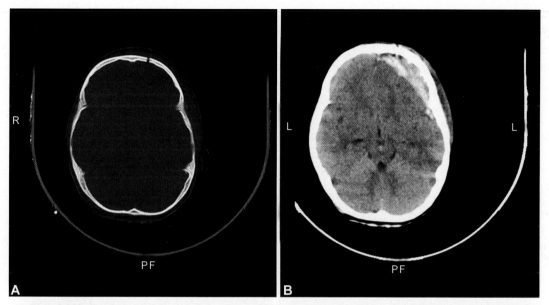

Figs 4.15A and B: Axial CT sections in bone window (A) and brain window (B) showing small subdural hematoma in left frontal region with linear non-depressed fracture of overlying frontal bone

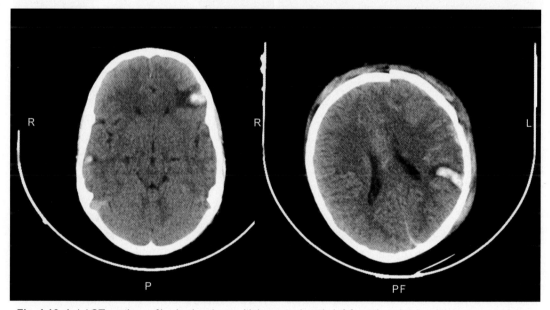

Fig. 4.16: Axial CT sections of brain showing multiple contusions in left frontal, parietal and right temporal lobes associated with mild perilesional edema. Note; depressed fracture of frontal bone

- Since the bleeding is often venous, these hematomas evolve slowly, and the clinical presentation of acute EDH in the young child can be less dramatic than in an adult.
- Unlike in adults, where the SDH is often unilateral, SDH in children is bilateral in up to 80% of cases.
- Often SDH in the pediatric age group is extensive, with involvement of the temporal, frontal and parietal regions. This results from the lack of adhesions in the subdural space that are present in the adult.

Intra-axial injuries include contusions (Fig. 4.16), diffuse axonal injury (DAI) (Figs 4.17A to D and 4.18) and intracerebral

hematomas. The imaging appearances of these abnormalities are similar to those in adults. However, skull is relatively smooth in children compared with adults, contusions are less common in the former.

Secondary Head Injury

Diffuse cerebral swelling (edema) results from:
- Increase in cerebral blood volume (hyperemia),
- Vasogenic edema, or
- An increase in tissue fluid (cytotoxic edema).

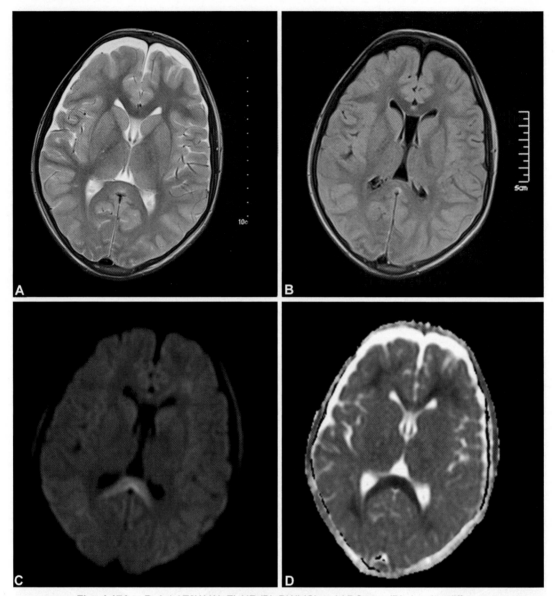

Figs 4.17A to D: Axial T2W (A), FLAIR (B), DWI (C) and ADC map (D) showing diffuse axonal injury involving the splenium of corpus callosum

Imaging features of cerebral edema include effacement of the cerebral sulci and cisterns, compression of the ventricles and loss of gray-white differentiation. The cerebellum and brainstem are usually spared in cerebral edema and may appear hyperdense (On CT) relative to the affected cerebral hemispheres.

Brain herniation occurs secondary to mass effect produced by other causes.

There are three types of herniation:
1. Subfalcine
2. Uncal
3. Transtentorial
   a. Descending
   b. Ascending

All types of herniation are a serious sign of cerebral injury accompanied by displacement of blood vessels and nerves.

Traumatic Ischemia-infarction

Infarctions may occur when cerebral swelling leads to transfalcine or transtentorial herniation that compresses the anterior or posterior cerebral arteries respectively. Cerebral ischemia can occur due to regional or global cerebral blood flow changes (Fig. 4.19).

Spinal Injuries

Spinal injuries in children are rare compared with similar injuries in adults. The prevalence of spinal injuries in children has been reported at less than 10% of all spinal injuries in several studies; however, the mortality rate of craniospinal injury in children is significantly higher than in adults. The cervical spine of young children is fundamentally different from that of adults and the type and outcome of spinal injuries in children also differs from adults.[16]

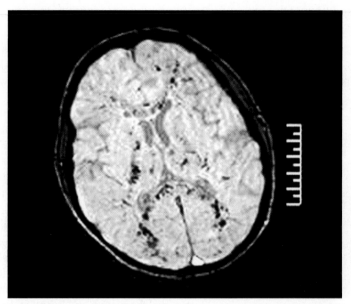

Fig. 4.18: FLASH MR image showing multiple foci of hemorrhages involving gray-white matter junctions and corpus callosum with blooming effect suggestive of diffuse axonal injury

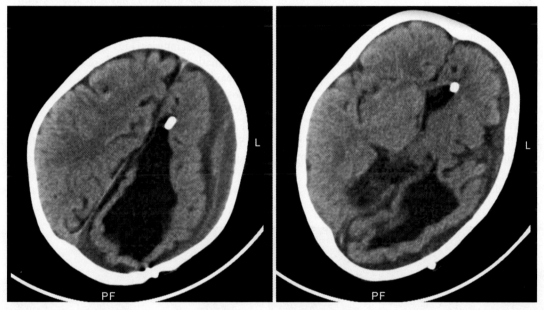

Fig. 4.19: Axial CT sections of brain showing atrophic changes in left cerebral hemisphere with ex-vacuo ventriculomegaly with VP shunt *in situ* and subdural hygroma, sequelae of post-traumatic brain injury

Anatomic differences in the pediatric cervical spine[3]
- Relatively larger head size, resulting in greater flexion and extension injuries
- Smaller neck muscle mass with ligamentous injuries more common than fractures
- Increased flexibility of interspinous ligaments
- Infantile bony column can lengthen significantly without rupture
- Flatter facet joints with a more horizontal orientation
- Incomplete ossification making interpretation of bony alignment difficult
- Basilar odontoid synchondrosis fuse at 3 to 7 years of age

- Apical odontoid epiphysis fuse at 5 to 7 years of age
- Posterior arch of C1 fuses at 4 years of age
- Anterior arch fuses at 7 to 10 years of age
- Epiphyses of spinous process tips may mimic fractures
- Increased preodontoid space up to 4 to 5 mm (3 mm in an adult)
- Pseudosubluxation of C2 on C3 seen in 40% of children
- Prevertebral space size may change because of variations with respiration.

Indications for imaging cervical spine include[19,20]
- Midline cervical tenderness
- Altered level of alertness

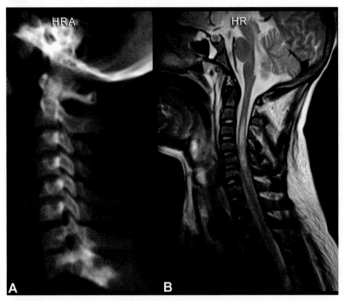

Figs 4.20A and B: Lateral radiograph of cervical spine (A) and sagittal T2W MR image (B) showing evidence of cord contusion without any obvious visible radiographic abnormality suggestive of SCIWORA

- Evidence of intoxication
- Focal neurologic deficits
- Presence of a painful distracting injury
- Significant head or facial injury

Indications for thoracolumbar CT [20]
- Motor vehicle crash at greater than 35 mph
- Falls of greater than 15 feet
- Automobile hitting pedestrian with pedestrian thrown more than 10 feet
- Assaulted with a depressed level of consciousness

- Known cervical injury
- Rigid spine disease

One should be very cautious in using these criteria in children younger than 2 years old, and also in children with congenital or acquired abnormalities (e.g. Down syndrome, juvenile rheumatoid arthritis, prior fracture).

When indicated, radiographic evaluation should routinely consist of three views: a cross-table lateral view, an anteroposterior view, and an open-mouth view to help visualize the odontoid process of C1. With these three plain film views of the cervical region, the sensitivity for detecting cervical fractures is 89% and the negative predictive value of these three views adequately done is nearly 100%.

CT with multiplanar reformatting has a crucial role in the assessment of cervical spine injury (CSI). MRI is the investigation of choice in the presence of neurological deficit or if there is concern for ligamentous injury as it provides direct evaluation of soft tissue abnormalities such as cord compression/contusion, hematoma, disk herniation and ligament disruption.

Types of cervical spine injuries [16]
1. Spinal cord injury without radiographic abnormality (SCIWORA), (Figs 4.20A and B)
2. Occiput–C1 injury
3. Atlantoaxial injuries (Figs 4.21A and B)
4. Traumatic spondylolisthesis of C2 (Hangman fracture)
5. Subaxial injuries (C3–C7)
6. Posterior ligamentous injuries
7. Wedge compression fractures
8. Facet dislocations

SCIWORA (Spinal Cord Injury Without Radiological Abnormality) is almost unique to the pediatric population and occurs as a consequence of a stretch or distraction injury to the relatively flexible spinal column that exceeds the tensile limits of

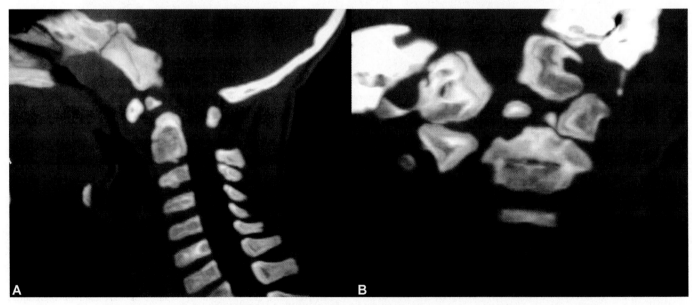

Figs 4.21A and B: Sagittal MPR (A) and coronal Thick MIP (B) images showing type1 fracture of dense of C2 vertebra and atlanto-occipital subluxation

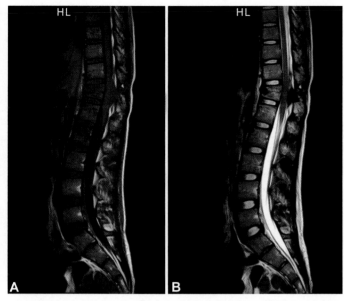

Figs 4.22A and B: Sagittal T1W (A) and T2W MR (B) images showing wedge compression fracture of D12 vertebral body with epidural hematoma. Cord shows normal signal intensity

the spinal cord. Because of increased musculoskeletal elasticity which serves to dissipate the kinetic energy transferred to the child's body during trauma thus preventing fracture or dislocation is not shared by the spinal cord, which may lead to the occurrence of spinal cord injury without radiological abnormality. There is another hypothesis that SCIWORA results from ischemia due to direct vessel injury or due to hypoperfusion of the spinal cord parenchyma.[16]

MRI can demonstrate a variety of neural and extraneural findings. The neural findings vary from cord edema, minor or major hemorrhage, to complete cord transection. The extraneural findings are more useful for assessing the stability of the spinal column and include ligamentous disruption, edema or hemorrhage in the paraspinal muscles, disk edema or herniation, or epidural/subdural hematomas.

Thoracic and Lumbar Spine Trauma

Approximately 30% of all spinal injury in children occurs in the thoracic region and 17–28% of spinal injury is seen in lumbar vertebrae. The most frequent fracture in the thoracolumbar spine is vertebral body compression fracture (Figs 4.22A and B), almost invariably due to a fall. Anterior wedging is seen on a radiograph. CT is essential to fully demonstrate the fracture extent.[16]

Normal radiographic parameters and variants: There are several normal anatomical variants that may be encountered during imaging of the pediatric cervical spine [16]

1. The atlanto-dens interval (ADI) is defined as the distance between the anterior aspect of the dens and the posterior aspect of the anterior ring of the atlas. This distance should be 5 mm or less in children. An ADI that exceeds 5 mm in lateral flexion and 4 mm in lateral extension indicates instability and is suspicious for ligamentous disruption.

2. Pseudospread of the atlas on the axis ('pseudo-Jefferson fracture') can be seen on anterior open-mouth radiographs. Up to 6 mm of displacement of the lateral masses relative to the dens is common in patients up to 4 years old and may be seen in patients up to 7 years old.

3. *Pseudosubluxation:* In children, it is seen most commonly at the C2–3 level, but can also be seen at the C3–4 level. This can be differentiated from true subluxation by the posterior cervical line described by Swischuk. The posterior cervical line is drawn along the posterior arches of C1 and C3, and in normal children the posterior arch of C2 lies within 1.5 mm of the posterior cervical line. An abnormal posterior cervical line measurement often indicates the presence of a bilateral pars interarticularis ('Hangman fracture') of C2.

4. The absence of lordosis, although potentially pathologic in an adult, can be seen in children up to 16 years of age when the neck is in a neutral position.

5. *Posterior interspinous distance:* It is a good indicator of ligamentous integrity and should not be more than 1.5 times greater than the interspinous distance one level either above or below the level in question.

6. *Vertebral body wedging:* In early infancy, cervical vertebral bodies have an oval appearance. These vertebrae take on a more rectangular appearance with advancing age. Anterior wedging of up to 3 mm of the vertebral bodies should not be confused with compression fracture.

7. *Retropharyngeal soft tissue buckling:* In pediatric patients, widening of the prevertebral soft tissues can be a normal finding that is related to expiration. When lateral radiography of the cervical spine in an infant with possible spinal injury shows wide prevertebral soft tissues, repeat lateral radiography in mild extension and in inspiration should be performed to determine if the apparent soft-tissue abnormality is real.

CONCLUSION

Imaging in pediatric trauma must use specific techniques with adapted protocols and algorithms taking the child's specific conditions into consideration. These differ from standard adult imaging strategies and protocols.

REFERENCES

1. Jaffe D. Emergency management of blunt trauma in children. N Engl J Med 1991; 324:1477–82.
2. Minin̆o A, Heron M, Smith B, et al. Deaths: final data for 2004. National vital statistics reports. Hyattsville (MD). National Center for Health Statistics.
3. Marx JA, Holberger RS. Rosen's emergency medicine: concepts and clinical practice. 5th ed. Mosby 2002; 267–81.
4. Kao SC, Smith WL. Skeletal injuries in the pediatric patient. Radiol Clin North Am 1997; 35:727-46.
5. Resnik CS. Diagnostic imaging of pediatric skeletal trauma. Radiol Clin North Am 1989; 27:1013-22.
6. Kellenberger CJ. Imaging children - what is special? Ther Umsch. 2009 Jan;66(1):55-9. Review.
7. AL Baert, et al. Imaging in Pediatric Skeletal Trauma: Techniques and Applications. 1st ed. Springer 2008; 1-11

8. Soudack M, Epelman M, Maor R, et al. Experience with Focused Abdominal Sonography for Trauma (FAST) in 313 pediatric patients. Journal of Clinical Ultrasound 2004;32:53–61.

9. Westra SJ, Wallace EC. Imaging evaluation of pediatric chest trauma. Radiol Clin North Am 2005; 43(2):267-81. Review.

10. Sanchez TR, Jadhav SP, Swischuk LE. MR imaging of pediatric trauma. Magn Reson Imaging Clin N Am 2009; 17(3):439-50.Review.

11. Stanescu LA, Gross JA, Bittle M, et al. Imaging of blunt abdominal trauma. Semin Roentgenol 2006;41(3):196–208.

12. Saladino RA, Lund DP. Abdominal trauma. In: Fleisher GR, Ludwig S, Henretig FM,et al.Textbook of pediatric emergency medicine. 5th ed. Philadelphia: Lippincott. Williams & Wilkins 2006; 1339-48.

13. Rose JS. Ultrasound in abdominal trauma. Emerg Med Clin North Am 2004; 22(3):581-89.

14. Bixby SD, Callahan MJ, Taylor GA. Imaging in pediatric blunt abdominal trauma. Semin Roentgenol 2008; 43(1):72-82.

15. Hussain, Barnes. Pediatric Skeletal Trauma—Plain Film to MRI: Imaging Techniques. Applied Radiology 2007; 36(8):24-33.

16. Cakmakci H. Essentials of trauma: Head and spine. Pediatr Radiol 2009; 39 Suppl 3:391-405.

17. Zimmerman RA, Bilaniuk LT. Pediatric head trauma. Neuroimaging Clin N Am 1994; 4:349-366

18. Schutzman SA, Greenes DS. Pediatric minor head trauma. Ann Emerg Med 2001; 37:65-74.

19. Daffner RH. Controversies in cervical spine imaging in trauma patients. Semin Musculoskelet Radiol 2005; 9(2):105-15.

20. Daffner RH, Hackney DB. ACR Appropriateness Criteria on suspected spine trauma. J Am Coll Radiol 2007; 4(11):762-75.

CHAPTER **5**

Neonatal Respiratory Distress

Akshay Kumar Saxena, Kushaljit Singh Sodhi

A newborn is considered neonate till the age of 28 postnatal days. Respiratory distress constitutes the commonest morbidity requiring admission of a neonate in an intensive care unit. Respiratory distress is defined by presence of at least 2 of the following three features:[1]

i. Tachypnea (respiratory rate >60 per minute),
ii. Retractions (intercostal, subcostal, sternal or suprasternal),
iii. Noisy respiration (grunt, stridor or wheeze).

Respiratory distress occurs in 11-14 percent of all live births.[2] Gestational age has pronounced effect on incidence of neonatal respiratory distress with incidence of respiratory distress on first day of life being higher in babies born at lesser gestation. Kumar and colleagues reported 60 percent incidence of respiratory distress in babies less than 30 weeks of gestational age which reduced to 5 to 6 percent in babies with gestational age more than 34 weeks.[2] There are several causes which can give rise to respiratory distress during the neonatal period. They can broadly be classified as follows:[3]

1. Causes affecting respiration at alveolar level: Hyaline membrane disease (HMD), pneumonia, meconium aspiration syndrome, pneumothorax, pulmonary hemorrhage, primary pulmonary hypertension, transient tachypnea of newborn etc.
2. Structural anomalies of the respiratory tract: Congenital lobar emphysema, congenital caustic adenomatoid malformation (CCAM), congenital diaphragmatic hernia, choanal atresia, tracheoesophageal fistula etc.
3. Extrapulmonary causes: Chest wall abnormalities, congenital heart disease, metabolic acidosis etc.

The management of neonatal respiratory distress depends upon clinical history, examination, radiology and laboratory data. The radiology of important causes of respiratory distress in neonatal period is discussed below.

MEDICAL CAUSES OF NEONATAL RESPIRATORY DISTRESS

Hyaline Membrane Disease (HMD)

HMD, also known as Respiratory Distress Syndrome (RDS), constitutes the most common cause of respiratory distress in the premature newborn infant accounting for up to 60 percent incidence in babies born at or before 29 weeks of gestation.[4] It is a manifestation of pulmonary immaturity and results from impaired surfactant production by Type 2 pneumocytes leading to formation of hyaline membranes within alveoli and terminal airways, hence the name. Oxygen therapy along with surfactant supplementation currently forms the cornerstone of treatment for HMD. Persistent barotraumas and oxygen toxicity in these neonates, due to intensive oxygen and ventilation therapy, can lead to bronchopulmonary dysplasia (BPD).[5]

The radiological evaluation of HMD has traditionally relied upon chest radiography. The radiographic findings in untreated HMD reflect the generalized acinar collapse that results from surfactant deficiency. Chest radiograph features in these babies demonstrate decreased expansion of lungs, symmetric generalized consolidation of variable severity, effacement of normal pulmonary vessels and air bronchograms (Figs 5.1A and B).[6] The commonly seen "reticulogranular" pattern of lung opacities in HMD represents the summation of collapsed alveoli, transudation of fluid into the interstitium from capillary leak and distension by air of innumerable bronchioles that are more compliant than surfactant deficient lung. This radiographic picture reaches maximum severity around 12–24 hrs of life. In severe cases, there may be complete bilateral "whiteout" of lungs due to extensive consolidation.[7]

The radiographic findings of HMD also depend on the timing of the administration of surfactant. Early on, despite prevention with surfactant, the lungs are hypoaerated and have a reticulo-granular pattern due to interstitial fluid and atelectatic alveoli. The administration of surfactant usually produces some clearing (Figs 5.2A and B), which may be symmetrical or asymmetrical; the asymmetry usually disappears in 2-5 days. Since the surfactant is not evenly distributed throughout the lungs, areas of improving lung alternating with areas of unchanged RDS are common finding.[8]

With positive-pressure ventilation usually given in these infants, the lung opacity decreases, and they appear radiographically improved. However, the positive pressure required to aerate the lungs can disrupt the epithelium, producing interstitial and alveolar edema. It can also cause the dissection of air into the interlobar septae and their lymphatics, producing pulmonary interstitial emphysema (PIE) (Fig. 5.3). Radiographically, PIE appears as tortuous, 1- to 4-mm linear lucencies that are relatively uniform in size and radiate outwards from the pulmonary hilum. The lucencies do not empty on expiration and extend to the periphery of the lungs.[9] PIE can be symmetrical, asymmetrical, or localized to one portion of a lung. Peripheral PIE can produce subpleural blebs

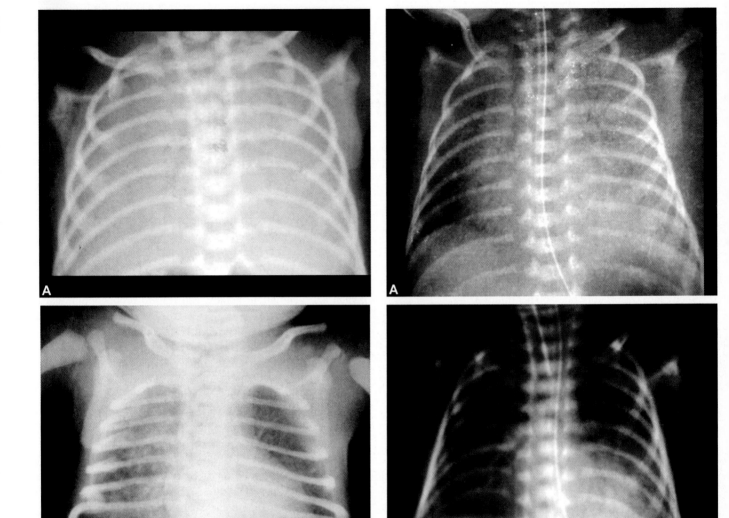

Figs 5.1A and B: (A) Chest X-ray AP view of a preterm neonate with respiratory distress soon after birth reveals low volume lungs with bilateral consolidation with "Whiteout" of lungs suggestive of HMD. (B) In another preterm neonate with respiratory distress soon after birth, consolidation is less extensive

Figs 5.2A and B: (A) Chest X-ray AP view of a preterm neonate with respiratory distress soon after birth reveals low volume lungs with bilateral consolidation with "Whiteout" of lungs suggestive of HMD. (B) 18 hours after surfactant administration, there is asymmetric clearing of upper zones

which can rupture into pleural space to produce pneumothorax or can extend centrally to produce pneumomediastinum or pneumopericardium.

Since, portable chest radiography imparts ionizing radiation and involves delay in availability of information to the clinician, alternative strategies in evaluation of HMD are desirable. A few studies have evaluated use of sonography in diagnosis of HMD.[10,11] Using the transabdominal approach for visualization of lung bases, these studies reported a typical pattern of increased retrodiaphragmatic hyperechogenicity (Figs 5.4A and B) which has high sensitivity and specificity for diagnosis of HMD. Another study by Copetti and colleagues,[12] tried transthoracic approach for evaluation of HMD. They suggested that a combination of white out lung, absence of areas of sparing and pleural line

abnormalities are 100 percent sensitive and specific for diagnosis of respiratory distress syndrome.

Sonography has also been used for follow-up of HMD and early prediction of BPD in neonates suffering from HMD.[13,14] In these studies, the incomplete clearance of retrodiaphragmatic hyperechogenicity was found to be a good predictor of later development of BPD. Avni and colleagues[13] suggested that Day 18 was the earliest day where the persistence of the abnormal retrodiaphragmatic hyperechogenicity was observed in 100 percent of the patients developing BPD at day 28. At that time, 95.2 percent of the patients without abnormal hyperechogenicity showed uncomplicated evolution and no BPD. They concluded that sonography can be a useful diagnostic tool to determine the occurrence of BPD and to predict as early as day 18 the prematures

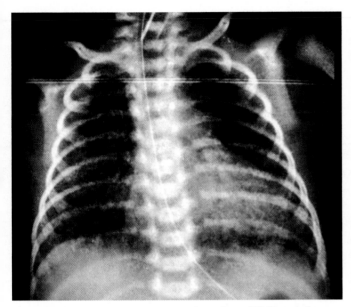

Fig. 5.3: Follow-up chest X-ray of a patient of HMD reveals lucent lesions suggestive of PIE

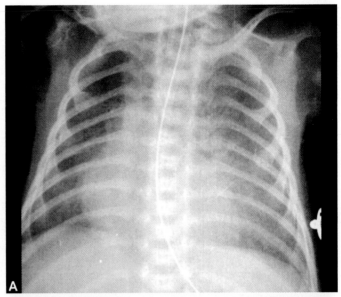

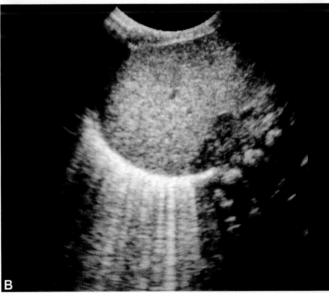

Figs 5.4A and B: (A) Chest X-ray AP view of a preterm neonate with respiratory distress soon after birth reveals low volume lungs with bilateral consolidation with "Whiteout" of lungs suggestive of HMD (B) Coronal transabdominal sonography reveals diffuse retrodiaphragmatic hyperechogenicity suggestive of HMD

at risk for the disease. In another similar study, Pieper et al[14] reported that Day 9 was the earliest day where persistence of abnormal retrodiaphragmatic hyperechogenicity was observed with the highest predictor values for the development of BPD. These preliminary studies suggest that sonography has a role in early identification of neonates who are at risk of developing BPD in future. However, there is some discrepancy regarding the exact postnatal age at which this can be achieved.

Transient Tachypnea of Newborn (TTNB)

Whereas HMD is a disease of premature neonates, TTNB affects term babies. In the fetal life, the lungs are distended with fluid. This fluid is cleared from the lungs during the squeeze through the birth canal while additional fluid is removed by pulmonary capillaries and lymphatics. The delay in clearance of pulmonary fluid leads to TTNB which is also known as "Wet Lung Disease". The risk factors include delivery by cesarean section; precipitous delivery; and very small, hypotonic or sedated babies. The babies present with mild or moderate respiratory distress soon after birth.[15] Typically, the disease is self-limiting with resolution of symptoms in 6-24 hours. Uncommonly, the symptoms may last 2-5 days when it becomes necessary to exclude alternative causes of respiratory distress.[3]

The radiographic features of TTNB include mild overaeration, mild cardiomegaly, small pulmonary effusion and prominent perihilar interstitial markings (Fig. 5.5). TTNB may mimic reticulogranular pattern of HMD but lacks the under aeration seen in HMD. The radiographic features may occasionally look similar to pulmonary edema or meconium aspiration syndrome.[15]

Copetti and Cattarossi[16] have recently evaluated the lung sonographic findings in TTNB and its clinical relevance. They reported that in neonates with TTNB, lung sonography revealed difference in lung echogenicity between the upper and lower lung

areas. There were very compact comet-tail artifacts in the inferior lung fields which were rare in the superior lung fields. They designated this finding the "double lung point". In this study, "double lung point" was not seen in healthy infants, infants with respiratory distress syndrome, atelectasis, pneumothorax, pneumonia, or pulmonary hemorrhage. Thus, the sensitivity and specificity of the "double lung point" was 100 percent for the diagnosis of TTNB. However, a recent report suggests that "double lung point" may be seen in pneumothorax as well.[17]

Neonatal Pneumonia

Pneumonia is an important cause of neonatal respiratory distress in India with all cases of neonatal respiratory distress being treated

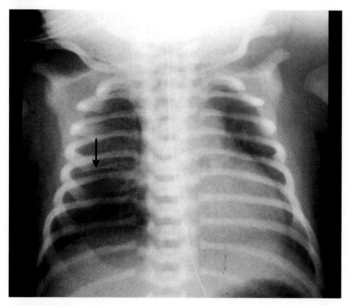

Fig. 5.5: Transient tachypnea of newborn: Chest X-ray of a term neonate born by cesarean section and respiratory distress soon after birth reveals normal volume lungs with perihilar infiltrate, prominent cardiac silhouette and pleural fluid in minor fissure (arrow)

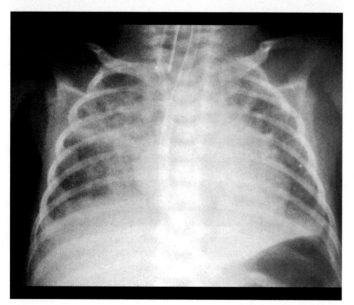

Fig. 5.6: Chest X-ray AP view of a neonate on ventilator with respiratory distress reveals patchy consolidation in right lung suggestive of pneumonia

as pneumonia at the first referral unit.[18] In a recent study which evaluated the causes of respiratory distress in outborn neonates brought to a referral unit, Mathur and colleagues[18] reported pneumonia to be the cause of respiratory distress in more than two third of cases. However, this study did not include patients having surgical causes of respiratory distress. The pneumonia may set in due to transplacental spread, lack of asepsis during delivery, aspiration of amniotic fluid or be acquired during hospital stay for other ailments. Ventilator associated pneumonia is the second commonest hospital-acquired infection amongst pediatric and

neonatal intensive care unit patients,[19,20] and is responsible for a very high mortality in neonatal intensive care unit patients. The majority of cases are of bacterial etiology.

Radiographically, pneumonia is characterized by pulmonary opacities (Fig. 5.6). However, similar appearance may be seen in hyaline membrane disease, transient tachypnea of newborn and meconium aspiration syndrome. Presence of pleural effusion is a helpful pointer towards pneumonia. Furthermore, some of these conditions may coexist with pneumonia.[15] The patients with positive radiograph who do not grow causative organism from blood culture are considered "probable pneumonia".[21] It is important to note that in some of the patients with pneumonia, chest X-ray may be normal and diagnosis is made on isolation of organism from blood culture.[18] Rarely, pneumonia may mimic mass lesion (Figs 5.7A to D).

Meconium Aspiration Syndrome

Meconium aspiration is a disease predominantly affecting term and postmature neonates. While, 10-15 percent of neonates pass meconium *in utero*, it is rare before 37 weeks.[21] Fetus manifests normal shallow regular respiratory movements during intrauterine life. Fetal hypoxia stimulates deep gasping respirations. In addition, it also leads to premature passage of meconium *in utero*. Meconium is sterile but locally irritant. It can cause obstruction of medium and small airways. In addition, it is a good medium for bacterial growth. The severity of meconium aspiration syndrome depends on several factors including consistency of meconium, adequacy of oropharyngeal suction, associated asphyxia, resuscitative measures etc.

The radiographic appearance in meconium aspiration is variable (Figs 5.8A and B). Incomplete bronchial obstruction leads to generalized overereation along with patchy areas of atelectasis secondary to complete bronchial obstruction. There may be subsequent development of pneumothorax and pneumomediastinum. The radiographic appearance may be further complicated by pulmonary edema (because of cerebral, myocardial or renal dysfunction secondary to ischemia), pulmonary hemorrhage, respiratory distress syndrome or pneumonia.[15] Some of the babies with meconium aspiration may eventually develop persistent pulmonary hypertension of newborn.[3]

Pneumothorax

Pneumothorax, defined as presence of air in the pleural cavity, is an uncommon but significant cause of neonatal respiratory distress.[18,22] Timely identification can be life saving. It can occur spontaneously or be secondary to infection, meconium aspiration, ventilation barotraumas (Fig. 5.9) or lung deformity. The incidence of spontaneous pneumothorax is more in premature babies (about 6%) as compared to term babies (1-2%). The radiographic diagnosis of pneumothorax, although of great clinical significance, can be missed on the X-rays as apicolateral accumulation of air is rather uncommon in the supine films. In the supine position, air preferentially accumulates in anteromedial and subpulmonic recesses.[23] The position of air collection is also modified by underlying lung disease. Subpulmonic pneumothorax presents as

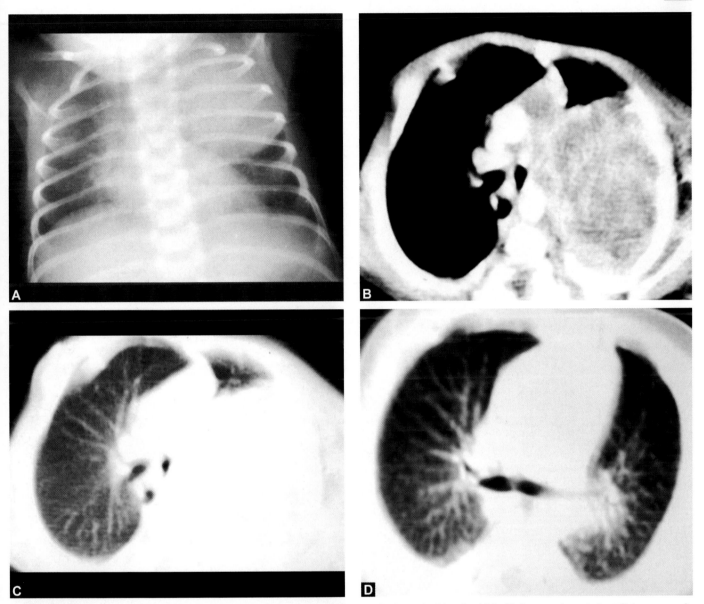

Figs 5.7A to D: Pneumonia mimicking mass lesion: (A) Chest X-ray AP view of a 3-week-old male child with fever and respiratory distress reveals mass like opacity in left upper zone. (B) Mediastinal and (C) Lung window of CECT scan confirm mass like consolidation in left upper lobe. (D) Lung window of repeat CECT scan after 4 weeks of antibiotics reveals resolution of opacity

a relatively lucent region in the left or right upper abdominal quadrant. Sometimes, the only radiographic sign of subpulmonic pneumothorax is deep lateral costophrenic angle (deep sulcus sign).[24]

Surgical Causes of Neonatal Respiratory Distress

Several conditions of neonatal chest require surgical procedure for management. Although listed here as causes of neonatal respiratory distress, it is to be remembered that they may present beyond the neonatal period. In addition, even if discovered during neonatal period, they may be managed conservatively initially. Some of these conditions, like diaphragmatic hernia, can be diagnosed antenatally. Conversely, some of these pathologies may

be discovered accidentally in later life and pose dilemma regarding the need for surgery.

Congenital Lobar Emphysema (CLE)

Congenital lobar emphysema or congenital lobar hyperinflation is a disease of multifactorial origin characterized by focal abnormality of a large airway. Unfortunately, the exact abnormality of large airway frequently remains a mystery as it is left inside the body of the patient proximal to the ligated bronchial stump. However, potential culprits include bronchomalacia, kinks, webs, mucosal webs and crossing vessels. Whatever the etiology may be, the result is impairment of bronchial function and hyperinflation of a pulmonary lobe.[25] Left upper lobe is the commonest site of involvement (40-50%) followed by right middle lobe (28-34%) and

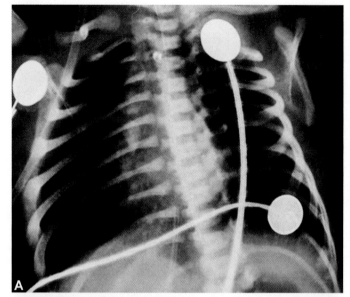

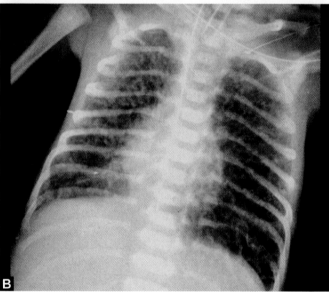

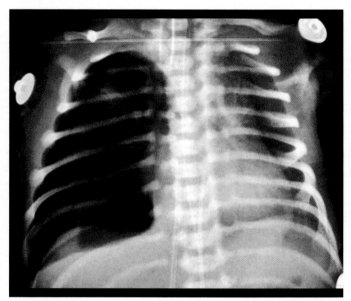

Fig. 5.9: Neonate on ventilator developed respiratory distress. Chest X-ray AP view revealed gross right pneumothorax

Figs 5.8A and B: (A) Term neonate with meconium aspiration. Chest X-ray AP view reveals bilateral hyperinflation. (B) In another neonate with respiratory distress and suspected meconium aspiration, chest X-ray AP view reveals bilateral pulmonary opacities. Pulmonary opacities in meconium aspiration may be due to atelectasis, chemical pneumonitis or super added pneumonia

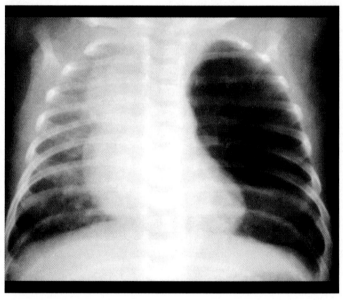

Fig. 5.10: Chest X-ray AP view of a neonate with respiratory distress reveals emphysematous left upper lobe with contralateral mediastinal shift suggestive of congenital lobar emphysema. Presence of vascular markings differentiate congenital lobar emphysema from pneumothorax

right upper lobe (20%).[26] The hyperinflated lobe causes mediastinal shift and atelectasis of the adjacent lobes.

Prenatal diagnosis is unusual in congenital lobar emphysema. Postnatally, the age of onset of symptoms and degree of respiratory distress may be variable. However, more than 50 percent become symptomatic within first week. Not all the symptomatic patients may require immediate surgery.[25,27] The postnatal chest radiograph, if acquired early in life, may reveal overdistended fluid filled lobe. Later on, the radiograph shows characteristic hyperinflation of a lobe with splayed pulmonary vessels, atelectasis of adjacent lobes and contralateral mediastinal shift (Fig. 5.10). The differential diagnosis is pneumothorax wherein the hyperlucent region will be

devoid of pulmonary vascular markings. If required, computed tomography scan (CT scan) can be performed to resolve the diagnosis. The findings seen on chest X-ray can all be seen on CT scan. Computed tomography can also reveal treatable extrinsic and intrinsic treatable cause of partial bronchial obstruction.[26]

Uncommonly, the lobar emphysema may affect two lobes. Either the lobes may be affected simultaneously or the second hyperinflated lobe may be detected after first thoracotomy. The bilobectomy procedure may be performed as one stage or two stage procedure.[27]

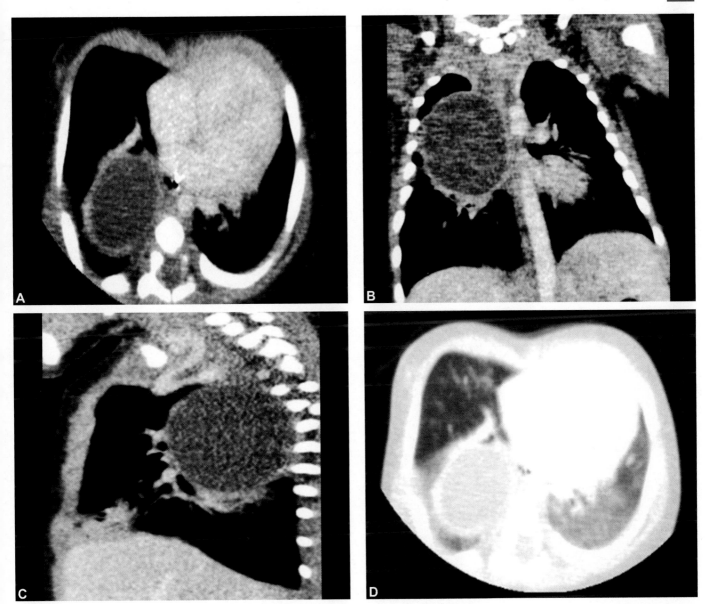

Figs 5.11A to D: A 3-day-old neonate with respiratory distress. Mediastinal window of contrast enhanced CT scan (A) axial (B) coronal reconstruction and (C) Right parasagittal reconstruction reveal a cystic mass lesion in right upper lobe. (D) Lung window additionally reveals bilateral pneumonia. This lesion can be CCAM or bronchogenic cyst. The patient was managed conservatively and is awaiting surgery

Congenital Cystic Adenomatoid Malformation (CCAM)

CCAM (also called CPAM-congenital pulmonary airway malformations) is a hamartomatous lesion believed to occur because of the failure of pulmonary mesenchyme into normal broncho-alveolar tissue.[15,26] On the basis of pathological findings, Stocker,[28] classified the CCAM into five types. However, radiological classification consists of three types:[26]

Type I: It constitutes 50 percent of CCAM patients and shows multiple or single large cysts which communicate with the bronchial tree of the affected lobe.

Type II: It constitutes 40 percent of CCAM and shows multiple cysts that rarely exceed 1.2 cm in diameter and communicate with the bronchial tree of the affected lobe.

About one-third of these patients have associated congenital anomalies.

Type III: It is least common type (10% of patients). It consists of multiple small (<0.5 cm) cysts and may appear solid on imaging. It usually causes mass effect on mediastinum.

Antenatal ultrasound may depict CCAM as a pulmonary mass with associated polyhydramnios or fetal anasarca. The disease is usually unilateral with single lobe involvement seen in 95 percent of patients. Bilateral disease is rare (2%). Neonatal respiratory distress occurs if the CCAM is large and causes mediastinal shift. The cysts may be detected radiographically in 90 percent of patients[26] and better characterized with computed tomography (Figs 5.11A to D) which also helps in excluding congenital lobar emphysema as differential diagnosis. It is to be noted that

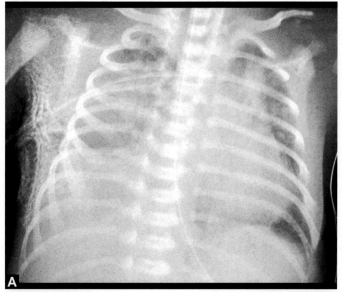

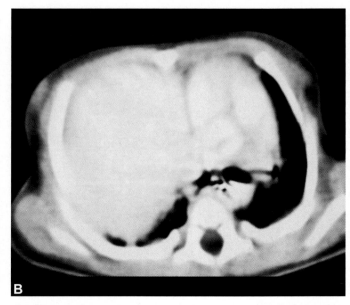

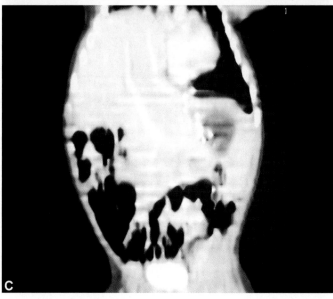

Figs 5.12A to C: One day old neonate with respiratory distress. (A) Chest X-ray AP view reveals high placed liver, right sided pneumonia and contralateral mediastinal shift. Contrast enhanced CT scan axial (B) and reconstructed coronal (C) images confirm herniation of liver through foramen of Morgagni

radiological classification of CCAM may not corroborate with pathological classification.[29] When the lesion abuts diaphragm, congenital diaphragmatic hernia needs to be excluded. This can be done through contrast study of the gastrointestinal tract. CCAM also needs to be differentiated from pneumatoceles. The diagnosis of pneumatoceles can be made if an earlier normal chest radiograph is available or when subsequent radiographs (or CT scan) show complete resolution of disease. Mesenchymal cystic hamartoma can mimic CCAM radiographically. Malignant masses may occasionally be seen within CCAM.[30,31]

Congenital Diaphragmatic Hernia (CDH)

Congenital diaphragmatic hernia (CDH) signifies intrathoracic herniation of abdominal contents through a defect in the diaphragm. Its incidence varies from 1:2000 to 1:5000 in live births. Many fetuses with the diaphragmatic hernia are stillborn. Amongst the live born, 28-50 percent may have associated anomalies. The diaphragmatic defect may be located anteromedially (Morgani hernia) (Figs 5.12A to C); posterolaterally (Bochdalek hernia) (Figs 5.13A to C) or in the central tendon of diaphragm.[26] The condition is being diagnosed increasingly during antenatal ultrasound which facilitates supervised institutional delivery. Bag and mask therapy during neonatal resuscitation may worsen the respiratory distress. Diaphragmatic hernia is accompanied by pulmonary hypoplasia, pulmonary immaturity, hypoplastic left heart and persistent pulmonary artery hypertension of the newborn.[32]

The radiographic appearance depends on the contents of hernia sac and distension of bowel. If radiograph is acquired early, the bowel may be fluid filled or collapse resulting is opacity of variable size in lower hemithorax with contralateral mediastinal shift. Subsequently, air can be identified in the herniated bowel loops making the diagnosis straight forward. However, in some cases, it may need to be differentiated from congenital cystic adenomatoid malformation. This may require a contrast study of the

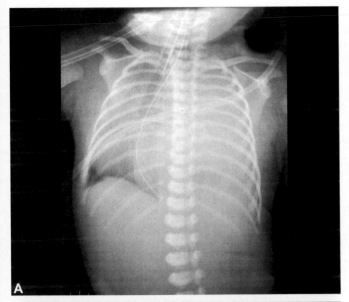

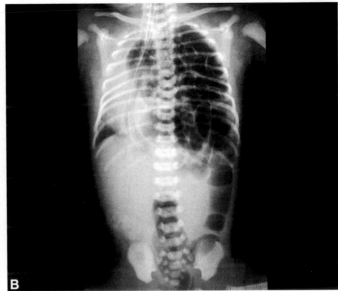

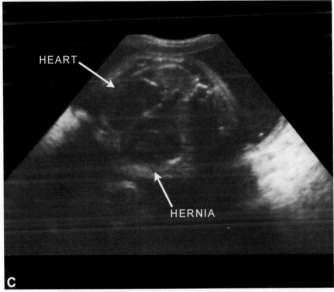

Figs 5.13A to C: Bochdalek hernia: One day old neonate with respiratory distress. Chest X-ray AP view (A) reveals large opacity in left hemithorax with contralateral mediastinal shift. X-ray of chest and abdomen. (B) was repeated 24 hours later which demonstrated thoracic herniation of bowel loops with paucity of bowel loops in abdomen. (C) Antenatal ultrasound for the same baby reveals hernia sac adjacent to heart

gastrointestinal tract to establish the diagnosis. After the diagnosis of diaphragmatic hernia is established, search should be made for associated congenital malformations using sonography (abdomen and head) and echocardiography.

Esophageal Atresia with Tracheoesophageal Fistula

Although western literature does not consider esophageal atresia with tracheoesophageal fistula a common cause of neonatal respiratory distress,[22] a recent Indian study reported it to be the commonest cause of neonatal respiratory distress which required admission in neonatal surgical intensive care unit.[33] Esophageal atresia can be diagnosed at birth with the baby pouring out oral secretions. The baby can develop respiratory distress due to aspiration pneumonia as also due to distended stomach. Antenatal sonography may reveal polyhydramnios. Postnatal diagnosis can be made by localizing the "gastric" tube coiled in the upper

esophageal pouch (Fig. 5.14). Small volume of non-ionic contrast can be injected through the tube before acquiring the radiograph for better localization.[3,26] However, spillage of contrast may make the situation worse.[33]

Miscellaneous Causes

Bronchogenic and esophageal duplication cysts[34] (Figs 5.15A to C) are congenital lesions which can cause neonatal respiratory distress by virtue of mass effect on surrounding structures or because of superadded pneumonia. If located in mediastinum, computed tomography is required to characterize the lesion and demarcate its size and extent. Careful scrutiny is required to exclude intraspinal communication to exclude neuroenteric cyst. Intrapulmonary bronchogenic cyst is difficult to differentiate radiologically from other congenital cystic lesions.

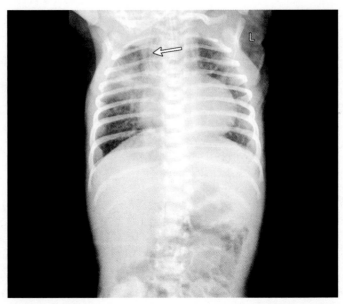

Fig. 5.14: One day old neonate with respiratory distress and pooling of saliva. Chest X-ray AP view reveals coiling of nasogastric tube in upper esophageal pouch (arrow) suggestive of esophageal atresia. Presence of air in abdomen confirms the presence of tracheoesophageal fistula

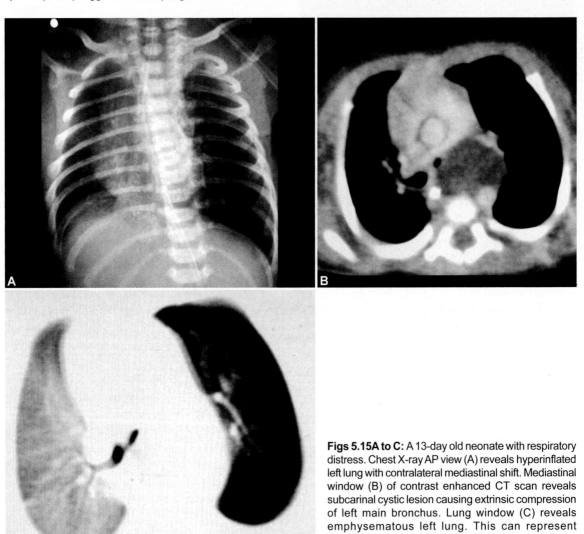

Figs 5.15A to C: A 13-day old neonate with respiratory distress. Chest X-ray AP view (A) reveals hyperinflated left lung with contralateral mediastinal shift. Mediastinal window (B) of contrast enhanced CT scan reveals subcarinal cystic lesion causing extrinsic compression of left main bronchus. Lung window (C) reveals emphysematous left lung. This can represent bronchogenic or esophageal duplication cyst. Note the absence of communication with the spinal canal

- To evaluate immunocompromised children with normal radiograph but with clinical suspicion of respiratory infection
- To guide the type and site of tissue sampling
- To assess the sequelae of respiratory infection (e.g post viral bronchiolitis obliterans).

Viral Pneumonia

Viral infection predominantly affects the mucosa of the airways resulting in bronchiolitis. The process may remain confined to the medium and small airways or may extend into the adjacent lung tissue resulting in peribronchiolar opacities. Respiratory syncytial virus is the most common cause, others being parainfluenza and adenovirus.[4] Most of these are acquired by inhalational route. Edema, increased mucosal secretions and necrotic debris in the lumen result in blockade of airways, more marked at the level of the bronchioles and cause air trapping. Children are more predisposed to air trapping and collapse in viral infection than adults due to the following reasons: (1) bronchi and bronchioles are smaller in diameter. (2) collateral pathways of ventilation, including pores of Kahn and channels of Lambert are not well developed. These do not mature until about 8 years of age. (3) mucus secretion is more in children.[2]

Radiographic signs of diffuse hyperinflation are hyperlucency, depression of the hemidiaphragm to more than 10 posterior ribs, flattening of the diaphragms, widening of intercostal spaces and increased retrosternal space. On the lateral view, findings of flattening of the hemidiaphragms and increased anteroposterior diameter, which often becomes more than the superior to inferior diameter, are often better evaluated (Figs 6.1 and 6.2A and B). When thick mucus inspissates resulting in complete plugging of the airway, there is segmental atelectasis. This is seen as wedge shaped areas of density, more common in the middle and lower lung (Fig. 6.3). Inflammation extending into the adjacent lung tissue

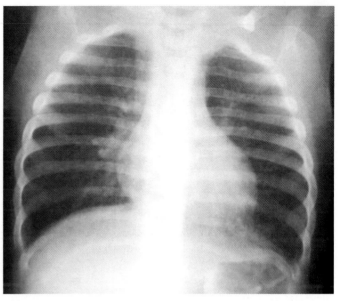

Fig. 6.1: Viral pneumonia. Frontal radiograph in a 4-month-old boy shows hyperinflation with increased peribronchial markings

can cause peribronchial edema and result in bronchopneumonia which manifests as bilateral, usually symmetrical peribronchial cuffing and thickening in the central perihilar location. On the lateral view, increased hilar size and density may be used as a marker for perihilar peribronchial thickening. Doughnut-like appearance on cross-section and tram-track line appearance of bronchi are seen radiating from the hilum.[2,4,5]

Although the central peribronchial thickening, hyperinflation and areas of segmental atelectasis are typical of viral infection in infants and small children, there are various pitfalls. Perivascular edema and reactive airway disease may simulate the appearance of

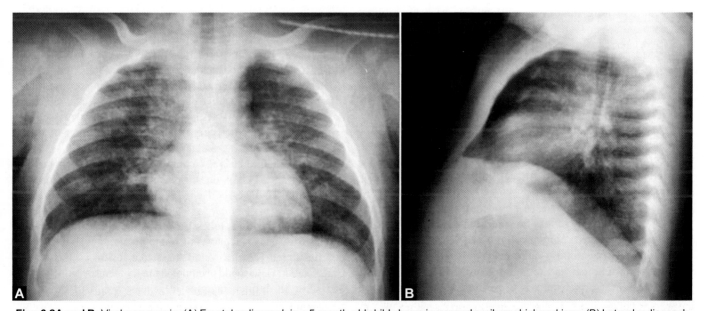

Figs 6.2A and B: Viral pneumonia. (A) Frontal radiograph in a 5-month-old child shows increased peribronchial markings. (B) Lateral radiograph shows prominent density and size of the hila, a supportive finding of increased peribronchial markings

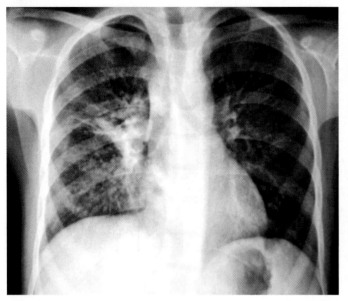

Fig. 6.3: Viral pneumonia. Frontal radiograph in a 4-year-old girl depicts prominent bronchovascular markings with triangular right perihilar area of atelectasis

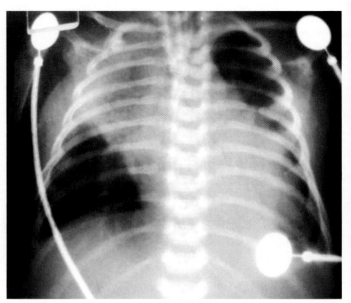

Fig. 6.4: Lobar pneumonia. Frontal radiograph in a 3-month-old infant shows consolidation of the right upper lobe suggesting a bacterial pneumonia

peribronchial thickening. Expiratory films may give the erroneous impression of peribronchial thickening. Sometimes, bacterial pneumonia like pertussis pneumonia (rare due to widespread immunization) mimics the appearance of viral pneumonia. Segmental atelectasis in viral pneumonia may be overinterpreted as consolidation in bacterial pneumonia. Secondary bacterial infection may develop in few cases of viral infection, related to altered immunity and ubiquitous pathogen, confounding the radiological picture.[4] Also, if bronchial wall thickening is present between bouts of acute illness, it suggests chronic airway disease such as asthma or cystic fibrosis, immunodeficiency or chronic aspiration.[3]

Although most infants recover uneventfully, viral pneumonias may result in long-standing complications of bronchiolitis obliterans and Swyer-James syndrome (unilateral hyperlucent lung) discussed later.[4]

Bacterial Pneumonia

Bacterial pneumonia is usually a result of *Streptococcus pneumoniae*, other common agents being *Hemophilus influenzae* and *Staphylococcus pneumoniae*. The usual route of spread is via the inhalational route. Air space pneumonia is classically the result of *Streptococcus pneumoniae* and *Klebsiella pneumoniae*. Inflammatory exudates and edema within the acini result in segmental or lobar consolidation (Fig. 6.4). This is usually unilateral in contrast to viral pneumonias. Air bronchograms, when seen are typical. There is usually little or no volume loss as the airways are not primarily affected. *Staphylococcus aureus*, gram negative bacteria and *Mycoplasma* usually result in bronchopneumonia that begins in terminal and respiratory bronchioles rather than alveoli. The disease then spreads to peribronchiolar alveoli that produce acinar filling and lobular consolidations. This results in patchy consolidation, loss of volume with absence of air bronchograms. When affected areas coalesce, the shadowing may

become more uniform and resemble lobar pneumonia. There may be accompanying pleural effusions, which are rarely associated with viral disease.

Sometimes, lobar consolidation may be difficult to distinguish from atelectasis seen in viral pneumonias. (In fact, these may coexist as superadded infection is common secondary to obstructed airway). It may be remembered that accompanying signs of volume loss like fissural distortion, mediastinal shift and compensatory hyperinflation, seen with atelectasis are unusual in consolidated lung.[4]

Although more gradual, the pneumonia generally resolves completely. Radiological improvement may lag behind clinical improvement by days or weeks, usually taking 1-2 weeks (Figs 6.5A and B). However, severity of the disease agent and underlying host factors may result in complications, like cavitatory necrosis, empyema and abscess formation.[4,5] Increase in antibiotic usage has led to increase in the incidence of complications.[4] Lung abscess is uncommon in children and suggests underlying aspiration and infection with gram negative bacilli or Staphylococcus. Multilobar consolidation with mixed flora in debilitated patients suggests aspiration as the underlying mechanism. Aspiration of gastric contents can also result in chemical pneumonitis.[4]

Round pneumonia is also common in young children, less than 8 years of age. This is due to paucity of collateral channels of ventilation as described earlier. This is most often due to *Streptococcus pneumoniae* and simulates a mass lesion.[2,5] These often involve the lower lobes, especially the superior segments. In a child with fever, diagnosis of round pneumonia should always be considered when a round mass like lesion is encountered (Figs 6.6A and B). Round pneumonia may contain air bronchograms and show ill-defined margins in at least a part of the border, suggesting the diagnosis. Follow-up radiography after antibiotic therapy is essential to rule out an underlying mass lesion, like bronchogenic cyst.[2]

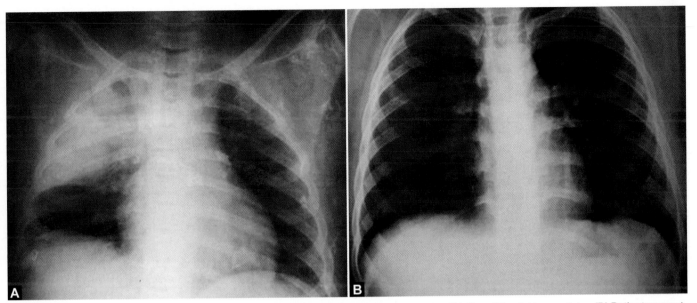

Figs 6.5A and B: Lobar pneumonia. (A) Frontal radiograph in a 2-year-old child shows consolidation of the right upper lobe. (B) Patient was put on antibiotics and radiograph obtained 2 weeks later shows complete radiological clearance

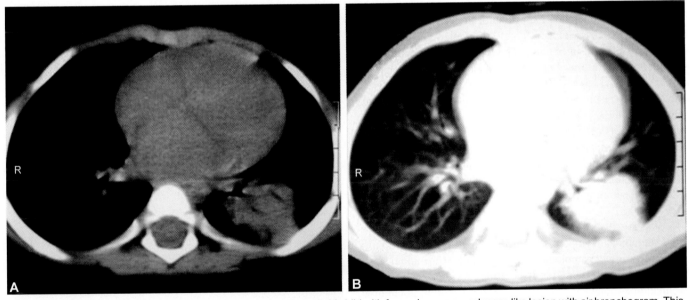

Figs 6.6A and B: Round pneumonia. Axial CT images in a 2-year-old child with fever shows a round mass like lesion with air bronchogram. This was a case of round pneumonia

Mycoplasma pneumoniae, which is an atypical cause of pneumonia, is a common cause of pneumonia in school-aged children. It is uncommon in children less than 3 years of age. It can have a broad spectrum of appearances which may simulate viral or bacterial pneumonia. The radiographic changes are more severe than the clinical symptoms. Hilar lymph nodes and pleural effusions can be associated.[2,6]

In most children with pulmonary infections, specific etiological agent is never documented. Invasive diagnostic procedures are usually not warranted and even when done, specific etiological agent is still not identifiable because of ongoing treatment with antibiotics.[5]

In a study by Bettenay et al,[8] it was suggested that both clinical and radiographic criteria overestimate the number of children with bacterial pneumonia by a significant proportion, owing to low positive predictive value. However, it was the high negative predictive value in the range of 80-90 percent of the clinical and radiographic findings that was useful in excluding bacterial pneumonia and affected the management decisions.

Few specific appearances pertaining to different bacterial agents may be mentioned here. Staphylococcal pneumonia presents with lobar or multilobar consolidation. Complications are most common with this organism. Pleural effusion is common which may develop into empyema. A frequent feature of

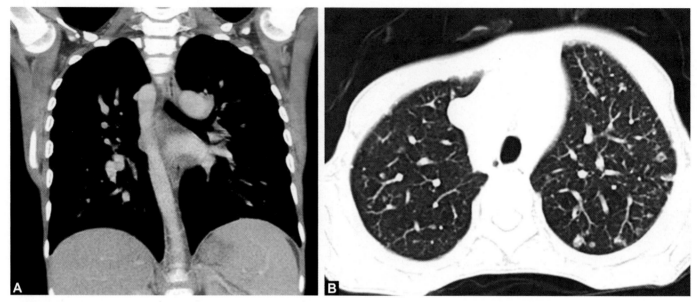

Figs 6.7A and B: Infective endocarditis with septic emboli. (A) Coronal reformatted CT image on mediastinal window settings shows right sided aortic arch in a case of ventricular septal defect with infective endocarditis. (B) Multiple nodular lesions, few showing feeding vessel sign, are seen on axial CECT at lung window settings

Staphylococcal pneumonia is pneumatocele formation, which is otherwise rare. It is seen as a round thin walled lucency due to collection of air in the interstitium. This may result in pneumothorax secondary to rupture. Although they generally disappear in days or weeks, few may persist for months.[6] Septicemic staphylococcal infection may result in multiple nodules which may also cavitate (Figs 6.7A and B).

In cases of infection with *Klebsiella pneumoniae*, a gram negative bacillus, there is homogenous opacification with copious inflammatory exudate which may result in an increase in the lung volume resulting in expansile pneumonia (Fig. 6.8) . Empyema and abscess are common complications.[6]

Exclusion of Other Pathologies

Since the clinical symptoms of pneumonia in children are fairly non-specific, other pathologies that may simulate pneumonia must be excluded. It is essential to look at the ribs and the airways to exclude other potential causes of respiratory distress in children. For example, rib erosions in cases of neuroblastoma (Figs 6.9A and B) and fractures in cases of child abuse are pointers to the correct diagnosis. Also, stridor due to vascular rings around the airway is common in children, compared to adults and warrants a careful look at the airways. Evaluation of the diameter of the airways should be stressed as a routine part of evaluation of pediatric chest radiographs.[2]

Nonresolving Pneumonia

In children, follow-up radiographs are usually reserved for those children who have persistent or recurrent symptoms or who have an underlying condition such as immunodeficiency, cystic fibrosis, or sickle cell anemia. These should also be considered in children with round pneumonia. When obtained, they should be done after

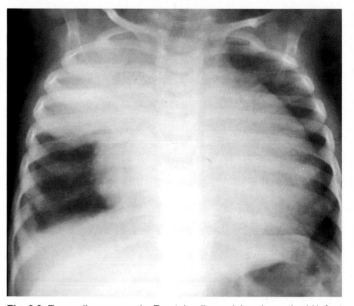

Fig. 6.8: Expansile pneumonia. Frontal radiograph in a 4-month-old infant shows lobar consolidation with bulging of the fissure suggesting expansile pneumonia

at least 2-3 weeks.[2] In patients with non-resolving pneumonia on antibiotic and other therapy, with non-contributory chest radiograph, contrast-enhanced CT is the modality of choice.

The various causes of recurrent or non-resolving pneumonia are enumerated below:[5,9-11]

- Aspiration syndromes—swallowing disorders due to neuromuscular disorders or immaturity, gastroesophageal reflux, H-type fistula, esophageal obstruction (foreign body, vascular ring).

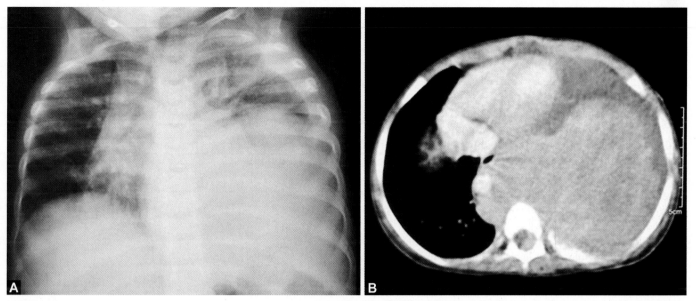

Figs 6.9A and B: Neuroblastoma.(A) Chest radiograph in a 2-year-old girl shows opacity in the left mid and lower zone with accompanying left pleural effusion. Note erosion and splaying of the left posterior 7th to 10th ribs differentiating neuroblastoma from pneumonia. (B) CT scan shows a posterior mediastinal mass displacing heart and aorta with extension into spinal canal

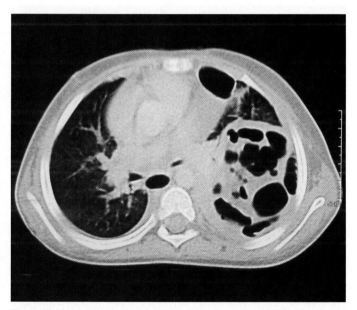

Fig. 6.10: Congenital cystic adenomatoid malformation. CT in a 3-year-old child with recurrent pneumonia shows multiseptated cystic mass with thickened walls in the left lower lobe. The diagnosis of CCAM was confirmed at surgery

- Underlying developmental lesions—like congenital cystic adenomatoid malformation (Fig. 6.10), bronchogenic cyst, sequestration.
- Bronchial obstruction – foreign body, neoplasm.
- Underlying systemic disorders – immunodeficiency (congenital and acquired), asthma, cystic fibrosis, immotile cilia disease.

Foreign bodies usually lodge in the bronchial tree and affect the lower lobes or the right middle lobe. Only large ones may lodge in the trachea. Children usually do not remember the episode or are too young to do so, hence present with pneumonia. This is usually chronic and develops slowly. Although the child may be very ill at presentation but without the toxicity of acute infection. Very small foreign bodies such as grass may migrate to the peripheral bronchi. Inorganic foreign bodies are usually inert and only result in mechanical obstruction, whereas organic foreign bodies such as peanuts also incite an inflammatory reaction in addition to the mechanical obstruction. Also, they may be fragmented and then spread into peripheral bronchi or bronchi of other lobes. Up to 85 percent are non-opaque on chest radiographs. When a foreign body is suspected, radiographic assessment should start with paired inspiratory and expiratory films or fluoroscopy. Decubitus film may be obtained if fluoroscopy is not available and expiratory film is difficult to obtain. Fluoroscopy can depict air trapping, mediastinal shift to affected side on inspiration and reduced diaphragmatic movement on the affected side. Distal atelectasis, especially in the lower lobes, pulmonary abscess, bronchiectasis and bronchiolitis obliterans are the complications that may be encountered. Stenosis of the bronchus can also result which predisposes to further infections.[6]

For assessment of swallowing mechanism, swallow should be done using solid food coated with barium, followed by thickened barium mixture and finally thin liquid barium. In case H-type tracheaesophageal fistula is suspected, tube esophageogram should be done, with patient in the prone position and using a horizontal beam. Combined bronchoscopy and endoscopy is the investigation of choice.[6]

Evaluation of Associated Complications

Suppurative complications of pneumonia may involve the pleura, lung parenchyma and rarely the pericardium.

Pleural Complications

A parapneumonic effusion (PPE) is a pleural fluid collection adjacent to infected lung. It may be simple or complicated depending on whether the infective organism is present or not within the collection. The term empyema is used when there is frank pus within the collection.[12]

Empyema in children is a different condition from that in adults. Although associated with significant morbidity, it is almost never fatal in contrast to adults, where mortality is nearly 20 percent, probably due to the higher incidence of premorbid conditions.[12]

The most common agents involved are *S. pneumoniae*, *S. aureus*, other streptococci (including *S. pyogenes*), *Hemophilus influenzae*, *Mycoplasma pneumoniae*, *Pseudomonas* spp, and *Mycobacterium tuberculosis*.[12]

Initially, there is pleural inflammation secondary to involvement of the subpleural lung. This leads to increase in pleural fluid production with influx of inflammatory cells resulting in simple parapneumonic effusion. There is consequent fibrin production, resulting in fibrinous septations, resulting in complicated PPE when fluid is thickened. Later there is pus formation, resulting in frank empyema. Eventually, a thick fibrous peel may trap the lung and may result in long-term restriction of lung function.[12]

Chest radiography and ultrasound are the imaging modalities of choice to detect effusions and guide drainage of complicated effusions. Chest radiography is usually the first investigation. The signs vary from obliteration of the costophrenic angle, meniscus of fluid tracking along the lateral chest wall in small effusions to complete opacification of the hemithorax with contralateral mediastinal shift in larger effusions (Figs 6.11 and 6.12). Pleural cap may be visualized. Loculated effusions tend to have a lenticular shape (Fig. 6.13). In cases of empyema, there may be scoliosis concave to the side of the collection, due to pain. On supine films, there may be homogenous haze of the affected hemithorax.

US is used to confirm the presence of effusion, characterize it and guide drainage. Effusions may be anechoic, or show fine internal echoes and fibrinous septations (Figs 6.14A to C). Ultrasound may also be used to characterize non-shifting nature of loculated fluid by scanning the patient in supine and sitting position. In cases of fibrous rind formation, pleural thickening is seen with lack of mobility of the underlying lung, suggesting entrapment. When a very organized collection is difficult to distinguish from the underlying consolidated lung, color Doppler may be used to demonstrate vessels in the consolidated lung in contrast to the avascular pleural collection.[12]

CT is reserved for special circumstances. As per the British Thoracic Society guidelines, CT should be reserved for failing tube drainage, and in immunocompromised individuals to detect associated parenchymal and mediastinal abnormalities. On CT, features of empyema include pleural thickening and enhancement, increased density and thickening of extrapleural fat, increased density of extrathoracic fat and lenticular shape suggesting loculation. Pleural thickening and enhancement is better appreciated in the parietal pleura, as the visceral pleura is difficult to differentiate from the underlying consolidated lung. Although septations are not readily appreciable on CT, their presence may

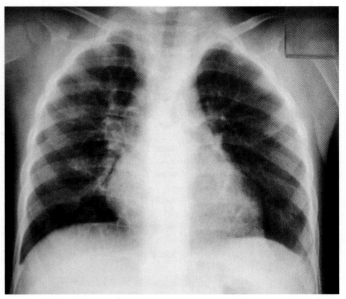

Fig. 6.11: Pleural effusion. Frontal radiograph of a child shows blunting of the left costophrenic angle suggesting effusion. This was confirmed on US

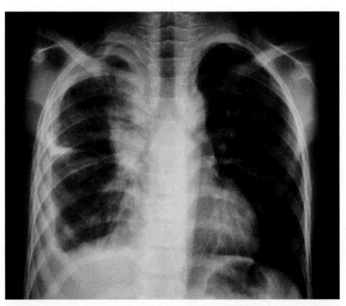

Fig. 6.12: Pleural effusion. Frontal radiograph of a 10-year-old child shows blunting of the right costophrenic angle with fluid tracking along the lateral chest wall and the horizontal fissure in addition to the opacities in the right lung

be inferred from air loculi within the pleural collection. This is due to air separating into tiny bubbles due to septations rather than forming an air-fluid level (Fig. 6.15).[12] CT can also be helpful in depicting malpositioned chest tubes (Figs 6.16A and B).

We have to remember that even an anechoic collection may contain frank pus. Therefore, imaging is not the basis for deciding whether the patient requires drainage. This decision is dependent on whether the collection is increasing in size or the patient is having respiratory embarrassment due to the collection.[12]

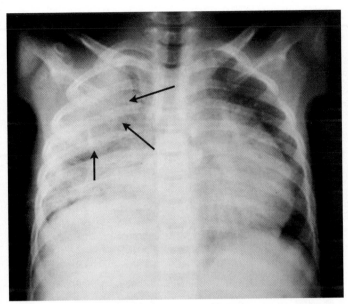

Fig. 6.13: Loculated pleural effusion. Frontal radiograph of a 10-year-old child shows lenticular shaped soft tissue opacity along the right upper lateral chest wall suggesting loculated pleural effusion (arrows). The underlying lung shows areas of consolidation and atelectasis

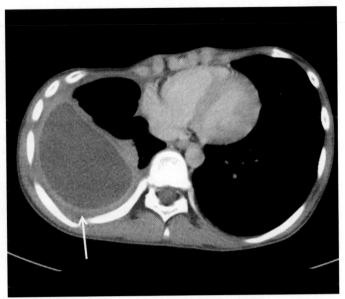

Fig. 6.15: Empyema. Axial CECT shows lenticular shape of the collection with pleural thickening and enhancement with increased thickness and density of extrapleural fat (arrow)

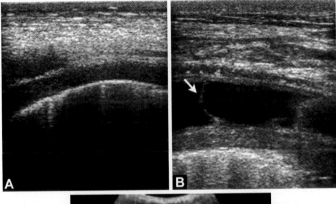

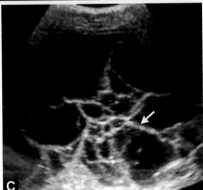

Figs 6.14A to C: Ultrasound in cases of pleural effusion may depict the clear nature of fluid (A) or show fine fibrinous septations (B,C)

Another clinical problem which may arise is whether we are dealing with empyema or a lung abscess. This is important because the treatment of abscess is primarily medical, and insertion of drainage tube increases the risk for bronchopleural fistula formation. While irregular thick wall and acute angle with chest wall favor the diagnosis of lung abscess, split pleura sign and compression of the adjacent lung favor the diagnosis of empyema.[12]

Lung Parenchymal Complications

The various complications include cavitatory necrosis, pulmonary abscess, pulmonary gangrene, pneumatocele and bronchopleural fistula. The names given to the suppurative process depends on several factors including the severity, distribution, and condition of the adjacent lung parenchyma and temporal relationship with disease resolution.[2,5,13-15]

Cavitatory necrosis is the most common complication encountered in children. *S. pneumoniae* and *S. aureus* are the frequent associated organisms. It is defined as a dominant area of necrosis with associated variable number of thin walled cysts. On CT, it appears as decreased contrast enhancement, lack of normal lung architecture, loss of lung pleura margin, multiple thin walled cavities filled with air or fluid with no peripheral enhancement (Figs 6.17A and B). The finding of decreased enhancement is indicative of pulmonary parenchymal ischemia, or impending cavitatory necrosis (Figs 6.18A and B). This is visualized on chest radiographs when air enters the cavities due to bronchial communication. Although associated with a protracted course, most patients are managed conservatively in contrast to adults.[5,15]

Lung abscess is fairly uncommon in immunocompetent children and is defined as collection of fluid or air within the lung parenchyma with a well defined enhancing rim (Figs 6.19A and B).[5,13-15] In early stages, pulmonary consolidation may show a low density center with no definite cavity formation.[7]

Pneumatoceles are seen as thin walled cysts on imaging and may represent a later or less severe stage of resolving or healing

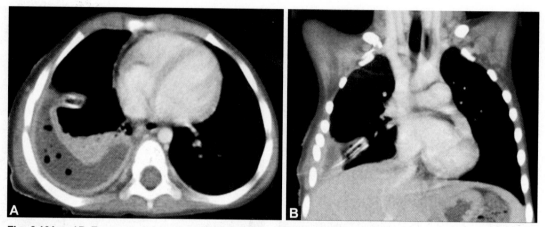

Figs 6.16A and B: Empyema. Axial and coronal reformatted CECT images depict the loculated right pleural collection with foci of air within. Note: is made of split pleura sign and underlying atelectasis. It is important to note the position of the chest tube which appears malpositioned

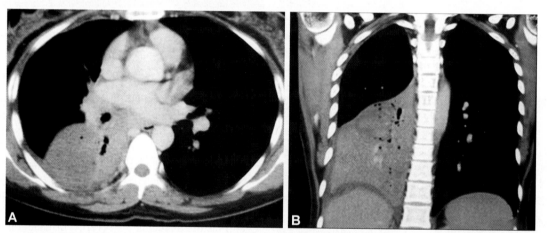

Figs 6.17A and B: Cavitatory necrosis. CT findings in a 7-year-old boy shows multiloculated cavity within consolidated lung

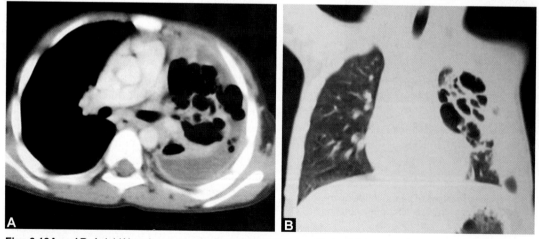

Figs 6.18A and B: Axial (A) and coronal reformatted (B) CT images of an adolescent with severe pneumonia shows consolidation of the right lower lobe with bulging of the lobe and areas of decreased parenchymal enhancement within (arrows), probably reflecting areas of ischemia and impending gangrene

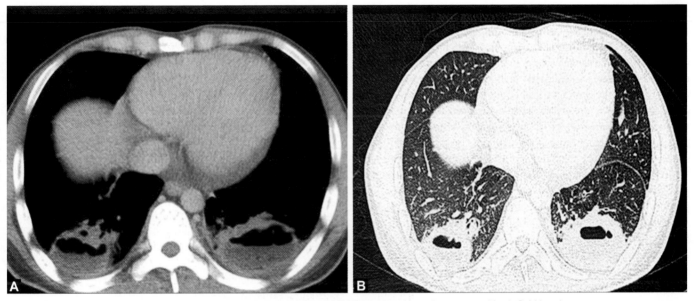

Figs 6.19A and B: Lung abscesses. Axial CECT images show abscesses with air-fluid levels in bilateral posterior dependent lungs suggesting aspiration as the probable cause

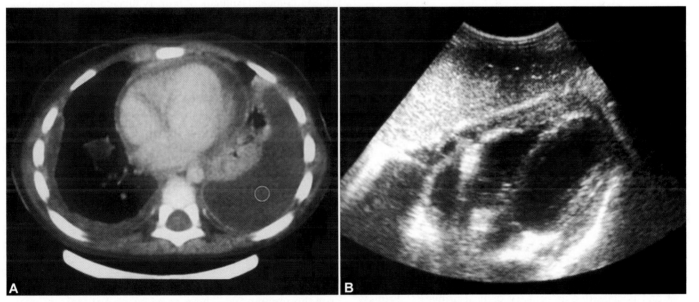

Figs 6.20A and B: Pericarditis. (A) Axial CECT image shows pericardial as well as pleural fluid in a case of pneumonia. (B) Correlative ultrasound image shows thick pericardial fluid with septations

necrosis.[2] Although pneumatoceles are most characteristic of staphylococcal pneumonia, other causes are *Pneumococcus, H. influenza, Streptococcus, M. tuberculosis* and *E.coli*. They are also known after hydrocarbon ingestion. When pneumatoceles develop in infected areas, inflammatory exudate may seep into them and produce air-fluid levels that simulate lung abscesses. However, true lung abscesses have a thicker and often somewhat shaggy wall.

Bronchopleural fistula is a communication between a bronchus and the pleural cavity. While it most commonly follows pneumonectomy, it may follow lung abscess, bacterial or fungal pneumonias and tuberculosis. Diagnosis is based upon increasing amount of sputum production, air in the pleural cavity which may be loculated.[6] CT may demonstrate direct communication between the pleural space and the bronchial tree in these cases.

Purulent Pericarditis

Pericardial fluid is not uncommonly encountered during US and CT of children with pneumonia. This may also result in cardiac tamponade when there is rapid accumulation. When the clinical features go unrecognized, the radiologist may be the first one to suggest the diagnosis (Figs 6.20A and B).[12]

Chronic Effects of Pneumonia

Most cases of pneumonia resolve completely. However, a few children may develop chronic complications. Increased susceptibility to infection in the same area of the lung may be a result of underlying damage to the airways in this area. Focal bronchiectasis is another complication that may occur in cases of infection with persistent collapse or foreign body aspiration. It usually affects the medium sized bronchi, as the proximal bronchi have more cartilage in their walls. Only allergic bronchopulmonary aspergillosis shows a tendency to attack the proximal bronchi. Diffuse bronchiectasis may also occur due to chronic recurrent pulmonary infection, particularly in cases of cystic fibrosis and primary ciliary dyskinesia syndromes.[3]

Bronchiolitis obliterans may result from a severe viral pneumonia. Swyer-James/McLeod syndrome is a form of post infectious obliterative bronchiolitis that has special features. It occurs following an insult to the developing lung (before the age of 8 years). The most frequently encountered scenario is postviral infection, in particular adenoviral and post mycoplasma infection. Non-infectious causes include hydrocarbon ingestion. The lung served by the affected bronchi and bronchioles remains inflated due to collateral air drift. Pulmonary tissue as well as pulmonary artery and its branches are hypoplastic. Patients are typically asymptomatic, presenting in adulthood or less commonly, may present with progressive exertional dyspnea or repeated respiratory infections. Disease on chest radiography is predominantly unilateral, giving rise to the key finding of unilateral transradiancy. This reflects hypoplasia of pulmonary vasculature as well as obliterative bronchiolitis. The hilum of the affected lung is small. The affected lung is small or normal in volume in contrast to congenital lobar emphysema. Ipsilateral air trapping is the key finding. CT changes are more complex than chest radiographs. It more commonly shows areas of bilateral abnormalities depicting areas of decreased attenuation. Air trapping can be confirmed on expiratory scans. Areas of cylindrical bronchiectasis may also be seen. There may be areas of collapse and scarring.[16]

TUBERCULOSIS (TB)

The pathological form is dependent on sensitivity of the infected host and is classified as primary or post-primary.[17] Primary tuberculosis, the most common form in childhood, is radiologically distinct from post-primary tuberculosis, the most common form occurring in adults. Due to difficulty in obtaining suitable sputum samples and low sensitivity of gastric washings, chest radiography plays an important role in evaluation for tuberculosis in pediatric cases.[18]

Primary Pulmonary Tuberculosis

Primary tuberculosis represents the reaction to first exposure and is often a subclinical condition. Incubation period varies from 2 to 10 weeks and ends when the patient becomes sensitized (i.e has a positive skin test). As the infecting bacteria are inhaled, it incites a local inflammatory reaction in the bronchiole/alveolus, usually peripherally in a subpleural focus, called the Ghon's focus. From this focus, lymphatic spread to the local hilar or mediastinal lymph nodes may occur.[17] The combination of a peripheral granuloma, involved lymphatics and lymph nodes is known as Ghon's or Ranke's complex. In most cases, the immune response is usually enough to limit the infection, which heals as a small granuloma. Primary focus is usually quite small as compared to the large lymph nodes. In young infants, or in cases with underlying illness or impaired nutrition resulting in impaired defenses, progressive primary disease may occur. Enlarging pulmonary focus of consolidation and caseation followed by liquefaction, occurs. This leads to cavitation and rupture into a bronchus, may result in acute tuberculous bronchopneumonia.[18] These children are usually quite ill with weight loss and failure to thrive.

Primary tuberculosis may be asymptomatic when the child is well and the disease is detected during a routine skin test. It may otherwise present in four major ways in childhood, in addition to a normal chest radiograph:
1. Lymphadenopathy
2. Lobar or segmental parenchymal disease
3. Pleural effusion
4. Miliary involvement

Lymphadenopathy; with or without parenchymal abnormaity, is the radiological hallmark of primary tuberculosis in childhood. The favored lymph nodal sites are right paratracheal, hilar, subcarinal and aortopulmonary window region. Children less than 3 years of age have shown a higher prevalence of lymphadenopathy than parenchymal changes as compared to older children. The reverse however does not hold true.[18,19] Contrast-enhanced CT may depict characteristic low attenuation nodes with rim enhancement (Figs 6.21A and B).

There is a tendency towards right sided parenchymal involvement, likely due to increased probability of inhalation of particles into the straighter right bronchus. No consensus has been reached regarding zonal predilection in primary tuberculosis.[18] The parenchymal involvement patterns described vary from ill defined parenchymal opacities to segmental or lobar consolidation.[18] Homogeneous, dense, and well defined air space consolidation is a typical appearance of primary tuberculosis (Fig. 6.22). Lymph nodes obstructing the adjacent bronchi can result in obstructive hyperinflation and atelectasis (Figs 6.23A to C). They may open into adjacent bronchi resulting in bronchopneumonia. There may be multifocal air space consolidation or diffuse nodularity. Bronchiectasis may be seen in areas of previous collapse. Evolution to cavitatory tuberculosis is uncommon in children. Cavitation may raise the possibility of previously unsuspected underlying immune disorder. Calcification occurs after caseation of the primary lesion and is seen earlier in infants (6 months after infection) than in older children (2 to 3 years after infection). Fibrotic and calcified lesions may persist. Single or multiple tuberculomas may develop in primary tuberculosis, but they are seen less frequently than in reactivation tuberculosis (Figs 6.24A and B).[3,7,20]

Pleural effusions usually occur due to direct extension from the parenchymal focus in cases of primary tuberculosis. Effusions are not a common feature of primary tuberculosis in young children and are more commonly encountered in adolescents and adults.[18]

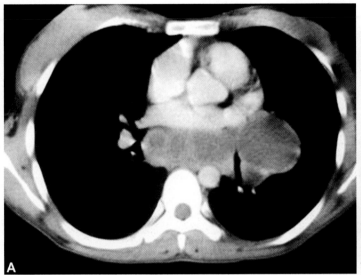

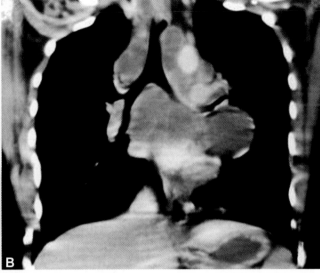

Figs 6.21A and B: Tuberculosis. Axial and coronal reformatted CECT images at mediastinal window settings depict large necrotic rim enhancing lymph nodes in a case of tuberculosis in a 5-year-old girl

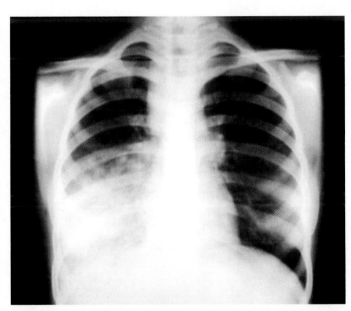

Fig. 6.22: Tuberculosis. Frontal radiograph in an 8-year-old child with proven tuberculosis shows right paratracheal lymphadenopathy with homogeneous consolidation in the right lower lobe

Hematogeneous spread occurs as a rule but is self-limited in primary tuberculosis. However, when an overwhelming number of mycobacteria are discharged into the blood stream, it can cause miliary infection of the lungs.[6,17] Infants are more susceptible to miliary tuberculosis, possibly due to low immunity at this age. CT can detect miliary disease earlier than chest radiographs (Figs 6.25A to C).[18]

Postprimary Tuberculosis

This is unusual in children and when seen in the pediatric age group, it is usually seen in adolescents. It results from reactivation of dormant residual foci. Reactivation tuberculosis is rarer in children who were infected with primary disease before the age of 2 years. It is much more frequent in children who were afflicted by the primary disease after the age of 7 years, especially near puberty.[3] It is characterized by parenchymal disease with an anatomic bias for the upper lung zones. Typically the lesions are located in the apical and posterior segments of the upper lobes and superior segments of the lower lobes, probably due to relatively higher oxygen tension and impaired lymphatic drainage.[18] However, no portion of the lungs has immunity. Bilateral and multilobar involvement is fairly frequent. Cavitation is a characteristic radiographic finding. Necrotic rim enhancing lymph nodes or calcified lymph nodes may be encountered (Figs 6.26 to 6.28). Fluid levels may be seen within cavities. Heavy seeding of the bronchial tree is likely, particularly in the presence of cavitation and widespread bronchopneumonia may result. Cicatrisation atelectasis is a common finding after post-primary tuberculosis. Bronchiectasis may be seen, either as a result of cicatricial bronchostenosis after local infection, or more commonly due to fibrosis of lung parenchyma with secondary bronchial dilatation (Figs 6.29A to C). Calcification is often seen coincident with increasing fibrosis.[6,17]

Miliary tuberculosis, due to hematogenous spread can be seen with both primary and post primary tuberculosis. Both well defined and poorly defined nodular opacities, 2-3mm in size are seen scattered randomly in both lungs. Coalescence of small nodules may form larger nodules or even consolidation. There may be reticulonodular opacities with thickening of the interlobular septa. Ground glass opacities may also be seen on HRCT when small granulomas below the resolution of the scan are superimposed on exudative changes of the lung.[6,17]

CT may be done when tuberculosis is suspected in children but the radiographic findings are inconclusive or when complications are suspected.[21]

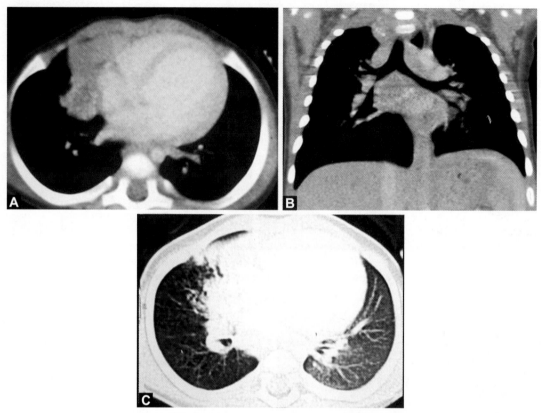

Figs 6.23A to C: Tuberculosis in a 1 year old child. CT images show right paratracheal, hilar and subcarinal node enlargement with foci of calcification. There is also collapse of the right middle lobe. This was probably due to the bronchial compression by enlarged lymph nodes

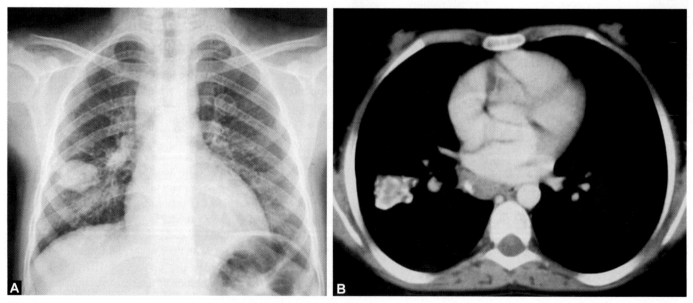

Figs 6.24A and B: Tuberculoma (A). Frontal radiograph of an 11-year-old child reveals prominence of the right paratracheal stripe and hilum with nodule in the right lung field. (B) Axial CECT image shows the calcified lymph nodes with granuloma in the right lung with foci of calcification

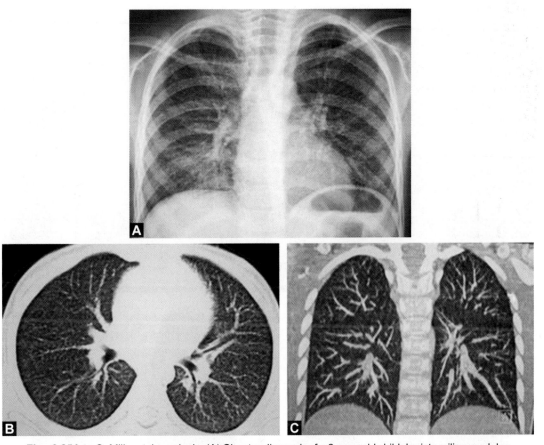

Figs 6.25A to C: Miliary tuberculosis. (A) Chest radiograph of a 6-year-old child depicts miliary nodules scattered in both lung fields. Axial CT image (B) with coronal MIP image (C) depicts the nodules well

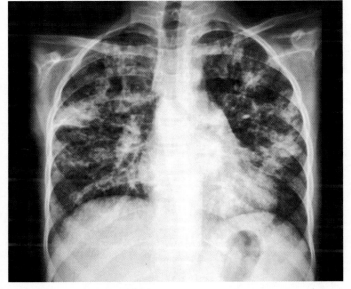

Fig. 6.26: Tuberculosis. In an adolescent with tuberculosis, frontal radiograph depicts multifocal area of consolidation in both lungs with an area of cavitation in the right upper lobe

Table 6.1: Radiographic characteristics of fungal and actinomyces infection[3]	
Infection	*Common radiographic patterns*
Actinomyces	Lung, nodal, pleural disease, chest wall involvement
Nocardia	Lung nodules, consolidation, cavitation, pleural disease
Blastomycosis	Consolidation, cavitation
Cryptococcosis	Consolidation, nodules
Invasive aspergillosis	Bronchocentric or angiocentric lesions, halo and air crescent signs
Coccidioidomycosis	Simulates tuberculosis, thin walled cavities
Histoplasmosis	Simulates tuberculosis

FUNGAL INFECTIONS

Although may occur in immunocompetent patients, these are mostly seen in immunocompromised patients. Necrosis, cavitation, calcifications, chronic inflammatory reaction, pleural disease may all occur. These resemble tuberculous lesions. There are no conclusive radiographic criteria that can distinguish mycosis from tuberculosis or one mycosis from another. Few common radiographic patterns are enumerated in Table 6.1. Other important features are highlighted in the following discussion.

Actinomyces

This anaerobic organism has both bacterial and fungal properties. *Acinomyces israelli* is the usual organism. It is mostly seen in neurologically impaired children with poor oral hygiene. Aggressive

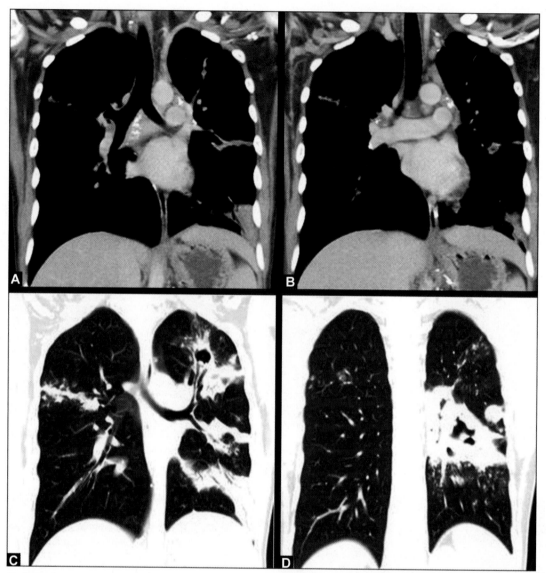

Figs 6.27A to D: Tuberculosis. In a 12-year-old girl, coronal reformatted CT images at mediastinal and lung window settings show mediastinal nodes with foci of calcification and multifocal patches of consolidation bilaterally with areas of cavitation and other centrilobular nodules

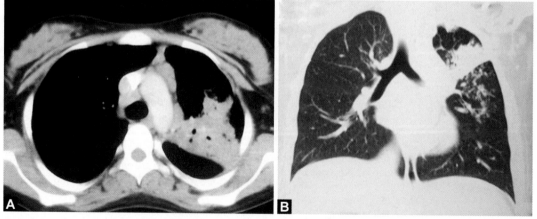

Figs 6.28A and B: Tuberculosis. In an adolescent, axial CECT image at mediastinal window (A) shows evidence of mediastinal lymph nodes with left upper lobe consolidation. Coronal reformatted CT image (B) at lung window depicts consolidation in the left upper lobe with few adjacent centrilobular nodules

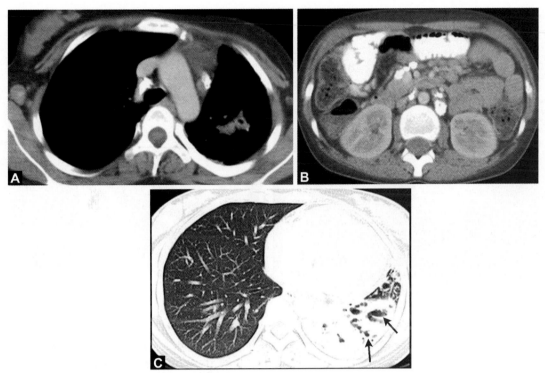

Figs 6.29A to C: In a 15-year-old boy, a follow-up case of tuberculosis, calcified lymph nodes are noted in the mediastinum (A) and abdomen (B) with varicose bronchiectasis in the left lung field (arrows in C)

invasion of the thoracic wall when present is characteristic and often distinguishes this from fungal infections other than mucormycosis.[3]

Aspergillosis

Aspergillus can produce four distinct patterns in children depending on immune status and patient's pre-existing disease.

Fungal balls can form in pre-existing cavities formed by tuberculous infection, bronchiectasis or fibrotic lung disease and are unusual in children. These are usually seen in the upper lobes or apical segments of lower lobes, because most of the cavities are caused by previous tuberculosis. Mobility can be demonstrated in most cases except when it nearly completely fills the cavity with no space to move around. In contrast, the air crescent sign of invasive aspergillosis usually does not have a background of fibrocavitatory disease. Pronounced associated inflammatory reaction may result in hemoptysis.[16]

Allergic bronchopulmonary aspergillosis is a hypersensitivity reaction to the presence of *Aspergillus fumigatus*. It is most commonly seen in association with asthma and cystic fibrosis. The immune reaction results in thick mucin plugging the bronchi. Radiographs may show gloved finger appearance due to mucin filled bronchi outlined because of collateral air drift. There may be patchy areas of atelectasis and emphysema. Central bronchiectasis may be seen. Aspergillus infection may be suggested in children with cystic fibrosis, when there are large patches of consolidation, often disproportionate to the magnitude of disease.

Invasive aspergillosis is invariably noted in immuno-compromised neutropenic patients with leukemia or after bone marrow or solid organ transplantation. It may be airway invasive or angioinvasive. The two forms may coexist and it is not always possible to distinguish between the two types. Multifocal bronchocentric or angicentric air space opacities may be seen. Peribronchiolar nodules, centrilobular micronodules (less than 5mm), ground glass opacities and consolidation may be seen. In the angioinvasive form, wedge shaped opacities can result from infarction as a consequence of hyphal invasion of blood vessels. Few non-specific but distinctive features are halo sign and air crescent sign. The halo sign represents hemorrhage surrounding the nodule due to vascular invasion. It is seen earlier and with greater frequency than the air crescent sign. The air crescent sign is seen in the recovery phase when neutrophillic count rises; retraction of the necrotic lung from the viable lung parenchyma results in a crescent of air collection, partially outlining the necrotic lung.[16] Semi-invasive aspergillosis is a less aggressive form seen in patients with underlying lung disease or with mild immuno-suppression.[3] This is also known as chronic airway invasive aspergillosis and may mimic reactivation tuberculosis. It usually starts as a focus of consolidation in the upper lobes, which may have cavitation and pleural thickening.

Histoplasmosis

This is endemic in many parts of the United States, especially in Ohio and Mississippi river valleys. The initial exudative phase simulates primary complex of tuberculosis; only the pulmonary foci are mostly multifocal. Ninty-five percent of patients are asymptomatic in the initial phase. The disease resembles tuberculosis in all phases.

Disseminated histoplasmosis may occur in an infant in the exudative phase, and resembles miliary tuberculosis. Massive

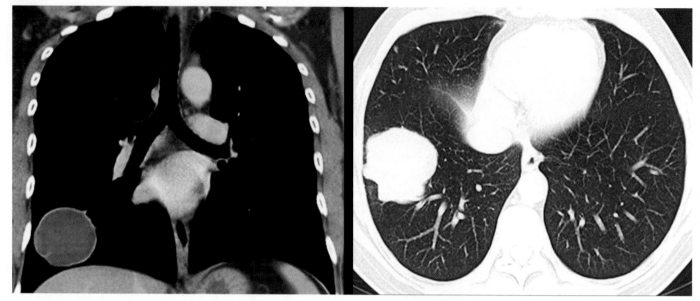

Figs 6.30A and B: Hydatid cyst. Homogeneous well defined rounded fluid attenuation mass lesion noted in the right lower lobe

hepatosplenomegaly may be seen with granulomatous or calcific foci.

A rare but serious complication is fibrosing mediastinitis, which may result in compression of the pulmonary artery, superior vena cava, airway and esophagus. In the west, chronic histoplasmosis is a frequent cause of mediastinal fibrosis in children.[3]

Coccidiodomycosis

Coccidiodomycosis, caused by *Coccidioides immitis*, is endemic in south western deserts of USA. The radiographic manifestations are similar to tuberculosis in all phases, including consolidation, lymph nodes, and pleural effusions. The primary complex lasts only a few weeks-duration being shorter than in tuberculosis. Residual calcifications may occur. Small thin walled cavities, commonly seen in adults are les common in children.[3]

PARASITIC INFESTATIONS

Hydatid Disease of the Lung

Hydatidosis, caused by larval stage of *Echinococcus granulosus*, is the most frequently encountered type of hydatid disease in humans. While in adults, hepatic involvement is more common than lungs, in children, the lungs are the commonest site of involvement. The lung facilitates the growth of the cyst due to compressible nature and the presence of negative pressure. Intact cysts are seen as sharply defined round to oval masses of variable size (Figs 6.30A and B). Lung cysts rarely calcify. Rupture or superimposed infection may result in varied appearances giving rise to air crescent sign, air bubble sign, water lily sign, mass within cavity sign and ring enhancement sign amongst others.[22]

Others

Few parasites including *Ascaris lumbricoides, Necator americanus, Ancylostoma duodenale, Strongyloides stercoralis*

may pass through lungs as a part of their life cycle. These may result in transient migratory pulmonary opacities without recognizable segmental distribution. Blood and sputum eosinophillia may be present along with pulmonary opacities (Loeffler's syndrome).[16]

Paragonimiasis is endemic in the Orient and is a common cause of necrosis and calcification in lungs and is difficult to distinguish from tuberculosis radiologically.

PULMONARY INFECTIONS IN HIV-POSITIVE CHILDREN

Most children are infected after vertical transmission from their mother, and majority develop AIDS early in life. Majority of perinatally infected children develop symptoms during the first 24 months of life. Children who develop HIV infection as a result of blood transfusion frequently are aysmptomatic for long periods of time, although immunological abnormalities may be seen. Respiratory infection is very common in children and more than 70 percent of patients with AIDS will suffer from at least 1 episode of respiratory infection in the course of their illness. In pediatric age group, lungs are often the site of life-threatening illness in these patients. As the radiographic appearance is not specific, the aim of imaging is to narrow the differential diagnosis based upon pattern recognition, clinical presentation, level of immunecompromise and current drug therapy such as HAART and PJP prophylaxis.[23,24]

Bacterial Pneumonias

Typical pneumonias (*S.pneumoniae, S. aureus*) occur as in immunocompetent children, but with increased frequency and severity. The radiological appearance is that of broncho-pneumonia and lobar pneumonia as in immunocompetent children but with an increased incidence of empyema and lung abscesses. Other uncommon pathogens include *Salmonella sp, Klebsiella spp. Pseudomonas spp, E.coli,* and other atypical organisms such as Mycoplasma. These can produce a wide variety of appearances; including bilateral patchy reticulonodular infiltrates and patchy or confluent air-space opacification. Also common are polymicrobial infections.[23]

Pyogenic infectious airway disease has been increasingly recognized in recent years in HIV population, including bronchitis, bronchiolitis and bronchectasis.

Mycobacterial Pneumonias

As CD4 lymphocytes, which play an important role in cellular immunity against mycobacterial infections, are the primary target of HIV infection, the risk of tuberculosis increases. Tuberculin test is less useful and treatment response is poorer in this subset of patients. Primary tuberculosis usually manifests as massive adenopathy, and pattern of consolidation similar to that in primary tuberculosis in immunocompetent children. Miliary pattern may also be encountered. Subcarinal group of lymph nodes are the most common. On MRI, lymph nodes have a strikingly low signal on T2 and STIR images. Pleural effusion is uncommon.[23,25]

Mycobacterium avium-intracellulare has also been observed in pediatric AIDS patients. Children tend to be older with lower CD4 lymphocyte counts (<50/mm^3) than the general pediatric HIV population. Children have non-specific features of air space opacification, nodular opacities, cavitation, bronchiectasis and mediastinal nodes.[23,25]

Fungal Pneumonias

P. jirovecii pneumonia remains the most common pulmonary pathogen in children with AIDS, although the incidence appears to decrease because of prophylactic treatment.[25] Children with PJP are usually younger than those with other pulmonary conditions, with a peak age incidence at 4-5 months. PJP can be fulminant, with a mortality rate as high as 40-50 percent. Most patients have a CD4 count less than 100 cells/mm^3. Radiographic findings include a normal radiograph, hyperinflation with prominent perihilar bronchovascular markings or air-space opacities. PJP needs to be included in the differential diagnosis of any infant with rapidly progressive pneumonia, even in those not known to have HIV infection as approximately 45 percent of children with PJP are not known to have HIV at the time of presentation. The use of PJP prophylaxis does not exclude the diagnosis. CT is the imaging modality of choice. CT features include patchy areas of ground glassing, especially in the perihilar location (Figs 6.31A and B). Interlobular septal thickening may be present. Other findings include lymphadenopathy, nodules and mass lesions. Pulmonary air cysts may be seen. Pneumothorax and pneumomediastinum may occur. Pleural effusion is uncommon and suggests other pathology.[23,25]

Infection with *Cryptococcus neoformans*, *Histoplasmosis*, *Mucormycosis*, and *Invasive aspergillosis* are the other fungal infections that may be encountered.

Viral Pneumonias

Viral pathogens include respiratory syncitial virus, parainfluenza, influenza, adenovirus, CMV, measles, varicella and herpes simplex

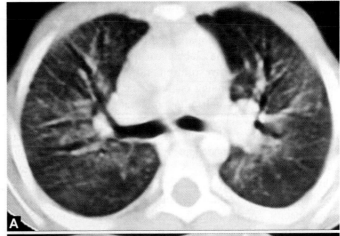
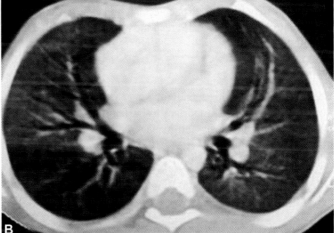

Figs 6.31A and B: PJP pneumonia. Areas of ground glass opacification are seen in bilateral lungs in a proven case of PJP pneumonia in a 6-year-old HIV positive boy

virus. Signs of consolidation are more common than wheezing in immunocompromised children.

Transmission of RSV is primarily via the hands contaminated with secretions from the mouth or nose. The radiographic findings are diffuse, patchy or nodular airspace opacities rather than interstitial infiltrates. Secondary bacterial infections are more common.[23]

CMV pneumonia usually presents when the CD4 counts fall below the level of 50 cells/mm^3. Chest radiographs may be normal, may show reticulonodular or air space pattern of disease. CT features include ground glass attenuation, nodules, consolidation and masses. Other feature may be cavitation, bronchiectasis, lymphadenopathy and pleural effusions.

Lymphocytic Interstitial Pneumonitis (LIP)

LIP is seen in 30-40 percent of patients with HIV infection. It is believed to be a response of the lymphoid system to circulating antigens of infectious agents (Epstein Barr virus) or to HIV itself. Patients tend to be a little older at diagnosis than those with opportunistic infections. It is most frequently diagnosed in children over 2 years of age. The course of the disease is relatively indolent compared to PJP. It presents with insidious development of respiratory distress and mild cough. Associated findings include generalized lymphadenopathy, salivary gland enlargement, hepatosplenomegaly and clubbing of fingers. It has a relatively good prognosis with resolution indicating severe immune suppression and impending opportunistic infections.[26]

Clinical features and radiographic appearance are usually sufficient to make the diagnosis. Chest radiographs range from mild prominence of bronchovascular markings to the more classical description of adenopathy and reticulonodular markings. Nodules may measure upto 2-3 mm in diameter. Lymphadenpathy may be massive but with no airway compression, in contradistinction to tuberculous adenopathy. On CT, diffuse ground glass opacity, poorly defined centrilobular nodules, interlobular septal thickening and thickening of the bronchovascular interstitium may be seen. Bronchiectasis and cyst formation may complicate the disease. LIP responds successfully to steroid treatment.[24,16]

CONCLUSION

Because of the high frequency of lower respiratory tract infections in children, it is important to be familiar with the role of imaging in the diagnosis and management of various pediatric pulmonary infections.

REFERENCES

1. Frush DP. Pediatric chest imaging. Radiol Clinics N Am 2005; 43:xi-xii.
2. Donnelly LF. Maximizing the usefulness of imaging in children with community acquired pneumonia. AJR 1999; 172:505-12.
3. Adler B, Effmann EL. Pneumonia and pulmonary infection. In Slovis TL (Eds): Caffey's diagnostic imaging (11th edn) Mosby-Elsevier 2008; 1184-7.
4. Markowitz RI, Ruchelli E. Pneumonia in infants and children: Radiological-pathological correlation. Semin in Roentgenol 1998; 2:151-62.
5. Donnelly LF. Imaging in immunocompetent children who have pneumonia. Radiol Clinics N Am 2005; 43:253-65.
6. Maeve McPhillips. Infection. In Carty H, Brunelle F, Stringer DA, Kao S (Eds). Imaging children (2nd ed). Elsevier Churchill Livingstone 2005; 1075-118.
7. Copley SJ. Application of computed tomography in childhood respiratory infections. British Medical Bulletin 2002; 61:263-79.
8. Bettenay FAL, de Campo JF, McCrossin DB. Differentiating bacterial from viral pneumonias in children. Pediatr Radiol 1988; 18:453-4.
9. Burko H. Considerations in the roentgen diagnosis of pneumonia in children. AJR Am J Roentgenol 1962; 88:555-65.
10. Kirkpatrick JA. Pneumonia in children as it differs from adult pneumonia. Semin Roentgenol 1980; 15:96-103.
11. Griscom NT, Wohl MB, Kirkpatrick JA. Lower respiratory*-+infections: How infants differ from adults. Radiol Clin North Am 1978; 16:367-87.
12. Calder A, Owens CM. Imaging of pleural effusions and empyema in children. Pediatr Radiol 2009; 39:527-37.
13. Donnelly LF, Klosterman LA. Pneumonia in children: Decreased parenchymal contrast enhancement – CT sign of intense illness and impending cavitary necrosis. Radiology 1997; 205:817-20.
14. Donnelly LF, Klosterman LA. The yield of CT of children who have complicated pneumonia and noncontributory chest radiography. AJR Am J Roentgenol 1998; 170:1627-31.
15. Donnelly LF, Klosterman LA. Cavitary necrosis complicating pneumonia in children: Sequential findings on chest radiography. AJR Am J Roentgenol 1998; 171:253-6.
16. Infections of the lungs and pleura. In Hansell DM, Armstrong P, Lynch DA, McAdams HP (Eds): Imaging of diseases of the chest (4th edn). Elseiver Mosby 2005; 183-276.
17. Santos JF. Tuberculosis in children. EJR 2005; 55:202-8.
18. Agrons GA, Markowitz RI, Kramer SS. Pulmonary tuberculosis in children. Semin Roentgenol 1993; 28(2):158-72.
19. Leung AN, Muller NL, Pineda PR, Fitzgerald JM. Primary tuberculosis in childhood: Radiographic manifestations. Radiology 1992; 182:187-91.
20. Lamont Ac, Cremin BJ, Pelteret RM. Radiological patterns of pulmonary tuberculosis in the pediatric age group. Pediatr Radiol 1986; 16:2-7.
21. Kim WS, Moon WK, Kim IO, et al. Pulmonary tuberculosis in children: Evaluation with CT. AJR 1997; 168:1005-9.
22. Turgut AT, Altinok T, TopcuS, Kosar U. Local complications of hydatid disease involving thoracic cavity: Imaging findings. EJR 2009; 70:49-56.
23. George R, Andronikou S, Theron S, et al. Pulmonary infection in HIV positive children. Pediatr Radiol 2009; 39:545-54.
24. Harty MP, Markowitz RI, Rutstein TM, Hunter JV. Imaging features of HIV infection in humans and children. Seminars in Roentgenol 1994; 29(3):303-14.
25. Marks MJ, Haney PJ, Mc Dermott MP, et al. Thoracic disease in children with AIDS. Radiographics 1996; 16:1349-62.
26. Theron S, Andronikou S, George R, et al. Non-infective pulmonary disease in HIV positive children. Pediatr Radiol 2009; 39:555-64.

CHAPTER 7

Chest Masses

Sanjay Thulkar, Arun Kumar Gupta

Thoracic masses in children may be located in mediastinum, lung or the chest wall. Majority of these are surgical conditions. The spectrum ranges from incidentally detected developmental lesions to aggressive malignant tumors. Chest radiography is the initial modality for their detection; however, most require further evaluation with CT or MRI. While obtaining the CT, special attention must be given radiation issues in children and dedicated pediatric CT protocols should be followed. Although MRI has the limitations of long imaging time often requiring general anesthesia as well as poor lung evaluation, it should be substituted for CT whenever possible.

LUNG MASSES

These can be classified as:

1. Congenital
   a. Abnormal lung bud development—congenital lobar emphysema; unilateral pulmonary agenesis/aplasia; pulmonary hypoplasia and hypogenetic lung syndrome (The conditions are described separately in this book)
   b. Abnormality of separation of lung bud: sequestration
   c. Hamartomatous lesions: congenital cystic adenomatoid malformation (CCAM); lung cysts; hamartoma
   d. Vascular anomalies: congenital arteriovenous malformation (AVM)
2. Inflammatory: lung abscess; hydatid cyst
3. Neoplastic: metastases; pulmonary sarcoma/blastoma.

Congenital Cystic Adenomatoid Malformation (CCAM)

This relatively rare entity is considered a focal pulmonary dysplasia and is defined as "a multicystic mass of pulmonary tissue in which there is proliferation of immature bronchial structures at the expense of alveolar development". Pathologically, the affected lobe is increased in volume and weight. The cysts are lined by cuboidal or columnar epithelium and the walls contain smooth muscle and elastic tissue. Type I is most common and contains one to four, varying sized air-filled large cysts over 2.0 cm in diameter. It may resemble congenital lobar emphysema especially if unilocular. Type II is characterized by numerous small to medium sized thin walled cysts of up to 2 cm in diameter, and prognosis is bad when associated with other congenital malformations. Type III is the least common. It is seen as a large solid lesion with multiple tiny fluid-filled cysts.[1]

CCAM may be seen in stillborn infant, with a classical triad of hydramnios, fetal ascites and cystic or solid mass in the fetal chest. The intrathoracic mass causes venous obstruction, which in turn is responsible for fetal ascites. On antenatal ultrasound, CCAM is seen as an echogenic intrathoracic mass, which may or may not have cysts. After birth, it presents with neonatal respiratory distress. In the older infant, it may cause pulmonary infection. The lesion is usually unilateral and occurs with equal frequency in both lungs with slight predilection for the upper lobes. CCAM usually involves an entire lobe or lung and produces mediastinal shift. The prognosis is usually poor due to large size and early *in utero* cardiovascular compromise.

Type I appears as a multicystic lesion with a tendency for recurrent infection in older children. Types II and III are usually associated with respiratory distress in the newborn, often with other congenital anomalies. Radiographically, in Types I and II demonstrate a multilocular air-filled bubbly mass. At this stage the differential diagnosis includes congenital diaphragmatic hernia (in which the abdomen will be gasless) and staphylococcal pneumatoceles (uncommon in the neonatal period). If one of the cysts becomes extremely large with very thin walls, it may resemble a pneumothorax or congenital lobar emphysema. Prenatal diagnosis may be made on ultrasound. Ultrasound is also helpful in the evaluation of fluid filled or solid appearing lesions. The solid lesions demonstrate highly reflective interfaces within due to the walls of the minute cysts. In uninfected CCAM, CT shows multilocular cystic mass with thin walls (Fig. 7.1) while in infected lesion, CT shows a complex mass with a mixture of solid and cystic lesions with variable definition and thick walls. The treatment is surgical excision even if the patient is asymptomatic. Type III lesion is seen as a solid pulmonary mass may be seen in the neonatal period.[2]

Pulmonary Sequestration

A bronchopulmonary sequestration is defined as a congenital mass of nonfunctioning lung tissue which contains both bronchial and alveolar elements but which lacks communication with tracheobronchial tree and receives blood supply from an anomalous systemic artery. Its venous drainage may be via the pulmonary veins, inferior vena cava or the azygos system. Sequestration occurs when a supernumerary lung bud develops caudal to the normal lung bud. If arrest occurs early in development, its communication with the foregut remains, sharing

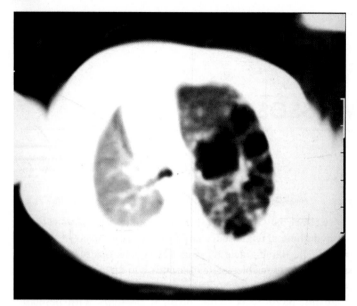

Fig. 7.1: CCAM: CT of chest shows a thin walled multicystic left lung mass

its blood supply. If arrest occurs later, sequestrated segment is connected with foregut through a fibrous band. This malformation has been further classified as intralobar in which the abnormal tissue is contained within the normal lung and its pleural covering and extralobar in which the sequestration is separate from the lung parenchyma and has its own pleural covering.

Intralobar sequestration predominantly occurs in lower lobes, usually on the left side. It tends to present later in life as an incidental finding on chest radiograph or because of recurrent infections. Patients may also present with hemoptysis if there is communication with bronchial tree. The sequestrated segment may communicate with the adjacent lung as a result of infection or occasionally cystic spaces in the lesion may communicate directly with bronchial tree.

On a chest radiograph and CT, the lesion appears as an oval, spherical or triangular basal opacity (Figs 7.2A to C). It is ill-defined and often contains multiple cysts of variable sizes, simulating CCAM. Indeed pulmonary sequestration may coexist with CCAM and then it is called as hybrid lesion of the lung. Other differential diagnosis includes pneumonia, bronchogenic cyst or pulmonary neoplasm. Most often, the abnormal vascular supply is a large vessel arising from the aorta either above or below the diaphragm. It is important to demonstrate the abnormal vascular channel on CT or MR angiography not only for diagnosis but also to avoid potential hemorrhage if surgery is contemplated.[3]

Extralobar sequestration occurs in contiguity with the left hemidiaphragm in 90 percent of the patients and is often seen incidentally as a basal soft tissue mass at or below the diaphragm with associated diaphragmatic hernia in almost 30 percent of patients. These masses enhance on CECT. Sometimes aeration may occur in this opacity. As it is completely separated from lung, there is less chance of secondary infection.

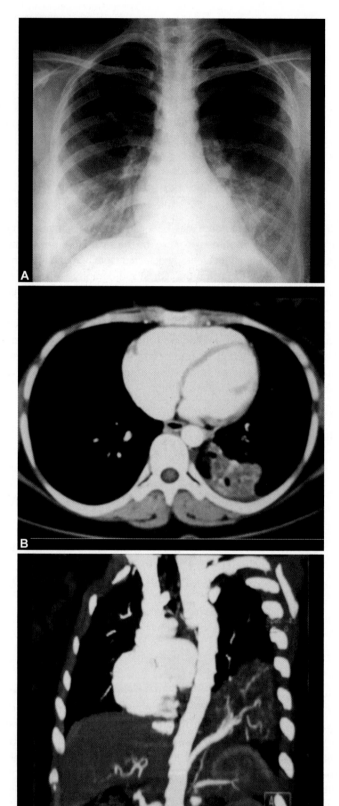

Figs 7.2A to C: Extralobar pulmonary sequestration: (A) Chest radiograph shows lung parenchymal opacity in left lower lobe, (B) CECT shows triangular consolidation with vascularity and cystic areas within, (C) CT angiogram shows arterial supply arising from the abdominal aorta

Bronchogenic Cyst

This congenital lesion presents after the newborn period. It arises as a result of anomalous supernumerary budding of the tracheal diverticulum of the ventral foregut. The cyst has a fibrous wall containing cartilage and is lined by respiratory epithelium and may be filled with air, mucoid or serous fluid or combination of this. The location of the cyst may be central (near hilum or mediastinum) or peripheral in the lung. Mediastinal bronchogenic cysts are more common and the usual locations are subcarinal, paratracheal and along the bronchi. Intrapulmonary cysts can be perihilar or peripheral. The central cyst is usually solitary and asymptomatic until infection occurs that produces hemoptysis, fever, cough or purulent expectoration. There is no direct communication of mediastinal bronchogenic cysts with the tracheobronchial tree. However, the mediastinal bronchogenic cysts may be attatched to major airways through a stalk. Rapid enlargement may be seen in infected cysts and respiratory distress may be profound. When peripheral, the cysts may be multiple and extensive. With multiple cysts, respiratory distress and even death may occur shortly after birth. Bronchial communication is common with peripheral cysts with air fluid levels and more rapid development of infection.

Chest radiograph shows round or oval, smooth, sharply marginated, thin walled, homogeneous water density mass or air-filled cyst in the mediastinal or perihilar location. Mass effect over the adjacent trachea, bronchus or esophagus may be demonstrable. An air-fluid level and thick wall may be seen in infected cysts. On CT, a hypodense, isodense or hyperdense mass lesion may be seen depending on the nature of fluid contents[4] (Fig. 7.3). The differential diagnosis on chest radiograph of a fluid filled intrapulmonary bronchogenic cyst includes round pneumonia, primary or metastatic pulmonary neoplasm, interlobar effusion. Air or air fluid-filled cyst should be differentiated from small congenital cystic adenomatoid malformation, pneumatocele and pulmonary abscess. Complications of bronchogenic cysts include infection, hemorrhage, spontaneous pneumothorax and rarely, development of malignancy.[5]

Vascular Lesions

Vascular malformations may be isolated or part of a congenital syndrome like hereditary telangiectasia. When multiple or large, they may cause high output cardiac failure and cyanosis from right to left shunting. A pulmonary AVM or varix may be seen on a radiograph as a well defined serpinginous or lobulated opacity. Calcification is rare.[6] Associated linear density representing a feeding vessel may be seen. If the feeding vessel is not apparent, the lesion may simulate a granuloma or metastasis. A thin-section CT pulmonary angiogram would demonstrate an arterial malformation to best advantage. Pulmonary angiography with and embolization is the treatment of choice.[7]

Lung Abscess

A lung abscess develops when necrosis, suppuration and cavitation occur in a localized infection of lung parenchyma. The necrotic cavity filled with purulent material may develop an air-

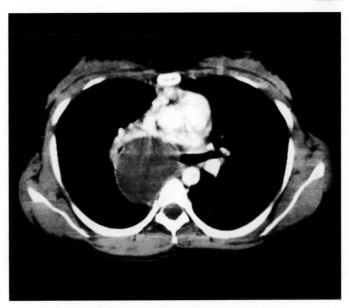

Fig. 7.3: Bronchogenic cyst: CT of chest shows a subcarinal fluid filled cyst

fluid level if erosion into the airway has occurred. Staphylococci, alpha and beta hemolytic streptococci, *Pseudomonas, Klebsiella* and aspirated anaerobic mouth flora are the common organisms for the lung abscesses. With advent of antibiotics and prompt therapy, incidence of primary lung abscess has markedly reduced. However, secondary abscess in an immunocompromised and severely ill patient has become more frequent.

The radiological appearance depends on the relative amount of necrosis, consolidation and presence of gas in the necrosis. In early stages, discrete pneumonic consolidation is seen on chest radiograph. CT at this stage may show low density center in the area of consolidation. There is absence of air-bronchogram within the abscess. When the cavity attains sufficient size and is filled with air after a bronchial communication, an air-fluid level will be seen. The abscess wall is enhancing, thick and shaggy (Fig. 7.4). Ultrasound is also useful to demonstrate lung abscess and to perform ultrasound guided aspiration.[8]

Cavitary necrosis is a more common complication of chest infection in children. It is seen as well demarcated area of necrosis filled with multiple small irregular cysts (Fig. 7.5). Affected part of the lung parenchyma does not enhance.[9] Round pneumonia is a localized infective pneumonia which appears as a rounded lung mass. This occurs in young children in whom collateral air circulation through pores of Kohn is not well developed. The consolidation remains localized and forms a mass like round opacity on chest radiographs. In children with clinical features of chest infection, round pneumonia is the most likely cause of lung mass on chest radiographs.[10]

Hydatid Cysts

This is caused by infestation with *Echinococcus granulosus* and *Echinococcus multilocularis*. As hydatid cyst grows, it compresses the adjacent lung tissue into a fibrotic capsule known as pericyst. The cyst itself has a thin smooth wall, consisting of

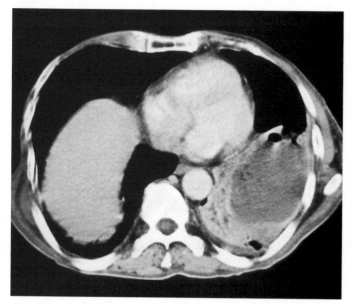

Fig. 7.4: Lung abscess: CECT shows a fluid filled rounded lesion with air lucencies within and thick enhancing wall

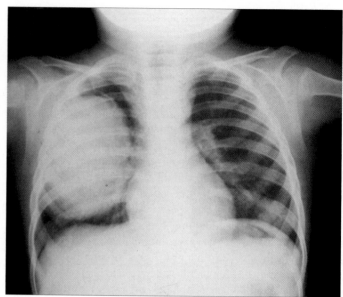

Fig. 7.6: Hydatid cyst: Chest radiograph shows a well defined homogeneous oval mass in right lung

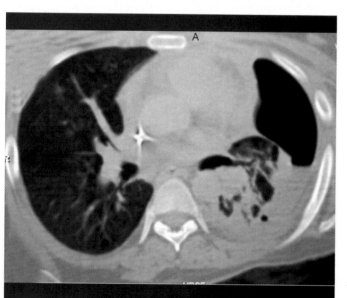

Fig. 7.5: Cavitary necrosis: CECT of chest of a leukemic man shows left lung consolidation with irregular cavites within. Variable sizes of the cavities help to distinguish it from air bronchogram. Associated hydropneumothorax is also seen

level results. Sometimes the cyst wall is seen crumpled up and floating in fluid which lies within the non-collapsed pericyst. This is described as water-lily sign or camalote sign. Fluid content is demonstrated on CT or MRI. With secondary infection, the membranes may disintegrate, walls thicken and the appearance is indistinguishable from bacterial lung abscess on chest radiograph. Sometimes all contents of the cyst may be expelled through the bronchial tree and resultant dry cyst is seen as air filled cavity.[11] Lesions abutting the chest wall or diaphragm can also be diagnosed on ultrasound which shows the characteristic cystic mass, with floating membranes.

Pulmonary Metastasis

Metastases are the most common malignant lesion of the lung in children. The common primary tumors that metastasize to lung include Wilms' tumor, osteosarcoma, Ewing's sarcoma, rhabdomyosarcoma, lymphoma, leukemia, germ cell tumors and neuroblastoma. The metastasis may be single or multiple, vary in size from a small nodule to large mass or a lymphangitis pattern may be seen. With a known primary malignancy, chest radiograph is always necessary to look for metastasis, and if present, further imaging studies may not be indicated. However, CT is routinely indicated in patients with normal chest radiographs in cancers with high incidence of lung metastases and whom the management would alter. Such cancers include most sarcomas, choriocarcinoma, and germ cell tumors. CT is also required if metastasectomy is considered. On CT, the metastases are seen as a round sharply defined nodules or masses with homogeneous attenuation. Deposits from Wilms' tumor, Hodgkin's disease and osteosarcoma may cavitate and when peripheral, these may cause a pneumothorax. Osteosarcoma is the most common cause of calcified metastases; it may also be associated with calcified

two adherent layers, the laminated ectocyst and thin lining endocyst. It grows rapidly and nearly two thirds may rupture either in the surrounding lung, bronchial tree or pleura.

Chest radiograph shows spherical or oval well-defined homogeneous opacity (Fig. 7.6). It may be single, multiple, unilateral or bilateral. Lung hydatids rarely calcify. When the pericyst ruptures into an airway and air dissects between pericyst and ectocyst, this gives rise to the characteristic meniscus or crescent sign. When the cyst ruptures into an airway, an air-fluid

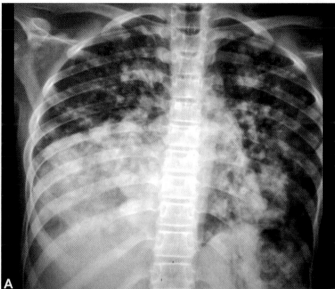

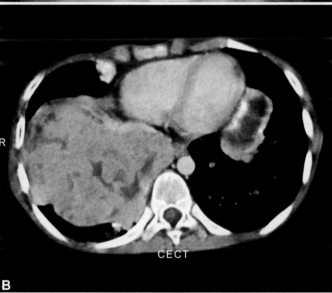

Figs 7.7A and B: Lung metastases from osteosarcoma: (A) Chest radiograph shows bilateral extensive nodules and masses, (B) CT shows a right lower lobe mass with multiple smaller bilateral nodules and masses with calcifications

mediastinal lymph nodes and calcified pleural deposits[12] (Figs 7.7A and B). Thyroid carcinoma causes miliary deposits with 2-5 mm nodules. Lymphoma and leukemia may also cause lung deposits. An air bronchogram within a lung nodule is a characteristic feature of the lymphomatous nodule.[21] Hilar adenopathy and interstitial disease may be associated. Lymphangitic spread on chest radiograph is seen as reticular or reticulo-nodular pattern. On HRCT, nodules are seen in continuity with a vessel. Also, there is beading and thickening of interlobular and interlobar septa and irregular thickening of bronchovascular bundles. It is important to note that in patients with known extrathoracic malignancies, large number of the lung nodules detected on CT as metastases are actually benign and may

represent granulomas.[13] This is especially common in areas with high incidence of tuberculosis or histoplasmosis.

Primary Lung Tumors

Primary pulmonary neoplasms in children are uncommon. The largest group of malignant tumors in childhood is grouped under the name *pleuropulmonary blastoma*. These occur in children as well as in adults; however, both are considered distinct entities. Pleuropulmonary blastoma of the childhood arises from primitive blastomatous tissues and develops in pre-existing congenital lung lesions like cystic adenomatoid malformation, sequestration or bronchogenic cysts.[14]

This tumor may be small and present as a solitary pulmonary nodule, or large and occupy the entire thorax. The lesion may be multicystic, cystic solid or entirely solid; with malignancy rate increasing in that order. The chest radiograph shows a large mass which may have features of local invasion (Figs 7.8A and B). CT and MR features are variable and ranges from fluid filled cysts with solid nodule, solid mass causing mediastinal shift and lung collapse, shows areas of necrosis within a heterogeneously enhancing mass. Pleural effusion may be present, however, chest wall invasion is uncommon.[15] Metastases may occur in liver and central nervous system. Prognosis is poor.

Mesenchymal sarcomas of childhood may be associated with developmental cystic lesions like bronchogenic cyst, cystic adenomatoid malformation or congenital pulmonary cyst. These include leiomyosarcoma, rhabdomyosarcoma and fibrosarcoma. Bronchogenic carcinoma is extremely rare but can occur in older children. Usual histologies include carcinoid tumor, adenocarcinoma, basaloid carcinoma and mucoepidermoid carcinoma. Initial diagnostic consideration is usually pneumonia in these children, resulting in delayed diagnosis.[16] Other rare primary lung tumors include hemangiopericytoma and Askin tumor.

Plasma cell granuloma, also called inflammatory pseudotumor, is a proliferation of plasma cells, histiocytes and granulocytes and could represent a reparative response to infection. On radiographs, a well-circumscribed mass, mostly uncalcified and of a large size is seen. On CT, central necrosis and peripheral contrast enhancement may be seen.

MEDIASTINAL MASSES

The primary thoracic masses in children are most commonly located in the mediastinum. The mediastinal masses represent a wide variety of congenital anomalies and cysts in addition to neoplasms. Children with mediastinal masses are frequently asymptomatic and most often chest X-ray is done for nonspecific symptoms like fever, malaise, cough. Airway compression, particularly before the age of one year is an important presentation. Respiratory distress results from easily compressible rings of the infant's trachea and bronchi. The risk of airway compression and high incidence of malignancy require prompt diagnosis and treatment for a child with mediastinal tumor.

Mediastinal masses can be classified as per their location into anterior, middle and posterior mediastinal masses. Since these

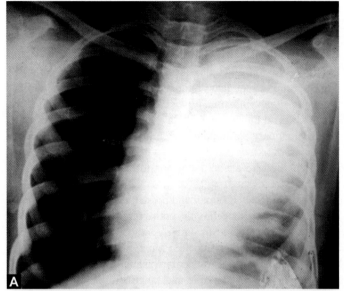

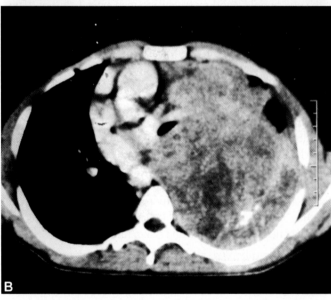

Figs 7.8A and B: Pulmonary blastoma: (A) Chest radiograph shows a large left lung mass with mediastinal shift to right side, (B) CT shows a large solid mass with areas of necrosis and calcifications with mediastinal and pleural invasion

compartments are not anatomical spaces, masses may often involve more than one compartment. In this situation, location of the center of the mass direction of displacement of adjacent structures, such as trachea and great vessels, is useful to suggest the likely region of origin.

Anterior Mediastinal Masses

Approximately 30 percent of mediastinal masses occur in anterior mediastinum. These include the four 'T's: teratoma (and other germ cell tumors), thymic tumor, thyroid tumor or cysts and 'terrible' lymphoma/leukemia. As thymus or thyroid tumors are rare in pediatric age group, important differential diagnosis of anterior mediastinal mass consists of germ cell tumor and lymphoma.

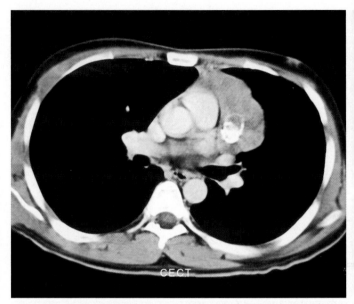

Fig. 7.9: Mediastinal germ cell tumor: CT shows an anterior mediastinal mass containing coarse calcification

Germ Cell Tumors

These include dermoid, teratoma, teratocarcinoma, chorio-carcinoma, embryonal carcinoma, seminoma, endodermal sinus tumors and mixed germ cell tumors. Most germ cell tumors arise in anterior mediastinum near thymus and few arise in other mediastinal compartments.

Teratomas may be benign (mature) or malignant (immature). Mature teratomas usually attain a large size before they present with symptoms. Both mature and immature teratomas are seen as lobulated anterior mediastinal soft tissue masses. Calcifications are common. On CT, teratomas are seen as complex solid or cystic solid masses with variable wall thickness. Calcification, teeth and fat densities are more readily visualized on CT[17] (Fig. 7.9). However, macroscopically demonstrable fat is unusual in malignant teratoma.

Seminoma arising in mediastinum is rare and metastatic seminoma in the mediastinum from occult gonadal lesion should always be excluded with USG of scrotum. Seminoma is seen as a bulky, homogenous anterior mediastinal mass on CT and may simulate lymphoma. Rarely, calcifications may be present. Involvement of adjacent structures is uncommon however; metastases to lymph nodes, lung or bone may be present. *Endodermal sinus tumor* (yolk sac tumor) is a poorly differentiated embryonal carcinoma, occurs often in males and patients usually have systemic symptoms and elevated serum alpha-fetoprotein. These tumors as well as most other non-seminomatous malignant germ cell tumors have nonspecific imaging features. On CT, these are seen as large irregular, heterogeneous mediastinal masses with areas of necrosis, cystic degeneration and hemorrhages.[18]

Lymphoma

Lymphomas are the most common cause of mediastinal masses in children. Both Hodgkin and non-Hodgkin (especially

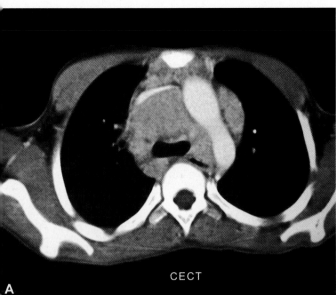

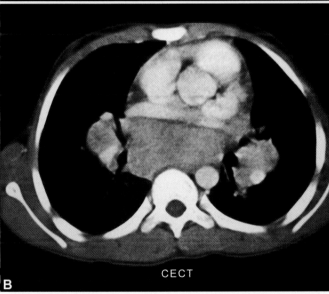

Figs 7.10A and B: Hodgkin's lymphoma: CT images at (A) Carinal and (B) Subcarinal levels show bilateral conglomerate homogeneous lymph node enlargement

lymphoblastic lymphoma) can present with large anterior mediastinal masses. However, the lymphadenopathy may be present anywhere in the mediastinum or the hila. CT is the modality of choice for evaluation and staging of lymphoma. On CT, mediastinal lymphadenopathy in lymphoma may be descrete, however, more often it produce conglomerate homogenous lymph node masses (Figs 7.10A and B). Mass effect such as vascular displacement, compression of trachea or obstruction of superior vena cava is common with large masses.[19] Necrosis and hemorrhages are rare but it may be seen in large masses of lymphoma. Calcification is also rare in lymphoma.

In Hodgkin's lymphoma, if transverse diameter of mediastinal lymph nodal mass measured on chest radiograph at T4-5 level exceeds transverse thoracic diameter, it is called as bulky disease.

It is denoted as suffix X to the stage and associated with inferior prognosis. It is uncommon for NHL to be limited to mediastinum only at the presentation. However, some NHL primarily involves anterior mediastinum. These include primary mediastinal large B-cell lymphoma and lymphoblastic lymphoma, the later is a T cell NHL. Both these are aggressive lymphomas seen in children and young adults. Patients usually present with dyspnea, stridor and SVC syndrome.[20] On imaging, large, often heterogeneous and infiltrative anterior mediastinal mass is seen.

Thymic Masses

Prominent but normal thymus is the most common pseudotumor of anterior mediastinum. On imaging, anterior mediastinal tumors displace the trachea and esophagus posteriorly and laterally in contradistinction to a normal enlarged thymus which does not displace adjacent structures.

Hyperplasia of thymus is uncommon and may occur in Graves' disease, lymphoma, leukemia and Langerhans' cell histiocytosis. It may also occur as a rebound thymic enlargement after chemotherapy.

Thymic cyst is of developmental origin, representing persistent tubular remnants of the third pharyngeal pouch. The cyst is usually asymptomatic and incidentally seen on chest radiograph. It is unilocular or multilocular and varies is size. CT is helpful in diagnosis.

Thymoma is rare in childhood. The association of thymoma and myasthenia gravis is also much less in children than in adults. On radiographs, thymoma is seen a variable sized lobulated soft tissue mass in anterior mediastinum. On CT, thymomas are generally seen as lobulated, homogeneously enhancing masses with smooth contour. They tend to grow asymmetrically to one side of the mediastinum. Calcifications may be present and this helps to differentiate thymoma from lymphoma. Rarely, thymoma may have pleural effusion with nodular pleural deposits or diffuse pleural thickening mimicking mesothelioma or pleural metastases.[21] On MRI, thymoma are homogenously isointense on T1 weighted images and heterogeneously hyperintense on T2 weighted images.[22]

Lymphangioma

Lymphangioma, also known as cystic hygroma, results from failure of primary lymphatic sac to establish drainage into the venous system. It is an uncommon cause of mediastinal masses in children. Most are caused by extension form other sites, such as neck or axilla, into the mediastinum.[23] Most are located in anterior or middle mediastinum but few may be seen in posterior mediastinum. It often presents as a large soft consistency mass and rarely causes airway obstruction. Pathologically these are lymphatic malformations macrocystic, microcystic or combined morphology. Chest radiograph shows well demarcated mass which may have a lobulated outline. On USG, macrocystic component is seen as cystic masses with internal echoes and septations. Mild vascularity may be seen on color Doppler. Microcystic component is highly echogenic. MRI is required to assess the

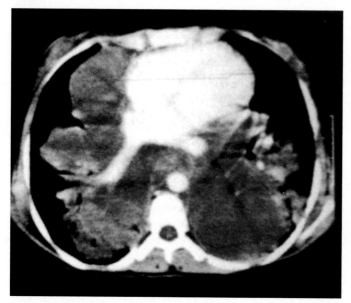

Fig. 7.11: Mediastinal lymphangioma: CT shows a multisepted, lobulated bilateral cystic mediastinal mass

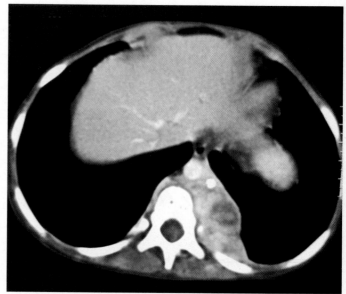

Fig. 7.12: Mediastinal neuroblastoma: CT shows enhancing left paravertebral mass with areas of necrosis and calcification

entire extent of lymphangioma. CT and MRI demonstrate a well circumscribed avascular cystic mass with septations and mild wall enhancement (Fig. 7.11). Areas of fat density may be demonstrated. Fluid-fluid levels may also be seen due to hemorrhages or protein contents. The septations show enhancement on contrast-enhanced MRI. The mass tends to envelop or mould to adjacent structures. The microcystic type may be seen as highly enhancing soft tissue mass on CE MRI.[24]

Pericardial Cysts

These are rare benign unilocular anterior mediastinal cyst containing clear fluid. Most are developmental in origin. On radiographs, these are seen as well defined, rounded or teardrop shaped mass in cardiophrenic angles abutting the heart. Most are seen on right side. On CT or MRI, these are seen as well demarcated nonenhancing cysts.

Middle and Posterior Mediastinal Masses

Common masses in middle mediastinum are enlarged lymph nodes or bronchogenic cyst. Lymph node enlargement may be in the paratracheal or hilar locations are mostly due to viral, tubercular or fungal infections, leukemia, lymphoma and histiocytosis. Massive adenopathy is seen in lymphoma and leukemia in which the nodes are confluent. Aneurysms of aorta, pulmonary artery or coronary artery are also rare causes of middle mediastinal masses. Bronchogenic cyst is discussed under congenital lung conditions. Almost 40 percent of mediastinal masses in children are located in the posterior mediastinum and majority of these are neurogenic tumors or cystic duplications.[25] Rare causes of posterior mediastinal tumors include hemangiomas and vascular malformations, extramedullary hematopoiesis, germ cell tumors, Ewing's sarcoma and rhabdomyosarcoma.

Neurogenic Tumors

These include ganglion tumors (ganglioneuroma, ganglio-neuroblastoma and neuroblastoma), nerve sheath tumors (neurofibroma and schwannoma) and paraganglioma.

Neuroblastoma and Other Ganglion Tumors

Ganglion tumors are derived from the sympathetic ganglia and include neuroblastoma (malignant), ganglioneuroma (benign) and ganglioneuroblastoma (having both components). They usually occur in the superior half of the posterior mediastinum and cannot be differentiated on the basis of imaging alone.

Neuroblastoma is the second most common solid tumor in children after brain tumors and represent 10 percent of all childhood cancers.[26] Thorax is the second most common site for neuroblastoma after the abdomen. It usually occurs in children less than two years of age but may rarely occur up to the age of 10 years. These may also be diagnosed on prenatal USG. Neuroblastoma is malignant but has a better prognosis in mediastinum when diagnosed under one year of age.

Patients with thoracic neuroblastoma have symptoms due to primary mass or the metastases. They present with respiratory distress or cord compression. Those with metastatic disease have pain, fever and weight loss. Rarely, neuroblastoma may be detected as a asymptomatic mass on chest radiograph. Usual appearance of neuroblastoma on chest radiograph is of a smooth elongated paraspinal mass with rib or vertebral erosion and characteristic splaying of ribs. Calcifications are seen in up to 30 percent cases.[27] On CT, a soft tissue mass with speckled, irregular and granular calcification is seen in the posterior mediastinum (Fig. 7.12). It shows mild contrast enhancement, occasionally with areas of necrosis and hemorrhages. Rib erosion and widened intervertebral foramina may be seen. Other bony

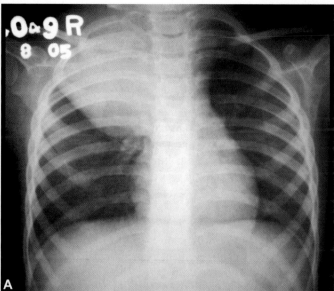

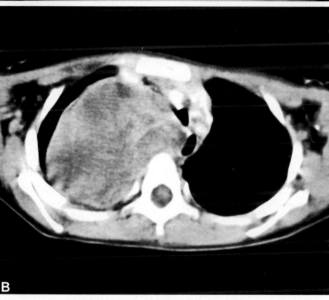

Figs 7.13A and B: Ganglioneuroblastoma: (A) Chest radiograph shows a large right mediastinal mass, (B) CT shows a large posterior mediastinal mass with displacement and compression of mediastinal structures

changes include pedicular flattening, spinal canal enlargement, posterior vertebral scalloping and localized kyphoscoliosis. Intraspinal extension is frequent even in absence of neurologic signs and symptoms. Vascular encasement and mediastinal lymphadenopathy may also be seen, though uncommonly. MRI is the modality of choice for staging because the intraspinal spread and spread along nerves and bone marrow involvement are better demonstrated by MRI. As bone metastases are common, radiographic skeletal survey and a bone scan using ⁹⁹ᵐTC-MDP or ¹²³I-MIBG is usually obtained as a part of imaging work up. Bony metastases are lytic or lytic sclerotic and have characteristic appearances.[28]

Median age for the diagnosis of ganglioneuroblastoma is 5 years and that for the ganglioneuroma is 10 years.[26] *Ganglioneuroblastoma* is more differentiated malignancy and has a good prognosis. These tumors are usually aysmptomatic until they invade or compress adjacent structures, metastasize to distant sites or produce unusual paraneoplastic syndromes. Nonspecific symptoms include fever, malaise, back pain or anemia. Lower limb weakness is present in lesions involving the spinal canal. The imaging features of ganglioneuroblastoma are similar to neuroblastoma. Twenty percent of ganglioneuroblastomas have calcification and show low homogeneous attenuation with minimal contrast enhancement (Figs 7.13A and B). *Ganglioneuroma* is a benign tumor which occurs in older children is seen as a large smooth spherical mass or small elongated sausage shaped mass which shows low homogeneous attenuation with minimal contrast enhancement. Differential diagnosis of neurogenic tumors includes malignant sarcoma arising from chest wall or inflammatory lesion such as actinomycosis.

Neurofibroma and Schwannoma

Neurofibroma and schwannomas are nerve sheath tumors. Schwannoma is encapsulated and do not contain nerve fibers while neurofibroma is uncapsulated and hence have nerve fiber within it. In thorax, these tumors arise from intercostals or sympathetic nerves. These tumors are mostly benign, asymptomatic and seen under 20 years of age. On imaging, neurofibroma and schwannoma are similar in appearance and seen as solid, well defined round or oval masses.[29] Neurofibroma usually occurs in patients with systemic neurofibromatosis rather than a solitary lesion. It is more often bilaterally located in posterior mediastinum. Chest radiograph in addition to this lesion shows 'ribbon like' rib deformities or scoliosis. On CT, the soft tissue mass is homogeneous with low attenuation and mildly enhances with contrast. It may extend to spinal canal, showing characteristic dumb-bell shape. In the plexiform variety, the mass may be confluent.

Paraganglioma

These are rare neurogenic tumors of the posterior mediastinum and actually represent extra-adrenal pheochromocytoma. These are derived from chromafin cells of the sympathetic nervous system. Imaging features are nonspecific but the diagnosis is usually established on the basis of excessive catecholamine secretions.

Duplication Cysts

Abnormal closure of ventral foregut results in formation of *bronchogenic cyst*. These are described above in congenital lung conditions. Abnormal closure of dorsal foregut results in enterogenic duplication cysts and these include esophageal duplication cyst and neuroenteric cyst. *Esophageal duplication cyst* constitutes almost 10 to 15 percent of all duplications of the gastrointestinal tract. In contrast to bronchogenic cyst which occurs in early age, the majority of children with esophageal duplications are over 10 years of age at the onset of symptoms. The lesion is smooth in outline, varies in size and usually impinges on a barium filled esophagus but rarely communicates with esophageal lumen. CT and MRI demonstrate the cystic and avascular nature of the lesion. These modalities clearly demonstrate precise size, location, its relation to adjacent organs and transdiaphragmatic extension. Technetium[99]m-pertechnetate scintigraphy demonstrates gastric mucosa in the cyst, thereby confirms the preoperative diagnosis.

The *neuroenteric cyst* results from incomplete separation of the foregut from notochord. These have a vertebral body cleft communicating with the spinal canal. It contains both neural and gastrointestinal element. It may be limited to the chest as a blind sac or may extend below the diaphragm where it either ends blindly or communicates with the intestinal tract. Most neuroenteric cysts are discovered in infancy because of esophageal and tracheobronchial compression.[30]

Anterior Thoracic Meningocele

Though rare, this entity is to be considered in the differential diagnosis of posterior mediastinal masses. It occurs due to spinal canal anomalies in which the leptomeninges herniate through the neural foramina. It is seen usually in patients of neurofibromatosis with kyphoscoliosis where the meningocele is at the apex of the convexity. MRI confirms the diagnosis.

Extramedullary Hematopoiesis

It is rarely seen in hematological disorders, most commonly in thalassemia. It is usually asymptomatic but may rarely cause cord compression. On imaging, it is seen as bilaterally symmetrical, well defined, lobulated lower thoracic paraspinal soft tissue mass.

CHEST WALL MASSES

Chest Wall Infections

Chest wall is the uncommon site for infections and abscesses as compared to the lungs. These are easily diagnosed clinically however; imaging is required to assess the deeper extent. Ultrasound is useful to detect and localize chest wall abscess. It is seen as cystic mass with debris. On CT, the abscess is seen as cystic area with wall enhancement. CT is especially useful to detect associated osteomyelitis of the rib and deeper extent of the abscess. Chest wall infection without the well formed abscess is seen as a heterogeneous, ill-defined mass on CT.

Lymphangioma

These are focal or diffuse masses that tend to involve subcutaneous tissues of neck, chest wall or axilla. These may extend into mediastinum. Imaging features are similar to those described above for mediastinal lymphangiomas.

Hemangioma

Hemangiomas are the most common soft tissue tumors in children. The usual sites are head and neck, chest and extremities. These are usually present at birth, however, after initial proliferation, majority of these disappear spontaneously. Small superficial hemangiomas have characteristic appearance and of no clinical significance. Large and extensive lesions may have mass effect. On color Doppler USG, large vascular channels with both arterial as well as venous flow are seen.[31] On MRI, hemangiomas are seen as lobulated masses iso and high signal intensity on T1 and T2 weighted images respectively, with areas of flow voids representing vascular channels. Diffuse enhancement following contrast administration. During involution, high T1 signal intensity is seen due to fatty replacement.

Venous malformations may have similar appearance, however, unlike hemangiomas, these are not tumors. On imaging, venous malformations tend to be solid without dilated vascular channels and on color Doppler, there is minimal or no detectable flow at all. Phleboliths are frequently seen as calcified focal lesions within the mass.

Neurofibroma

Neurofibroma and *schwannoma* may also involve chest wall. Extensive chest wall involvement by plexiform neurofibromatosis may be seen in children with NF1. These tumors may cause secondary bony abnormalities in the form of ribbon appearance of the ribs, scalloping of the vertebral bodies and kyphoscoliosis.

Benign Osseous Masses

Fibrous dysplasia of the rib is the most common osseous lesion of the chest wall. These are frequently seen as incidental findings on imaging. Radiographically, it is seen as a focal, well defined, expansile lytic lesion of the rib. Alternatively, there may be diffuse fusiform enlargement of the rib with ground glass matrix. *Osteochondromas* (or exostosis) are benign bony outgrowths with cartilage cap on the surface. These usually occur in long bones; however, ribs, sternum, scapula, clavicle or spine may also be involved. Most are asymptomatic and detected incidentally while others may be symptomatic due to mass effect on adjacent structures. Malignant transformation is rare. On radiography, osteochondroma is seen as a bony outgrowth with both cortex and medulla that are continuous with the host bone. CT and MRI show similar features and cartilage cap is better evaluated on these modalities. Irregularity or thickening of the cartilage cap more than 2 cm is suspicious for malignant transformation into chondrosarcoma.[32] *Enchondroma* of the rib usually occurs in adults and uncommon in children. It is seen as a well defined, expansile lytic lesion of the rib with endosteal scalloping. Calcifications may also be present.

Mesenchymal hamartoma of the chest wall is a rare benign tumor of the infancy. It is a mature mesenchymal tumor containing bone, cartilages, fat and fibrous tissues. On imaging, it is seen as a large complex cystic solid soft issue mass along with destruction of one or several contiguous ribs. Intense enhancement is seen in solid parts of the mass.[33]

Primitive Neuroectodermal Tumor (PNET)

These include Ewing's sarcoma of the bone and PNET of the chest wall (Askin's tumor). Clinically, these present a large painful soft tissue masses, often associated with cough and dyspnea. On chest radiographs, large thoracic soft tissue mass with or without associated rib destruction is seen (Figs 7.14A and B).

Rhabdomyosarcoma

It is the second most common malignancy of the chest wall in children.[35] Chest wall rhabdomyosarcomas are more aggressive than those occurring in head and neck or genitourinary tract. On radiographs, soft tissue mass is seen with or without rib destruction. CT and MR features are nonspecific and similar to those of PNET.

Miscellaneous Malignant Chest Wall Masses

Both Hodgkin and non-Hodgkin's lymphoma may secondarily involve the chest wall by direct extension from mediastinal or pleural disease. Most common pattern is of homogeneous parasternal chest wall mass contiguous with anterior mediastinal lymphadenopathy. Rib or sternum may be eroded or appear normal in spite of large chest wall mass. Uncommonly, descrete and isolated chest wall may also be seen with lymphoma. Neuroblastoma may involve the chest wall as a direct extension from posterior mediastinal tumor.[36] MRI is most useful to evaluate the extent of chest wall as well as spinal involvement by neuroblastoma. Osteosarcoma of the rib is uncommon in children. It is seen as destructive lesion of the rib with new bone formation. Associated soft tissue component is also present although not as massive as PNET.

Other rare malignant chest wall tumors in children include congenital fibrosarcoma, mesenchymal chondrosarcoma and malignant peripheral nerve sheath tumor (MPNST). Their imaging features are nonspecific.

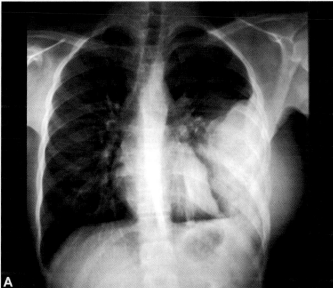

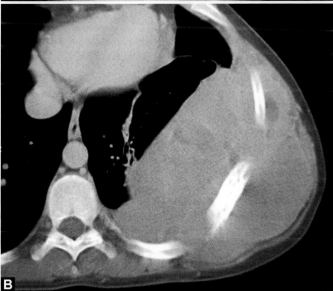

Figs 7.14A and B: PNET of chest wall: (A) Chest radiograph shows a large left sided chest wall mass with both intra- and extrathoracic components, (B) CT show lytic sclerotic rib within the mass

CT demonstrates large extrapleural mass with heterogeneous contrast enhancement and rib destruction. The extraosseous soft tissue mass component is disproportionately larger than the bone lesion. Very large tumors may occupy most part of the hemithorax and cause lung collapse and mediastinal shift to the contralateral side. Pleural effusion may be present but it is usually not massive. Incidence of lung metastases is high and hence, careful lung evaluation should also be done on CT. MRI appearance is similar to CT. These tumors may also have skip lesions along the intercostal nerves. These tumors are usually treated with chemoradiotherapy followed by surgery; however, the prognosis is poor.[34]

REFERENCES

1. Stocker JT, Madewell JE, Drake RM. Congenital cystic adenomatoid malformation of the lung: classification and morphologic spectrum. Hum Pathol 1977; 8:155-71.
2. Winters WD, Effaman EL. Congenital masses of the lung: prenatal and postnatal imaging evaluation. J Thorac Imaging 2001; 16:196-206.
3. Lee EY, Siegel MJ, Sierra LM, et al. Evaluation of architecture of pulmonary sequestration in pediatric patients using 3D MDCT angiography. AJR Am J Roentgenol 2004; 183:183-8.
4. Reed JC, Sobonya RE. Morphologic analysis of foregut cysts in the thorax. AJR Am J Roentgenol 1974; 120:851-60.
5. McAdams HP, Kitejczyk WM, Rosado-de-Christensen ML, et al. Bronchogenic cysts: imaging features with clinical and histopathologic correlation. Radiology 2000; 217:441-6.
6. Paterson A, Imaging evaluation of congenital lung abnormalities in infant and children. Radiol Clin N Am 2005; 43:303-23.
7. Abushaban L, Uthaman B, Endrys J. Transcatheter coil closure of pulmonary arteriovenous malformations in children. J Interven Cardiol 2004; 17:23-6.
8. Yang P, Lih K, Lee Y, et al. Lung abscesses: ultrasonography and ultrasound guided transthoracic aspiration. Radiology 1991; 180:171-5.
9. Donnely LF. Practical issues concerning imaging of pulmonary infections in children. J Thorac Imaging 2001; 16:238-50.
10. Rose RE, Ward BH. Spherical pneumonias in children simulating pulmonary and mediastinal masses. Radiology 1973; 106:179-82.

11. Erdem CZ, Erdem LO. Radiological characteristics of pulmonary hydatid disease in children: less common radiological appearances. Eur Radiol 2003; 45:123-8.

12. Rastogi R, Garg R, Thulkar S, et al. Unusual thoracic CT manifestations of osteosarcoma: review of 16 cases. Pediatr Radiol 2008; 38:551-8.

13. Aquino SL. Imaging of metastatic disease to the thorax. Radio Clin N Am 2005; 43:481-95.

14. Maniwell JC, Priest JR, Watterson J, et al. Pleuropulmonary blastoma: the so called pulmonary blastoma of childhood. Cancer 1988; 62:1516-26.

15. Orazi C, Inserra A, Schingo PM, et al. Pleuropulmonary blastoma, a distinct neoplasm of childhood: report of three cases. Pediatr Radiol 2007; 37:337-44.

16. Lal DR, Clark I, Shalkow J, et al. Primary epithelial lung malignancies in pediatric population. Pediatr Blood Cancer 2005; 45:683-6.

17. Brown LR, Muhm JR, Aughenbaugh GL, et al. Computed tomography of benign mature teratomas of the mediastinum. J Thorac Imaging 1987; 2:66-71.

18. Lee KS, IM JG, Han CH, et al. Malignant primary germ cell tumors of the mediastinum: CT features. AJR Am J Roentgenol 1989; 153:947-51.

19. Arya LS, Narain S, Tomar S, et al. Superior vena cava syndrome. Indian J Pediatr 2001; 69:293-7.

20. Shukla NN, Trippett TM. Non Hodgkin lymphoma in children and adolescents. Curr Oncol Rep 2006; 8:387-94.

21. Thomas CR, Wright CD, Loeherer PJ. Thymoma: state of art. J Clin Oncol 1999; 17:2280-89.

22. Santana L, Givica A, Camacho C. Best cases from AFIP: thymoma. Radiographics 2002; 22:95-102.

23. Sumner TE, Volberg FM, Kiser PE, et al. Mediastinal cystic hygroma in children. Pediatr Radiol 1981; 11:160-62.

24. Konez O, Borrows PE. Magnetic resonance of vascular anomalies. Magn Reson Imaging Clin N Am 2002; 10:363-88.

25. Mea MP, Benson M, Slovis TL. Imaging of mediastinal masses in children. Radiol Clin N Am 1993; 31:583-604.

26. Lonergan CJ, Schwab CJ, Suarez ES, et al. Neuroblastoma, ganglioneuroblastoma and ganglioneuroma: radiologic-pathologic correlation. Radiographics 2002; 22:911-34.

27. Softka CM, Semelka RC, Kelekis NL, et al. Magnetic resonance imaging of neuroblastoma using current techniques. Magn Reson Imaging 1999; 17:193-8.

28. Hiorns MP, Owens CM. Radiology of neuroblastoma in children. Eur Radiol 2001; 11:2071-81.

29. Laurent F, Latrabe V, Lecesne R, et al. Mediastinal masses: diagnostic approach. Eur Radiol 1998; 8:1149-59.

30. Strollo DC, Rosado-de-Christenson ML, Jett JR. Primary mediastinal tumours. Part II: tumors of the middle and posterior mediastinum. Chest 1997; 112:1344-57.

31. Paltiel HJ, Burrows PE, Kozakewich HPW, et al. Soft tissue vascular anomalies: utility of US for diagnosis. Radiology 2000; 214:747-54.

32. Lee KC, Davis AM, Cassar-Pullicino VN. Imaging the complications of osteochondromas. Clin Radiol 2001; 57:18-28.

33. Groom KR, Murphy MD, Howard LM, Mesenchymal hamartoma of the chest wall: radiologic manifestations with emphasis on cross sectional imaging and histopathological comparison. Radiology 2002; 222:205-11.

34. Fefferman NR, Pinkney LP. Imaging evaluation of chest wall disorders in children. Radiol Clin N Am 2005; 43:355-70.

35. Shamberger RC, Grier HE. Chest wall tumours in infants and children. Semin Pediatr Surg 1994; 3:267-76.

36. Wyttenbach R, Vock P, Tschappeler H. Cross sectional imaging with CT and/or MRI of pediatric chest tumours. Eur Radiol 1998; 8:1040-9.

CHAPTER 8

Pediatric Airway

Ashu Seith Bhalla

Diseases affecting the airway, extrinsic or intrinsic, are much more common in children than in adults. Also, the smaller airway caliber coupled with the greater collapsibility of the airway in infants and young children, leads to early and more symptomatic airflow disturbances, even with minor amounts of airway edema and mucus. Clinically, the presentation of these disorders may be acute or chronic. In their acute form, the airway disorders can be life threatening. "Always look at the airway" is a lesson that must be emphasized in pediatric radiology.[1-4]

The airway is referred to as the upper airway (above the thoracic inlet) or lower airway being below it. While the predominant presentation of upper airway obstruction is inspiratory stridor, that of lower airway obstruction is expiratory wheeze.[1-4] Other clinical presentations include feeding difficulty, respiratory distress, tachypnea, nasal flaring, chest wall retractions, hemoptysis, fever, failure to thrive and even no symptoms.[4] Diseases affecting the pediatric airway are broadly classified in Table 8.1.

Imaging Modalities

The purpose of imaging is to delineate: location of the abnormality, if the involvement diffuse or focal and extrinsic or intrinsic. If the lesion is an intrinsic process, is it mural or intraluminal and is the obstruction fixed or dynamic.[4] The radiographic evaluation of airways in infants and young children is challenging due to inability to obtain motionless end-inspiratory and end-expiratory images. The resultant artifacts are especially noticeable in HRCT images. Also the caliber of airways of young children is small and difficult to detail in infants and small children.

Plain Radiographs

Plain radiographs are the primary and often only imaging modality used in evaluation of children with airway obstruction. The evaluation should include frontal and lateral high kV radiographs of the upper airways, and frontal and lateral views of the chest. When an endobronchial foreign body is a consideration, decubitus chest views may be helpful. Expiratory radiographs aid in demonstrating air trapping.

Fluoroscopy

Fluoroscopy of the airway demonstrates dynamic airway collapse during expiration in children with tracheobronchomalacia.[4] Decubitus fluoroscopy may be performed in cases of suspected foreign body in infants and young children.

Barium Swallow

A barium swallow may be useful for demonstrating gastro-esophageal reflux in patients with chronic aspiration simulating asthma . This study is also helpful for establishing the diagnosis of vascular rings and slings, although cross-sectional imaging is eventually required for better anatomic delineation.

MDCT

Relative to MRI, CT has the advantage of rapid scan times enabling performance of the examination without sedation, it has the disadvantage of radiation exposure and need for using contrast. *Dynamic CT* can be obtained as a paired inspiratory- expiratory scan in older cooperative children.

In uncooperative children, some authors have reported a controlled ventilation CT (CVCT). CVCT uses positive pressure feedback ventilation. The child is sedated but otherwise breathing on his her own; and images are acquired during hyperventilation-induced transient respiratory pause. The technique does not require intubation or general anesthesia and provides motionless inspiratory and expiratory phase images. In this technique, several sequential inspirations are augmented by face-mask ventilation which induces hypocarbia. Hypocarbia (through Hering-Breuer reflex) results in brief apneic periods during which images can be acquired.[3,4] CT images can be acquired at desired degrees of airway distention.

In those uncooperative children in whom even the controlled-ventilation technique is not feasible or not available, cine CT can be used. *Cine-CT* involves rapid acquisition of images of the airway throughout the respiratory cycle during free breathing. Once the site of suspected airway stenosis or malacia is localized, CT images are rapidly and sequentially acquired at the same axial level. Cine CT technique can provide multiple images of the airway during inspiration and expiration, even in tachypneic patients.

Multiplanar and 3D volume-rendered image reconstructions further enhance the accuracy of MDCT in delineating the level of narrowing, degree of obstruction, segment length and distal airway.[5]

MRI

MRI can demonstrate abnormal airway motion in addition to anatomic causes of obstruction. The protocol includes axial and sagittal T1 weighted as well as STIR images.

Dynamic (cine) MRI studies can be used to evaluate airway motion in real time. Sagittal midline MR cine (fast gradient echo

Table 8.1: Diseases affecting the pediatric airway

Upper Airway Obstruction

Acute

Croup

Epiglottitis

Retropharyngeal cellulitis and abscess

Exudative tracheitis

Foreign body

Chronic

Space occupying lesions	- Adenoidal enlargement
	- Enlarged pharyngeal tonsils
	- Juvenile nasopharyngeal angiofibroma
Fixed airway narrowing	- Stenosis/stricture
Congenital	- Micrognathia
	- Macroglossia
	- Laryngeal malacia
	- Laryngeal cysts

Lower Airway Obstruction

Central airways

Extrinsic: Congenital	- Vascular compression, Vascular malformations
	- Bronchopulmonary foregut malformations - Bronchogenic cyst
	- Thoracic deformity
Inflammatory	- Lymph nodes
	- Mediastinal abscess/cellulitis
Masses	- Hemangioma
	- Lymphoma
	- Germ cell tumor

Intrinsic

Wall abnormality:

Congenital	- Tracheobronchomalacia
	- Tracheal stenosis
	- Bronchopulmonary foregut malformations - Bronchial atresia, Tracheoesophaegeal fistula
	- Tracheobronchial branching anomalies
Inflammatory	- Exudative tracheitis, tuberculosis
	- Fibrotic stricture
Post-intubation stricture	
Intraluminal	- Foreign body
	- Masses: hemangioma, carcinoid

Peripheral airway abnormalities

Asthma

Bronchiectasis

Bronchiolitis/Small airway disease

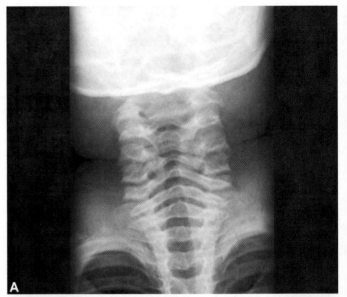

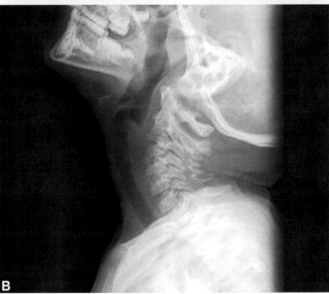

Figs 8.1A and B: Normal frontal (A) and lateral (B) radiographs neck of a 5-year-old child

UPPER AIRWAY OBSTRUCTION

Normal Anatomy (Plain Radiographs) (Figs 8.1A and B)

Epiglottis: The normal epiglottis has very thin borders. Epiglottis may appear artefactually thickened if imaged obliquely- this is due both the left and right sides being imaged next to each other. This is referred to as the "omega" appearance.[1,2]

Aryepiglottic folds: Aryepiglottic folds are mucosal folds which extend from the epiglottis superiorly to the arytenoids cartilages, posteroinferiorly. On a lateral radiograph, these appear thin and convex inferiorly.

Subglottic trachea: On frontal views subglottic trachea appears rounded with lateral convexities or "shoulders". On the lateral view it should not be narrower than the airway above or below it.

imaging) is performed. Axial MR Cine images are obtained craniocaudally at the level of mid-tongue in those with obstructive sleep apnea.[2] The use of cine MR imaging during coughing for evaluation of tracheal collapsibility in patients with suspected tracheomalacia has been described.[6]

Retropharyngeal soft tissues: Normally, the soft tissues between the posterior aspect of the aerated pharynx and anterior aspect of the vertebral column, should not be more than the anteroposterior diameter of the vertebral bodies. However, "pseudothickening" of the retropharyngeal soft tissues may be seen if the radiographs are obtained in a flexed position of the neck, especially in infants with short necks. The radiographs should hence be performed with adequate neck extension. The thickness of soft tissues is measured transversely somewhere between the level of adenoids superiorly to base of epiglottis inferiorly, below which these are normally thicker due to the presence of esophagus.

Tonsils/Adenoids: At less than 6 months of age, the adenoids are rarely visible on radiography. There is rapid proliferation during infancy with peak size reaching between 2-10 years. A size up to 12 mm is considered normal. Subsequently, during the second decade there is reduction in size.

ACUTE OBSTRUCTION

The commonest causes of acute upper airway obstruction are inflammatory, followed by foreign body. Ingestion of corrosive/caustic substances is another cause.[1, 2]

Croup (Acute Laryngotracheobronchitis)

Croup is a benign, self-limiting acute inflammatory condition of the upper airways. It results from viral infection, and is the commonest cause of upper airway obstruction in young children and infants.[1, 2] (6 months to 3 years of age). Affected children present with "croupy" (barky) cough and inspiratory stridor.

The purpose of obtaining radiographs in a suspected case of croup is to exclude secondary causes such as foreign body. It, however, has characteristic findings – on frontal radiographs there is loss of the normal shoulders (lateral convexities) of the subglottic trachea due to subglottic edema. The subglottic trachea becomes elongated, extending below the level of the pyriform sinuses. The appearance is referred to as a "church steeple" or "inverted V" appearance. Lateral radiographs may reveal similar narrowing of the subglottic trachea with loss of its wall definition.[1]

Epiglottitis

Unlike croup, epiglottitis is a life-threatening condition requiring emergency intubation. The most common organism responsible is *Haemophilus influenzae.* Affected children present with abrupt onset fever, dysphagia, stridor and worsening of respiratory distress in recumbent position. The 'classic' mean age of presentation is 3-5 years (older than croup). Now with availability of vaccination the incidence of this entity has significantly declined, and patients may present at a later age (13-14 years).[1,2]

Diagnosis is made on basis of presentation and physical examination. If not, a single lateral radiograph of neck may be obtained. This reveals markedly thickened epiglottis ("thumb" appearance). The pathological thickening of epiglottis can be differentiated from "omega" appearance, due to associated thickening of aryepiglottic folds in the former. The thickened aryepiglottic folds appear convex superiorly.

Retropharyngeal Cellulitis and Abscess

Retropharyrgeal space inflammation is usually of pyogenic origin, following upper respiratory tract infection. Patients present with fever, dysphagia, a stiff neck and occasional stridor. It is commonest between 6 to 12 months of age.

Lateral radiographs reveal thickening of the retropharyngeal soft tissues. On radiographs, the only conclusive finding differentiating cellulitis from abscess is the presence of gas within the latter. Contrast-enhanced CT scans can aid in the distinction of cellulitis from a drainable fluid collection. An abscess appears as a well-defined, low-attenuation area with an enhancing rim[1] (Figs 8.2A and B).

Exudative Tracheitis

Exudative tracheitis is also referred to as membranous laryngotracheobronchitis or membranous croup. It is a purulent infection of the trachea characterized by formation of exudative plaques along the tracheal walls. Patients are older than croup, typically 6-10 years of age, and are also more ill. The causative organism may be *Staphylococcus aureus*, or the infections may be multimicrobial.

The characteristic finding on radiographs is a linear soft tissue filling defect (membrane) seen within the airway. A plaque-like irregularity of the tracheal wall is also suggestive. Other findings include narrowing of subglottic trachea (symmetric or asymmetric) with loss of its wall definition. The older age of the patient (> 3 years) aid distinction from croup.

Foreign Body

Post aspiration most foreign bodies lodge in the lower airway. Foreign bodies in the larynx or trachea are much less common, and the patients present with sudden onset stridor and respiratory distress. Foreign bodies if lodged in the esophagus may also present with respiratory symptoms. Radiographs reveal either a radiopaque foreign body or soft tissue density within the airway or loss of definition of the airway wall[1] (Figs 8.3A to C).

CHRONIC OBSTRUCTION

Obstructive Sleep Apnea (OSA)

The clinical presentation in children with chronic upper airway obstruction differs from that of acute obstruction. While these children may present with stridor, symptoms of sleep apnea or snoring are more common.[1, 2] Sleep apnea may be seen in up to 3 percent of children.[3] The various causes include any space occupying lesion or fixed narrowing, which maybe congenital, inflammatory or neoplastic in etiology.

At various levels the causes are:
Nasal cavity/Nasopharynx: Adenoidal enlargement, choanal atresia, juvenile angiofibroma.
Oropharynx: Micrognathia with posterior displacement of tongue, macroglossia, glossoptosis.
Hypopharynx: Hypopharyngeal collapse.
Larynx: Laryngomalacia, congenital cysts.

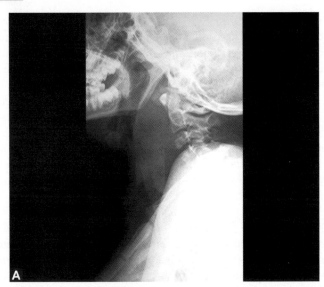

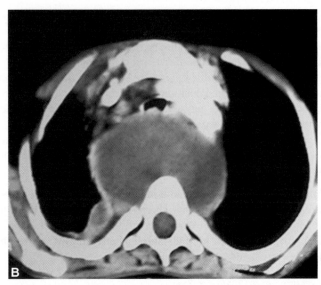

Figs 8.2A and B: Retropharyngeal and mediastinal abscess: (A) Lateral radiograph neck of an 8-year-old boy with low grade fever, respiratory distress and dysphagia reveals widening of the retropharyngeal soft tissues. (B) Contrast-enhanced CT scan at the level of the thoracic inlet shows a large prevertebral abscess compressing the trachea

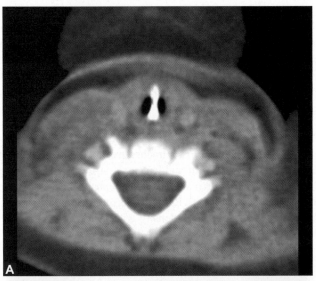

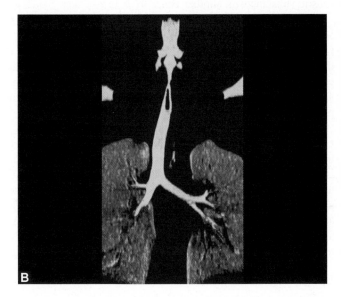

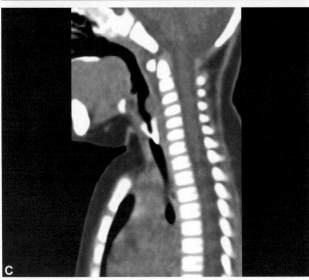

Figs 8.3A and C: Foreign body: Axial CT scan (A) of a 7-month-old infant with sudden onset stridor reveals a radiopaque foreign body lodged in the trachea. Coronal minIP (B) and sagittal MPR (C) demonstrate the object well.

Large hemangiomas/vascular malformations can cause airway obstruction at any level.

MRI is useful in evaluation of patients with OSA. Indications for dynamic MR sleep imaging include persistence of OSA despite tonsillectomy and adenoidectomy, OSA with predisposition to obstruction at multiple sites (craniofacial anomalies, Down syndrome), evaluation of OSA before any complex airway surgery and obesity.

Enlarged Tonsils/Adenoids

The commonest cause of chronic upper airway obstruction is enlargement of adenoids and palatine tonsils. Enlargement of lingual tonsils results in OSA only uncommonly. On a lateral radiograph, enlarged adenoids appear as convex soft tissue mass (>2 cm) in the posterior nasopharyx narrowing or obliterating the nasopharyngeal air lucency. CT also demonstrates tonsillar adenoidal enlargements well (Figs 8.4A to C). Enlarged palatine tonsils appear as soft tissue mass projecting on the posterior aspect of soft palate.[1] On T2W and STIR images adenoids and tonsils appear hyperintense.

Glossoptosis

Glossoptosis means abnormal posterior motion of the tongue during sleep and is associated with underlying hypotonia, macroglossia or micrognathia. Macroglossia and micrognathia may be diagnosed on lateral radiograph. However glossoptosis can be demonstrated on dynamic sleep fluoroscopy or cine MRI.

Hypopharyngeal Collapse

Hypopharyngeal collapse refers to cylindrical collapse of the hypopharynx; with its anterior, posterior and lateral walls all moving centrally. It is associated with disorders of decreased muscular tone. This can be diagnosed on cine fluoroscopy or MRI.

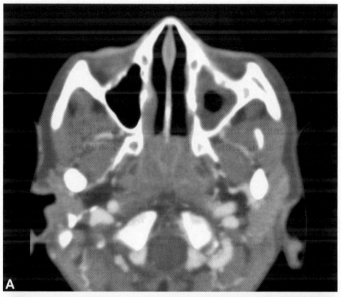

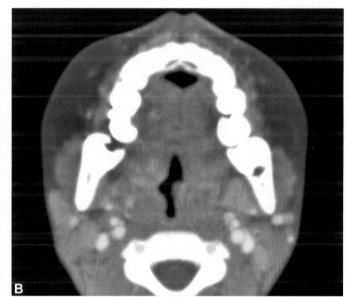

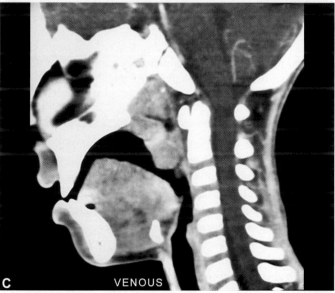

Figs 8.4A to C: Enlarged adenoids and tonsils: CECT of a 9-year-old boy with history of snoring reveals enlarged adenoids (A) and palatine tonsils (B). Sagittal MPR (C) shows narrowing of the nasopharyngeal airway

Subglottic Obstruction

Subglottic Stenosis

Short segment subglottic stenosis is often congenital in origin (Figs 8.5A and B).

Post-intubation Stenosis

Prolonged intubation can lead to either tracheomalacia or airway stenosis, particularly with oversized endotracheal tubes or balloon cuffs. Airway stenosis consequent to prolonged intubation usually occurs at the level of cricoid cartilage, which is the narrowest part of the upper airway[7] (Figs 8.6A to C).

Subglottic Hemangioma

Hemangiomas located in the soft tissues of the neck may extend into the subglottic airway. Large hemangiomas or vascular malformations can cause obstruction at any level (Figs 8.7 and 8.8). These present in infancy, often at less than 6 months of age; and may be associated with hemangiomas of the face or trunk.

Plain radiographs reveal asymmetric subglottic narrowing with associated soft tissue. On cross-sectional imaging, the lesions show intense contrast enhancement which may be nodular. These lesions are unilateral or bilateral, but often asymmetric and occasionally circumferential. On T2W images, as elsewhere hemangiomas appear hyperintense.[2] Although a benign lesion with a natural history of proliferation and involution, complications of bleeding and airway obstruction can be life threatening. Spontaneous regression is typical. Endoscopy confirms the diagnosis. When the presentation demands active management, as in patients with symptomatic airway compromise, treatment options include systemic or intralesional corticosteroids, laser ablation, interferon therapy or surgical excision.[4,8]

LOWER AIRWAY OBSTRUCTION

Central Airways

Small airway diseases such as asthma and bronchiolitis are more common than central causes of obstruction. The central causes may be extrinisic or intrinsic (involving either the wall or lumen).

Investigations include frontal and lateral radiographs of the airway and chest. The neck radiographs help to exclude upper airway obstruction. Chest radiographs should be evaluated for tracheal caliber, cardiac size, position of the aortic arch, mediastinal widening, asymmetric lung aeration, lung collapse or consolidation and radiopaque foreign body. The length of tracheal narrowing and involvement of anterior/posterior walls should be noted. If the radiographs are suggestive of an intrinsic cause of obstruction, then one can proceed with fiberoptic bronchoscopy. If the suspected cause is extrinsic then further cross-sectional imaging is indicated.

The choice between CT and MRI is not clearly defined. While MRI has the advantage of being radiation free and not dependent on intravenous contrast, its main drawback is the long scanning times. The need for sedation especially in a child with airway compromise often negates the advantages of MRI, making CT the

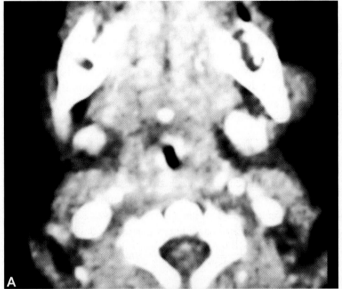

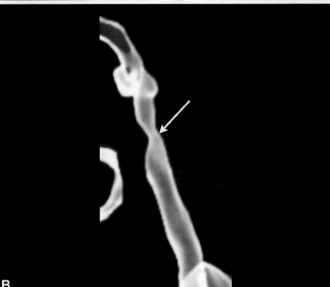

Figs 8.5A and B: Subglottic stenosis: CECT of a newborn with stridor. Axial (A), sagittal VRT (B) images show a short segment, smooth subglottic stenosis (arrow)

preferred modality. Both modalities offer good contrast between the central airway and surrounding structures, while the lungs are better visualized on CT.

Extrinsic Causes

Any mass lesion of the mediastinum such as nodes and cysts include the non-vascular causes of airway compression. Chest wall deformities may similarly result in airway compromise.

The classical vascular causes include double aortic arch, anomalous left pulmonary artery (pulmonary sling) and innominate artery compression syndrome. However, several other vascular causes such as dilatation of pulmonary artery (Figs 8.9A to C), enlargement of ascending aorta, midline descending aorta and right arch with aberrant left subclavian artery can also result in airway compression. A vascular ring encircling the airway occurs as a

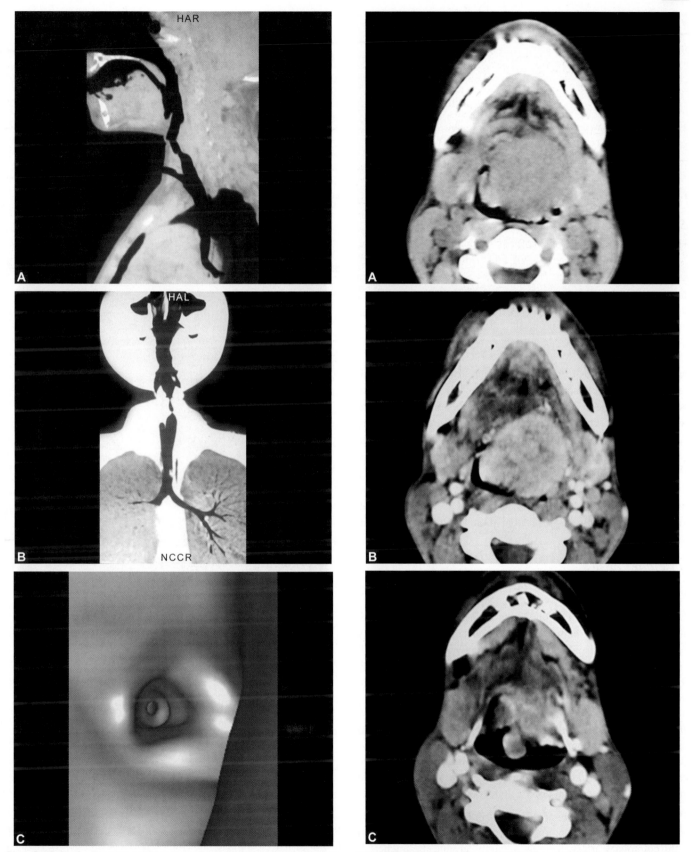

Figs 8.6A to C: Post-intubation stenosis: A short segment, smooth subglottic stenosis is seen on sagittal MPR (A), coronal minIP (B) and VB (C) CT images of a child with history of prolonged intubation *(For color version Fig. 8.6C see plate 1)*

Figs 8.7A to C: Hemangioma: NCCT (A) and CECT (B, C) image reveal an enhancing, well defined soft tissue mass significantly narrowing the oropharyngeal and subglottic airway

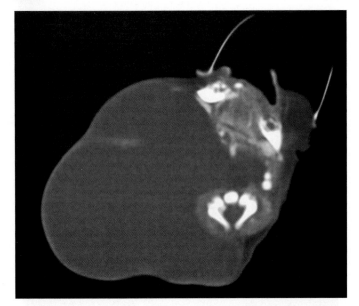

Fig. 8.8: Lymphangioma: CECT neck of a neonate showing a large multiseptated, multicompartmental cystic lesion obliterating the oropharyngeal airway

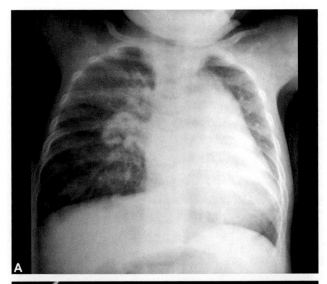

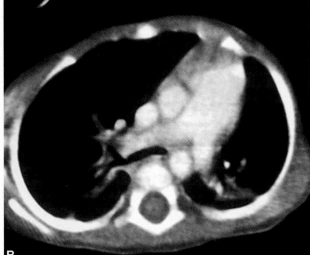

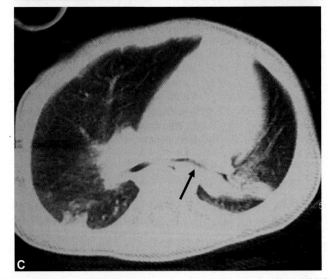

Figs 8.9A to C: Vascular compression : Chest radiograph (A) and CECT (B and C) of a 5-month-old infant with ventricular septal defect, showing enlarged central pulmonary arteries with volume loss of the left lung. There is compression of the bilateral main bronchi by the enlarged pulmonary arteries, especially the left main bronchus (arrow)

result of the failure of primitive vascular structures to fuse and regress normally during the development of the aortic arch, pulmonary arteries, and/or ductus arteriosus. Patients with vascular rings may have wheezing, stridor, feeding difficulties, choking episodes, or even aspiration pneumonia; depending on the degree of tracheal and esophageal narrowing.[4]

Plain radiographs and barium swallow cannot reliably distinguish among the types of vascular ring. Cross-sectional imaging, either with CT or MR, is helpful in delineating the anatomy and aiding in presurgical planning and postsurgical assessment.[4,9,10]

Vascular Causes

Vascular Rings

Double Aortic Arch: Double aortic arch is a congenital arch anomaly, and is the commonest vascular ring to cause airway compression. It is usually an isolated anomaly. Both right and left arches are seen to arise from the ascending aorta and join to form the descending aorta. Right arch is commonly larger and posterosuperior.[1,2]

The two arches surround and compress the trachea anteriorly, and esophagus posteriorly. The level of compression is mid to lower thirds of intrathoracic trachea.[1,2]

On radiography, lateral tracheal indentations are seen. On cross-sectional imaging, it is important to determine the dominant arch (side), as the surgical approach differs accordingly.

Pulmonary sling: Pulmonary sling refers to a pulmonary artery anomaly wherein the left pulmonary artery arises from the proximal right pulmonary artery, forming a "sling" around the trachea. It subsequently passes between the trachea and esophagus as it courses towards the left lung. It may be associated with congenital heart disease and complete tracheal rings, worsening the airway compromise.[1,2]

Frontal radiograph reveals asymmetric lung inflation. On lateral radiograph, there is posterior compression of the trachea with anterior esophageal impression. It is the only vascular ring to course between the trachea and esophagus, to be associated with asymmetric lung inflation and also the only one to cause anterior indentation on the esophagus.[1,2]

Innominate artery compression syndrome: Innominate artery (Brachiocephalic) crosses the trachea anteriorly, just below the thoracic inlet. In infants, it arises more to the left than adults. In addition the presence of a large thymus in the mediastinum and lack of rigidity of infantile trachea results in tracheal compression. The range of symptoms vary from none to stridor and dyspnea resulting from severe compression. Most children outgrow the disease and surgery is reserved only for those with severe compression.

Lateral radiographs reveal focal anterior indentation of the trachea. CT and MRI detail the severity of the compression and exclude other causes.[1, 2]

Right arch with aberrant left subclavian artery: This is an arch anomaly wherein the aortic arch is located to the right of trachea. The left subclavian artery (LSA) originates from the proximal descending aorta and courses to the left behind the esophagus. In 60 percent cases there is dilatation of origin of the LSA (aortic diverticulum of Kommerell). It is commonly an asymptomatic finding with only 5 percent patients having symptoms.[2] However, this anomaly may be associated with a constricting left ligamentum arteriosum, forming a vascular ring and causing airway compression. If the ligamentum arteriosum connects to LSA it forms a loose vascular ring, while if it extends to the aortic diverticulum of Kommerell, a tight ring is formed.

On frontal radiograph there is aortic arch indentation on the right wall of the trachea with tracheal deviation to the left (Figs 8.10A to C). Right sided descending aorta may also be seen. Lateral view reveals indentation on the posterior aspect of trachea. On barium swallow, frontal views show a filling defect coursing from right inferior to left superior. On lateral view, there is posterior esophageal indentation. Cross-sectional imaging is indicated when there is clinical or radiographic evidence of airway compression.

Midline descending aorta: In this anomaly the descending aorta is positioned immediately anterior to the vertebral body, instead of the normal left paravertebral location. It may be an isolated lesion or be associated with hypoplastic right lung and hence mediastinal shift; or aortic arch anomalies.

Malposition may result in airway compression due to crowding of structures. Radiographs are often normal, cross-sectional imaging reveals the diagnosis.

Vascular Malformations

Vascular malformations may be venous, lymphatic, or mixed venolymphatic. Although these lesions are usually soft and compressible, giant malformations of the neck and/or chest can compress airway.

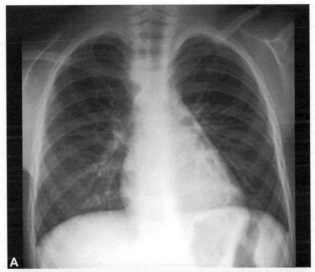

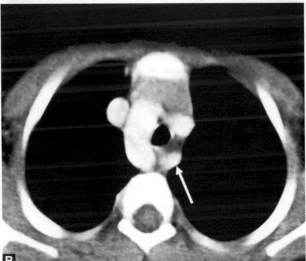

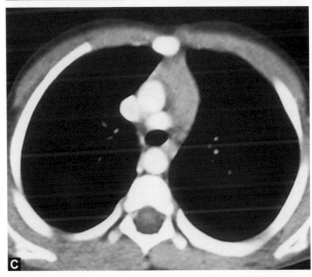

Figs 8.10A to C: Right sided aortic arch: Chest radiograph (A) of a 5-year-old boy reveals a right sided aortic arch with hyperlucent left lung. CECT chest (B) shows indentation on the right wall of the trachea by the arch with an aberrant left subclavian artery (arrow).The descending aorta is in midline (C)

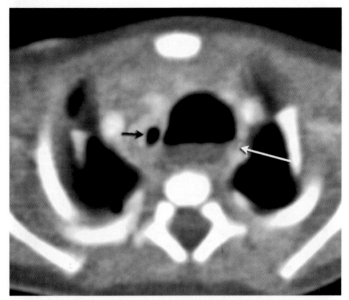

Fig. 8.11: Esophageal atresia: CECT of a neonate with esophageal atresia, performed to evaluate respiratory distress shows the dilated proximal esophageal pouch (white arrow) causing significant compression of the trachea (black arrow)

Bronchopulmonary foregut malformations: Bronchogenic cysts are among commonest cystic lesions in the pediatric chest. The commonest location is around the carina. Hence, when large, these result in compression of the proximal bronchi. They can occur anywhere along the respiratory tract.[4]

The dilated proximal esophageal pouch in patients of esophageal atresia can also exert a mass effect on the adjoining airway[4] (Fig. 8.11).

Inflammatory causes: Deep neck space infections,when they spread into the mediastinum, can compress the airway. Large paravertebral abscesses, even tubercular may result in significant airway compression (Fig. 8.2).

Mediastinal lymphadenopathy, tubercular or fungal infections can also narrow the airway by mass effect (Figs 8.12A to D).

Masses: Lymphoma is the commonest childhood neoplasm to cause symptomatic airway compromise in children.[11] Other neoplasms that tend to narrow the airway by extrinsic mass effect include infantile hemangiomas, germ cell tumors, rhabdomyosarcomas and neurogenic tumors (Figs 8.13A and B).

Intrinsic Causes

Intrinsic causes include those involving the wall which may be dynamic (tracheomalacia) or fixed (stenosis) and intraluminal lesions.

Wall Abnormalities

Tracheomalacia: Tracheomalacia refers to abnormal softening of the trachea due to abnormality of the cartilaginous rings. This results in intermittent (expiratory) collapse of the trachea. The narrowing of the tracheal lumen is most marked during forced expiration, coughing, or the Valsalva maneuver.[4] It may be primary

or secondary to compression by masses or vascular structures. Similar condition may involve the proximal bronchi. It may be congenital associated with syndromes such as cystic fibrosis, or even result from chronic inflammation, chronic extrinsic compression or prior intubation. The characteristic clinical presentation is of an expiratory wheeze.

The diagnosis cannot be made on the basis of a single radiograph. Fluoroscopy, and typically fibreoptic bronchoscopy can demonstrate the characteristic dynamic collapse of the trachea. Airway fluoroscopy done in a lateral projection is the traditional radiographic method of diagnosing tracheomalacia. However, bronchomalacia is difficult to diagnose on fluoroscopy, and controlled-ventilation CT, cine CT, or cine MR imaging are preferred methods for this entity.[4] On a single phase inspiratory CT the diagnosis is difficult, although the trachea may demonstrate an abnormal shape being flattened slightly posteriorly in the membranous part[1,2] (Figs 8.14A to C). Paired inspiratory-expiratory MDCT/cine MDCT is more sensitive to demonstrate the expiratory collapse, and require the measurement of the area of trachea in both the phases.[12]

Stenosis: Fixed trachea stenosis may be congenital or acquired. Congenital tracheal stenosis results from absence of the membranous portion of the trachea resulting in complete or near complete cartilaginous tracheal rings. The various patterns of tracheal stenosis include generalized stenosis, carrot- or funnel-shaped segmental stenosis, and focal stenosis. Focal stenosis usually involves the lower trachea. A tight focal stenosis causes more severe symptoms than a long, mild stenosis. It may be associated with congenital heart disease, pulmonary sling, TEF, or skeletal abnormalities.[2,4] On axial imaging, trachea appears as a round or complete circle (O-shaped). Other findings include: circumferential narrowing of the entire length of the trachea and fusion of the cartilaginous tracheal rings posteriorly.[4,13]

Congenital tracheal web is a rare entity. The web is usually not associated with deformity of the tracheal cartilage or the tracheal wall. CT reveals a weblike structure traversing and narrowing the tracheal lumen,[14] which is well demonstrated on coronal reformatted images and virtual bronchoscopy.[4]

Bronchopulmonary foregut malformations: Bronchopulmonary foregut malformations include a wide spectrum of disorders such as: tracheal agenesis, tracheal stenosis, tracheal fistula, branching anomalies, bronchial stenosis, or lung agenesis and hypoplasia; as well as bronchogenic cysts are also included in this group.[3] These anomalies may present with respiratory distress in the newborn, recurrent pulmonary infections or mass lesions later in life. This chapter deals with anomalies affecting the major bronchi.

Bronchial atresia and sequestration: Bronchial atresia most often involves the left upper lobe. On CT, a mucocele is identified as a hypo- or fluid-attenuating branching structure distal to the atretic bronchus near the hilum. The pulmonary parenchyma distal to the atretic segment is often lucent and demonstrates air trapping. The affected region may even be outlined by pseudofissures.[4]

Bronchial atresia may be isolated or associated with a retained systemic vascular connection, when it is referred to as intralobar

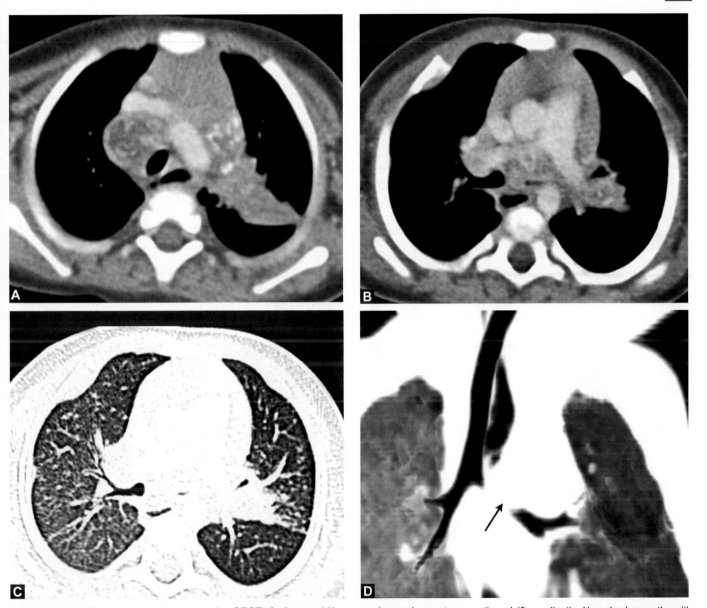

Figs 8.12A to D: Tubercular lymphadenopathy: CECT of a 6-year-old boy reveals conglomerate, necrotic, calcific mediastinal lymphadenopathy with left upper lobe consolidation (A). A more caudal section mediastinal window (B), and lung window (C) and minIP (D) show narrowing of the left main (arrow) and upper lobe bronchii.

sequestration. The imaging appearance is virtually identical to that of isolated bronchial atresia, except that the atretic bronchus is ectopically located at the margin of the lung. Rarely, such ectopic bronchi may not be atretic but have a connection with the gastrointestinal tract, usually the esophagus. Such cases are usually accompanied by bronchiectasis and accumulated secretions from impaired clearance of lung parenchyma. It is hence important to look for airway abnormalities, pulmonary parenchymal abnormalities, retained systemic vascular connections, anomalous pulmonary venous drainage, and airway communication with the gastrointestinal tract in patients with suspected bronchopulmonary foregut malformations.[4, 15,16]

Tracheo-esophageal fistula (TEF): Esophageal atresia with or without TEF is believed to result from a faulty separation of the embryonic trachea and esophageal remnants. The commonest type of these is proximal esophageal atresia with distal TEF (up to 80–90%). H-shaped TEFs with no atresia constitute up to 5–8 percent.[4] Typical clinical presentation includes failure to pass a feeding tube in a newborn with a history of polyhydramnios at prenatal US, excessive secretions from the mouth, and respiratory distress.[4] Chest radiograph demonstrates the feeding tube catheter ending/coiling in the proximal thoracic esophagus. The presence of air in the distal gastrointestinal tract confirms the presence of a distal TEF. In such patients, it is important to observe the airway as there is frequently associated tracheomalacia.[17] Also, a dilated proximal esophageal pouch can result in airway compression. Patients with H type fistula may present with recurrent aspiration or small airway disease. While contrast esophagogram is the

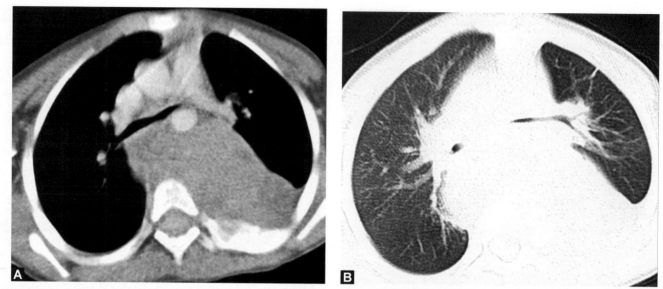

Figs 8.13A and B: Neuroblastoma: CECT (A) showing a large posterior mediastinal mass lesion causing displacement and compression of the major bronchi, especially the left main bronchus. Lung window (B) reveals a hyperlucent left lung

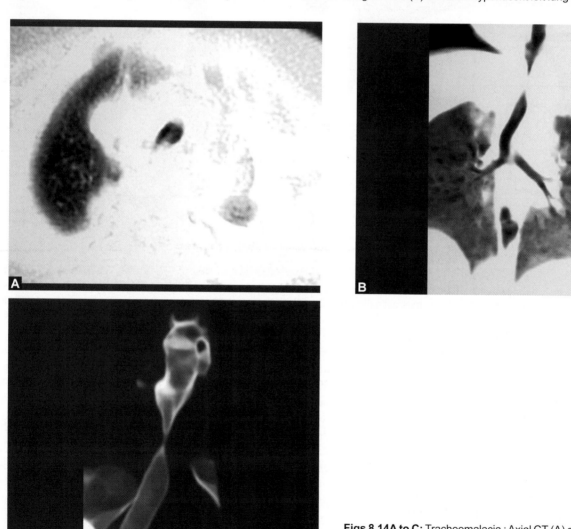

Figs 8.14A to C: Tracheomalacia : Axial CT (A) of a neonate with stridor showing slight posterior flattening of the trachea. min IP (B) and VRT images (C) show narrowing of subglottic trachea. On bronchoscopy, this narrowing was found to be dynamic

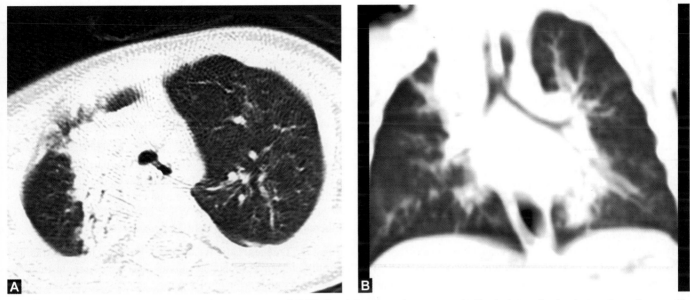

Figs 8.15A and B: Tracheoesophageal fistula (TEF): Axial CT (A) of an infant reveals a communication between the trachea and esophagus with right upper lobe consolidation. Coronal MPR (B) also demonstrates the fistula

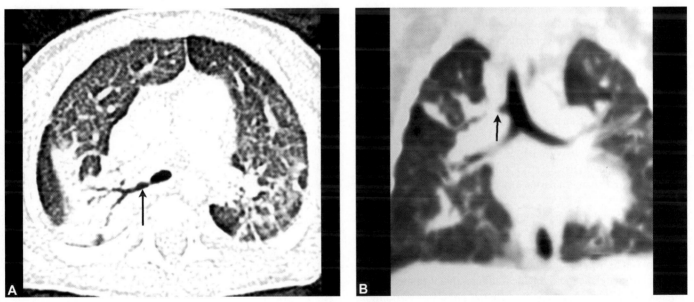

Figs 8.16A and B: Tracheal bronchus: Axial lung window (A), coronal MPR (B) reveal an accessory bronchus arising from the trachea and aerating the posterior segment of right upper lobe (arrows)

investigation of choice, CT scan may demonstrate the fistula (Figs 8.15A and B).

Tracheobronchial branching anomalies: Tracheobronchial branching anomalies may be seen as an isolated finding or accompanying heterotaxy syndromes, pulmonary sling, and conditions associated with pulmonary underdevelopment (agenesis, aplasia or hypoplasia). The commonest amongst these is the tracheal bronchus or "pig bronchus" (Figs 8.16A and B). A tracheal bronchus arises from the trachea or mainstem bronchus and aerates either the entire upper lobe or a segment.[4,18] An accessory cardiac bronchus or tracheal diverticulum are also

relatively common anomalies. An accessory cardiac bronchus arises from the medial wall of the right mainstem bronchus or bronchus intermedius, grows toward the pericardium terminating as a blind-ending stump or branching further.[19] Tracheal diverticula is seen arising with a narrow stalk from the right posterolateral wall of the trachea near the thoracic inlet.[4] Other abnormal branching patterns include tracheal trifurcation, bilateral right-sided isomerism or bilateral left-sided isomerism. A detailed classification of tracheo-bronchial branching anomalies has been given in "Imaging of the tracheobronchial tree" in AIIMS-MAMC-PGI Imaging Course Series, Diagnostic Radiology-Chest and Cardiovascular Imaging 3rd edition.[20]

Metabolic conditions: Hunter syndrome (a mucopolysaccharidosis) may cause the deposition of mucopolysaccharides in the walls of the major airways results in progressive airway narrowing due to wall thickening and anteroposterior collapse.[4, 21]

Acquired: Acquired tracheal or bronchial strictures usually result from *chronic inflammation*, often tubercular (Figs 8.17A to E). Another cause of acquired airway strictures is *posttraumatic* sequelae.

Intraluminal Causes

A foreign body (FB) is the most common cause of bronchial obstruction. Soft tissue masses of the trachea and bronchi are rare.

Foreign body: Foreign body aspiration is most often seen in infants and toddlers (8 months-3 years). The bronchi are the most common site of lodgement (76%), while laryngeal (6%) or tracheal (4%) lodgement is far less common. Right bronchus is more common (58%), than the left (42%).[2] The clinical presentation may be acute, while more often the symptoms remain indolent. The symptoms and signs can mimic asthma, upper respiratory infection, or pneumonia. The history of aspiration is often not elicited. Foreign body may lead to partial ("ball-valve" effect) or complete obstruction, resulting in hyperinflation or collapse respectively. Chest radiograph findings include asymmetric lung aeration, lung consolidation or atelectasis, and even pneumothorax or pneumomediastinum[1] (Figs 8.18 and 8.19). Metallic foreign bodies can be identified on plain radiographs (Fig. 8.18). However, commonly aspirated airway foreign bodies are food products, particularly nuts, and seeds, which are not radio-opaque enough to be identified at conventional radiography (Figs 8.20A to D). These organic materials can swell following absorption of water and then rapidly change a partial airway obstruction to a complete obstruction.[4]

Inspiratory radiographs alone may be normal in up to a third of patients (14-35%) with foreign bodies.[1,2] The lung volume of the affected lung/segment may be normal, increased or decreased.[1,2] Majority (up to 97%) of the foreign bodies are non-radiopaque.[1]

The characteristic radiographic finding is that the lung volume remains static with no change in different phases of respiration. This can be demonstrated by obtaining paired inspiratory - expiratory radiographs in cooperative children. In infants and uncooperative children bilateral decubitus radiographs of the chest or fluoroscopy can demonstrate the same finding.[1,2] The differential diagnosis of an asymmetric, lucent lung include Swyer-James syndrome and pulmonary hypoplasia.[1,2] However, air trapping may be seen in partial obstruction.

CT is not routinely advocated in evaluation of a bronchial foreign body. It may, however, be performed as work-up for non-resolving pneumonia or collapse, or even stridor (Fig. 8.20). CT is also a good option when the clinical setting does not strongly warrant bronchoscopy or if bronchoscopy is not readily available.[4] On CT, foreign bodies are well demonstrated as filling defects in the bronchus, besides detailing the changes in the distal lung. It can identify both opaque and non-opaque foreign bodies. Kosucu

et al reported a 100 percent sensitivity and specificity of CT in the evaluation of endobronchial foreign bodies.[22] Applegate et al while evaluating low-dose helical CT found a sensitivity of 83 percent and specificity of 89 percent for visualizing plastic pieces in the airway. Peanuts however were not well visualized in the same study.[23]

Even esophageal foreign bodies can present acutely with symptoms related to airway compression or with complications consequent to perforation and neck and/or mediastinal infection.[4]

Inflammatory: Tuberculosis- Occasionally, enlarged lymph nodes erode into the bronchus and result in endobronchial fibrosis or luminal occlusion. Intraluminal granulomas may occur in the trachea or bronchi.[4,24] In a series by Weber et al, airway involvement in tuberculosis was seen in upto 30 percent cases.[25]

Tumors: Tracheal soft tissue tissue masses include tracheal papilloma; while bronchial masses may be carcinoid tumors.[1] Carcinoid tumor is the most common amongst these. Rare lesions include adenoid cystic carcinoma, mucoepidermoid carcinoma, inflammatory myofibroblastic tumor, juvenile xanthogranuloma, and metastasis.[4]

Carcinoid tumors comprise about 80 percent of endobronchial neoplasms in children and adolescents. These present in children or young adults and may be associated with neuroendocrine secretion.[3, 26] Most carcinoid tumors occur in the mainstem or lobar bronchi, and patients present with dyspnea, wheezing, cough or hemoptysis. CT reveals typically intensely enhancing, ovoid lesions with a long axis parallel to the bronchovascular bundle.[4] These lesions may have intraluminal, mural, and extrabronchial components. Associated collapse, consolidation, or air trapping is often seen (Figs 8.21A to C). They are relatively slow growing masses, and complete surgical resection offers the best chance of cure.[27,28]

Peripheral Airways

Bronchiolitis/Small Airway Disease

Acute: Acute inflammation of the bronchi and bronchioles is common in children, and is most often infective in etiology. Plain radiographs reveal hyperinflation with increased perihilar markings. This entity is covered in detail in the chapter on Pulmonary Infections.

Chronic: The causes of chronic, small airway disease in children include: constrictive bronchiolitis, extrinsic allergic bronchiolitis, diffuse panbronchiolitis, follicular bronchiolitis and lung disease of prematurity.[3]

The chest radiograph and even CT findings are often non-specific though the underlying etiologies may be quite variable. CT scan reveals ground glass opacities with mosaic attenuation and air trapping. Mild bronchiectasis with bronchial wall thickening may be seen (Figs 8.22 and 8.23).

Constrictive bronchiolitis or bronchiolitis obliterans: Although constrictive bronchiolitis may present as a unilateral hyperlucent lung (Swyer James Syndrome), it is more often bilateral. There are

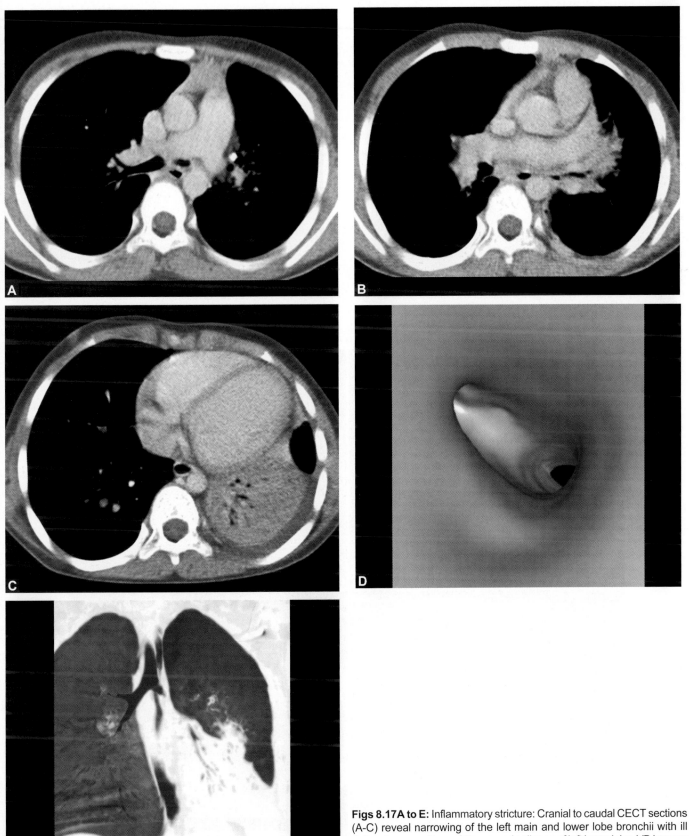

Figs 8.17A to E: Inflammatory stricture: Cranial to caudal CECT sections (A-C) reveal narrowing of the left main and lower lobe bronchii with ill defined surrounding soft tissue and collapse of left lower lobe. VB images (D) also confirm the main bronchus stricture with non-visualization of the distal airway. Coronal min-IP (E) shows a long segment involvement *(For color version Fig. 8.17D see plate 1)*

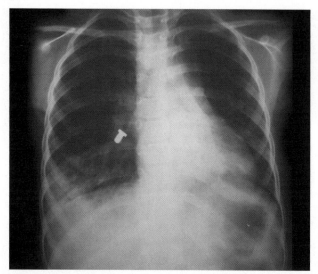

Fig. 8.18: Foreign body: Chest radiograph demonstrates a radiopaque foreign body in the right lower lobe bronchus with consolidation in the distal lung

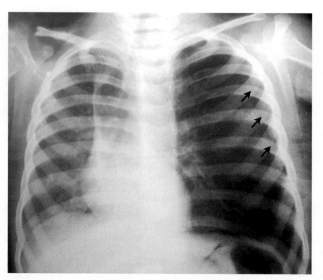

Fig. 8.19: Foreign body: Chest radiograph of a 2-year-old boy with history of foreign body aspiration and sudden onset respiratory distress reveals a hyperinflated left lung with spontaneous pneumothorax (arrows) and extensive subcutaneous emphysema

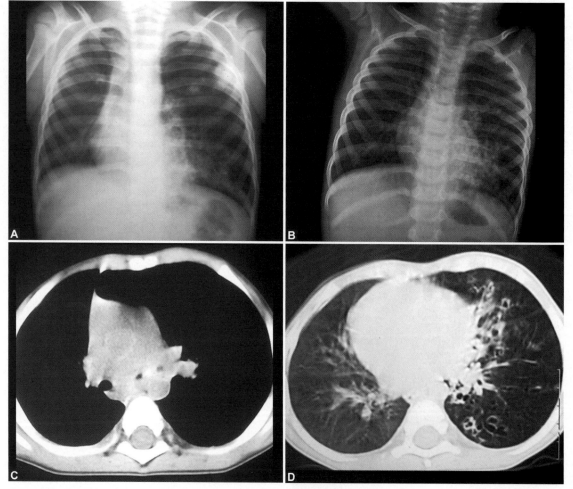

Figs 8.20A to D: Foreign body: Chest radiograph (A) of a toddler with history of recurrent high grade fever reveals a hyperinflated left lung with tram-track lesions in the left lower zone. A subsequent chest radiograph (B) shows progression in the lung parenchymal lesions with decrease in the hyperinflation. CT scan (C,D) reveals abrupt cut-off of the left main bronchus with intraluminal contents, and distal bronchiectasis. A "neem fruit ball" was removed from the left main bronchus on bronchoscopy

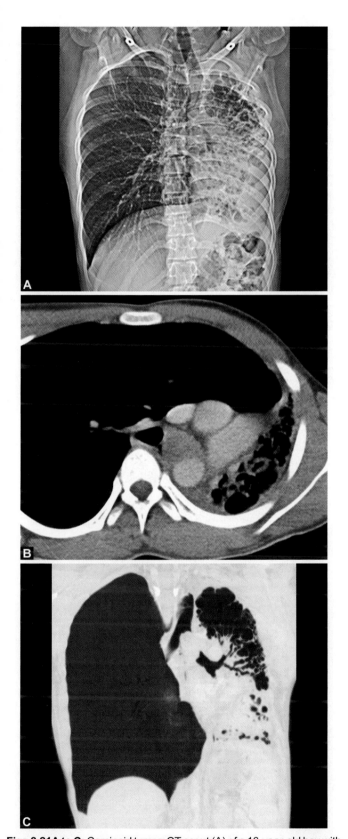

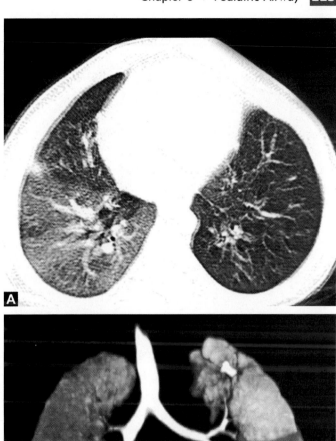

Figs 8.22A and B: Chronic bronchiolitis : Axial CT lung window (A) and minIP (B) of a 3-year-old girl with history of dyspnea reveals prominent mosaic attenuation with air-trapping and mild bronchiectasis

Figs 8.21A to C: Carcinoid tumor: CT scout (A) of a 16-year-old boy with history of recurrent pulmonary infections reveals volume loss of left lung with extensive consolidation and bronchiectasis. Axial CECT (B) shows a homogeneous mass in the left main bronchus with mediastinal shift to left. minIP (C) demonstrates the entire extent of the mass with distal lung changes. Histopathology revealed a carcinoid tumor

several causes of this entity including infection (viral or mycoplasma), toxic and fume exposure, collagen vascular diseases such as Rheumatoid arthritis; and complication of bone-marrow or heart-lung transplant.[3,29]

HRCT reveals a prominent mosaic attenuation with bronchial abnormalities including bronchiectasis; and air-trapping[3, 30] (Figs 8.22A and B). The pattern is similar to severe asthma or cystic fibrosis.

Extrinsic allergic alveolitis: Extrinsic allergic alveolitis or hypersensitivity pneumonitis is a form of cellular bronchilitis. In the acute stage CT reveals multiple, ill-defined centriliobular nodules; while in the subacute or chronic stage mosaic alternation with expiratory air trapping are seen[3, 29] (Figs 8.23A and B). Areas of fibrosis may also be present.

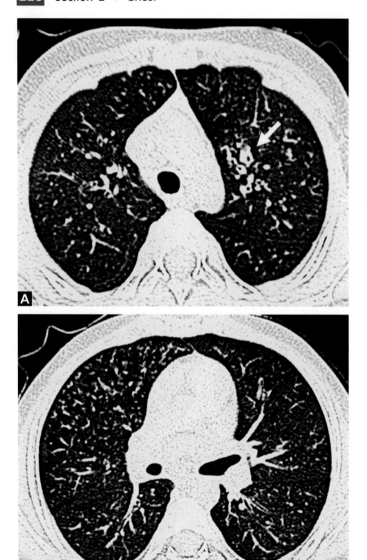

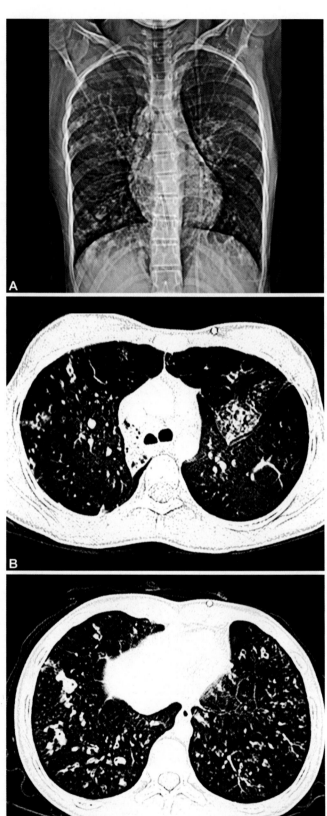

Figs 8.23A and B: Chronic bronchiolitis : HRCT (A and B) of 8-year-old child reveals multiple, ill-defined centriliobular nodules and bronchial wall thickening (arrow)

Diffuse pan-bronchiolitis: Diffuse pan-bronchiolitis is an exudative form of bronchiolitis seen in Eastern and South-Eastern Asia. CT reveals multiple small centrilobular nodules and linear opacities diffusely distributed in both the lungs.[3]

Follicular bronchiolitis: Follicular bronchiolitis or lung hyperplasia of the bronchus associated lymphoid tissue is also a cause chronic obstructive diffuse lung disease. In addition to expiratory air trapping, CT reveals areas of ground glass opacity.[3, 31]

Lung Disease of Prematurity

This is a unique form of airway disease seen in premature infants with bronchopulmonary dysplasia. It is a destructive diffuse lung disease occurring in a background of rapid alveolar growth. CT helps in excluding other causes of chronic respiratory distress such as central airway lesions.[3]

Figs 8.24A to C: Cystic fibrosis: CT scout (A) of a 16-year-old girl showing tubular, branching opacities in the right lung with paratracheal adenopathy. CT scan (B and C) reveals areas of fibrosis, bronchiectasis, bronchial wall thickening, air trapping and mucus plugging

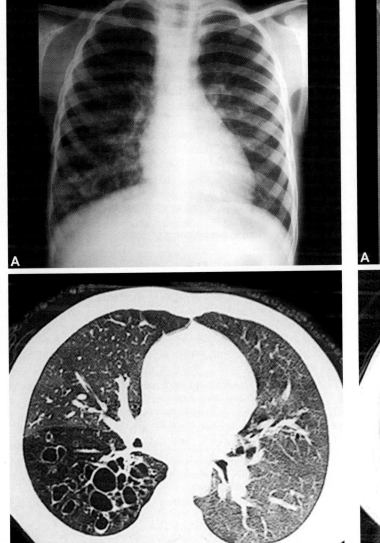

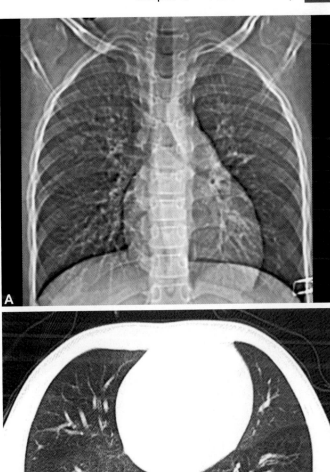

Figs 8.25A and B: Bronchiectasis: Chest radiograph (A) showing cystic lucencies with air-space nodules in the right lower zone suggesting secondary infection. CT scan (B) at a different date shows tubular and cystic bronchiectasis in right lower lobe with air trapping

Figs 8.26A and B: Asthma: CT scout (A) showing relative hyperlucency of left lower zone. CT scan (B) shows multiple areas of air trapping

Bronchiectasis

Bronchiectasis is a common cause of respiratory symptoms in children.[28] It is often the result of chronic inflammation causing damage to the supporting structure of the airways. Also, chronic or recurrent inflammation due to immunodeficiency states may cause bronchiectasis. Other etiologies include, abnormal mucus as in cystic fibrosis and abnormal mucociliary clearance in children with ciliary dyskinesias (Figs 8.24A to C). Proximal bronchial obstruction due to an intrinsic or extrinsic cause may also lead to bronchiectasis in the distal lung. Aspiration secondary to gastroesophageal reflux due to its chronic, recurrent nature has also been postulated as a cause of bronchiectasis.[3,32]

Patients typically present with recurrent infections. Chest radiographs are relatively insensitive in detecting early changes,

with HRCT being the imaging modality of choice.[3] Chest radiographs reveal multiple cystic, ring or tram-track lucencies with bronchial wall thickening. In case of secondary infection mucous plugging, air-fluid levels, bronchial wall thickening and even enlarged draining nodes may be seen (Figs 8.24 and 8.25).

Asthma

The peak age of prevalence of asthma in children is 6 to 11 years, with a male predominance. Thirty percent of these persist into adulthood.[2] Chest radiographs are usually normal and are indicated in case of poor response to therapy, suspected complications or suspicion of an alternate diagnosis.[2]

Radiographs reveal hyperlucency of lungs or foci of atelectasis. The differential diagnosis includes viral bronchiolitis. CT is seldom indicated in asthma and reveals non-specific findings of small airway disease (Figs 8.26A and B). Findings of secondary allergic

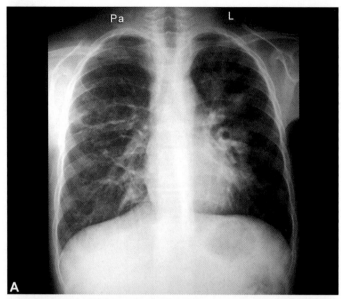

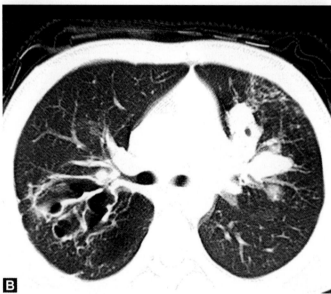

Figs 8.27A and B: ABPA: Chest radiograph (A) of a 16-year-old asthmatic boy showing multiple tubular, branching opacities in bilateral lung fields giving a "finger-in-glove" appearance. CT scan (B) confirms the presence of bilateral tubular bronchiectasis with bronchoceles

bronchopulmonary aspergillosis (ABPA) may be seen (Figs 8.27A and B).

Complications are more frequent in younger children as their bronchi are smaller and more easily occluded in an exacerbation. Complications include: lobar collapse, segmental or subsegmental atelectasis, pneumonia, air leaks (pneumomediastinum, subcutaneous emphysema and rarely pneumothorax or pulmonary interstitial emphysema (PIE).

In conclusion, it is critical to evaluate the airway in all children presenting with acute, chronic or recurrent respiratory symptoms. Multiphasic imaging is essential. Plain radiographs and fluoroscopy form the initial methods of evaluation, with CT being required often for a complete diagnosis.

REFERENCES

1. 'Airway' in Fundamentals of Paediatric Radiology LF Donnelly 2001 Saunders, Philadelphia, USA.
2. 'Airway' in Diagnostic imaging Paediatrics. LF Donnelly (Ed). Amirsys, Utah, USA, 2005.
3. Long FR. Paediatric airway disorders : Imaging evaluation. Radiol Cl N Am RCNA 2005; 43:371-89.
4. Yedururi S, Guillerman R P, Chung T, et al. Multimodality Imaging of Tracheobronchial Disorders in Children Radiographics 2008; 28(3):e29.
5. Dinesh Kumar, S, Ashu Seith, Raju Sharma, et al. Unpublished data AIIMS, Postgraduate Thesis - Evaluation of tracheobronchial lesions by multi-detector row CT" 2003-06.
6. Suto Y, Tanable Y. Evaluation of tracheal collapsibility in patients with tracheomalacia using dynamic MR imaging during coughing. Am J Roentgenol (AJR) 1998; 171:393-4.
7. John SD, Swischuk LE. Stridor and upper airway obstruction in infants and children. Radiographics 1992; 12:625-43.
8. Bitar MA, Moukarbel RV, Zalzal GH. Management of congenital subglottic hemangioma: trends and success over the past 17 years. Otolaryngol Head Neck Surg 2005; 132:226-31.
9. Choo KS, Lee HD, Ban JE, et al. Evaluation of obstructive airway lesions in complex congenital heart disease using composite volume-rendered images from multislice CT. Pediatr Radiol 2006; 36:219-23.
10. Swischuk LE. Cardiovascular system: imaging of the newborn, infant and child. 5th ed. Philadelphia, Pa: Lippincott Williams & Wilkins, 2003; 303-17.
11. Glick RD, La Quaglia MP. Lymphomas of the anterior mediastinum. Semin Pediatr Surg 1999; 8:69-77.
12. Lee EY, Litmanovich D, Boiselle PM. Multidetector CT evaluation of tracheobronchomalacia Radiol Clin N Am 2009; 47(2):261-69.
13. Berrocal T, Madrid C, Novo S, Gutierrez J, Arjonilla A, Gomez-Leon N. Congenital anomalies of the tracheobronchial tree, lung, and mediastinum: embryology, radiology, and pathology. Radiographics 2004; 24:e17.
14. Legasto AC, Haller JO, Giusti RJ. Tracheal web. Pediatr Radiol 2004; 34:256-8.
15. Langston C. New concepts in the pathology of congenital lung malformations. Semin Pediatr Surg 2003; 12:17-37.
16. Newman B. Congenital bronchopulmonary foregut malformations: concepts and controversies. Pediatr Radiol 2006; 36:773-91.
17. Swischuk LE. Alimentary tract, imaging of the newborn, infant and child. 5th ed. Philadelphia, Pa: Lippincott Williams & Wilkins, 2003; 350-6.
18. Ghaye B, Szapiro D, Fanchamps JM, Dondelinger RF. Congenital bronchial abnormalities revisited. Radiographics 2001; 21:105-119.
19. McGuinness G, Naidich DP, Garay SM, Davis AL, Boyd AD, Mizrachi HH. Accessory cardiac bronchus: CT features and clinical significance. Radiology 1993; 189:562-6.
20. Ashu Seith Bhalla, Raju Sharma. Imaging of the tracheobronchial tree in AIIMS-MAMC-PGI Imaging Course Series, Diagnostic Radiology-Chest and Cardiovascular Imaging, 3rd edn, Jaypee Publishers, New Delhi 2009; 90-116.
21. Davitt SM, Hatrick A, Sabharwal T, Pearce A, Gleeson M, Adam A. Tracheobronchial stent insertions in the management of major airway obstruction in a patient with Hunter's syndrome (type-II mucopolysaccharidosis). Eur Radiol 2002; 12:458-62.
22. Kosucu P, Ahmetoglu A, Koramaz I, et al. Low-dose MDCT and virtual bronchoscopy in pediatric patients with foreign body aspiration. Am J Roentgenol AJR 2004; 183:1771-7.

23. Applegate KE, Dardinger JT, Lieber ML, et al. Spiral CT scanning technique in the detection of aspiration of LEGO foreign bodies. Pediatr Radiol 2001; 31:836–40.

24. Sima Mukhopadhyay, AK Gupta, Ashu Seith. Imaging of tuberculosis in children in essentials of tuberculosis in children 3rd edn, Vimlesh Seth, SK Kabra (Eds) Jaypee Brothers, New Delhi 2006; 375-404.

25. Weber AL, Bird KT, Janower ML. Primary tuberculosis of childhood with particular emphasis on changes affecting the tracheobronchial tree. Am J Roentgenol AJR 1968; 103:123-32.

26. Ferretti GR, Thony F, Bosson JL, et al. Benign abnormalities and carcinoid tumors of the central airways:diagnostic impact of CT bronchography. Am J Roentgenol AJR 2000; 174:1307-13.

27. Curtis JM, Lacey D, Smyth R, Carty H. Endobronchial tumours in childhood. Eur J Radiol 1998; 29:11-20.

28. Kothari NA, Kramer SS. Bronchial diseases and lung aeration in children. J Thorac Imaging 2001; 16:207-23.

29. Hansell DM. Small airways disease: detection and insights with computed tomography. Eur Respir J 2001; 17:1294-1313.

30. Lau DM, Siegel MJ, Hildebolt CF, et al. Bronchiolitis obliterans syndrome: thin section CT diagnosis of obstructive changes in infants and young children after lung transplantation. Radiology 1998; 208:783-8.

31. Kinane BT, Mansell AL, Zwerdling RG, et al. Follicular bronchitis in the paediatric population. Chest 1993; 104:1183-6.

32. Patterson PE, Harding SM. Gastroesophageal reflux disorders and asthma. Curr Opin Pulm Med 1999; 5:63-67.

CHAPTER **9**

Developmental Anomalies of Gastrointestinal Tract

Alpana Manchanda, Sumedha Pawa

Derangement of embryological development can lead to malformations at any point along the gastrointestinal tract (GIT) from the oropharynx to the anorectum. Most of these abnormalities manifest clinically with GIT obstruction and present with vomiting and abdominal distention. Bile-stained vomiting occurs when the obstruction is below the ampulla of Vater, whereas vomiting of clear gastric contents indicates obstruction above the second part of the duodenum. Abdominal distention indicates a low level of obstruction. However, one must remember that both vomiting and abdominal distention may occur in conditions like sepsis, increased intracranial pressure, etc. in the absence of anatomic abnormality of the GI tract.[1] Infants who have undergone resuscitative efforts, or infants on continuous positive airway pressure, may swallow an excessive amount of air, leading to clinically significant abdominal distention. Since the distention is by air only, the walls of the distended loops on the abdominal radiograph are razor-sharp. Pathological conditions, involving the gut, such as ileus and obstruction, are characterized by dilatation with both air and fluid.[2] Developmental lesions of the neonatal gastrointestinal tract can be grouped as follows:[1]

Anatomical

Attributed to embryological maldevelopment
- Esophageal atresia with or without fistula
- Antropyloric atresia
- Antral diaphragm
- Duodenal atresia
- Duodenal stenosis
  - Intrinsic: Windsock duodenum
  - Extrinsic: Annular pancreas
  - Midgut malrotation with peritoneal bands
- Anorectal atresia.

Attributed to *in utero* catastrophic (ischemic) complication
- Jejunoileal atresia
- Colonic atresia or stenosis
- Complicated meconium ileus.

Functional

- Meconium plug syndrome and its variants
- Megacystis-microcolon-intestinal hypoperistalsis.

Combined Anatomical-Functional
- Hypertrophic pyloric stenosis
- Midgut volvulus (complicating midgut malrotation)
- Uncomplicated meconium ileus
- Colonic aganglionosis (Hirschsprung's disease).

IMAGING MODALITIES

The imaging methods available to investigate the gastrointestinal tract in the neonate include, plain film radiography, ultrasonography and contrast studies of the GI tract. Nuclear scintigraphy, computed tomography and magnetic resonance imaging are uncommonly required in infants.[1]

Plain Film Radiography

It is the simplest, usually the first and sometimes the only examination performed. An anteroposterior supine radiograph may be sufficient only if the purpose is to evaluate a palpable mass or the presence of calcification. If obstruction is suspected, additional films are required. A cross-table lateral projection with the infant in supine position is best in terms of leaving the patient virtually undisturbed. However, a left-lateral decubitus view with a horizontal beam has the advantage of better identification of free gas over the liver and better anatomical definition of bowel loops in a frontal projection. If only one film is desired, a prone radiograph will give the most information regarding free gas as well as defining the level of obstruction. Occasionally, a prone lateral film is valuable for detection of gas in the rectum.[1]

Within seconds after birth, air enters the gastrointestinal tract and it can be seen radiographically in the stomach. Air is seen in the small bowel within the first hour, it reaches the cecum within 3 to 4 hours, and appears in the sigmoid colon by 11 hours. Gas fluid levels are generally absent except in the stomach and occasionally in the right colon. The normal bowel gas pattern in neonates is quite different from that seen in older children and adults. It is characterized by gas throughout the small and large bowel and little fluid with respect to air, so that bowel-air interfaces are thin and sharp, with few if any loops identified; rather, the gas distribution is one of multiple, closely apposed, rounded or polyhedral structures. Small and large bowel cannot be distinguished.[2]

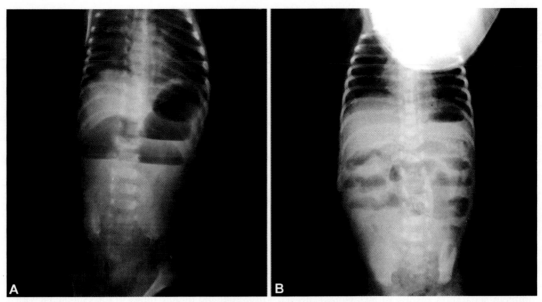

Figs 9.1A and B: Plain X-ray abdomen erect view reveals (A) few (three) air-fluid levels in proximal small bowel with absence of distal air diagnostic of a high small bowel (jejunal) obstruction in a newborn presenting with bilious vomiting. (B) In contrast, multiple air-fluid levels seen in another neonate with abdominal distention, is indicative of a low small bowel (ileal) obstruction

A gasless abdomen after the first few hours of life is occasionally seen in normal infants as well as in those with uncontrollable vomiting, continuous gastric aspiration, severe dehydration, esophageal atresia without a fistula and deficient air swallowing, secondary to CNS depression. Obstruction is manifested by distention of portion of the GI tract proximal to the obstruction, with little or no gas below. By observing the number and distribution of distended bowel loops and air fluid levels, one can estimate the approximate level of obstruction (Figs 9.1A and B).

Contrast Studies

Air is the cheapest, easiest and most commonly available contrast medium. The presence of gas within the bowel can be very useful in delineating abnormalities, particularly a proximal high atresia. Occasionally, one may require to inject air to delineate the bowel better and it can be instilled by nasogastric tube or per rectum.[3]

Barium is not used in the following circumstances: (i) suspected perforation, where preferably a non-ionic contrast medium should be used; (ii) instances of lower small-bowel obstruction when retained fluid proximally is likely to cause oral barium suspension to precipitate and degrade the images; (iii) when a cleansing effect is also desired, as in attempted reduction of meconium ileus or meconium plug.

Ionic water-soluble contrast media are ideal for stimulating evacuation of retained thick tenacious intestinal contents by virtue of their high osmolarity, which increases the intraluminal fluid and bulk. This, however, may cause water and electrolyte imbalance and appropriate patient hydration and electrolyte homeostasis should be carefully maintained. Ionic contrast media are contraindicated when investigating esophageal problems because aspiration may cause pulmonary edema. Non-ionic contrast media

are ideal for most of the circumstances. In suspected Hirschsprung's disease, in which the rate of evacuation has some potential diagnostic value, barium should be preferred. The radiologist should modify the routine use of contrast as needed in a particular case.

Ultrasonography (US)

Ultrasonography has been found to be highly accurate in the diagnosis of hypertrophic pyloric stenosis. It is useful in the diagnosis of gastric and duodenal duplications and in the detection of duodenal dilatation accompanying intrinsic or extrinsic duodenal obstruction, such as duodenal atresia and stenosis. Although duodenal dilatation is non-specific and additional contrast studies may be required to identify the specific cause, US is an excellent screening technique for localization of the site of obstruction. Ultrasound is valuable in the investigation of abdominal distention or palpable mass lesions because of easy and accurate detection of ascites as well as meconium peritonitis and intraperitoneal cystic lesions such as intestinal duplications and mesenteric or omental cysts.[1]

ESOPHAGUS

Esophageal Atresia and Tracheoesophageal Fistula (TEF)

Esophageal atresia with or without tracheoesophageal fistula is the most common congenital abnormality of the esophagus, manifesting itself during the neonatal period, occurring in about 1 in 2500 to 4000 live births.[4] It is usually sporadic and its etiology is uncertain.[3] No definite familial tendency has been documented in esophageal artesia, but more than one case in the same family has been noted.

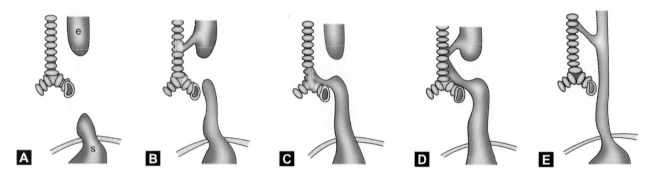

Fig. 9.2: Types of esophageal atresia/tracheoesophageal fistula. The plain radiographs
for types A and B are similar as in case for types C and D

Embryology

The trachea and esophagus develop from the common foregut during the early first trimester. During the fifth and sixth weeks of gestation, the common foregut divides into trachea and esophagus. Incomplete separation results in esophageal atresia with or without associated tracheoesophageal fistula. Because separation of the trachea and esophagus occurs cranial to tracheal branching of the carina, T-E fistulas generally present above the carina.[5]

Clinical Features

The presentation is usually in the first few hours of life, with the newborn having excessive oral secretions, choking and sometimes even cyanosis. Typically, symptoms become more pronounced during the first feed. The abdomen may be distended due to air passing through the distal fistula into the stomach or may be scaphoid or gasless in patients who have atresia without a fistula or atresia with a proximal fistula. Patients with an H-fistula usually present later with history of choking while feeding, cough, cyanosis, recurrent or chronic pneumonias and a distended abdomen from tracheal gas passing through the fistula into the esophagus and stomach.[5]

Esophageal atresia may be diagnosed by antenatal ultrasound. It is suspected on the basis of maternal polyhydroamnios with an absent fluid filled stomach, the proximal esophageal pouch seen as a central anechoic area in the fetal neck or upper chest. The presence and size of the tracheoesophageal fistula determines the amount of fluid in the stomach and gastrointestinal tract. Associated anomalies in the other systems may be identified. The atresias may be multiple and involve the esophagus, duodenum and anus.

Classification

Esophageal atresia and tracheoesophageal fistula have been classified based on their anatomical and radiographic appearance, i.e. on the basis of presence (and location) or absence of a tracheoesophageal fistula (Fig. 9.2). They have been variously designated as types A to E (or 1 to 5) as follows[3]

Type A—Esophageal atresia without fistula (7.8%)
Type B—Esophageal atresia with proximal fistula (0.8%)
Type C—Esophageal atresia with distal fistula (85.8%)

Type D—Esophageal atresia with fistula in both the pouches (1.4%)
Type E—H-type fistula without atresia (4.2%)

In the majority of patients, the atresia occurs between the proximal and middle thirds of the esophagus with a gap of varying length between the atretic pouches.[3]

Most commonly, there is a proximal esophageal atresia with a distal tracheoesophageal fistula. This occurs in approximately 85.8 percent of cases. Next most common, occurring approximately in 7.8 percent cases, is isolated esophageal atresia. H-type fistula occurs in approximately 4.2 percent of cases. Esophageal atresia with proximal tracheoesophageal fistula or with both proximal and distal tracheoesophageal fistulas are quite rare.[6]

Approximately 50-70 percent of patients with esophageal atresia have additional anomalies. The VACTERL syndrome is seen in 15 to 30 percent of patients. "V" is for vertebral and vascular abnormalities. Of these, a right-sided aortic arch is seen in 5 percent cases. "A" is for anal and auricular malformations. "C" is for cardiac abnormalities like ventricular septal defects, patent ductus arteriosus and complex cyanotic heart disease. "TE" is for tracheoesophageal fistula and esophageal atresia. "R" represents renal abnormalities. "L" is for limb malformations.[7]

Imaging Features

Plain film of the chest taken soon after birth reveals proximal esophageal pouch distended with air, thereby indicating the diagnosis on plain radiographs. In unequivocal cases, a thin soft rubber nasogastric tube is passed into the proximal pouch and about 5 cc of air is injected. A frontal radiograph of the chest showing dilated proximal esophageal pouch with round distal margin and coiled nasogastric tube within is diagnostic. The distended air filled proximal esophageal pouch may make visualization of the lower cervical and upper dorsal spine more clear. A lateral radiograph though not routinely indicated, if obtained, shows considerable anterior bowing and narrowing of the trachea by the dilated blind esophageal pouch.[3] Plain radiograph of the chest should include the abdomen to evaluate the presence of air in the gastrointestinal tract. The presence of air in the stomach and the small bowel indicates esophageal atresia with a distal tracheoesophageal fistula. Absence of air in the stomach eliminates the possibility of a distal fistula. The

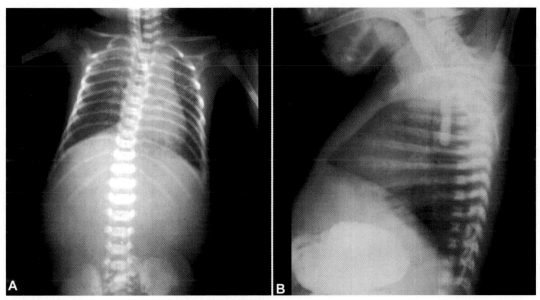

Figs 9.3A and B: Esophageal atresia: (A) Frontal radiograph of chest and abdomen showing a catheter in the proximal pouch. The abdomen is gasless. (B) Lateral film shows the tip of the nasogastric tube at the level of 4th dorsal vertebra

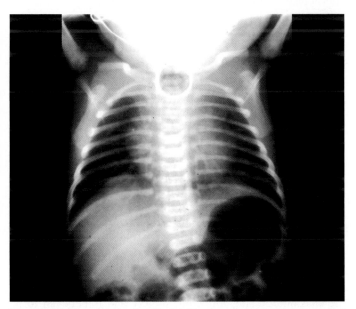

Fig. 9.4: Esophageal atresia with distal tracheesophageal fistula: Coiled nasogastric tube is seen in the proximal esophageal pouch. Air is seen in the stomach and bowel

possibility of proximal tracheoesophageal fistula, however, cannot be eliminated (Figs 9.3A, B and 9.4).

Air confined to the stomach raises the possibility of associated duodenal atresia and necessitates a follow-up plain film examination.

Routine contrast examinations are not required in the neonate with esophageal atresia and TEF.[3] Use of radiopaque contrast in the proximal pouch should be avoided, owing to the possibility of aspiration. Swallowed air or air through nasogastric tube is usually adequate for the diagnosis and to demonstrate the extent of the proximal pouch. If positive contrast examination is needed then isotonic nonionic contrast medium should be used in minimal

amount under fluoroscopic monitoring. Immediately after the study, contrast should be aspirated out.

Through H-type fistulas can be at any level, most are at the thoracic inlet, between C_7 and T_2 vertebral bodies. The connection is angulated superiorly from the esophagus to the trachea, thus accounting for the more precise but less popular appellation of the N-type fistula. (Fig. 9.5) The best way to demonstrate H-type tracheoesophageal fistula is with careful injection of contrast medium via a nasogastric tube, first placed at GE junction and then gradually withdrawing the nasogastric tube with simultaneous injection of contrast under fluoroscopic guidance at various levels of the esophagus. The main reason that the H-type TEF is inconstantaly patent is that the normal esophageal mucosa is quite redundant and usually occludes the esophageal side of the fistula. Normal active swallowing may not distend the esophagus sufficiently to allow passage of contrast into the fistula.[8] The patient should be viewed in the lateral or steep prone oblique projection with the right side down. Care should be taken to separate tracheal and esophageal lumens during the study so that fistula is readily identified between them. If the contrast appears in the trachea or lungs, it is very important to be certain if the contrast went through a fistula or was aspirated. If in doubt, then the investigation must be repeated once the trachea is cleared of the contrast.

The side of the aortic arch should be determined. This information is important to the surgeon because the surgical approach to the mediastinum for repair of esophageal atresia with a distal TEF is from the side opposite to the aortic arch. When plain radiograph fails to indicate the side of the arch, computed tomography or a cardiac ultrasound can localize the arch.

H-type fistulas are commonly demonstrated by contrast studies.[3] However, bronchoscopy and endoscopy are more sensitive methods and may be indicated to confirm the diagnosis, especially in a symptomatic older child where the contrast esophagogram is normal.

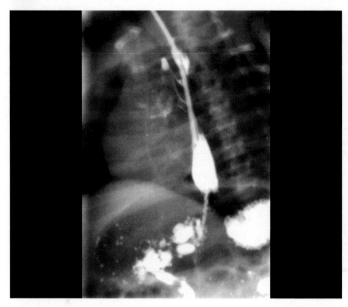

Fig. 9.5: Contrast esophagogram demonstrating an oblique tract of an H-type tracheoesophageal fistula arising from the anterior wall of the esophagus and passing cephalad to the posterior tracheal wall, with contrast filling the tracheobronchial tree

Computed tomography (CT) is occasionally used in the preoperative evaluation of neonates with TEF and has proved to be a noninvasive and quick investigation. As compared with conventional bronchoscopy or catheterization, CT does not require any general anesthesia. The improved spatial and temporal resolution of new generation of scanners facilitates assessment of such small defects such as TEF. Either direct sagittal acquisition or axial acquisition with multiplanar reconstruction may help in demonstrating the precise location of fistula and the length of the gap between esophageal segments. Alternatively, length of the atretic segment can be assessed by passing a feeding tube from above and a metal bougie from below, via a gastrostomy.

The knowledge of the origin of the fistula is helpful to the surgeon not only in deciding the side of the thoracotomy (right or left), but also in anticipating the gap to be bridged. The most important advantage of CT is that both esophagus and trachea are seen in their natural (unstretched) positions, and the interpouch gap can be measured accurately.[9]

High resolution CT scan on a 64-slice CT scanner has shown to provide definitive diagnosis and help in surgical planning in a critically ill neonate with H-Type TEF by distending the esophagus with air (by means of nasogastric feeding tube) during CT acquisition. Such a maneuver has proved to be very useful in optimizing the visualization of the fistula which may be totally or partially closed by a valve like mucosal flap or by a spasm of the muscular layer of the esophagus.[10]

When there is a proximal fistula, it is located in the anterior wall of the esophagus. In esophageal atresia with a distal fistula, primary repair is possible as the length of the gap between the esophageal segments is usually short. When there is atresia with no distal fistula, there is usually a long gap (of the order of about five vertebral bodies) between the proximal and distal esophageal segments. The growth of the esophageal segments during the first few months of life tends to lessen the gap, thereby making a delayed primary repair feasible. A gastrostomy is established for feeding in the meantime.

Radiological Evaluation of Postoperative Complications

Most patients of isolated esophageal atresia and tracheoesophageal fistula do well following surgical repair. Nevertheless, complications following surgery do occur and can be grouped under early and late complications. The *early complications* include: (i) leakage at the anastomotic site (14-16%), (ii) esophageal stricture and (iii) recurrent fistula. Oral feeding is not started for 1 to 2 weeks following surgery, till the edema subsides. A contrast study of the esophagus should be performed prior to the institution of oral feeds. A low-osmolal nonionic contrast should be used as leakage at the anastomotic site and is the most commonly identified early complication of surgical repair. Anastomotic leak increases the risk of esophageal stricture in the future. Donnelly et al found that the appearance of an extrapleural fluid collection after esophageal atresia repair performed via an extrapleural approach was associated with a high incidence of anastomotic leakage.[8] If an anastomotic leak is left untreated, it may eventually lead to diverticulum formation. Most anastomotic leaks have been seen to close spontaneously.

Stricture is another common complication which can occur following esophageal atresia repair. Most often, the stricture or narrowing is slight at the site of anastomotic repair and may persist for years, even though the patient has no functional problem (Figs 9.6A and B). Those with true stricture at anastomotic site are symptomatic and generally respond to bougie dilatation, with reoperation generally not required. However, if a stricture is associated with gastroesophageal reflux, the stricture may not respond to dilatation if it continues to be exposed to the acidic gastric contents. Hence, patients with postoperative strictures should be evaluated for reflux by upper gastrointestinal series or pH monitoring.

A tracheoesophageal fistula can recur (3-14% cases) again at the anastomotic site, following surgery and is believed to be related to anastomotic leakage with erosion into trachea caused by local inflammation.

The *late complications* which can occur following repair of an esophageal atresia are dysmotitily, gastroesophageal reflux, tracheomalacia, rib fusion and scolosis. Dysmotility is present in nearly all patients who have had esophageal atresia.

Gastroesophageal reflux is also commonly associated and has been reported in 40 to 70 percent of cases. Reflux is thought to be related to the shortening of the intra-abdominal portion of the esophagus, or occur secondary to the surgical repair. Reflux may lead to peptic esophagitis and is likely to be the cause of more distal strictures in those who have had a history of repaired esophageal atresia.

Tracheomalacia is thought to occur due to chronic intrauterine compression of trachea by a distended upper esophageal pouch.

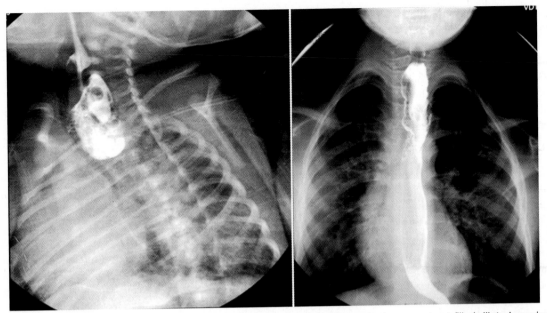

Figs 9.6A and B: (A) Esophageal atresia with distal TEF in a neonate. Lateral radiograph shows contrast filled dilated proximal esophageal pouch bowing the trachea anteriorly. (B) Barium swallow following primary anastomosis of esophageal atresia demonstrates slight narrowing at the anastomotic site (D4 vertebral level). The child had mild respiratory distress with dysphagia

STOMACH

Microgastria

Congenital microgastria is an extremely rare anomaly in which fetal rotation of the stomach fails to occur. There is no differentiation into fundus, body, antrum and pyloric canal and the lesser and greater curvatures also do not develop.[8] It is believed to occur as a result of atresia of normal foregut development in the fifth week of embryonal development.

Microgastria is often accompanied by other congenital anomalies such as malrotation, asplenia, renal, limb, vertebral and cardiac anomalies (VACTERL syndrome).[4] The common association between microgastria and upper extremity limb reduction defects, has led to the term microgastria-limb reduction complex.[8]

The clinical presentation of microgastria depends on the stage at which gastric development has been arrested. On prenatal ultrasound it may mimic esophageal atresia due to failure to visualize a distended stomach. Postnatally, microgastria presents with postprandial vomiting, failure to thrive, developmental delay, growth retardation, malnutrition and aspiration pneumonia. Most of the symptoms are due to secondary gastroesophageal reflux (GER).[4]

An upper GI study shows a small tubular stomach in the midline. The esophagus is dilated and appears to take over the storage function of the small capacity stomach. The gastroesophageal junction is incompetent and GER is present. There is associated esophageal dysmotility, secondary to its massive dilatation.[4]

The treatment of microgastria depends on its severity. The less severe forms may be treated conservatively, with surgery reserved as the first line of treatment in severe cases. The surgical treatment consists of creation of a Hunt-Lawrence pouch as a gastric reservoir, which allows for the secondary esophageal changes to resolve.[4]

DEVELOPMENTAL OBSTRUCTIVE DEFECTS

Congenital gastric obstruction is rare, as unlike the esophagus, the stomach undergoes little alteration in form during development. Gastric obstruction in the newborn may be due to:
1. Gastric atresia
2. Pyloric stenosis
3. Pyloric/prepyloric membrane/Antral web.

Gastric Atresia

Isolated gastric atresia is very rare and accounts for less than 1% of all congenital obstructions.[11] Almost all gastric atresias occur at the pylorus or antrum. They are thought to be due to localized vascular occlusion in fetal life and not to failure of recanalization of the intestinal tract.[3] Gastric atresia is classified into three types:[12]
a. Complete atresia with no connection between the stomach and duodenum
b. Complete atresia with the fibrous band connecting the stomach and duodenum, and
c. A gastric membrane or diaphragm producing atresia.

Gastric atresia may be familial or associated with epidermolysis bullosa. The newborn presents mainly with regurgitation of non-bilious vomitus within the first few hours after birth. As obstruction is complete, a plain radiograph of the abdomen reveals a "single bubble appearance" with marked dilatation of the stomach, proximal to the obstruction and absence of gas in the small bowel and colon. This appearance is diagnostic and most patients are taken directly to surgery without any contrast imaging.[11]

Pyloric Stenosis or Prepyloric Membrane or Antral Web

A pyloric stenosis or prepyloric membrane or antral web is a rare cause of symptomatic gastric obstruction in the newborn.[2] Patients with webs or stenosis of the pylorus, rather than complete atresia may present later in life or even in adulthood because the obstruction is incomplete.[8] The most common presenting symptoms are cyclic postprandial vomiting and episodes of transient vomiting.[9] Radiographically, the stomach is dilated with varying degrees of distal air, the extent of which depends on the degree of obstruction. In patients with incomplete obstruction, webs are more common than stenosis.[4]

It is difficult to diagnose an antral web on imaging studies. On UGI barium studies, a web is seen as a thin, 2-3 mm, linear circumferential filling defect traversing the barium column producing a reduction in the antral lumen, with a normal pyloric canal.[11] On ultrasound, the membrane may be visible if the stomach is filled with clear fluid and appears as echogenic band extending centrally from the lesser and greater curvatures in the prepyloric region. A mucus strand may be mistaken for an antral membrane. On the basis of clinical and radiographical findings, the definitive diagnosis of antral web can be made endoscopically.[2]

Ectopic Pancreas

Ectopic pancreas is an uncommon anomaly in which pancreatic tissue is found in the antropyloric region, less commonly in the duodenum. It is seen as an incidental finding. Less commonly it can cause symptoms of pain, GI bleeding or obstruction.[8] An upper GI study shows a smooth, dome shaped filling defect, 1-3 cm in diameter on the greater curvature of stomach, with central umbilication at times. Ectopic pancreatic tissue may produce intermittent obstruction if it prolapses into the pylorus.[11]

Hypertrophic Pyloric Stenosis (HPS)

Hypertrophic pyloric stenosis (HPS) is a common developmental condition affecting young infants. The incidence of HPS is approximately 3 in 1000 live births and boys are affected four to five times more commonly than girls. There is a familial disposition. Affected patients usually present between 2 to 6 weeks of age, with projectile non-bilious vomiting. Other conditions that can manifest with non-bilious vomiting include pylorospasm, hiatus hernia and preampullary duodenal stenosis.[13] HPS is never seen beyond 3 months of age, except reported in premature infants, in whom, enteral feeding has been started late.[14]

Diagnosis can be made on appropriate history and palpation of an 'olive' mass in the subhepatic region of an infant. The mass is reported to be seen in up to 80 percent of cases. Antral peristaltic waves can also be observed.[3]

HPS is characterized by hypertrophy of pyloric circular muscle and redundancy of the pyloric mucosa. However, its etiology is unknown. Possible causes include hypersecretion with

resulting duodenal irritation and pylorospasm. There is a constant association with hyperplasia of the antral mucosa.[3] Recent work has confirmed that the pylorus is abnormally innervated, and suggested that a lack of nitric oxide synthetase may be responsible for the pylorospasm that leads to gastric outlet obstruction and muscular hypertrophy.[5]

In most cases, a clinical diagnosis can be confidently made. However, further investigation may be required when the diagnosis remains in doubt. The diagnosis of HPS can be established by either barium studies or US. Ultrasonography has replaced barium examination being non-invasive and its ability to visualize the pyloric muscle directly to obtain measurements of muscle thickness.[15,16]

Ultrasonography (US)

Ultrasonography is the imaging modality of choice in an infant suspected of having pyloric stenosis, with a reported accuracy approaching 100%.[13] The examination is typically performed with a high frequency linear transducer (>5MHz) as the stomach, pylorus and duodenum are very superficial in an infant.[17] The gall bladder which is adjacent to the pylorus, serves as a good landmark.[3] Longitudinal and transverse images through the pylorus are obtained with the infant in the right posterior oblique position while scanning the right upper quadrant just off the midline. In this position, any fluid in the fundus of the stomach moves into the antrum and pyloric region, distending these regions. The stomach should not be emptied prior to the examination as this makes identification of antropyloric area difficult. If there is inadequate distention of the antrum, the infant may be given a glucose solution or water, orally or via a nasogastric tube. If fluid is administered, it should be removed at the end of the examination to prevent further vomiting and the risk of aspiration. In addition, if there is lot of gas, scanning the baby in the prone position may help in visualization of the pyloric region.[17]

The US evaluation of HPS includes assessment of both morphological and quantitative features. The classic findings are of a thickened echo-poor pyloric muscle and an elongated pyloric canal.[15,16,18] The thickened muscle is seen as two curved bundles of mixed but generally low reflectivity bulging into the base of the duodenal cap and gastric antrum. The mucosal echoes are seen as one or two central bright lines. On transverse images the hypertrophic pylorus has a doughnut appearance, representing the reflective central mucosa and submucosa surrounded by echo-poor muscle. The hypertrophic muscle may look non-uniform on transverse scanning of the pylorus. This is related to the sonographic artifact of anisotropic effect because of the orientation of the muscle fibers.[3] Other signs include exaggerated peristaltic waves that terminate at the pylorus, esophageal reflux and little if any gastric emptying.

An experienced examiner can frequently make the diagnosis just by qualitative assessment of the thickness of the pyloric wall. The exact measurements that separate a normal pylorus from a hypertrophic one, are controversial.[16,18-20] However, as a general guide, a pyloric canal length greater than 15 mm, muscle thickness

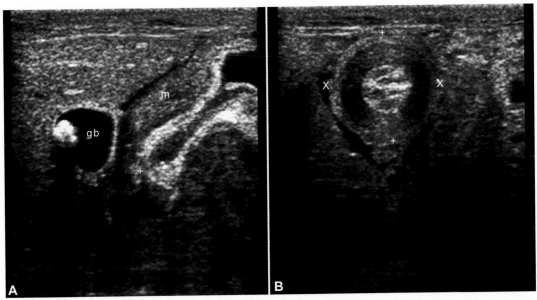

Figs 9.7A and B: (A) Hypertrophic pyloric stenosis: Longitudinal ultrasound image showing an elongated thickened pylorus seen as two curved bundles of low reflectivity (m). The mucosal echoes are seen as central bright lines. gb – gallbladder shows sludge within. Minimal fluid is present around the stomach. (B) Transverse section shows the muscle thickness as an echo poor rim – "Bull's eye" sign. Serosa to serosa measures 15 mm (cursors)

greater than 3.0 mm, and transverse serosa-to-serosa diameter greater than 15 mm is consistent with HPS. (Figs 9.7A and B). At least two values should be positive. A muscle thickness less than 2.0 mm is unequivocally normal. A muscle thickness between 2 and 2.9 mm is abnormal but non-specific, and can be seen in gastritis and pylorospasm as well as in HPS. Though pylorospasm may mimic HPS on sonography as there is some pyloric muscle thickening and/or slight elongation of the pyloric canal, pylorospasm is transient and generally resolves in 30 minutes. An important pointer for diagnosing pylorospasm is that there is considerable variation in measurement or image appearance with time during the study.[21] Borderline muscle thickness measurements are more likely to occur in premature than in term infants.

A number of ancillary sonographic signs of HPS have been described.[17]

• "Shoulder sign" – refers to an indentation upon the gastric antrum produced by hypertrophy of the pyloric muscle
• "Double tract sign" – this refers to fluid, trapped in the mucosal folds in the center of an elongated pyloric canal seen as two sonolucent streaks in the center
• "Nipple sign" is produced due to the evagination of redundant pyloric mucosa into the distended portion of the antrum.

Color Doppler evaluation of the pylorus may reveal hyperemia within the muscle and mucosal layers.

False negative diagnosis may be made if the stomach is overdistended, because it can displace the pylorus posteriorly, making it difficult to visualize the pyloric canal. If the scan is not in the midline, or is tangential to the antrum, the antral wall can simulate a thickened pyloric muscle, leading to a false positive diagnosis.

Barium Study

A barium study should be performed if ultrasound is inconclusive or gastroesophageal reflux is suspected.[21] If gastric distention is severe, a nasogastric tube should be passed and the stomach emptied. With the patient in the prone oblique position, the tube is placed in the antrum and adequate barium is injected via the tube under fluoroscopic control and spot films are taken.

Most of the infants, with and without HPS, show some degree of pylorospasm. In HPS, generally barium will pass through the antropyloric region within 1 to 10 minutes, but may be delayed as long as 20 to 25 minutes. The pyloric canal is narrowed (the "string sign") and elongated and almost always curved upward posteriorly (Fig. 9.8). Combination of narrowing and elongation is the hallmark of HPS on barium study. Barium may be caught between folds overlying the hypertrophied muscle and parallel lines (the "double string sign") may be seen (Fig. 9.9). The enlarged muscle mass looks much like an "apple-core lesion", with undercutting of the distal antrum and proximal duodenal bulb. The "beak sign" is noted as the thick muscle narrows the barium column as it enters the pyloric canal. Virtually all of the above signs can be seen transiently in infants especially those with some degree of spasm. The study should be continued sufficiently long to document the persistence of the findings in order to assure the diagnosis of pyloric stenosis. Occasionally, an associated antral web or diaphragm may be identified.

Adult Idiopathic Hypertrophic Pyloric Stenosis (AIHPS)

It is a mild form of HPS which may rarely present later in adult life. Its exact incidence is not known, as majority of these patients are asymptomatic for years. Around 80 percent of patients with

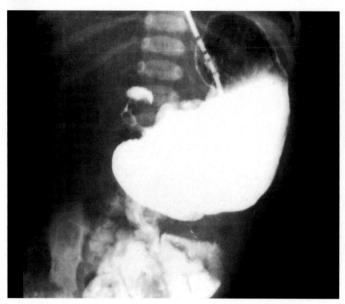

Fig. 9.8: Upper GI barium study in a child with pyloric stenosis. The markedly narrowed pylorus curves upward and posteriorly to the duodenal bulb which shows an impression of the hypertrophied muscle in the base

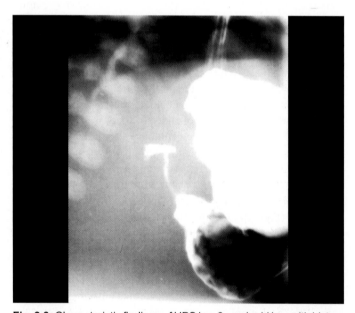

Fig. 9.9: Characteristic findings of HPS in a 6-week-old boy with history of vomiting: The pyloric canal is narrowed and elongated and the base of the duodenal bulb is stretched by the pyloric mass

the adult form of the disease are men which is in concordance with the male preponderance of congenital HPS. The primary form of AIHPS should be differentiated from the secondary form which is caused by diseases such as peptic ulcer disease, hypertrophic gastritis or malignancy.[23]

In AIHPS, the pylorus is bulbous or fusiform with its thickest portion at the pyloroduodenal junction. Patients present with symptoms of delayed gastric emptying not associated with any pain.

The radiologic and endoscopic studies may be non-specific. However, the diagnosis should be suspected if there is elongation of the pyloric canal and is accompanied by marked dilatation of the stomach.

In AIHPS, the "string sign" may be seen as an extremely thin line of barium on an upper GI study. A marked thickening of the pyloric muscle may produce a convex indentation at the base of the duodenal bulb, causing a mushroom-like deformity ("Kirklin's sign"). The presence of a barium filled cleft between the hypertrophied muscle and the fibers of the pylorus can project into either one or both sides of the pylorus, proximal to the base of the bulb ("Twining's sign"). However, none of these signs are pathognomic and presence of two or more of them strengthens the radiologic diagnosis. Endoscopy may be useful and the classic finding that has been described is the "donut" or the cervix sign which consists of a fixed narrow pylorus with a smooth border.

In the congenital type of HPS, pyloromyotomy is the preferred treatment. Normal emptying of the stomach occurs within 2-3 days after the procedure. However, muscle thickness gradually regresses to normal and may even take 6-8 weeks.[3] In contrast, in AIHPS, pyloroplasty and recently, laparoscopic pyloromyotomy have been tried with successful results.[22]

An increased incidence of renal anomalies like pelviureteric junction obstruction, primary megaureter, duplex kidney, renal agenesis or ectopia and horseshoe kidney have been reported in patients with HPS.[23]

DUODENUM

Duodenal obstruction is a relatively common form of intestinal obstruction in the newborn. It may be complete (duodenal atresia) or incomplete. Complete duodenal obstruction is seen more frequently than congenital gastric obstruction.[11] Incomplete obstruction may be intrinsic, such as duodenal stenosis caused by a web or "windsock" membrane; or it is more often extrinsic, e.g. duodenal compression from bands, annular pancreas, etc. Intrinsic and extrinsic obstructions may coexist.

Table 9.1: Causes of duodenal obstruction in the newborn	
Intrinsic	*Extrinsic*
Duodenal atresia	Ladd's bands
Duodenal stenosis	Midgut volvulus with malrotation
Duodenal web or diaphragm	Annular pancreas
	Duplication
	Preduodenal portal vein

Duodenal Atresia and Stenosis

Atresia is much more common than stenosis, but the etiology is the same. Atresia or stenosis occurs when the duodenum, which is a solid tube till about 3 to 6 weeks' gestation, fails to recanalize partially or completely. Unlike jejunal and ileal atresia, it does not appear to be related to intrauterine ischemia.[11] Atresia and stenosis almost always occur in the region of the ampulla of Vater (about 80% are just distal to the ampulla); thus they are frequently

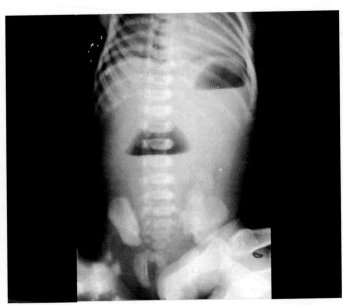

Fig. 9.10: Duondenal atresia : Erect film of the abdomen demonstrating the "double bubble" sign

accompanied by abnormalities of the bile duct and pancreas. Annular pancreas occurs in 20 percent of patients with duodenal atresia or stenosis. It may contribute to the duodenal obstruction but is seldom or never found without intrinsic obstruction of the duodenum.

Duodenal atresia and stenosis may be associated with other congenital anomalies, like intestinal atresia and congenital heart disease and may be part of VACTERL association. About 30 percent of the patients have Down's syndrome.[24-26]

Duodenal atresia and stenosis occur with equal frequency in boys and girls. Prematurity and maternal polyhydramnios are common. Bilious vomiting in the first few hours of life is the cardinal symptom but those with duodenal stensois can present at variable times, because the clinical findings depend on the degree of stenosis. Bilious vomiting is a feature in 80 percent of neonates with duodenal atresia as the atresia is present distal to the ampulla of Vater. In the remaining 20 percent, the vomitus is non-bilious.[3]

Imaging Features

In newborns with duodenal atresia, the abdominal radiograph is usually diagnostic. Air is present in the stomach and proximal duodenum, but there is no air distally in the gastrointestinal tract. Erect film shows two gas-fluid levels in which the higher, larger bubble to the left is the stomach and the other bubble is the dilated proximal duodenum which is seen above the region of obstruction.[11] Thus, the typical appearance of a "double-bubble sign" represents air, or air and fluid filled distended stomach and duodenal bulb (Fig. 9.10).

In duodenal stenosis, the stomach and duodenal bulb usually are distended, but air is present in the distal bowel.

In newborns with evidence of complete duodenal obstruction on abdominal radiograph, there is mostly no need for further radiologic investigation. If enough air is not present to adequately demonstrate the obstruction, one can introduce through a naso-gastric tube.[12] However, a contrast enema in patients with complete duodenal obstruction may be done to exclude additional, more distal atresia.[7] A microcolon implies that there is a distal atresia or atresias.

The newborn with congenital duodenal obstruction, complete or partial, requires surgery and is frequently taken to surgery without any more radiological investigation other than the plain film. However, further radiological study is required for making a preoperative diagnosis, specifically to distinguish between a cause of partial obstruction for which operation may be delayed, such as duodenal stenosis, from midgut volvulus, which requires emergent surgery. In these cases, when the infant is clinically stable, an upper gastrointestinal (UGI) series may be very useful. On UGI study, duodenal stenosis appears as dilatation of the duodenum proximal to the point of obstruction with abrupt caliber change.[3]

Duodenal Web

In patients with duodenal webs, the findings on UGI vary. In some, the appearance is of complete obstruction, in others there is narrowing of the duodenum. In the latter, a web is indistinguishable from simple duodenal stenosis. The most diagnostic appearance of a web is that of a thin, convex, curvilinear defect extending for a variable distance across the lumen of the duodenum. The "wind sock" appearance that a duodenal web may have in an adult or older child, the so called intraluminal duodenal diverticulum, is not seen in newborns. This appearance is probably due to stretching and redundancy of the web caused by years of peristalsis, proximal to an incomplete obstruction.[27]

Annular Pancreas

Annular pancreas is due to anomalous pancreatic tissue encircling the second part of duodenum. It is believed to result from the failure of normal pancreatic tissue to rotate around the duodenum. The duodenal obstruction may be total at the time of birth if a complete ring is formed. If the ring is incomplete, the obstruction may occur later in life or may never produce symptoms.[11] With severe obstruction, patient presents as a neonate. Presenting symptoms with delayed presentation are usually pain and vomiting. Radiographs are normal. On upper GI studies, a persistent waist is seen, partially obstructing the second part of duodenum.[3]

Preduodenal Portal Vein

Preduodenal portal vein is rarely the sole cause of duodenal obstruction and is rarely diagnosed preoperatively. It is thus important for the surgeon to be aware of the association of this anomaly with the other congenital lesions causing duodenal obstruction.[3]

A preduodenal portal vein (persistent left vitelline vein) results from normal situs asymmetry and is commonly seen in patients with heterotaxy. The resultant portal vein courses anterior to the pancreas and duodenum. The condition is diagnosed by

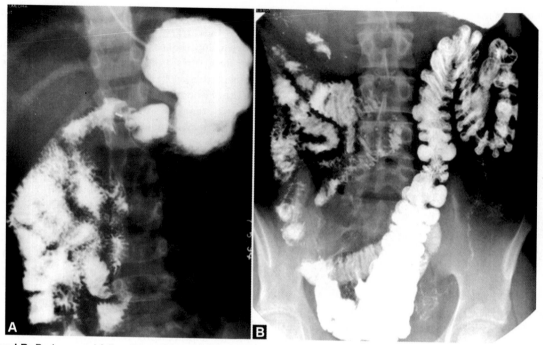

Figs 9.11A and B: Barium meal follow through study shows (A) jejunal loops on the right side of the abdomen and (B) colon and cecum on the left side, with the ileum seen crossing the midline from right to left – Non-rotation

identifying the prepancreatic course of the portal vein on sonography, CT and MR imaging. It is now believed that in most cases of duodenal obstruction associated with a preduodenal portal vein, the obstruction is due to a primary, obstructing duodenal lesion such as intraluminal membrane or web and such a lesion should be suspected in these patients if duodenal obstruction is present.[21]

SMALL BOWEL

Anomalies of Rotation and Fixation

Embryology

At approximately sixth week of gestation, the primitive midgut herniates into the extraembryonic coelom in the umbilical cord. The proximal and distal portions of the midgut elongate and rotate 270 degrees anticlockwise around the axis of the superior mesenteric artery. By the end of the third month of gestation, the bowel loops return to their final position in the abdominal cavity. Fixation of the duodenojejunal junction or the ligament of Treitz in left upper quadrant occurs. The cecum is the last part of the GIT to be fixed and it normally comes to lie in the right lower quadrant. When all or part of the physiological rotation of bowel fails to occur, a wide variety of anomalies of intestinal rotation and mesenteric fixation occurs which consist of nonrotation, malrotation or reversed rotation.[12]

i. **Nonrotation** – It is an asymptomatic condition in which the small bowel lies entirely on the right side and the colon on the left side. It is demonstrated incidentally on barium studies in older children or adults. (Figs 9.11A and B). The bowel is not very mobile and volvulus is not a common complication of nonrotation of the bowel.

ii. **Malrotation** – In malrotation of the bowel, final position of the GI tract is somewhere between normal and complete nonrotation.[12] Malrotation is a general term that includes a wide spectrum of anomalies that occur when this intestinal rotation and fixation occurs in an abnormal fashion. It can also be referred to as "malfixation". Most commonly, there is incomplete rotation, which leads to a shortened mesenteric root which may have a narrow rather than a broad base that has a tendency to twist on its axis. This leads to extrinsic compression of the bowel, causing bowel obstruction, and if the twist persists, it may lead to occlusion of the mesenteric vessels. This twist of malfixed intestines around the short mesentery is called a **midgut volvulus**. (Figs 9.12A to C). In patients with malfixation of the bowel, in addition to the absence of a normal mesentery, frequently there are aberrant peritoneal bands (**Ladd's bands**). These bands extend from the malpositioned cecum across the duodenum and attach to the hilum of the liver, posterior peritoneum or abdominal wall and can cause extrinsic duodenal obstruction[24] (Figs 9.13A & B and 9.14).

iii. **Reversed intestinal rotation** – It is a rare rotational anomaly which renders the hepatic flexure and left transverse colon posterior in position. These portions of the colon lie behind the descending duodenum and the superior mesenteric artery. The cecum is usually malrotated and medially placed and the small bowel is more right-sided than normal. Obstructing bands and midgut volvulus can occur.[12]

Clinical Features

Two-thirds of patients who are symptomatic present with an acute onset of bilious vomiting in the first month of life with many of them presenting in the first week of life. Fifteen to twenty percent

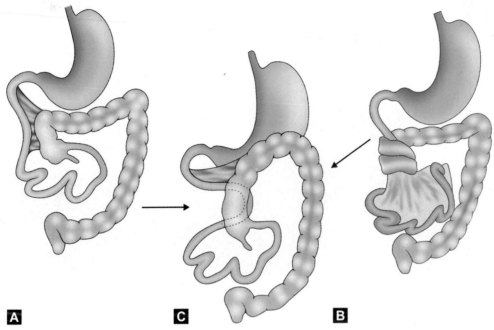

Figs 9.12A to C: Illustration of midgut volvulus. Narrow mesenteric attachment of nonrotation (A) or incomplete rotation (B) may lead to midgut volvulus (C)

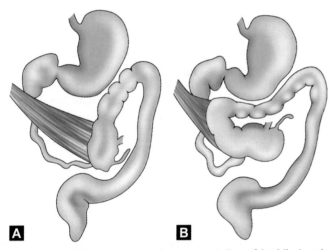

Figs 9.13A and B: Diagrammatic representation of Ladd's bands causing duodenal compression in patients with malrotation. The cecum is left sided (A) and mid-line (B) in position and has dense peritoneal bands crossing over the duodenum

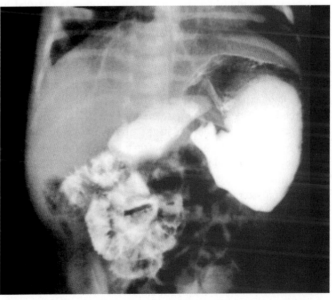

Fig. 9.14: Midgut malrotation with Ladd's bands: Barium study shows distended proximal duodenum with tapering at the level of obstruction indicative of extrinsic compression. The small intestine, distal to the usual site of the ligament of Treitz lies below the duodenum and to the right

of patients present in late infancy or early childhood. In the remaining patients, malrotation is seen as an incidental finding.

The bowel obstruction may be caused by the volvulus, by Ladd's bands, or both. The sudden onset of bilious vomiting in a newborn who has been normal for the first few days of life should be considered to be due to a midgut volvulus until proved otherwise.

Imaging Features

Plain radiographs may show feature of duodenal obstruction due to partially obstructing Ladd's bands. The duodenal bulb dilatation

is less than that seen with duodenal atresia. There may be little distal bowel gas. When there is a volvulus, the plain films may show features of distal bowel obstruction. Bowel-wall thickening and pneumatosis may be present due to volvulus-induced ischemia. The fluid-filled bowel loops associated with volvulus can simulate an abdominal mass. The abdomen may be gasless, which may be due either to proximal obstruction or to diffuse

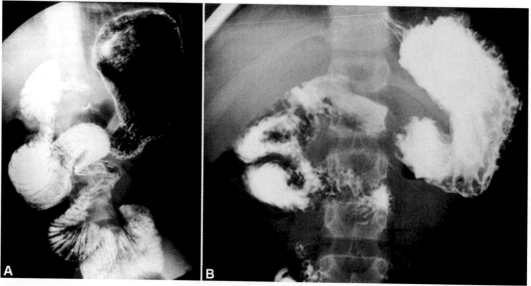

Figs 9.15A and B: Upper GI barium study in two different patients showing classic "corkscrew" appearance of the duodenum in midgut volvulus

bowel necrosis in midgut volvulus. Of all the congenital anomalies that result in bilious emesis, only malrotation is likely to produce a normal abdominal film.[24]

Upper gastrointestinal barium examination is performed to document the location of ligament of Treitz and to evaluate for duodenal obstruction. Normally, the duodenojejunal junction lies to the left of the body of the first or second lumbar vertebra at the level of the duodenal bulb. In malrotation, it is located lower and to the right of normal. It is important to remember that the duodenojejunal junction is mobile in children and may be pushed inferomedially by an overdistended stomach, chronic bowel dilatation, enlarged spleen or in the presence of a nasojejunal tube.[3] A lateral view of the contrast filled duodenum is an important additional view in the upper GI study when evaluating for malrotation. Normal duodenum being a retroperitoneal structure, on lateral views is seen to lie behind the level of the stomach, with the fourth part of the duodenum superimposed on the second part of duodenum. This superimposed relationship is lost in case of malrotation of duodenum as it is seen to course anteriorly. An abnormal position of the duodenojejunal flexure may be the only indication of malrotation, as in 16% of cases cecum occupies its normal position.

In addition, in malrotation the jejunum is usually on the right side of the abdomen. However, this should not be taken as an indication of malrotation as the jejunum in a normal child is relatively mobile and may be seen to the right of the spine.[3]

When volvulus occurs, there may be complete or partial duodenal obstruction. With complete obstruction, a beaked tapering of the obstructed duodenum may be seen. More commonly, the volvulus is intermittent with incomplete bowel obstruction with contrast filling the proximal small bowel. Occasionally, the pathognomonic corkscrew pattern of the twisted duodenum and jejunum is seen due to their clockwise twisting around the superior mesenteric artery (Figs 9.15A and B). In

malrotation, the cecum and right colon may have abnormal mobility. The cecum is in the right upper quadrant or in midline in malrotation. A colonic beak may be present in the right colon on barium enema in the presence of volvulus.[24] In the past, a contrast enema was the first investigation performed to evaluate for malrotation.[3] This has been replaced by an upper GI study due to its greater sensitivity and specificity for malrotation. The cecum may be mobile in neonates and may be seen in the right upper quadrant in the absence of malrotation.

A barium meal upper GI study should be done for suspected malrotation since a normal barium enema does not exclude malrotation. The position of the cecum may be normal in a significant number of patients with malrotation.[21] Hence, the upper GI study is the investigation of choice for the diagnosis of malrotation.

Ultrasound may be useful in the early detection of midgut malrotation as well as complicating midgut volvulus. A distended proximal duodenum with a tapered end in front of the spine is consistent with malrotation in the proper clinical set-up. If in addition, one finds peritoneal fluid and edematous bowel loops on the right, the diagnosis of volvulus can be made. A normal anatomical relationship, however, in no way excludes the possibility of malrotation. A UGI series is mandatory if this diagnosis must be confirmed or excluded prior to surgery.

Ultrasound and CT scan may be helpful in suggesting the diagnosis of malrotation owing to abnormal superior mesenteric artery (SMA) or superior mesenteric vein (SMV) anatomy. The SMV normally rests to the right and anterior to the SMA. When the SMV is to the left of the SMA, this is highly suggestive of volvulus. When the SMV is anterior to the SMA, this is suggestive of malrotation with possible volvulus. Color Doppler US demonstrates '**whirlpool' sign** due to clockwise spiralling of the mesentery and superior mesenteric vein around the superior mesenteric artery. Inversion of the mesenteric vessels or the SMV

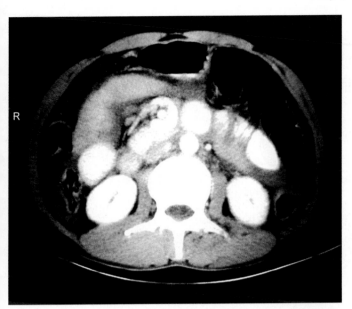

Fig. 9.16: Axial CECT of the abdomen showing characteristic "whirlpool" sign of clockwise twisting of the SMV and mesentery around the SMA

rotation sign is not a sensitive screening test, because it may be present in normal population, patients with situs inversus and patients with abdominal masses. Other CT findings of midgut malrotation complicated by midgut volvulus are: (1) the `whirl' sign of small-bowel loops revolved around the SMA; (Fig. 9.16) (2) a dilated, fluid-filled, obstructed stomach and proximal duodenum; (3) thick-walled loops of ischemic right-sided small bowel loops with potential pneumatosis intestinalis and mesenteric edema; and (4) free intraperitoneal fluid.

Jejunoileal Atresia and Stenosis

Small bowel atresias (i.e. jejunal, jejunoileal or ileal) are more common than duodenal or colonic atresia. They are more common in the proximal jejunum and distal ileum than in the intervening small intestine.[24] Jejunal atresias comprise around 50 percent of small bowel atresias and may be associated with other jejunal and ileal atresias.[2]

Embryology

Most jejunal and ileal atresias and stenoses, except those that are familial, are thought to be secondary to ischemic injury to the developing gut. The ischemia may be due to primary vascular accident, usually in the mid second trimester or secondarily to a mechanical obstruction, as may occur in case of an *in utero* volvulus.[24] There is no solid core phase in the development of jejunum and ileum, so recanalization is not thought to be involved. Jejunoileal atresia may involve the bowel anywhere from the ligament of Treitz to the ileocecal valve, with the majority of cases of atresia occurring at the extremes of the small bowel. The devascularized bowel becomes necrotic and is resorbed leaving an atretic area of varying length with its attached mesentery. Several forms of atresia have been described surgically, but it is not possible to differentiate them by imaging studies.[4]

Clinical Features

Antenatal diagnosis of small bowel atresia may be suggested on ultrasound by the presence of polyhydramnios and dilated fluid filled bowel loops. These findings are non-specific and the diagnosis is usually not confirmed until after birth.[3] Proximal atresia may present with bilious vomiting; whereas more distal atresias present with abdominal distention. There may be failure to pass meconium. It is commonly associated with prematurity. Meconium may be passed if atresia is located in the jejunum or occurred later in intrauterine life.

Classification

Small bowel atresia usually occurs as an isolated anomaly of the gastrointestinal tract. There are four types of small bowel atresia[3] (Figs 9.17A to D):

Type 1—Membranous or web-like atresia, composed of mucosal and submucosal elements with no interruption of the muscularis.

Type 2—Atresia with a solid fibrous cord connecting the atretic bowel ends, but the mesentery is intact. All the three layers of the intestinal wall are interrupted.

Type 3—Complete absence of a segment of bowel (total atresia) as well as a portion of the mesentery (V-shaped defect in the mesentry)

Type 4—The familial form of multiple atresias

There are two unusual forms of atresia that are inherited.[24] They are:

  i. "Apple peel" or "Christmas tree" atresia
  ii. A syndrome of multiple intestinal atresias

"Apple peel" or "Christmas tree" atresia is a rare variant of Type 3 atresia which consists of proximal jejunal atresia with absence of the distal superior mesenteric artery, shortening of the small bowel distal to the atresia and absence of the dorsal mesentery. This type of atresia is probably caused by prenatal occlusion of the SMA, distal to the origin of the midcolic artery. The distal small intestine spirals around its vascular supply giving the characteristic apple peel appearance (Fig. 9.17D). The result is a very short intestine with a propensity towards necrotizing enterocolitis.[28]

The syndrome of multiple intestinal atresias with intraluminal calcification is transmitted as an autosomal recessive pattern. There are multiple atresias from stomach to rectum. The radiological hallmark of this syndrome is extensive calcification of intraluminal contents between the areas of atresia. Nonhereditary bowel atresias may also demonstrate intraluminal calcification.[24]

Imaging Features

Plain radiograph of the abdomen demonstrates typical findings of small-bowel obstruction. The site (jejunal or distal ileal) of the atresia can be suspected by the number and location of gas-filled loops of bowel.[3] (Fig. 9.18). Proximal jejunal atresia may have a few markedly dilated loops, the so-called triple bubble sign, more distal atresia typically has a more uniform dilatation of small bowel with associated air-fluid levels. The loop just proximal to the site of atresia is frequently disproportionately distended, with

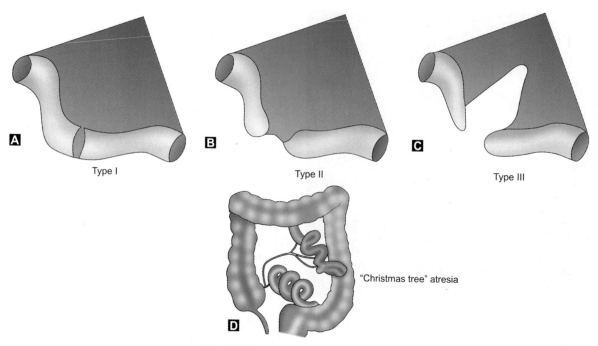

Fig. 9.17: Types of small bowel atresia

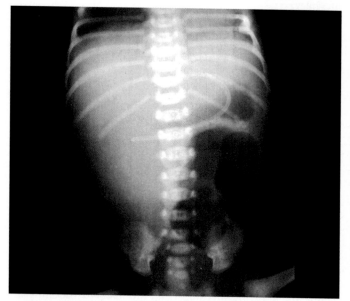

Fig. 9.18: Small bowel atresia. Air is seen in the stomach and dilated part of the jejunum proximal to the atresia

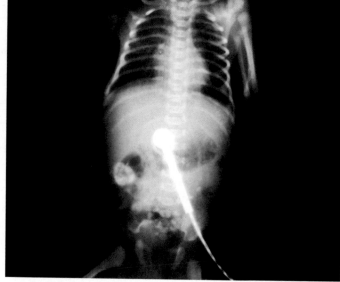

Fig. 9.19: Plain radiograph of the abdomen in a case of meconium peritonitis shows curvilinear calcification in the right flank

a bulbous end. If the ischemic event that produced the atresia caused a perforation, there may be evidence of meconium peritonitis which is a chemical peritonitis occurring as a result of extruded bowel contents producing an intense peritoneal inflammatory reaction. It leads to the formation of dense fibrotic tissue which often calcifies, resulting in characteristic intraperitoneal calcifications. Peritoneal calcifications may be identified on plain films as a consequence of meconium peritonitis, wherein they are seen as linear or flocculent areas of calcification within the peritoneal cavity. (Fig. 9.19) The most frequent finding is a linear calcification under the free edge of

the liver, though any or all portions of the peritoneum may be involved.[4] The calcification may extend into the scrotum through a patent vaginal process to produce a calcified mass in the scrotum.[28] The association of meconium peritonitis with small bowel obstruction is virtually diagnostic of small bowel atresia.[4]

Ultrasound depicts the calcifications of meconium peritonitis as highly echogenic linear or clumped foci in the abdomen or pelvis. The appearance of meconium peritonitis on US may be either generalized or cystic. In the generalized condition, highly echogenic material spreads throughout the abdomen and around the bowel loops to produce a characteristic "snowstorm"

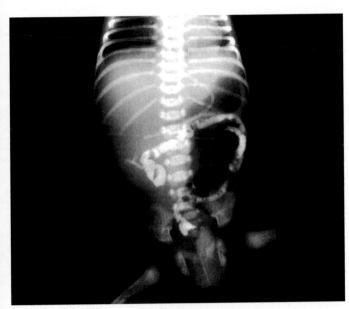

Fig. 9.20: Small bowel atresia. Contrast enema demonstrates a microcolon

appearance. Encysted collections of meconium show a variable appearance from homogeneous to heterogeneous echogenicity and may be ill-defined or well defined.

Sonography may also be useful in differentiating ileal atresia from meconium ileus. In ileal atresia, the bowel contents are echopoor while in meconium ileus, the dilated bowel loops are filled with echogenic material.[21]

Additional imaging is not required in the presence of a high intestinal obstruction. A contrast enema is required for further evaluation for low bowel obstruction to distinguish between a large or distal small bowel obstruction, as the differentiation of the two on plain radiographs may be difficult or impossible. The most common causes of neonatal distal small bowel obstruction are ileal atresia and meconium ileus.[3]

Contrast enema should be performed with water soluble low osmolar contrast media introduced via a soft rectal catheter. Care must be taken to perform the enema as the distal blind pouch is prone to perforation. The one diagnostic finding to be looked for in the contrast enema performed in a setting of low bowel obstruction, is the presence or absence of a microcolon (Fig. 9.20). A microcolon is a colon of very small caliber, generally less than 1cm diameter, and the entire colon must be involved. (i.e. not a portion as in small left colon syndrome). Normally, colonic measurements are not needed for diagnosing microcolon as it is usually obvious on inspection. The colon is small owing to lack of use rather than anatomic or functional abnormality. The more distal the small bowel obstruction, the smaller the colon. A microcolon or unused colon occurs when no or little intestinal juices (succus entericus) reaches the colon and is highly suggestive of a distal small bowel obstruction (meconium ileus or ileal atresia). A normal sized colon almost always excludes these diagnoses.[24]

It is important to remember that the presence of microcolon is diagnostic of long standing distal small bowel obstruction, but a normal colon does not exclude it in all cases. Also, microcolon on contrast enemas may be seen in premature infants and occasionally, in total colonic aganglionosis (long segment Hirschsprung's disease). The rectum is distensible in distal ileal atresia, thereby distinguishing it from the microcolon of long segment Hirschsprung's disease.[3]

Jejunal atresia does not lead to a microcolon because the remaining small bowel, distal to the atresia produces sufficient succus entericus to give a colon of normal caliber. Hence, a microcolon in the presence of a high bowel obstruction indicates a second, more distal atresia.[3]

Surgical treatment involves resection of the atretic portion of the intestine with reanastomosis. The proximal dilated bowel may remain dilated for sometime in the post operative period, showing delayed motility with delayed passage of contrast across a widely patent anastomosis.

Meconium Ileus

Meconium ileus is a low intestinal obstruction caused by inspissation of abnormal meconium in the distal ileum.[24] It is almost always associated with cystic fibrosis and is a presenting feature of cystic fibrosis in 5 to 10 percent of these patients.[24] The lack of normal pancreatic enzymes leads to thick, tenacious meconium that collects in the distal ileum and cecum, occluding its lumen and resulting in high grade distal small bowel obstruction.

Meconium ileus can be complicated or uncomplicated, with complicated meconium ileus being seen in up to half of the patients which include intestinal atresia, volvulus of the distal intestinal loop and perforation with meconium or pseudocyst formation.[3]

Imaging Features

Meconium ileus is the most common mimic of small bowel atresia clinically and on plain films.[4] Plain radiograph may demonstrate a distal bowel obstructive pattern with air-fluid levels. Bowel loops may vary in size, a finding seen less often in atresia. The dilated small-bowel loops that contain air can mimic colon loops in size and course. In addition, some air mixes with the viscid meconium and results in a bubbly appearance in the right lower quadrant. This "soap bubble appearance" is not specific and a similar fecal pattern can be seen with any cause of distal intestinal obstruction like ileal atresia, colonic atresia, aganglionosis of the terminal ileum and meconium plug syndrome.[28] Patients with meconium ileus have fewer air-fluid levels than patients with small-bowel atresias. Meconium peritonitis may occur and be associated with peritoneal calcifications. However, this differential point is not specific in all cases. A localized perforation forms a meconium pseudocyst which may have peripheral curvilinear calcifications seen on plain radiographs. The term pseudocyst is also used to refer for a mass of necrotic, fluid-filled bowel loops with a fibrous wall which may be seen as a mass on radiographs.[3]

Ultrasound can detect abnormal bowel dilatation and echogenic bowel contents in infants with meconium ileus. Ultrasound can also pick up complications of meconium peritonitis or pseudocyst which is seen as echogenic material lying outside the bowel loops, with or without associated calcification.

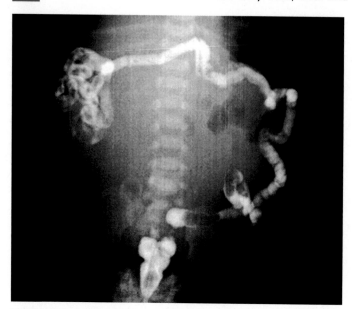

Fig. 9.21: Meconium ileus: Water soluble contrast enema showing a microcolon. Filling defects due to meconium are seen in colon and distal ileum

The colon of babies with meconium ileus is often said to be the smallest of all colons, and is empty except for a few occasional pellets of meconium. The distal 10 to 30 cm of ileum appears dilated due to meconium within and may even displace the right colon to the left.[24]

Definitive diagnosis is made with a low osmolal water soluble contrast enema which demonstrates a microcolon with inspissated meconium pellets identified in the collapsed distal ileum with dilated small bowel proximal to the obstruction (Fig. 9.21).

Uncomplicated cases of meconium ileus may be treated with multiple contrast enemas, i.e. one or two enemas per day. The aim is to introduce the contrast into the dilated small bowel, proximal to the obstructing inspissated meconium. But care must be taken not to overdistend the meconium. This leads to mechanical loosening of the meconium pellets. The patient should be well hydrated if high osmolarity agents are used because of fluid shifts. The therapy is largely mechanical and the osmotic load probably plays little role. Repeated enemas may be used only if progress is seen in decreasing the obstructing pellets. In premature infants, isotonic non-ionic contrast medium is used. Enema has a success rate of about 50 to 60 percent in treating meconium ileus.[3] If signs of obstruction are not relieved or perforation/peritornitis develop, further attempts at therapeutic enema should be abandoned. Surgery in such patients often reveals complicated meconium ileus.

Megacystis-microcolon-intestinal Hypoperistalsis Syndrome (Berdon Syndrome)

Megacystis-microcolon-intestinal hypoperistalsis syndrome is a pseudoatresia. There is a functional small bowel obstruction with a microcolon, malrotation and a large unobstructed bladder. There is four-to-one female predominance with associated genitourinary and congenital heart malformation in up to 14 percent cases.

Upper GI contrast study shows hypomotility of small bowel with retrograde peristalsis. Ultrasound reveals a dilated bladder with bilateral hydroureteronephrosis.[21] The prognosis is poor for long-term survival.

Meckel's Diverticulum

Meckel's diverticulum is a congenital blind pouch in the small bowel which results from an incomplete obliteration of the proximal part of the vitelline duct (omphalomesenteric duct) during the fifth week of gestation. It results in a true diverticulum arising from the antimesenteric border of the distal ileum.[29] For Meckel's diverticulum, the common rule by which it is known is the "rule of twos," i.e.–it is found in 2 percent of the population, twice as common in males, most frequently found in those less than 2 years of age and usually 2ft from the ileocecal valve. It may contain ectopic mucosa, usually gastric mucosa which is responsible for the adjacent ulceration in the ileum.

Meckel's diverticulum usually does not give rise to symptoms. Bleeding is the most common complication in children reported in over 50% of cases, while it is seen in only around 12% cases in adults. Bleeding is usually minor, resulting in chronic anemia.[22] It may present with malena due to ulceration of ectopic gastric mucosa in its wall. In 20-30 percent of patients, it may give rise to symptoms such as inflammation, and or perforation which may often be indistinguishable from acute appendicitis. Obstructive symptoms have been seen to occur more frequently than hemorrhage in patients with Meckel's diverticulum presenting in adulhood. The obstruction may occur due to intussusception, volvulus, inflammatory adhesions. The diverticulum may get obstructed with resulting diverticulitis, may present as a mass and initiate intussusception in childhood.

Preoperative evaluation of a Meckel's diverticulum is difficult, and routine and special radiological studies such as plain abdominal radiograph, barium meal follow through, arteriography and computed tomography are often non-diagnostic and often of limited diagnostic value. The diverticulum is seldom recognized on a small bowel follow-through study because there is no significant hold-up, and the barium residue remaining in it is very small because of its wide neck.[29,30] In suspected symptomatic Meckel's diverticulum, preoperative evaluation includes [99m]Tc (technetium -99m pertechnetate) scanning which relies on the presence of ectopic gastric mucosa. In this study, ^{99m}Tc is injected intravenously, and over time it accumulates in the gastric mucosa.

As symptoms such as bleeding is caused by the ectopic gastric issue, ^{99m}Tc scanning may help in the diagnosis in symptomatic cases. In children, the scan has a sensitivity of 85 percent and specificity of 95 percent, but in adults the sensitivity is 62.5 percent and the specificity 9 percent. The accuracy of the scan can be improved with the use of pentagastrin or cimetidine. In patients with non diagnostic scan or with nonbleeding presentation, ultra-sonography could prove to be useful in achieving a diagnosis.

Enteric Duplication

Gastrointestinal duplications are uncommon congenital abnormalities that may occur anywhere in the gastrointestinal tract. But the most common locations are the distal ileum (35%),

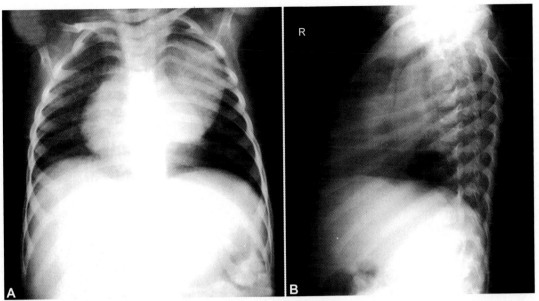

Figs 9.22A and B: Esophageal duplication – chest PA showing a well-defined soft tissue mass in the left hemithorax (A) lying posteriorl in the lateral film (B). There is associated hyperinflation of the let lung. The vertebral bodies appear normal

distal esophagus (20%) and stomach (9%) followed by duodenum and jejunum. Colonic and rectal duplications are rare. Multiple duplications may be present in 15-20% cases.[21] Enteric duplication occurs in the late first or early second trimester owing to abnormal canalization of the bowel. The duplication has smooth muscle in its wall with gastrointestinal mucosal lining. The wall thickness is 3 to 5 mm as seen in normal bowel. It is usually adjacent to and in most instances, does not communicate with the gastrointestinal tract. In most cases of hemorrhage or ulceration, gastric mucosa is present. Esophageal duplications are located at the posterior aspect of the esophagus. Gastric duplication is found along the greater curvature of the stomach interposed between the stomach and the transverse colon. Duplications may be spherical or tubular. Tubular duplication is more likely to communicate with the adjacent bowel. They typically occur along the mesenteric border of the intestine and share a common blood supply. Thus the tubular type of duplication may complicate bowel-sparing surgery because of difficulty in preserving the enteric blood supply. Unlike neurenteric cysts, duplication cysts are usually not associated with vertebral segmental anomalies.[29]

Clinical Features

Duplications can present with a variety of symptoms and signs depending on the site of duplication and its size. Upper esophageal duplications present with symptoms due to tracheal compression. Other symptoms include nausea and vomiting. In the presence of heterotopic gastric mucosa, patients may present with gastrointestinal hemorrhage or even perforation. Patient may also present with distention, ulceration, volvulus, an abdominal mass lesion or with obstruction, particularly when the duplication is in the region of the ileocecal valve or duodenum.

Forty percent of patients with enteric duplication present by one month of age, with 85 percent diagnosed during the first year of life.

Malrotation, genitourinary anomalies and jejunal or ileal atresias are also seen. Duplications are more common in boys except for gastric ones, which occur without gender predominance.

Imaging Features

Plain radiographs may demonstrate a mass lesion, especially in the chest in the case of esophageal duplication, (Figs 9.22A and B). The bowel gas pattern may suggest an obstruction, particularly with duodenal or ileal duplications. Enteric duplication cysts may reveal mural calcifications.

Occasionally, duplication may get filled with barium suspension during gastrointestinal examinations. In most cases, however, the duplications are not demonstrated in this manner. Barium study usually reveals extrinsic compression (Figs 9.23A and B) of the bowel or an obstruction.

On ultrasonography, a duplication cyst appears as a well-defined, unilocular anechoic mass with good through transmission (Fig. 9.24). Rarely the contents are reflective or contain septations secondary to hemorrhage or inspissated material within the lumen. A highly reflective mucosa and a surrounding echo poor muscular wall may be seen as the duplication is of gastrointestinal origin.[31,32] This is most easily identified in the dependent portion of the cyst.[21] The presence of this double layered appearance ("gut wall signature") is relatively specific for the diagnosis of duplication cyst and is useful to exclude other cystic masses, such as mesenteric or omental cyst, choledochal cyst, ovarian cyst, pancreatic pseudocyst or abscess. The reflective lining may be absent as a result of extensive mucosal ulceration by gastric enzymes.

Radionuclide studies may be useful in 30 percent of patients where the enteric duplications have gastric mucosa. Free pertechnetate is taken up and secreted by gastric mucosa, thus localizing the enteric duplication.[5]

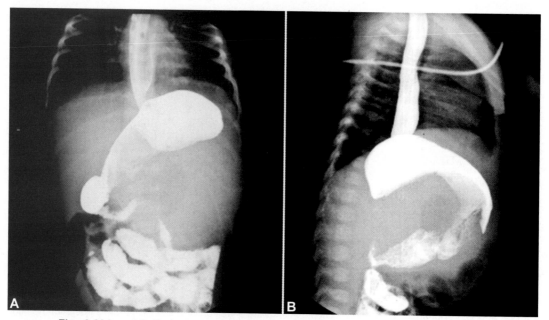

Figs 9.23A and B: Barium study shows extrinsic impression on the body of the stomach with effacement of the mucosa in AP and lateral views in a case of gastric duplication

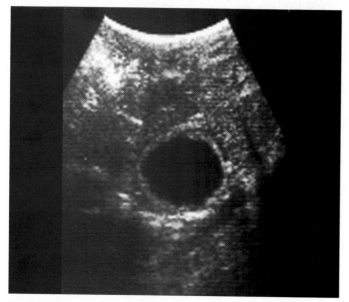

Fig. 9.24: Ultrasound abdomen reveals a well-defined, smooth rounded cystic lesion with inner echogenic mucosal stripe and outer hypoechoic muscle layer–Enteric duplication

CT or MRI may be useful in further characterizing the nature of enteric duplication cysts when the diagnosis is unclear, wherein they are seen as well-marginated, smooth walled masses of fluid attenuation/signal not showing any contrast enhancement. (Figs 9.25A and B).

LARGE BOWEL

Colonic Obstruction

Obstruction of the colon in the newborn may be either anatomical or functional. The first type includes atresia of the colon, anorectal atresia, and with a functional element, aganglionosis or Hirschsprung's disease. A group of poorly understood disorders like meconium plug, neonatal small left colon syndrome, etc. cause transient self-limited functional obstruction.

Colonic Atresia

Colonic atresia is quite rare as compared to atresias of the small bowel.[24] It is thought to be secondary to vascular insult. Multiple atresia syndromes may involve the colon in addition to small bowel. Proximal location is more common than distal, with atresias beyond the splenic flexure being unusual. If atresia is located in the ascending colon, it may often be indistinguishable from obstruction of the distal ileum.[28] The classification system based on the anatomic appearance is same as with jejunoileal atresia. Type I represents a diaphragmatic occlusion, type II represents a complete atresia with a blind, solid cord extending between the two ends of atretic segment; and type III represents a complete atresia with complete separation and an associated V-shaped mesenteric defect.

Clinical Features

Patients present with distension and failure to pass meconium. Presentation may be delayed up to 48 hours, if the atresia is proximal.

Imaging Features

Prenatal sonography may demonstrate dilatation of the colon proximal to the atresia.

Plain radiograph may demonstrate a distal obstruction with multiple air-fluid levels and may be nonspecific. Occasionally, a hugely and disproportionately dilated loop of bowel may be present and render the plain film evaluation highly suggestive of the diagnosis.[2] A "soap-bubble" appearance of retained meconium

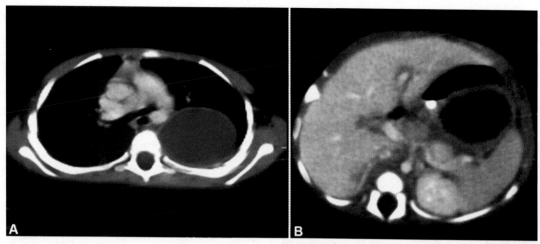

Figs 9.25A and B: CECT images of esophageal and gastric duplications of the two patients of the same case as in Figures 9.22 and 9.23 show sharply marginated, non-enhancing, homogeneous mass of water attenuation in the (A) posterior mediastinum and (B) along the greater curvature of stomach.

may be seen. There is dilatation of the proximal colon up to the level of the atresia, unless multiple atresias are present.

Contrast enema shows a microcolon, distal to the atresia with obstruction to the retrograde flow of barium at the site of atresia. The colon may have a hook or question-mark appearance at the site of atresia. The colon is often non-fixed or malpositioned in the midline. The distal colon segment may perforate into the peritoneal cavity during a contrast enema because often the blind end is covered with only mucosa.

Hirschsprung's Disease (Aganglionosis of the colon)

Hirschsprung's disease is a condition caused by absence of normal ganglion cells in a segment of the colon, leading to a form of low intestinal obstruction. It accounts for around 15-20 percent of cases of neonatal bowel obstruction.[28]

Embryology

In normal intrauterine development, neuroenteric cells migrate from the neural crest to the upper end of the gastrointestinal tract by 5 weeks and then proceeds in a caudal direction. These cells reach the rectum by 12 weeks and commence the intramural migration from Auerbach's (myenteric) plexus to the submucosal plexus. Hirschsprung's disease is caused by abnormal neural crest cell migration, resulting in arrested distal migration of these cells.[3] As the normal migration is continuous from proximal to distal, the part of the GI tract distal to the site of arrest is aganglionic.[8]

In the majority of cases (75-80%), the aganglionic segment is limited to the rectosigmoid region (short segment aganglionosis). The aganglionosis always involves the anus and internal sphincter and extends proximally for a variable distance. The transition from innervated to aganglionic bowel is found in the rectosigmoid region in 73 percent of patients, the descending colon in 14%, and more proximal colon in 10 percent, according to Swenson et al.[8] Total colon aganglionosis involves the entire

colon and part of the terminal ileum. It can very rarely involve the large as well as whole of the small bowel, which is incompatible with life. At the other end of the spectrum is ultrashort segment Hirschsprung's disease which is also rare. In this type, the aganglionosis is limited to the region of the internal sphincter.[3] The ultrashort segment can only be diagnosed by manometry (not biopsy or imaging) and is usually not diagnosed in the neonatal period.[4] Skip lesions in Hirschsprung's disease are believed to be unlikely to exist if one accepts the concept of neuronal migration down the GI tract. It is likely that such areas represent areas of intrauterine ischemic insult leading to destruction of ganglion cells.[12]

However, according to recently published literature, skip lesions in Hirschsprung's disease, though a controvertial condition, is a definite entity, with 24 cases reported till date. Skip lesions have been found to occur predominantly in patients with total colonic aganglionosis (92%). The presence of a skip area of normally innervated colon in total colonic aganglionosis may influence the surgical management, enabling the surgeons to preserve and use the ganglionated skip area during pull through operations.[33]

Hirschsprung's disease may be associated with certain congenital anomalies like intestinal atresia, malrotation. Down's syndrome is present in 2-3 percent cases.

Clinical Features

The absence of ganglion cells interrupts the normal propagation of colonic peristalsis. Patients with Hirschsprung's disease fail to pass meconium in the first 48 hours of life. They may present with abdominal distention, bilious vomiting, or enterocolitis. Over 80 percent of patients present within the first 6 weeks in life. Hirschsprung's disease is about three to four times as common in boys as in girls. Older children may present with chronic constipation. Hirschsprung's disease can be complicated by life threatening enterocolitis which presents with diarrhea, abdominal distention and fever and may progress to perforation with peritonitis.[3]

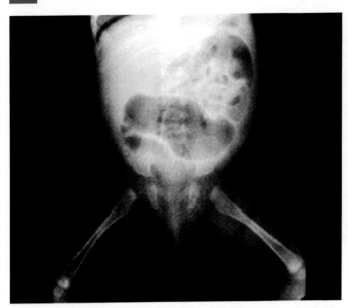

Fig. 9.26: Plain X-ray abdomen showing a dilated proximal sigmoid colon with a smaller distal sigmoid with relatively little rectal gas in a neonate with Hirschsprung's disease

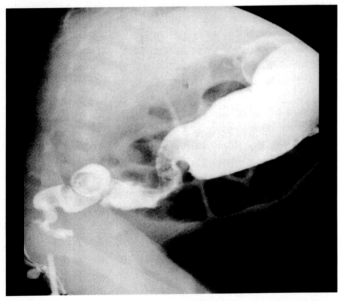

Fig. 9.27: Hirschsprung's disease: Barium enema shows an abrupt transition from the narrow caliber rectosigmoid (aganglionic) to the larger caliber more proximal sigmoid colon

Imaging Features

Plain films may demonstrate features of distal bowel obstruction. However, a dilated colon proximal to the distal and smaller aganglionic segment is the more typical finding (Fig. 9.26). A small gas-filled rectum can be seen, especially on prone films and may help in the diagnosis. The absence of rectal gas is not specific for Hirschsprung's disease as it is commonly seen in infants with sepsis and necrotizing enterocolitis.[21] At times, the bowel pattern may appear normal. Less commonly (4%), pneumoperitoneum

may be seen in patients with long segment or total colonic disease secondary to colonic perforation.

The radiographic diagnosis is made by contrast enema and is directed towards identifying the transition zone which is the most specific sign of Hirschsprung's disease. This is where the normal-sized, distal aganglionic bowel changes in caliber to join the proximal ganglionic bowel.[3] This findings may not be obvious in the newborn, hence, careful attention should be given to the technique of performing barium enema.

Barium enema is performed on an unprepared patient by inserting a straight-tipped catheter to a point just beyond the anal sphincter. Balloon catheters are not used to avoid expanding a narrow segment of aganglionic colon, and may thus obscure the diagnosis. There is also risk of perforation of the stiff aganglionic rectum.[24] Barium contrast should be prepared with normal saline to avoid possibility of water absorption from the large surface area of dilated colon.[29] With the patient in the lateral position, barium suspension is introduced slowly by gravity drip infusion, under fluoroscopic monitoring. The infusion is stopped and restarted as serial spot radiographs are obtained. As filling progresses into the descending colon, the patient is rolled into the supine position. If the examination is positive, the diagnosis in most cases is made by the time the barium fills the proximal descending colon. Rapid infusion of barium suspension can distend and mask the transition zone. When the transition zone is observed, the examination should be discontinued because filling of the more proximal dialated bowel beyond the transition zone may lead to impaction. However, the distention of the bowel, proximal to the aganglionic segent is gradual, and a transition zone is seen in only 50% of neonates during the first week of life.[28]

The transition zone generally is funnel-shaped and it is an important diagnostic feature. In some instances, the transformation from dilated bowel to narrowed bowel is abrupt (Fig. 9.27). In other cases, the funneling of the bowel occurs incrementally over a long segment of bowel to appear almost imperceptible because of the gradual change in caliber. In long segment Hirschsprung's disease, a variable portion of the colon proximal to the sigmoid colon is aganglionic (Fig. 9.28). The pathological transition zone is usually somewhat more proximal than the radiographical one. Under fluoroscopic visualization, irregular saw-toothed mucosal pattern may be seen due to disordered contractions in the aganglionic colon (Fig. 9.29). Another radiographic appearance of Hirschsprung's disease that has been described in neonates and young infants in whom the rectosigmoid region appears normal, is the presence of straight transverse bands in the involved segment of colon. These bands are thought to represent areas of persistent spasm.[12]

The rectosigmoid index can be used in the diagnosis of Hirschsprung's disease confined to the rectum. This compares the ratio of the rectal diameter to the sigmoid diameter and is considered abnormal if the sigmoid colon is more dilated than the rectum (R/S index <1).[3]

The immediate postevacuation film may be useful in identifying the collapsed distal aganglionic segment. Delayed

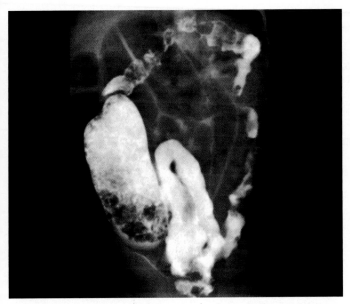

Fig. 9.28: Barium enema reveals a colon of reduced caliber from rectum to hepatic flexure with markedly dilated colon (cecum and ascending colon) proximal to it—Long segment aganglionosis

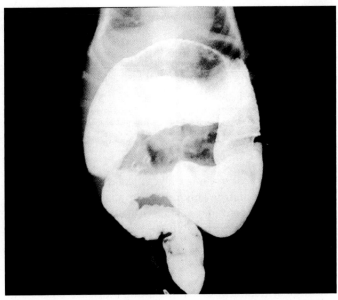

Fig. 9.29: Colonic aganglionosis with transition zone in sigmoid colon showing irregular mucosal outline/contractions

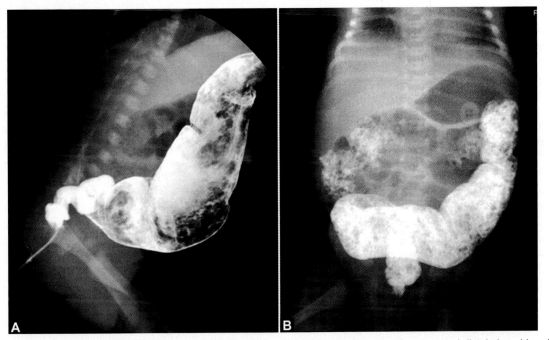

Figs 9.30A and B: (A) Short segment Hirschsprung's disease with aganglionosis of rectum and distal sigmoid and marked dilatation proximal to it. (B) 24 hours film showing significant retention of barium

radiographs taken after 24 hours may show prolonged retention of barium, which is a strong indicator of Hirschsprung's disease when enema findings have been inconclusive (Figs 9.30A and B). Other signs observed in Hirschsprung's disease is contrast media mixed with stool or a more obvious transition zone than seen on immediate films.[3]

In total colonic Hirschsprung's disease, barium enema may be non-diagnostic with no discordant sizes in the distal large bowel. A useful sign is a colon that is shortened with flexures

pulled down and rounded in appearance (question mark colon) A true microcolon appearance similar to that seen in distal ileal atresia is rare.[5]

Confirmation of Hirschsprung's disease is by means of a suction biopsy which should be taken 2 cm above the dentate line, as below this line the normal anus shows relative hypoganglionosis. Contrast enema can be safely performed 24 hours after a suction biopsy, though ideally the enema should precede a biopsy.[3]

Table 9.2: Differentiating features between small left colon syndrome and Hirschsprung's disease		
Points of difference	Small left colon syndrome	Hirschsprung's disease
1. Change in caliber/transition	Usually at splenic flexure, with proximal distended right colon and transverse colon	Transition usually more distal, most commonly at rectosigmoid
2. Type of transition	Abrupt change in caliber	Cone shaped and gradual change
3. Caliber of involved segment	Left colon is usually smaller in caliber than normal colon	Near normal caliber of aganglionic colon
4. Rectum	In most patients rectum is quite distensible	The aganglionic colon is of uniform caliber to the anus.

In equivocal cases, further investigation which may help is anorectal manometry. This relies on anal sphincter reflex relaxation in response to distention of the rectum and is absent in patients with Hirschsprung's disease.

Enterecolitis is a major cause of death in patients with Hirschsprung's disease, with enema contraindicated in these patients.

Surgical treatment of Hirschsprung's disease consists of resection of the aganglionic segment, confirmation of ganglia in the proximal bowel and reanastomosis of the bowel.

Functional Immaturity of the Colon/Neonatal Functional Colonic Obstruction

Functional immaturity of the colon is a common cause of neonatal obstruction, especially in premature babies. It comprises of several entities, most common being *small left colon syndrome* and *meconium plug syndrome*.[28] Its exact etiology is not known and it is thought to be associated with functional immaturity of the ganglion cells of the colon. The babies are frequently infants of diabetic mothers or mothers who have received magnesium sulphate for eclampsia.

Clinical Features

In general, babies with functional immaturity of the colon are not sick as compared to other babies presenting with low intestinal obstruction.[24]

Most infants present within the first 24-36 hours of life with abdominal distention, biliary emesis and failure to initiate the normal passage of meconium. This is due to transient colonic inertia with failure of normal peristalsis in a normally innervated colon.[12]

Plain radiography findings are non-specific, showing distal bowel obstruction with no gas seen in the distal colon or rectum.[3] Both the conditions causing neonatal functional colonic obstruction will be dealt separately.

Meconium Plug Syndrome

This is the most frequent cause of delayed passage of meconium in infants. Contrast enema performed is both diagnostic and therapeutic in such infants. Low osmolal contrast should be used with careful attention of hydration of the neonate.

The colon is usually of normal caliber. The meconium plug occupies the rectosigmoid region, but may extend throughout the colon. A normal evacuation pattern is established following stimulation of rectum by enema or occasionally digital examination.[3]

Meconium plug syndrome needs to be differentiated from meconium ileus. The term meconium ileus is reserved for bowel obstruction secondary to inspissated meconium in the distal small bowel and proximal colon, most often seen in patients of cystic fibrosis.[3]

Small Left Colon Syndrome

In this, the contrast enema demonstrates a distended right and transverse colon with transition to a very small diameter descending and rectosigmoid colon, occurring near the splenic flexure, with the rectum being quite distensible. Typically, there is improvement in the clinical and radiological finding over the next few hours or days. The condition may mimic Hirschsprung's disease, but there are several findings which help in differentiating the two[2] (Table 9.2).

It is important to follow the patients closely because if they have Hirschsprung's disease, they will return with intestinal problems like constipation or diarrhea.[12] At times, distinction between the two is not possible and a rectal biopsy should be performed in those children in whom the symptoms do not resolve.[24]

CONCLUSION

Imaging plays an important role in most neonatal as well as childhood developmental lesions of the gastrointestinal tract, which usually present with obstruction. The role of imaging may vary from establishment of diagnosis, evaluation of associated abnormalities, surgical planning or therapy for some conditions. Plain radiographs and contrast examinations serve as primary imaging modalities. CT and MR imaging help in more complex cases as they provide excellent anatomical detail.

Plain radiographs are often diagnostic in neonates with complete gastric and duodenal atresia and generally do not require any further radiological investigation. An upper GI contrast study should be performed in all patients presenting with incomplete intestinal obstruction. Ultrasound is useful in evaluating developmental lesions such as hypertrophic pyloric stenosis, entertic duplication cysts, midgut malrotation, meconium ileus and meconium peritonitis.[21]

It is important to be familiar with the role and usefulness of various imaging modalities so that they can be used judiciously. The aim of every radiological study is to obtain maximum possible information while avoiding unnecessary radiation exposure and minimizing patient discomfort.

REFERENCES

1. Silverman FN, Kuhn (Eds). The gastrointestinal tract. Caffey's Pediatric X-ray Diagnosis: An Integrated Imaging Approach Mosby, 1993.

2. Hernanz-Schulman M. Imaging of neonatal gastrointestinal obstruction. Radiol Clin North Am 1999; 37:1163.

3. Donohue V, Twomey EL. The neonatal and non-neonatal gastrointestinal tract. Carty H, Brunelle F, Stringer DA Kazo Simon CS (Eds): Imaging children Volume 2 Second edition. Elsevier Churchill Livingstone 2005; 1305-1528.

4. Leonidas J C, Singh SP, slovis T L. Congenital Anomalies of the Gastrointestinal tract. Kuhn Jerald P, Slovis Thomas L, Haller Jack O (Eds): In Caffey's Pediatric Diagnostic Imaging Volume 1, Tenth Edition, Mosby 2004; 113-62.

5. McAlister WH, Kronemer KA. Emergency gastrointestinal radiology of the newborn. Radiol Clin North Am 1996; 34:819.

6. Ein SH, Shandling B. Pure esophageal atresia: A 50-year review. J Pediatr Surg 1994; 29:1208.

7. Iuchtman M, Brereton RJ, Spitz L, et al. Morbidity and mortality in 46 patients with the VACTERL association. Isr J Med Sci 1992; 28:281.

8. Schlesinger AE, Parker BR. Abdomen and gastrointestinal tract. Kuhn JP Slovis TL, Haller JO (Eds): In Caffey's Pediatric Diagnostic Imaging volume 2 Tenth Edition Mosby. Section VI 2004; 1421-690.

9. Ratan SK, Varshney A, Mullick S, Saxena NC. Evaluation of neonates with esophageal atresia using chest CT Scan. Pediatr. Surg Int 2004; 20:757-61.

10. Ou P, Seror E, Layouss W, Revillon Y, Brunelle F. Definitive diagnosis and surgical planning of H- type tracheesophageal fistula in a critically ill neonate : First experience using air distension of the esophagus during high-resolution computed tomography acquisition. J Thorac Cardiovase Surg 2007; 133:1116-7.

11. Berrocal T, Torres I, Gutierrez J, Prietio C, del Hoyo ML, Lamas M. Congential Anomalies of the upper gastrointestinal tract. Radiographics 1999; 19(4):855-72.

12. Swischuk, LE. Alimentary tract. Swischurk LE (Ed) In Imaging of the Newborn, Infant and Young child, 5th edition Lippincott Williams and Wilkims 2004; 341-482.

13. Schulman MH. Infantile hypertrophic pyloric stenosis. Radiology 2003; 227:319-31.

14. Chung E. Infantile hypertrophic pylotic stenosis : genes and environment. Arch Dis Child 2008; 93:1003-4.

15. Haller JO, Cohen HL: Hypertrophic pyloric stenosis: Diagnosis using ultrasound. Radiology 1986; 161:335.

16. Hayden CK Jr, Swischuk LE, Lobe TE, et al. Ultrasound: The definitive imaging modality in pyloric stenosis. Radiographics 1984; 4:517.

17. Amodio J, Fefferman N. Ultrasound of pediatric abdominal and scrotal emergencies. Applied Radiology 2007; 36(12):22-9.

18. Blumhagen JD, Maclin L, Krauter D, et al. Sonographic diagnosis of hypertrophic pyloric stenosis. Am J Roentgenol 1988; 150:1367.

19. Hernanz-Schulman M, Sells LL, Ambrosino MM, et al. Hypertrophic pyloric stenosis in the infant without a palpable olive: Accuracy of sonographic diagnosis. Radiology 1994; 193:771.

20. O'Keeffe FN, Stansberry SD, Swischuk LE, et al. Antropyloric muscle thickness at US in infants: what is normal? Radiology 1991; 178:827.

21. Gupta AK, Guglani B. Imaging of Congenital Anomalies of the Gastrointestinal Tract. Indian J Pediatr 2005; 72(5):403-14.

22. Vaos G, Misiakos E P. Congenital Anomalies of the Gastroinestinal Tract Diagnosed in Adulthood – Diagnosis and Management J Gastrointest Surg 2010; 14:916-25.

23. Atwell JD, Levick P. Congenital hypertrophic pyloric stenosis and associated anomalies in the genitourinary tract. J Pediatr Surg 1981; 16:1029.

24. Buonomo C. Neonatal gastrointestinal emergencies. Radiol Clin North Am 1997; 35:845.

25. Bailey PV, Tracy TF, Connors RH, et al. Congenital duodenal obstruction: A 32 - year review. J Pediatr Surg 1993; 28:92.

26. Fonkalsrud E, de Lorimier A, Hays D. Congenital atresia and stenosis of the duodenum: A review compiled from the members of the surgical section of the American Academy of Pediatrics. Pediatrics 1969; 43:79.

27. Pratt A. Current concepts of the obstructing duodenal diaphragm. Radiology 1971; 100:637.

28. Berrocal T, Lamas M, Gutierrez J, Torres I, Prieto C, del Hoyo ML. Congenital Anomalies of the small Intestine, Colon and Rectum. Radiographics 1999; 19(5):1219-36.

29. Thomas KE Owens C M. The Pediatric Abdomen. Sutton D (Ed) In Textbook of Radiology and Imaging Volume 1. Seventh Edition Churchill Livingstone 2002; 849-84.

30. Macari M, Balthazar EJ. The acute right lower quadrant: CT evaluation. Radiol Clin North Am 2003; 41:1117.

31. Macpherson RI. Gastrointestinal tract duplications: Clinical, pathologic, etiologic and radiologic considerations. Radiographics 1993; 13:1063.

32. Barr LL, Hayden CK Jr, Stansberry SD, et al. Enteric duplication cysts in children: Are their ultrasonographic wall characteristics diagnostic? Pediatr Radiol 1990; 20:326.

33. O' Donnell A M, Puri. Skip segment Hirschsprung's disease: a systematic review. Pediatr Surg Int. published online 17th Aug. 2010.

CHAPTER 10

Imaging of Anorectal Anomalies

Arun Kumar Gupta

Anorectal anomalies (ARA) are rare with an incidence of approximately 1 in 5,000 births. They have a male preponderance.

Embryology of the Cloaca Related to ARA

Embryology of the cloaca can be described under internal and external cloaca.

Internal Cloaca

It is an endodermal reservoir which is in contact with the surface ectoderm at the cloacal membrane. At present, there is a general agreement that the division of internal cloaca occurs in two stages (Tourneux's method), i.e. a combination of craniocaudal extension of the urorectal septum and lateral ingrowths of the mesenchyma. Most of the ARA can be explained by this mechanism of combined division.

External Cloaca

On the other hand external cloaca refers to the partitioning of the proctodeal pit, the perineum and the genital folds. Essentially, the rectal group of ARA consists of those abnormalities which are intrinsic in the partitioning of the internal cloaca, whereas aberrations in the external cloacal division results in the anal group of malformations.

Classification

Two major classifications presently in use are the following:
1. International classification, 1970 (Table 10.1)
2. Wingspread classification, 1984 (Table 10.2)

International classification was considered by some to be too detailed and too complex. A simplified version of it was, therefore, considered and is known by the name of Wingspread classification (so called because the meeting to decide it was held at the Wingspread convention center in Racine, Wisconsin).

In the author's experience, if one is dealing with a large number of ARA in a major hospital, then use of international classification is essential. On the other hand for general teaching and occasional encounter with these patients, Wingspread classification should be adequate.

Information Required in a Patient of ARA

Four major answers, one is looking for, are the following:
1. Level of the blind terminal bowel and of any fistula, if present.
2. Levator muscle mass status.

3. Associated congenital anomalies.
4. Nerve supply status to the levator muscle group.

The last one is assessed by clinical tests while the rest are evaluated by imaging.

Clinical Clues

Males

Perineum should be carefully scrutinized for any orifice. Visible orifice suggests an anal translevator anomaly (exception—rectal atresia). External orifice may be located anywhere from the normal anal site to the tip of penis.

In the absence of a perineal orifice, level of the anomaly is difficult to predict although the majority will be rectal lesions. In these patients, urine may be examined next (after collection and not catheterization) for meconium or squamous epithelial cells. In the absence of meconium an invertogram should be done while presence of meconium in urine requires a defunctioning colostomy.

Females

Non communicating anomalies occur rarely in females. Careful examination for the site and number of orifices must be made.

If only one orifice is present, then it indicates a cloacal anomaly with a common cloaca for the urethra, vagina and rectum. Colostomy is required.

If two orifices are visible in the vulva with no anal orifice, then one of them is of the urethral, while the other one is of the vaginal orifice. Meconiun would come from the latter due to the associated recto-vaginal fistula. Colostomy is again indicated.

If three orifices are visible, then two of them are respectively, of the urethra and the vagina, both at their normal site, while the third one is the bowel which could be at the normal anal site, or it might open as a fistulous track anteriorly at an abnormal site—either in the perineum or in the vestibule.

Imaging Work-up

During the imaging of a case with ARA, one or more of a number of investigations can be carried out— invertography; contrast opacification of the urinary tract, fistula or colon; ultrasound; CT and MRI scan. All these investigations are complementary, providing information regarding different facets of the complex problem of ARA.

Table 10.1: Anorectal anomalies: international classification (1970)

Level	Male	Female

High anomalies	1. Anorectal agenesis:
	  a. Without fistula
	  b. With fistula:
	    i. Rectovesical
	    ii. Rectoprostatic urethral
	      (including H or N type)
	2. Rectal atresia
		1. Anorectal agenesis
		  a. Without fistula
		  b. With fistula:
		    i. Rectovesical
		    II. Cloacal anomalies
		    iii. Rectovaginal (high)
		2. Rectal atresia

Intermediate anomalies	1. Anal agenesis
	  a. Without fistula
	  b. With fistula:
	    i. Rectobulbar
	
	2. Anorectal stenosis
		1. Anal agenesis
		  a. Without fistula
		  b. With fistula:
		    i. Rectovaginal (low)
		    ii. Rectovestibular
		2. Anorectal stenosis

Low anomalies	1. At normal anal site:
	  a. Covered anus, complete
	  b. Anal stenosis
	2. At perineal site:
	  a. Anterior perineal anus
	  b. Anocutaneous fistula
		1. At normal anal site:
		  a. Covered anus, complete
		  b. Anal stenosis
		2. At perineal site:
		  a. Anterior perineal anus
		  b. Anocutaneous fistula
		3. At vulvar site:
		  a. Anovestibular fistula
		  b. Vulvar anus
		  c. Anovulvar anus

Table 10.2: Anorectal anomalies: Wingspread classification

Level	Male	Female

High anomalies	1. Anorectal agenesis:
	  a. Without fistula
	  b. With rectoprostatic urethral fistula
	2. Rectal atresia
		1. Anorectal agenesis:
		  a. Without fistula
		  b. With rectovaginal fistula
		2. Rectal atresia

Intermediate anomalies	1. Anal agenesis without fistula 2. Rectobulbar urethral fistula	1. Anal agenesis without fistula 2. Rectovaginal fistula 3. Rectovestibular fistula
Low anomalies	1. Anocutaneous fistula 2. Anal stenosis	1. Anovestibular fistula 2. Anocutaneous fistula 3. Anal stenosis
Cloacal malformations	Rare	Rare

Invertography

Invertography was first described by Wangensteen and Rice in 1930.[1]

Technique: Six to eight hours after the birth, a newborn baby with ARA should be held upside down for at least 3 minutes, and then a strict lateral view (in this upside down position) is taken with the thighs of the baby flexed at hip, and beam accurately centered on the greater trochanter. Anal dimple and the natal cleft should be outlined by barium paste. In a correctly taken radiograph: (i) both the ischial bones would accurately superimpose, and (ii) the terminal blind bowel will be rounded and well-distended. Interpretation of an invertogram should be attempted only, if both these features are present otherwise it may be fallacious.

Interpretation: Basic purpose of invertography is to identify the relationship of the gas bubble in the blind pouch to the bony pelvis, which in turn indicates the relation to the levator ani muscle complex. Information contained in an invertogram can be interpreted in two ways.

1. By using three lines, a concept which was first put forward by Stephens and Smith (1971).[2] The three lines are: (i) PC

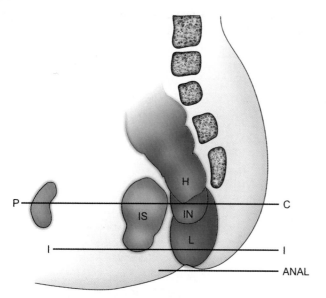

Fig. 10.1: Line drawing showing high (H), intermediate (IN) and low (L) anomalies and their relationship to PC and I lines

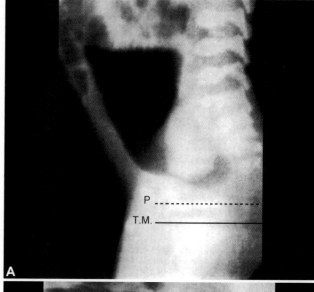

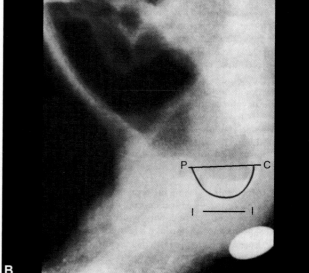

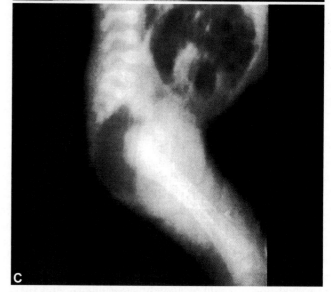

Figs 10.2A to C: Examples of high (A), intermediate (B) and low (C) anomalies on invertography

(pubococcygeal) line, (ii) the I (ischial) line or I point, and (iii) the anal pit line (Fig. 10.1). A gas bubble situated above the PC line is designated "high" anomaly, one located between the PC and I line or point "Intermediate" anomaly and if it extends below the I line (point), then it is called "low" anomaly (Figs 10.2A to C).

2. However, Cremin (1971)[3] did not find PC line very accurate. They proposed a "M line" or "M point", which is located at the junction of upper two-third and lower one-third of the ischium (Figs 10.2A to C). Anomalies are then divided into "high" and "low" types with no intermediate category.

Accuracy of invertography to differentiate supralevator (gas bubble above the I line or point) and infralevator lesions (gas bubble below the I line or point) has been reported to range from 60 to 87 percent. One must be aware of the potential pitfalls of this technique in order to avoid misdiagnosis. Some of the common reasons are listed below:

1. Insufficient time for the gas to reach the terminal bowel.
2. Meconium blocking the terminal segment.
3. In a crying child, puborectalis sling may move significantly up or down giving erroneous results.
4. Gas may escape through a fistula.
5. Improper technique—in positioning, centering or marker placement.

Besides the conventional upside down invertography described above, two more methods have been described to obtain the same information. They are as follows:

1. Prone cross table lateral view (Narasimharao et al, 1983).[4]
2. CT invertography (Leighton and de Campo, 1989).[5]

During the reading of an invertogram, besides evaluating the level of bowel gas, one should also look for the following:

1. *Spine* Congenital anomalies of the spine are common.
2. Presence of gas in the region of urinary bladder and vagina, which would indicate an underlying fistula.

Contrast Studies

Purpose of any contrast study is:
    i. To confirm the level of blind bowel pouch, and
    ii. To document the presence (or absence) and level of the fistula between the GI (gastrointestinal) and the GU (genitourinary) system.

Contrast Studies in Males

1. *Retrograde urethrography (RGU)/micturating cysto-urethrography (MCU)*: Prior to or even after the colostomy, RGU is a good technique to demonstrate the fistula. If negative, then RGU is followed by MCU in the same sitting to demonstrate the possible fistula.
2. *Distal cologram*: Once colostomy has already been done, then distal cologram, in the author's experience, is a reliable technique to demonstrate the fistula. Fluoroscopy with image intensifier, use of water-soluble contrast media and raising the intraluminal pressure in the distal colon to fill the fistula more consistently are some of the prerequisites in this technique. In a case with colostomy, distal cologram should be done first, and only if it is negative in demonstrating the fistula, then RGU/MCU should be done in the same sitting.

   Sometimes the fistula is not documented inpite of all the efforts but on RGU, an acute backward angulation of the posterior urethra and on colography an anteroinferior "beaking" of the blind rectal pouch is seen (Figs 10.3A and B)—these findings suggest the presence of fistula or adhesion.
3. *Direct catheterization*: If a patient has a cutaneous fistula, then direct catheterization and retrograde injection of contrast into the fistula should be carried out. However, urethra and bladder should be first outlined with a catheter (filled with radiopaque contrast) *in situ*.

ARA IN MALES

These are discussed under high, intermediate and low anomalies.

High Anomalies

In these patients, the imperforate bowel or its fistulous connection lies above the puborectalis sling of the levator ani muscle. Various types described under this group are the following:

Anorectal Agenesis without Fistula

Anorectal agenesis without fistula is uncommon. Invertography and contrast studies would show the blind rectal pouch lying at or cranial to the PC line with no suggestion or demonstration of a fistula.

Anorectal Agenesis with Rectoprostatic Urethral Fistula

Anorectal agenesis with rectoprostatic urethral fistula is the most common type in this group. Most common site of fistulous opening is at the level of the verumontanum, but rarely it may open either more cranially closer to the bladder neck or more distally just above the bulb (Figs 10.4A and B).

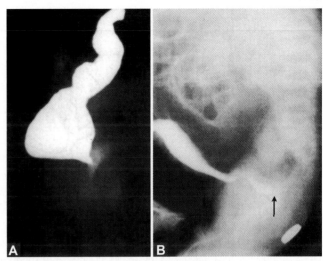

Figs 10.3A and B: "Beaking" from anteroinferior angle of blind rectal pouch on colography (A) and "acute backward angulation" (arrows) of posterior urethra on RGU (retrograde urethrography) (B) without actually filling the fistula, indicating presence of underlying fistula or adhesion

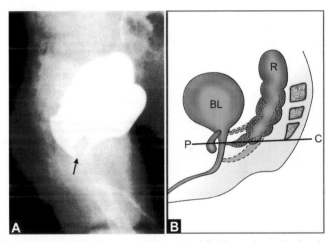

Figs 10.4A and B: Rectoprostatic urethral fistula—schematic drawing (A) and a case (B). As indicated by dotted lines fistula may enter either more cranial or distal to verumontanum (arrow—fistula)

H or N Type of Rectoprostatic Urethral Fistula

H or N type of rectoprostatic urethral fistula is extremely rare. This entity was not even described in the original International classification. There is a H or N-shaped fistulous connection between the prostatic urethra and the anterior wall of the rectum just cranial to the valves. Characteristically, urethra distal to the site of fistula is usually stenotic (Figs 10.5A and B).

Rectovesical Fistula

Rectovesical fistula is also rare. Fistulous tract usually enters close to the bladder base. During contrast injection into the distal colon via colostomy site, urinary bladder would fill first (Figs 10.6A and B) without opacifying the urethra, thereby, excluding a urethral fistula. This sequence of events must be carefully monitored and specifically looked for real time on the image intensifier. It is very

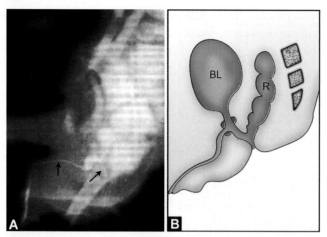

Figs 10.5A and B: H or N fistula is extremely rare—note the patent anal canal and the microcaliber of the penile urethra (arrowhead—fistula, arrow—narrow penile urethra)

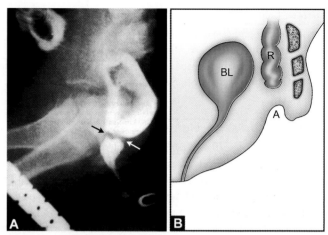

Figs 10.7A and B: Rectal atresia—opacification was done from both ends of the site of atresia. One cm metallic scale helps in accurately measuring the distance of atretic bowel (arrows—atretic segment)

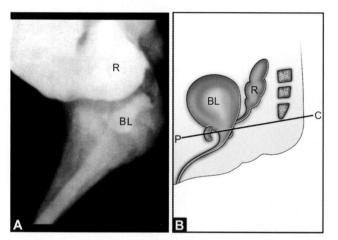

Figs 10.6A and B: Rectovesical fistula—another rare type filling on distal colography—note the filling of urinary bladder immediately after opacification of the rectum (arrowhead—fistula)

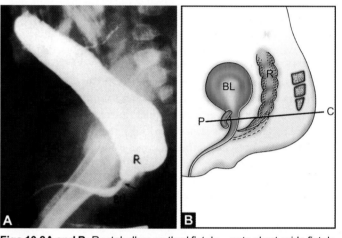

Figs 10.8A and B: Rectobulbar urethral fistula—note short, wide fistula entering directly into the posterior wall of bulb of urethra. Other variety is long and narrow which enters into the under surface of penile urethra

important to differentiate this type of fistula from the rare more cranially located rectoprostatic urethral fistula by the observations described above.

Rectal Atresia

It is a rare and an unusual condition. In these patients, the terminal bowel ends blindly at varying levels. Anus and the anal canal are normal and the bowel in between these two segments is deficient (either a short membranous or a long, string-like) (Fig. 10.7A). Its etiopathogenesis is believed to be a vascular insult after the formation of a normal rectum. Complete documentation in such cases require contrast injection from both ends (i.e. distal cologram + anal canal opacification) simultaneously (Fig. 10.7B).

Intermediate Anomalies

Intermediate anomalies are termed so due to a complex relationship to puborectalis muscle. Thus, the blind terminal bowel is lying on (i.e. above) the puborectalis sling muscle, a feature of "high" anomalies, but the fistulous track when present is within or through the sling, a criterion for diagnosing "low" anomalies. Thus, features of both the "high" and the "low" anomalies are present in this group of anomalies.

Anal Agenesis without Fistula

Invertography and distal cologram would reveal the blind bowel pouch to lie between the PC line and the I point without demonstrating a fistula.

Anal Agenesis with Rectobulbar Urethral Fistula

Two types are described (Fig. 10.8A)—either the fistula is short, wide and enters the posterior surface of the bulb directly (Fig. 10.8B), or it is long, thin, passing distally within the cavernous tissues of the penis in midline to enter on the undersurface of the urethra.

Anorectal Stenosis

Anorectal stenosis is rare. It is generally agreed that "anal stenosis" should be classified under the low anomalies while stenosis

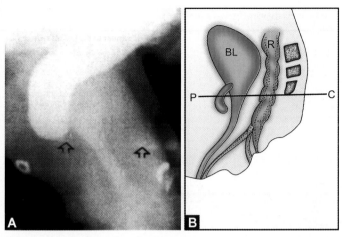

Figs 10.9A and B: Rectocutaneous fistula (arrowheads)—fistula, as shown in schematic drawing, can open anywhere from near the anal opening to the tip of penis

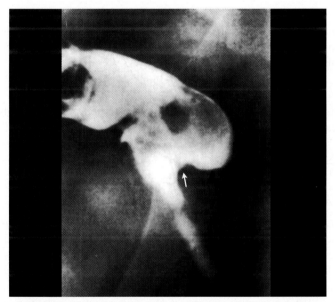

Fig. 10.10: Anterior perineal anus demonstrated on barium enema—note removal of cannula and posterior shelf (arrowheads)

occurring up to 4 cm within the anus are more appropriate to be termed "anorectal stenosis". Mechanism of its formation is postulated to be ischemic and is thus similar to rectal atresia described earlier.

Low Anomalies

These are essentially "anal deformities". Various types are listed below:

1. Anocutaneous fistula (covered anus, incomplete)
2. Anterior perineal anus
3. Covered anal stenosis
4. Anal membrane stenosis
5. Covered anus, complete
6. Imperforate anal membrane

The entire group of low anomalies can be readily appreciated on the clinical examination itself, and imaging is usually not indicated. First two subtypes are briefly described below.

Anocutaneous Fistula

In this condition, the anal canal is of normal caliber till the level of anal valves beyond which it is suddenly reduced to a tube of small caliber and runs forward covered by skin to open anywhere from the ventral surface of the penile shaft to an area adjacent to the anal site (Figs 10.9A and B). Although fistulogram is not necessary, but if required it can be readily carried out.

Anterior Perineal Anus

In this condition, anus is normal in appearance but is located more anteriorly than the normal site close to the posterior or membranous urethra. This is an important differential in the list of causes of constipation in children. On per rectal examination, "posterior shelf"—a characteristic finding of this condition might be felt which can also be demonstrated on barium enema examination (Fig. 10.10). Cannula may distort the anal anatomy due to sheer mechanical pressure. Therefore, the catheter/cannula should be removed before the film is taken in strict lateral view at the time of barium defecation.

ARA IN FEMALES

Anorectal anomalies are divided into high, intermediate and low types.

High Anomalies

Anorectal Agenesis without Fistula

Anorectal agenesis without fistula is rare and is similar to that seen in males, i.e. the blind terminal bowel lies above the PC line without any fistula.

Anorectal Agenesis with High Rectovaginal Fistula (Without a Urogenital Sinus Defect)

The vagina, urinary bladder and urethra are normal. Rectal fistula enters the posterior (dorsal) wall of the vagina (Fig. 10.11A). Rectovaginal fistulae have been classified as "high" or "low" depending on the level of the terminal bowel, and these terms do not refer to the level of entry of fistula into the vagina.

Vaginogram or distal cologram following colostomy would readily demonstrate these fistulae (Fig. 10.11B).

Cloacal Anomalies

This is a very large and one of the the most complex group of anomalies which is beyond the scope of this text. In these anomalies, there is only a single orifice for the urethra, vagina and rectum. A large number of subtypes based on the internal anatomy have been described. Retrograde injection of contrast through the external orifice as well as colography would delineate the internal anatomy (Figs 10.12A and B). Some of the most severe forms may present immediately after birth with acute respiratory distress due to a hugely dilated vagina.

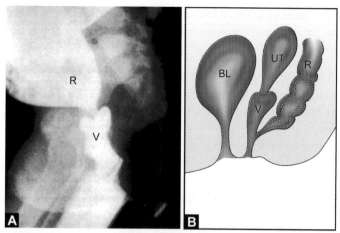

Figs 10.11A and B: Rectovaginal fistula demonstrated on vaginogram. Difference in "high" and "low" rectovaginal fistulae lies in the level of blind bowel pouch and not on the site of entry of fistula into the vagina (R—rectum, V—vagina, BL—bladder, UT—Uterus)

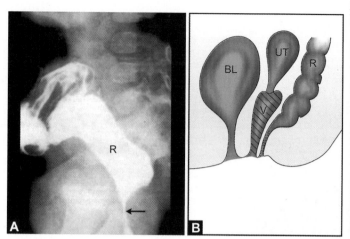

Figs 10.13A and B: Rectovestibular fistula—demonstrated on retro-grade contrast injection—note the long, narrow fistulous track (arrow)

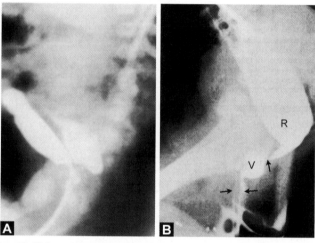

Figs 10.12A and B: Cloacal anomalies—two different cases:(A) retro-grade injection showing urethra and rectum only with absent vagina, and (B) One of the variants in which common channel leading into urethra and vagina (arrows) while rectum opening into the vagina (arrowheads)

Rectovesical Fistula

Rectovesical fistula is extremely rare in females. On documentation the appearance is similar to that seen in males.

Rectal Atresia

Rectal atresia is similar to the lesions seen in males.

Intermediate Anomalies

Anal Agenesis without Fistula

Anal agenesis without fistula is easy to diagnose by inverted plain films of the abdomen specially taken in lateral views.

Rectovestibular Fistula

From the anterior wall of the rectum arises a fistula which opens in the vestibule. Usually, it is thin and long (more than 1 cm)

(Fig. 10.13A). Diagnosis is evident on clinical examination by noting three orifices in the vestibule and combining it with a gentle probe test. Retrograde injection of contrast would readily opacify the fistula and the rectum (Fig. 10.13B).

Low Rectovaginal Fistula

Low rectovaginal fistula is very rare. Its difference from the high type has already been discussed earlier.

Low Anomalies

These are again designated as "anal deformities".

Anovestibular Fistula

Like rectovestibular fistula, it opens in the vestibule. However, its length is very short (less than 1 cm) and well formed anal canal extends quite low down close to the skin at the anal site (Fig. 10.14). A probe would pass not only upwards parallel to the vagina, but to some extent, it can be turned posteriorly just beneath the perineum. The latter maneuver cannot be achieved in rectovestibular fistula. Contrast study, if at all done, demonstrates the anatomy clearly.

Anocutaneous Fistula/Anterior Perineal Anus

Anocutaneous fistula/anterior perineal anus is similar to those observed in males.

Anal Stenosis

Anal stenosis is similar to the lesions in males.

Investigations

As the first step, a careful and detailed clinical examination is absolutely essential. This may provide a number of clues pointing to a specific type of the anomaly. This has been discussed earlier.

Invertography: Its role is similar to that described earlier in males.

Contrast studies: Non communicating anomalies are rare in females. Communication of the bowel may be either to the

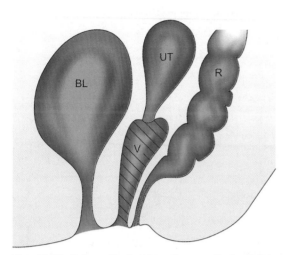

Fig. 10.14: Schematic drawing of anovestibular fistula

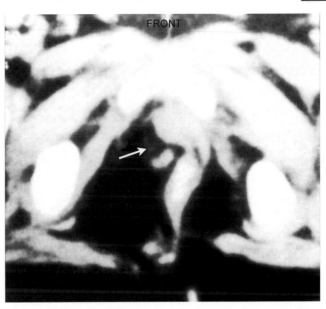

Fig. 10.16: Pelvic CT, postoperative—fat has been drawn along with the neorectum (arrow) which was the cause of incontinence

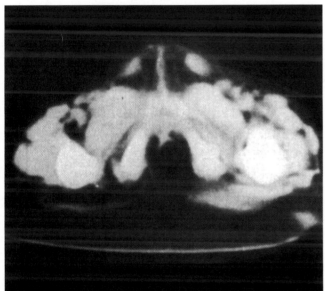

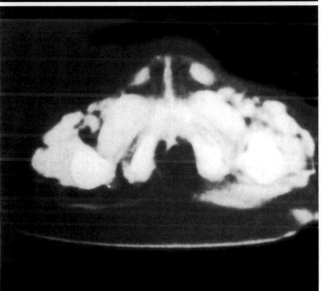

Figs 10.15A and B: Pelvic CT, preoperative—puborectalis sling and external anal sphincter are very poorly formed

exterior and, therefore, visible as an abnormal orifice or internally into one of the pelvic viscus. Contrast studies can be carried out to demonstrate both the types.

Other Investigations

Besides the invertography and the conventional contrast studies, other newer imaging modalities have also an important role to play prior to as well as after the surgery.

Ultrasound

In spite of being an ideal imaging modality in the pediatric age group, i.e. its painless, requires no, contrast or sedation and without ionizing radiation—yet ultrasound has still not been established as a reliable technique. Reason is obvious—high incidence of fallacies and operator dependence. However, probably ultrasound still has potential in this clinical problem, and one should explore it before deciding its fate. It is, however, routinely used in screening the abdomen for the detection of congenital malformations, especially of the upper urinary tracts.

CT Scan

CT has established an important place in the work-up of ARA. It is used preoperatively to demonstrate the thickness of muscles (puborectalis sling and external anal sphincter) (Figs 10.15A and B).

In the postoperative period, it demonstrates the relationship of the pulled-through bowel (neorectum) to the above muscles (i.e. whether neorectum is central, eccentric or even outside the sling) and any evidence of fat drawn into the sling (Fig. 10.16)—all of these may be the reason for the incontinence in the postoperative period.

MRI Scan

With the introduction of MRI, not only has the visualization of the sphincter muscles become easy and better, but they can also

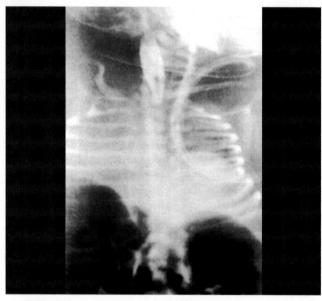

Fig. 10.17A: Associated anomalies—esophageal atresia

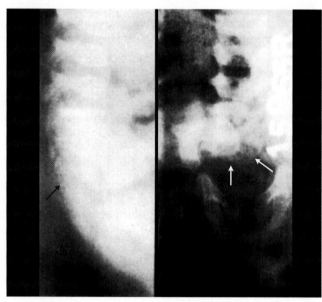

Fig. 10.17B: Associated anomalies—gross spinal abnormalities (partial agenesis of sacrum arrows)

be seen in multiple planes (axial, coronal and sagittal)—thereby allowing better understanding of the relationship of the bowel with the muscles. MRI has a tremendous potential in demonstrating the pelvic muscle anatomy with a very high degree of sensitivity and is used for obtaining the same information for which CT is otherwise used.

Relationship of Sacral Development and Levator Muscle Development

In order to determine the levator muscle mass prior to surgery, CT and MRI are routinely used. However, if these modalities are not

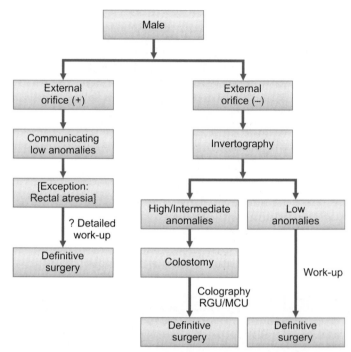

Fig. 10.18: Diagnostic algorithm in a male ARA (anorectal anomalies)

available, then a good indicator is the development of the sacrum as seen on plain radiographs. It has been observed that:

i. If sacrum is normal then muscle mass and innervation are also normal;

ii. If S4, S5 are absent then muscle and innervation are usually still normal;

iii. If S3–S5 are absent then there is variable degree of deficiency of the muscle mass, and patient is usually incontinent;

iv. If S1–S5 are absent then muscles are markedly hypo-plastic, and all the patients are incontinent.

Associated Anomalies

ARA are frequently associated with other congenital anomalies. Its incidence varies from 20 to 70 percent depending upon the efforts put in to find the anomalies. Almost any system may be affected, but the spine, genitourinary, gastrointestinal and the cardiac systems are more frequently affected (Figs 10.17A and B). Supralevator, i.e. high and intermediate anomalies are much more likely to have the associated anomalies than the infralevator lesions.

Diagnostic Algorithm

Diagnostic algorithms in a new case of ARA are shown in (Figs 10.18 and 10.19) for male and female respectively. A combination of the clinical findings and the information provided by invertography are used to make the crucial decision on day 1.

Anorectal anomalies are rare complex congenital malformations which need a teamwork between the pediatrician, pediatric

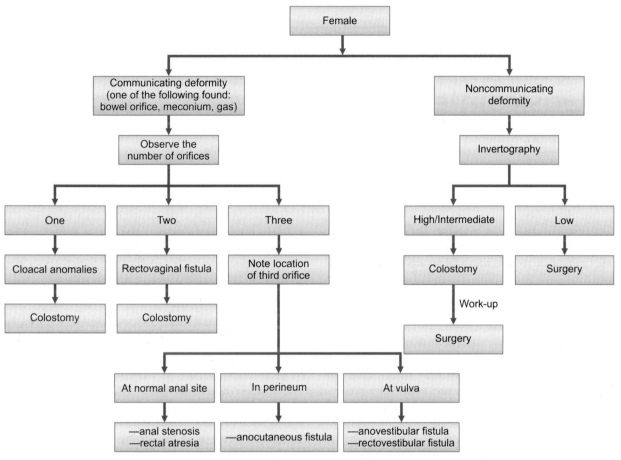

Fig. 10.19: Diagnostic algorithm in a female ARA (anorectal anomalies)

surgeon and the pediatric radiologist with an aim to deliver the best possible management, utilizing the available investigations and resources in a planned and judicious manner.

REFERENCES

1. Wangensteen OH, Rice CO. Imperforate anus—a method of determining the surgical approach. Ann surg 1930; 92:77.
2. Stephens FD, Smith ED. Anorectal Malformations in Children Chicago: Year Book Medical Publishers, 1971.
3. Cremin BJ. The radiological assessment of anorectal anomalies. Clin Radiol 1971; 22:239.
4. Narasimharao K, Prasad G, Katariya S et al. Prone cross table lateral view—an alternative to the invertogram in imperforate anus. AJR 1983; 140:227–29.
5. Leighton DM, de Campo M. CT invertograms. Pediatr Radiol 1989; 19:176–78.
6. Willital GH. Advances in the diagnosis of anal and rectal atresia by ultrasonic echo examination. JPS 1971; 6:454–57.
7. Schuster SR, Teele RL. An analysis of ultrasound scanning as guide in determination of "high" or "low" imperforate anus. JPS 1979; 14:798–800.
8. Oppenheimer DA, Carroll BA, Schuchat SJ. Sonography of imperforate anus. Radiology 1983; 148:127–28.
9. Ikawa H, Yokoyama J, Sanbonmatsu T. The use of computerized tomography to evaluate anorectal anomalies. JPS 1985; 20:640–44.
10. Kohda E, Fujioka M, Ikawa H et al. Congenital anorectal anomaly—CT evaluation. Radiology 1985; 157:349–52.
11. Silverman F (Ed). Caffey's Pediatric X-Ray Diagnosis (8th ed) Chicago: Year Book Medical Publishers 1985; 2:1863–73.
12. Harris RD, Nyberg DA, Mack LA et al. Anorectal atre-sia—prenatal sonographic diagnosis. AJR 1987; 149:395–400.
13. Sato Y, Pringle KC, Bergman RA et al. Congenital anorectal anomalies—MR imaging. Radiology 1988; 168:157.
14. Stephens FD, Smith ED, Paul NW. Anorectal malformations in children—update 1988. Birth Defects 1988; 24(4).
15. Taccone A, Martucciello G, Fondelli P et al. CT of anorectal malformation—a postoperative evaluation. Pediatr Radiol 1989; 19:375–78.
16. Vade A, Reyes H, Wilbur A et al. Anorectal sphincter after rectal pull-through surgery for anorectal anomalies—MRI evaluation. Pediatr Radiol 1989; 19:179–83.
17. Arnbjornsson E, Laurin S, Mikaelssan C. CT of anorectal anomalies—correlation between radiologic findings and clinical evaluation of fecal incontinence. Acta Radiol 1989; 30:25–28.

CHAPTER 11

Gastrointestinal Masses in Children

Arun Kumar Gupta

The diagnostic evaluation of a gastrointestinal tract (GIT) mass in an infant or child is a challenging problem. The role of diagnostic imaging is to identify the precise location, the organ of origin and the extent of pathologic process with a minimal number of imaging procedures.

GIT masses in children include:
- Masses arising from the GIT, i.e. esophagus to rectum
- Mesenteric and omental masses.

Clinically, the patient may present with either a **palpable** abdominal lump as in hypertrophic pyloric stenosis, large GIT tumors, mesenteric masses or the mass may be clinically **non-palpable,** e.g. gastrointestinal polyps and these latter group of patients may present with other abdominal symptoms like abdominal pain, distension, bleeding or occasionally with the symptoms related to the mass effect on other organs.

Imaging modalities available for the evaluation of GIT masses in children are:
- Plain radiographs
- Contrast studies
- Ultrasonography (US)
- Computed tomography (CT)
- Magnetic resonance imaging (MRI)
- Angiography

The presenting symptoms of a patient govern to a large extent, the type of initial investigation performed. Thus, in a child with an abdominal lump, US is the initial investigation of choice whereas in patients presenting with nonspecific abdominal symptoms without a palpable abdominal mass, an abdominal radiograph or contrast study may be done initially.

PLAIN RADIOGRAPHS

Plain radiographs do not have any significant role in the diagnostic evaluation of patients with GIT masses. However in certain clinical situations, where a patient presents with atypical features, plain radiographs may be obtained to exclude an acute process such as small bowel obstruction and bowel perforation. Also in masses with calcification, e.g. teratoma, plain radiographs are diagnostic.[1]

CONTRAST STUDIES

Clinical circumstances of the patient determine which contrast study to be performed and in what fashion. Over the years, with advancements in the imaging technology and increasing experience with newer modalities, the diagnostic algorithms have changed dramatically in most diseases. The role of barium studies in the evaluation of GIT masses in children has declined significantly in most situations except for conditions like polyposis where they continue to be the initial investigation of choice.

ULTRASONOGRAPHY

US is the screening modality of choice in a child suspected to have an intra-abdominal mass.[2] It is quick, easy to perform, rarely requires sedation, requires no patient preparation and is non-ionizing. Lack of intra-abdominal fat in infants and children allows better visualization of intra-abdominal structures when compared with adults. It can yield information about intraperitoneal fluid, presence and location of mass, nature of mass, i.e. whether cystic or solid, presence or absence of adenopathy, etc.

COMPUTED TOMOGRAPHY

CT is an extremely accurate and fast imaging modality, and is playing an increasing role in the radiological evaluation of GIT masses in children. It can provide information about the bowel wall, mesentery, lymph node status, peritoneum, omentum and solid organs. It is useful in assessing the extent of mass lesion. Optimal and uniform opacification of bowel loops is required along with intravenous contrast in a dose of 2 ml/kg. Short sedation may be required especially in children between 4 months to 4 years of age. Relative disadvantage of CT is the radiation exposure. Spiral CT further decreases the scan time and allows the use of 3D reconstruction algorithms.

MAGNETIC RESONANCE IMAGING

MR imaging offers exquisite soft tissue resolution, excellent delineation of vascular structures, multiplanar ability, absence of ionizing radiation but because of expense, limited availability, motion artifacts from bowel peristalsis and frequent need for sedation, it is usually reserved only for equivocal cases. Also the total scan time is considerably longer than in CT and claustrophobia is a real issue in paediatric patients. MR compatible anaesthesia equipment is another important requirement.

ESOPHAGEAL MASSES IN CHILDREN

In general, the appearance of the normal esophagus in infants and children is similar to that in adults, except for the following variations:

- Air is more often noted in the esophagus in neonates and children than in adults and is a normal finding due to aerophagia from feeding or crying.
- In children <5 years of age, thoracic esophagus may lie slightly to the right of the spine. This variation must be borne in mind in these young patients so that the esophagus is not mistaken for adenopathy.

Masses arising from the esophagus are very rare in children. They can be broadly classified into:

- Congenital
- Neoplastic

Congenital Masses

Esophageal duplication cysts[3] occur most commonly in the distal third of esophagus. Duplication cyst (DC) is a spherical/tubular structure that is lined by alimentary tract epithelium, has smooth muscle in its wall, and is usually attached to the GI tract. They share a common muscular wall and blood supply with the adjacent bowel. Ectopic gastric mucosa can be seen in all locations of enteric duplication cysts but is most common in esophageal duplications where autodigestion of pulmonary tissue can lead to massive hemoptysis.

Clinical Presentation

- Patient may be asymptomatic and DC is diagnosed incidentally on a chest radiograph
- Dysphagia or dyspnea may be present due to compression of the esophagus or tracheobronchial tree, respectively, especially if located in upper 2/3rd of esophagus.
- Rarely, *pain* from peptic ulceration or *hemoptysis* if the cyst ruptures into the tracheobronchial tree, may be the presenting features.

Associated anomalies include gastric duplication and partial pericardial absence.

Imaging Features

Plain radiograph: A well-defined posterior mediastinal mass with displacement of the trachea/bronchus may be seen depending upon the site and size of mass.

Barium swallow: Extrinsic compression of the esophagus by the mass may be appreciated.

US: Using a high frequency transducer through posterior chest wall an esophageal DC located in the posterior mediastinum and abutting the posterior chest wall can be diagnosed based on the wall characteristics.

The cyst is typically anechoic, but the presence of echogenic contents represents either hemorrhage or inspissated secretions.

CT and MRI are helpful in demonstrating the relationship of the cyst to the surrounding structures. DC appears as a homogeneous, round, sharply outlined, fluid filled mass located adjacent to the esophagus. If mucoid material or calcium is present within, then higher attenuation values of the fluid will be noted.

Technetium 99m pertechnetate scan confirms the presence of ectopic gastric mucosa within the DC.

Neuroenteric cysts arise due to incomplete separation of foregut from the notochord. They can have residual communication with the spinal canal either via a sinus tract or a fibrous band. They contain both the GI and neural elements in the wall. Radiographic appearance is similar to that of enteric duplication cyst except for the presence of associated vertebral anomalies.

Presence of dorsal vertebral anomalies in association with a posterior mediastinal mass on a frontal chest radiograph (Fig. 11.1) in a child suggests the diagnosis of neuroenteric cyst.[3,4] MRI can help to delineate the associated intraspinal anomalies.

Neoplasms

Primary esophageal tumors are extremely rare in children. Most of those that do occur are benign tumors like leiomyoma, neurofibroma, fibroma, hemangiomas and polyps. Of the malignant esophageal tumors, secondary tumors, especially lymphomas and rarely metastasis are more likely to affect children than a primary neoplasm.

Esophageal lymphomas account for <1 percent of total GIT lymphomas in children.

GASTRIC MASSES IN CHILDREN

Gastric masses can be broadly classified into:

- *Congenital:* Duplication cyst
- *Acquired outlet obstruction of stomach:* Hypertrophic pyloric stenosis
- *Neoplasms:* Both benign and malignant.
- *Miscellaneous:* Bezoars

Significant differences occur in the radiographic appearance and investigation of gastric masses in younger children as compared with adults:

- Distended, air-filled stomach is commonly seen in normal infants because they swallow a large amount of air while crying/feeding.

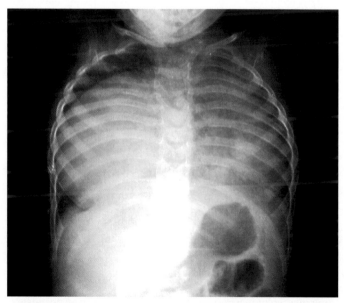

Fig. 11.1: Neuroenteric cyst, Frontal chest radiograph: Large right posterior mediastinal mass with congenital dorsal vertebral anomalies

- Because ulcers and mucosal diseases are relatively rare in children, single contrast barium studies are usually more helpful than double contrast studies.
- In single contrast studies, gastric emptying may normally be slow in infancy, and this should not be confused as indicative of hypertrophic pyloric stenosis.

Congenital

Gastric duplication cysts are rare accounting for only 3.8 percent of all gastrointestinal duplications. A female preponderance has been noted. Duplication cysts usually occur in the antral region along its greater curvature.[4,5] Gastric DC may have associated multiple duplications in the bowel.

Clinical Presentation

Gastric DC usually presents in early infancy with one or more of the following:
- Vomiting, fever, pain, anemia. Vomiting may be related to partial or complete small bowel or pyloric obstruction. Larger cysts may also be palpable clinically.
- Complications such as perforation, hemorrhage, fistula from ulceration due to aberrant pancreatic or gastric tissue may be present.

Imaging Features

Barium studies: In its typical location along the greater curvature gastric DC impinges on the stomach causing its upward displacement while in the late films of the same follow through study transverse colon is displaced downwards. This combination of gastric and colonic displacements in the same study is reported to be a specific finding in an appropriate clinical setting.

Ultrasonography: Gastric DC are typically anechoic on US but the presence of echogenic contents represents either hemorrhage or inspissated secretions.

Due to its location gastric DC may simulate pseudopancreatic cyst on US but a more specific diagnosis can usually be made using a high frequency, usually linear, transducer probe by observing the characteristic appearance of bowel wall, i.e. echogenic mucosal stripe surrounded by hypoechoic line of muscle wall.

US is usually more than sufficient to diagnose cystic duplication.

Computed tomography: On CT scan DC is seen as a fluid filled mass with an enhancing well defined rim or wall.

Acquired Outlet Obstruction of Stomach

Hypertrophic pyloric stenosis (HPS) is the most common cause of gastric outlet obstruction in infants. There is hypertrophy and hyperplasia of the circular muscle of pylorus with thickening and lengthening of pylorus gradually progressing to gastric outlet obstruction.[4]

Etiology

Etiology is unknown but several mechanisms have been postulated, two important ones are:

- Abnormal nerve cells of myenteric plexus. Electron microscope studies have disproved this hypothesis.
- Hyperacidity causing prolonged pylorospasm leading to muscle hypertrophy.

Clinical Presentation

Typically, the child presents at 3 weeks of age with nonbilious, projectile vomiting. There is a male predominance with a ratio of 4:1. Usually, the baby is well at birth and vomiting begins at 2nd to 3rd week of life with progression from regurgitation to projectile vomiting after every feed. On clinical examination a lump (olive) may be palpable in the epigastrium in about 80 percent of cases. Exaggerated peristaltic wave may be seen travelling from LUQ across the epigastrium. Presentation before 1st week and after 3 months of age is rare.

Diagnosis of classical HPS is based on clinical history and finding of a hypertrophied mass on abdominal palpation.

For confirmation of clinical findings nowadays ultrasonography is the modality of choice. Only in equivocal cases barium study should be done.

Imaging Features

Plain radiograph if done, may show increased gastric distention with air and little amount of small bowel or colonic air.

US[6-12]

Technique
- A high frequency linear transducer probe (7-10 MHz) should be used.
- Child is positioned in supine or RPO position.
- Adequate amount of gastric fluid is essential to provide the ultrasonic window and identification of anatomical structures. By placing a nasogastric tube and filling of saline through it keeps the whole procedure under control.
- On transverse section, the upper pole of right kidney is identified and the transducer is moved towards the xiphoid process. When pyloric canal is located, the transducer is angled to align it to the long axis of pyloric canal. *The lumen of pylorus is always a straight line in HPS in the longitudinal plane.* This is important because scanning in tangential plane can produce false positive results.

Findings on US
- Thickness of muscle is the most sensitive and specific measurement. It is measured from the outer edge of echogenic mucosa to the outer edge of muscle on both longitudinal and transverse scan and these measurements should be in close agreement. Normal wall thickness of pyloric canal is <2 mm. Earlier workers had proposed that thickness >4 mm is abnormal but recently it has been agreed that the critical value should be decreased and presently if pyloric wall thickness is >3 mm then it is considered abnormal (Fig. 11.2A).
- Total pyloric canal length (TPL) is more variable than muscle thickness. Length >17 mm is considered abnormal, whereas

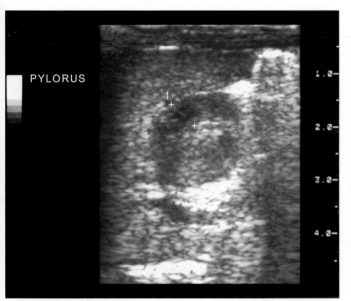

Fig. 11.2A: Hypertrophic pyloric stenosis (HPS): Ultrasonography, transverse view shows significant wall thickening of the pyloric canal

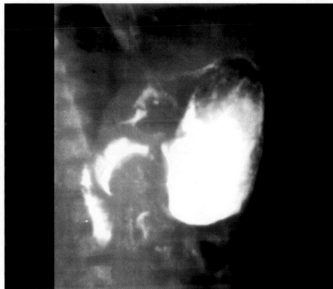

Fig. 11.2B: Hypertrophic pyloric stenosis (HPS): Barium UGI study: Pyloric canal is narrow and elongated. Note indentations on the duodenal cap and the antrum by the hypertrophied muscle. Gastric emptying is delayed

<14 mm is felt to be unequivocally normal. However, diagnosis should not be made on pyloric canal length alone.

Increase in wall thickness and TPL are the two main diagnostic features.

Other findings which may be present are:

- "Empty cervix sign": Hypertrophic muscle mass indents the duodenal bulb and bulges into the antrum, an appearance resembling that of empty cervix.
- "Mucosal nipple sign": Redundant pyloric mucosa may protrude into the antrum.
- Hyperperistalsis of stomach with failure of gastric contents to pass into the duodenum.
- Overdistended, fluid filled stomach and also the squared off rather than rounded configuration of the end of stomach can provide indirect clues to the diagnosis of HPS.

Barium Study[4]

It is always advisable to put a nasogastric tube so that gastric filling with barium is better. Findings could be:

- Delayed gastric emptying.
- Elongated and narrowed pyloric canal — "string sign". This is one of the most important finding for diagnosis of HPS on barium study (Fig. 11.2B).
- "Double track" of barium may be seen if the hypertrophied muscle squeezes the lumen into separate compartments.
- Indentation of the gastric antrum and duodenal bulb producing "shoulder sign"
- "Beak sign" is produced as the barium column enters the narrowed pylorus.
- Hyperperistaltic waves seen stopping at the pylorus.

Diagnosis of HPS cannot be based only on delayed gastric emptying because delay could be due to pylorospasm and gastritis as well.

After the completion of the barium study residual barium should be drained via the nasogastric tube before tube removal in order to prevent aspiration of barium into the lungs.

Treatment

Ramstedt pyloromyotomy Postoperatively the normal gastric emptying is usually resumed within 2-3 days. Muscle thickness may remain abnormal on US for up to 6 weeks. Most important is to assess the gastric emptying in postoperative period preferably with barium.

HPS is not an emergency. *False positive diagnosis must be avoided. Since HPS is a progressive disease* borderline cases must be re-examined in a day or two to avoid unnecessary surgeries.

NEOPLASTIC MASSES

These could be **benign** or **malignant.**

Benign Masses[4,13]

Polyps may be present in isolation or may be associated with several polyposis syndromes like Peutz-Jeghers, juvenile polyposis syndromes as well as familial polyposis coli. They are commonly hamartomatous polyps. Barium upper gastrointestinal study readily detects these as well circumscribed filling defects that interrupt the normal mucosal pattern.

Benign gastric tumors are rare in children. They are usually derived from mesenchymal tissue. Two relatively common masses are teratoma and leiomyoma.

Gastric Teratoma[1,4,14,15]

Stomach is a rare site for development of teratoma. They have a benign clinical course. These usually occur in infants <1 year of age. A strong male preponderance is observed. Most common site is along the greater curvature.

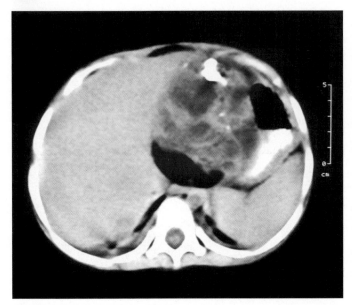

Fig. 11.3: Gastric teratoma, CT abdomen: A heterogeneous mass with areas of calcification is seen in the lesser omentum displacing the stomach down and outwards

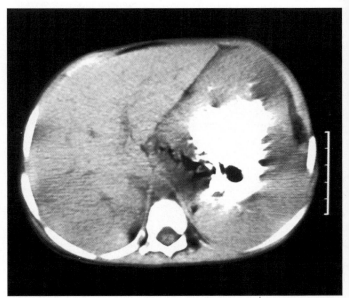

Fig. 11.4: Ossified gastric leiomyoma. NCCT abdomen shows a densely ossified mass in the epigastrium. Note extension of gas into the center of the mass from its medial side. Tumor had communication with the gastric lumen

Clinical presentation: They are often large in size and presents as a palpable abdominal mass. GI bleeding and proximal GIT obstruction may be the other presenting features.

Imaging features: On both US and CT a large solid mass with areas of cystic component is seen in the epigastric region, usually along the greater curvature. Calcification is seen in nearly half the cases (Fig. 11.3). Abdominal radiographs would show an epigastric soft tissue mass with areas of calcification.

Gastric Leiomyoma[4,16-19]

Gastric leiomyomas are extremely rare in children.

Imaging features: Barium is a smooth, rounded, well-circumscribed filling defect in the stomach with or without central ulceration may be seen on barium study.

CT: A homogeneous soft tissue mass with uniform contrast enhancement is seen on CT. Very large myomas may contain necrotic areas. CT provides excellent delineation of exophytic component of the mass which is otherwise difficult to assess on barium studies. Calcification is uncommon. A rare case of ossified leiomyoma (Fig. 11.4) has also been reported.[16]

Other benign tumors are teratoma, leiomyoma, lipoma,[20] fibroma, neurogenic tumor, hemangiomas.

Malignant Gastric Tumors

Adenocarcinoma of Stomach

Adenocarcinoma of stomach is a disease of adults but cases have occasionally been reported in children.[21] Clinical presentation is as a chronic gastric ulcer. Detection is usually late (Fig. 11.5) and is associated with a poor prognosis. Endoscopy should therefore be undertaken in any patient with persistent chronic gastric ulcer symptoms.

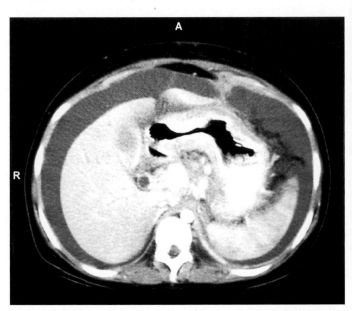

Fig. 11.5: Gastric adenocarcinoma. CT shows significant thickening of gastric walls with luminal narrowing and ascites

Gastric Lymphoma

Gastric lymphoma is the most common malignancy of stomach in children.[4,22-24] Stomach is the second most common site of primary GIT lymphomas in children after ileum. This is in contrast with adults where stomach is the commonest site of primary GIT lymphomas and accounts for approximately 80 percent of all cases.

Clinical presentation: Patient may present with abdominal pain, abdominal mass, weight loss.

Imaging features: Barium studies may show an intraluminal mass with ulceration, fold thickening, or narrowing of lumen.

CT usually demonstrates gastric wall thickening with smoothly lobulated outer border. CT is particularly valuable in the diagnosis of gastric lymphoma since the disease originates in the submucosa and endoscopic biopsy may yield limited information especially in early stages.

Gastric Leiomyosarcoma

Gastric leiomyosarcoma is an exceedingly rare condition.[17] It is usually seen in children <1 year of age but can occur at any age. *Carneys triad* has been described, i.e. gastric leiomyosarcoma, pulmonary chondromas and extraadrenal paraganglioma. It usually affects young females with an average age of 19 years. Mortality rate is almost 20 percent mostly due to paraganglioma.

Gastric Gastrointestinal Stromal Tumors (GISTs)

GIST are a subset of GI mesenchymal tumors. About 60-70 percent of total GIST occur in the stomach.[27] Histologically and on imaging they resemble leiomyoma group. However for definitive diagnosis presence of CD34 and CD117 is essential.[25-27] About 10-30 percent are malignant but majority are benign.[27] Factors indicating higher probability of malignancy are: extraintestinal location, size more than 5 cm, central necrosis, extension into adjacent organs and presence of metastases.[27]

BEZOARS[4,28]

A bezoar is a mass of ingested, non-opaque foreign material in the stomach. At one time they were mainly a problem of older children and for most part were trichobezoars (hair) and phytobezoars (vegetable matter). Recently, lactobezoars have become common especially in premature infants, due to the formation of dense milk coagulum when powdered milk is mixed with inadequate quantities of water.

Trichobezoars is the most common and is due to chronic hair swallowing by mentally disturbed children especially young females. Over a period of time an intraluminal mass develops representing matted hair, trapped food particles and air taking the shape of stomach. It may extend into the duodenum and even small bowel.

Clinical Presentation

Patient may present with a mass or with history of gastric outlet obstruction. A palpable mass in the LUQ or epigastrium is common. Limited mobility is typically seen in smaller masses. Complications like gastric outlet obstruction, perforation, hemorrhage and ulceration may also be cause for presentation.

Imaging Features

Plain abdominal radiograph may show a mottled epigastric mass often rimmed by gas. This can mimic food residue. Therefore, it is important to know when the child ate last and a delayed fasting film can sort out problem cases.

Barium studies: Bezoar produces a filling defect. After the free barium has been expelled from the stomach, barium that has adhered to the surface of the bezoar forms a mottled shadow of increased density. Delayed films may show extension of the bezoar into the duodenum or jejunum.

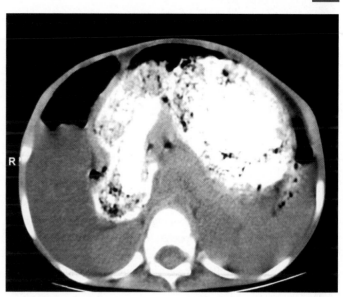

Fig. 11.6: Gastric bezoar. CT with oral contrast demonstrates a heterogeneous mass filling and distending the gastric and duodenal lumens (also jejunal in lower sections). Pockets of air and positive contrast are trapped within the mass

On US a curved broad band of increased echogenicity is seen with distal acoustic shadowing produced by air inside and around the bezoar. No details of the mass can be appreciated.

On CT an intragastric mass with entrapped air, debris and contrast is seen (Fig. 11.6).

Lactobezoars usually disappear after formula adjustment and increased water intake.

Tricho and phytobezoars require surgical removal to prevent complications.

SMALL BOWEL MASSES IN CHILDREN

Masses can be classified into:
• *Congenital:* Enteric duplication cysts.
• *Infectious:* Abdominal Koch's
• *Neoplastic:* Both benign and malignant
• *Miscellaneous:* Intussusception, intramural hematoma.

Congenital

Enteric Duplication Cyst[4,29-32]

Embryologically DC arise from abnormalities of development, separation and recanalization of primitive foregut during the late first or early second trimester. Spherical duplications usually do not communicate with the GIT while the much less common tubular type frequently does communicate. Although they can occur anywhere in the GI tract, the most common site is the distal ileum followed by esophagus. Approximately 40 percent of the patients present by first month of age while 85 percent present during the first year of life.

Duodenal duplication cysts are rare. They may present with gastric outlet obstruction and on imaging can mimic pseudopancreatic cyst. Ileal DC lie on the mesenteric border of normal small bowel and their muscular wall is often intimately attached to the muscular wall of the normal bowel. Therefore, surgical removal is often impossible without resecting the adjacent loop of bowel. Very rarely, persistent fibrous connection to the spinal cord can exist. In such cases anterior vertebral body segmentation anomalies can be seen. Most are solitary, but they can be multiple. Transdiaphragmatic extension into chest has been reported.

Clinical presentation: Patient may present with abdominal pain, abdominal mass, vomiting or abdominal distention secondary to intestinal obstruction. Presence of ectopic gastric or pancreatic mucosa may result in complications such as bleeding or perforation.

Imaging features: US is the modality of choice in the initial examination of any child suspected to have DC. It shows a well-defined, usually unilocular, cystic anechoic mass. The characteristic appearance of bowel wall showing "rim-sign" with echogenic inner-rim of mucosa surrounded by a relatively hypoechoic layer representing gut muscle is diagnostic (Fig. 11.7). Unfortunately, not all duplication cysts have this sign either because the mucosal layer has been enzymatically destroyed or the duplication is tubular and communicating type and so is not always fluid filled. Also, rimming may be seen in any cyst where bleeding occurs and fibrin is deposited along the cyst wall, most often in the ovarian cyst. ^{99m}Tc pertecheatate scan then becomes useful since ectopic gut mucosa usually takes up ^{99m}Tc pertecheatate. Another interesting finding of duplication cyst is the presence of peristalsis in the cyst wall which may be appreciated in real time scanning.

CT would show a cystic mass with sharp, enhancing wall.

Differential diagnosis includes mesenteric cyst, omental cyst, ovarian cyst, choledochal cyst and pancreatic pseudocyst.

Infection

Abdominal tuberculosis, particularly involving the *ileocecal* region and *tubercular peritonitis* can present as an abdominal mass in children.[4,33-35]

In ileocecal TB, the ileocecal (IC) valve may be so thick that it mimics a mass in the RIF. The patient may present with nonspecific complaints and a RIF mass and both CT and US would demonstrate adherent bowel loops, gross bowel wall thickening, thickened mesentery and large regional nodes producing a soft tissue mass centered around the IC junction. Barium may demonstrate contracted, coned, irregular cecum; gaping, incontinent IC valve; narrowed, rigid terminal ileum; matted, fixed bowel loops with or without strictures.

Loculated ascites, as may be seen with tuberculous peritonitis (*wet form*), may present as an abdominal mass in children. It may contain septations, debris. US appearance of loculated ascites can mimic mesenteric or omental cyst.

In the d*ry form of* tuberculous peritonitis, bowel, omentum or mesentery may be clumped together (Fig. 11.8) due to multiple caseous nodules on the surface and adhesions, often becoming palpable and may present as a mass. On US a very characteristic "Swiss-Cheese" appearance is noted.

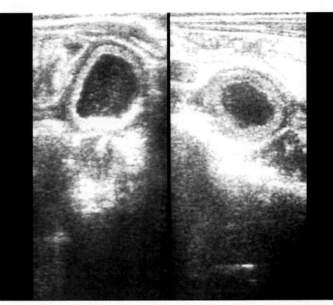

Fig. 11.7: Duplication cyst. Ultrasonography shows the typical wall characteristics of duplication cyst

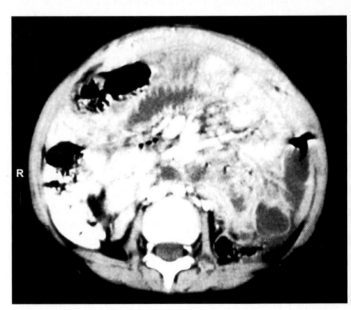

Fig. 11.8: Abdominal tuberculosis. On CECT abdomen matted bowel loops, mesenteric nodes and small pockets of fluid are seen

NEOPLASTIC MASSES

Neoplastic masses could be benign or malignant.

Benign

Benign small bowel tumors,[4,36] which include hemangiomas,[37] lipomas, leiomyomas (Fig. 11.9), neurofibromas and fibromas are rare in children.

Polyps of small bowel are usually seen in association with polyposis syndromes especially Peutz-Jeghers and juvenile gastrointestinal polyposis.

Clinical presentation: Patient may be asymptomatic and detection is incidental. Most common clinical presentation is

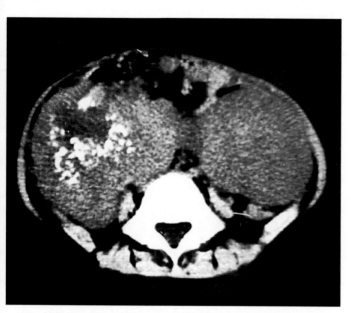

Fig. 11.9: Small bowel leiomyoma. NCCT abdomen shows a large bilobed soft tissue mass with areas of calcification

crampy abdominal pain and bloody stools due to recurrent entero-enteric intussusception.

Imaging features: If the presentation is not acute, the polypoidal mass or masses are readily identified in most cases as filling defects on barium follow through. If the condition presents as intussusception, the lead point may be seen as a polypoidal mass on barium meal follow through studies.

Malignant Small Bowel Masses

Malignant masses of the small bowel include lymphoma, adenocarcinoma, leiomyosarcomas and carcinoid. Of these, lymphoma is the commonest tumor. All the benign tumors have their malignant counterparts. Also patients with polyposis syndromes can develop GI malignancies.

Small Bowel Lymphoma[4,17,23,38]

Although relatively rare in childhood *lymphomas constitute the most common small bowel malignancy in children.* Those under 8 years of age are at greatest risk. Burkitt lymphomas, which has a strong male predominance, is the commonest type of lymphoma.

In children, GI lymphomas account for 19 percent of total lymphomas and *majority occur in ileum* followed by stomach and jejunum. This is in contrast with adults in whom primary GI lymphomas occur in only 4-12 percent cases and the most common site is stomach.

Clinical presentation: Nausea, vomiting, abdominal pain, altered bowel habits, GI bleeding, small bowel obstruction, a palpable abdominal mass or features of intussusception are some of the features with which a patient may present. Approximately *25 percent patients present with intussusception. Burkitt lymphoma is the most common lead point in children of > 4 years of age presenting with ileocolic intussusception.*

Imaging features: The investigations performed would depend upon the clinical presentation. Plain abdominal radiograph is usually nonspecific and may be normal, show a soft tissue mass or may show features of intussusception with small bowel obstruction.

Barium meal follow through (BaMFT) may be the initial investigation performed if the patient presents with unusual abdominal pain or features of subacute intestinal obstruction. BaMFT may demonstrate a stricture, mass or features of intussusception. Findings are similar to that seen in adult lymphomas and six radiological patterns have been described on barium: Aneurysmal (Fig. 11.10A), nodular, ulcerative, constrictive, mesenteric and sprue patterns.

The appearance on BaMFT may mimic Crohn's disease or tuberculosis and differentiation may be difficult based only on imaging.

If there is a suspicion of an abdominal mass, then US is the most appropriate initial imaging study. On US an atypical target is seen, i.e. a hypoechoic mass due to bowel wall thickening, usually in the RIF, with a central irregular echogenic area due to the bowel lumen (Fig. 11.10B). Also, enlarged nodes and ascites may be frequently seen.

CT is crucial to demonstrate the full extent of the mass and any associated lesions.

CT findings include one or more of the following:
- Marked bowel wall thickening
- Luminal narrowing
- Aneurysmal dilatation (Fig. 11.10C)
- Bulky mesenteric and RP nodal masses with loop separation
- Intussusception
- Small bowel obstruction.
- Omental, mesenteric, peritoneal dissemination.

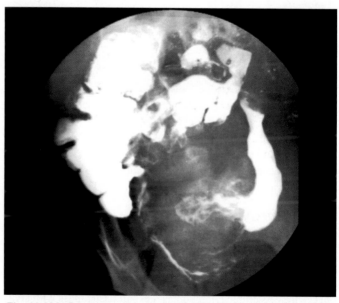

Fig. 11.10A: Small bowel lymphoma: BaMFT shows dilated bowel with irregular outline, narrow lumen and significant wall thickening

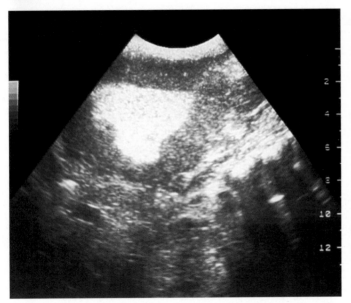

Fig. 11.10B: Small bowel lymphoma: US—aneurysmal dilatation of affected bowel loop with marked thickening of wall

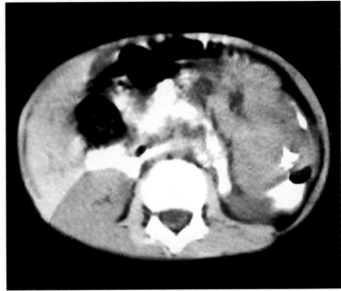

Fig. 11.11: Small bowel leiomyosarcoma. On CT a soft tissue mass on the left side of abdomen with a contrast opacified bowel loop located eccentrically

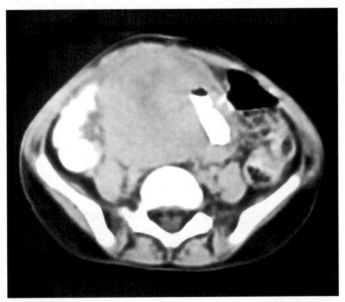

Fig. 11.10C: Small bowel lymphoma: CT with oral contrast: A large soft tissue mass with a contrast containing bowel within it

- Ascites and pleural effusion
- Renal, hepatic, splenic and pancreatic lesions
- Calcification, uncommon in untreated cases.

Leiomyosarcomas[36]

Leiomyosarcomas can also rarely occur in small bowel especially in <1 year age group. Most commonly they present with small bowel obstruction, perforation, intussusception, bleeding, and anemia. Obstruction in a newborn can cause meconium peritonitis. On CT they resemble leiomyomas, i.e. soft tissue mass with areas of necrosis (Fig. 11.11) and may be even calcification. Intestinal leiomyosarcomas in children are smaller at diagnosis than in adults

and majority are resectable and have a slightly better prognosis. Metastases have been reported in regional lymph nodes, lung, liver, bone.

GIST[27]

These tumors are similar to those in stomach. Small bowel GIST account for 20-30 percent of total cases.[27] Large mass with areas of necrosis are common CT findings.

Adenocarcinoma

Adenocarcinoma of the small bowel is extremely rare in children. Most cases occur in the second decade. *Clinical presentation* may be nonspecific and includes nausea, vomiting, small bowel obstruction. On *barium follow through* study tumor is seen as a short segment narrowing (Fig. 11.12), an appearance which may simulate tubercular stricture of small bowel.

Generally, the prognosis is poorer than in adults because of late diagnosis since symptoms are nonspecific and there is a low index of suspicion.

Intussusception

Intussusception is the prolapse of one portion of bowel into the other. The segment of intestine that prolapses is called the *intussusceptum* while the receiving segment is the *intussuscipiens*.[4] Ileocolic intussusception is most commonly seen (90%) in children. Ileoileocolic, colocolic and ileoileal intussusceptions are rarer. It commonly affects children < 2 years of age and is more frequent in boys.

Unlike in adults where majority of intussusception are due to pedunculated polypoidal tumor (80%, mostly lipoma), in children only 5 percent cases are due to identifiable lead points such as Meckel's diverticulum, duplication cysts, lymphoma, polyps,

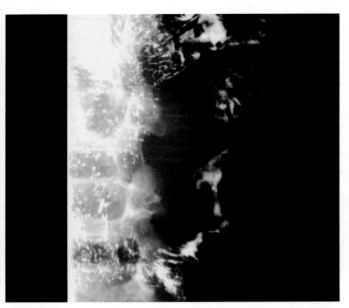

Fig. 11.12: Small bowel adenocarcinoma. BaMFT shows marked degree of narrowing, irregularity and loss of normal fold pattern in a segment of small bowel

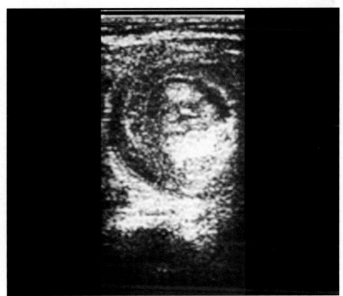

Fig. 11.13A: Intussusception: US transverse view demonstrates concentric ring pattern. Note the characteristic eccentric echogenic mesenteric fat

hematoma. Lead points are more frequent in children less than 1 month or more than 4 years of age where approximately 50 percent of cases may be caused by lead points.

Clinical Presentation

The classical triad of abdominal pain, currant jelly stools and palpable abdominal mass is seen in <50 percent cases. Diagnosis may be difficult and delay may be life-threatening due to bowel necrosis and complications. Therefore, imaging modalities play a vital role in diagnosing or excluding intussusception.

Imaging Features

Although US is the initial investigation of choice, plain abdominal radiograph[39] and barium enema may be done in equivocal cases during the course of evaluation.

Ultrasound features are:[40-42]

- A mass with either an atypical target or a concentric ring appearance in transverse section (Fig. 11.13A) and sandwich/pseudokidney appearance in sagittal plane.
- Since any condition causing bowel wall thickening, e.g. inflammation, edema, hematoma, etc. may mimic intussusception on US, an extremely useful differentiating sonographic feature is the characteristic appearance of *eccentric, semilunar, echogenic mesenteric fat* on transverse section that is pulled along with the vessels and lymph nodes into the intussusception.
- US may be able to depict lead point and detect other intraabdominal lesions unrelated to intussusception.
- On color Doppler imaging absence of blood flow might indicate the presence of ischemia or necrosis and that vigorous attempts at reduction in such patients should be avoided.

Plain radiographs: If done might show:[39]

- Soft-tissue mass in the region of cecum or transverse colon with meniscus sign (due to the presence of rim of gas around the intussusceptum).
- Absence of caecal gas or stool.
- Features of small bowel obstruction.

The sensitivity of plain abdominal radiographs in diagnosing intussusception is low. *The best positive predictor is the presence of a soft tissue mass in the abdomen and the absence of cecal gas even in prone position. The only way to exclude intussusception is the presence of cecal gas.* However, misidentification of air can lead to false negative results.

Diagnostic barium enema had been the gold standard for the diagnosis till mid 80's when it was realized that sonography could be highly accurate in the diagnosis of intussusception. Since about 50 percent of patients with clinical suspicion of intussusception turn out to be normal on barium enema, US rather than barium enema should be done initially in all patients with suspected intussusception. When used appropriately, a negative US obviates unnecessary diagnostic enemas and the use of enema can be limited to therapeutic purpose only. On a diagnostic barium enema study an intussusception is seen as a convex intraluminal filling defect (Fig. 11.13B). Coiled spring appearance may be produced as the contrast insinuates between the intussusceptum and the intussuscipiens.

Reduction can be attempted using either dilute barium/water soluble contrast (hydrostatic) or more recently using air (pneumatic) each under either fluoroscopic or US guidance.[43-46]

Procedure for reduction using barium enema:

- Hydration status and vitals should be checked, an intravenous line should be established, procedure is explained to the parents and their written consent is obtained.

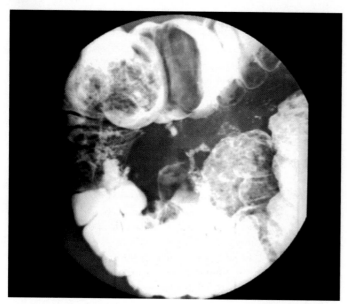

Fig. 11.13B: Intussusception: Barium enema shows a filling defect due to intussusceptum head in the proximal transverse colon

- Anal opening is occluded using an appropriate sized Foley's catheter.
- 25 percent w/v barium or a diluted (1:3 or 1:4) water soluble contrast is used, latter is preferred in young infants with long duration of symptoms.
- Rule of three's is followed, i.e.
  - Reservoir is kept at 3 ft high from the table (5 ft in case of water soluble contrast)
  - Reduction attempt is maintained for 3 minutes
  - A maximum of 3 attempts are made.

For air enema reduction pressure between 85 and 120 mm Hg is safe.

Successful reduction is marked by free flow of contrast into the terminal ileum with disappearance of soft tissue mass.

Some workers prefer air enema under fluoroscopy than barium reduction because it is quicker, easy, less messy and exposes patient to lower amount of radiation. Recent studies have shown that US with saline reduction is safe with comparable results. Pneumatic reduction under US guidance has been tried and might have fewer complications but is much more cumbersome.

The only contraindications to enema reduction are clinical features of *peritonitis, shock*[43] and radiological features *of perforation.*

Relatively lower rates of successful reduction are obtained in the following situations:
- Symptoms for >24 hours
- Presence of associated small bowel obstruction or rectal bleeding
- Presence of lead points
- Position of intussusceptum, e.g. those located distally are more difficult to reduce
- Ileoileal and ileoileocolic types are more difficult to reduce.
- US appearance of an atypical target indicating more tight intussusception is less likely to be reduced than one with

concentric ring appearance suggesting a more loose type of intussusception, though this criteria is not considered reliable now.

Major complication of enema reduction is perforation. Perforation rates in both hydrostatic and pneumatic reduction are comparable and is <1 percent, provided air pressures are not exceeded and proper technique is followed.

Increased risk of perforation is noted in infants <6 months of age, >36 hours duration of onset and absent flow on color Doppler imaging.

There is 5-10 percent recurrence rate after successful hydrostatic or pneumatic reduction. Most recur within 72 hours. Children with recurrent intussusception appear to be *no more* likely to have a lead point than those with single episode.

MESENTERIC MASSES IN CHILDREN

Mesenteric masses[47-49] may be classified as:
- Cystic
- Neoplastic

Mesenteric cysts, omental cysts and lymphangiomas are believed to be different manifestations of a common problem, i.e. malformation of lymphatic system in which the lymphatic vessels of the mesentery fail to establish communication with the central lymphatic system resulting in the formation of large masses with dilated fluid filled lymphatic spaces. They may adhere to the adjacent organs but do not invade them. Rarely, they may be associated with lymphatic malformation elsewhere.

Clinical Presentation

Most of these patients present in the first few years of life but rarely in the newborn period. Presenting features include:
- Abdominal distension, pain, abdominal mass or features of small bowel obstruction.
- Rarely, diffuse lymphangiomas may extend via patent processus vaginalis and present as an inguinal hernia
- Diffuse lymphangiomas can produce protein losing enteropathy.

Imaging Features

Plain radiograph may show a soft tissue mass displacing the gas filled bowel loops. Mesenteric mass would displace the bowel loops around it while an omental mass would displace the bowel loops posteriorly (Fig. 11.14). Features of small bowel obstruction may also be seen.

US features include:
- Cystic anechoic mass which is usually unilocular but may show fine septations. Presence of echoes within suggest blood, chyle or purulent material.
- Mesenteric and omental cysts are solitary and occasionally multiloculated, whereas abdominal lymphangiomas are more widespread and multicystic.
- Mesenteric cysts are usually mobile and changes shape.

CT: On CT a large, thin walled cystic, sometimes multiseptate, mass is seen which displaces the bowel loops posteriorly (Fig. 11.15). Mural calcification is rare.

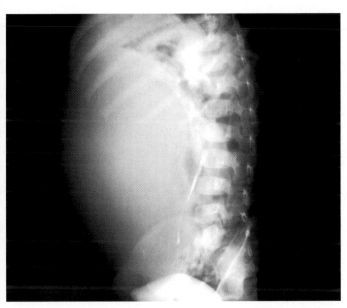

Fig. 11.14: Lateral view of an excretory urography shows a large omental mass displacing the bowel loops posteriorly

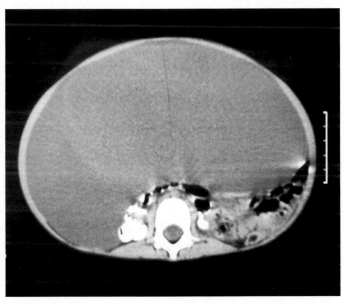

Fig. 11.15: Omental cyst on a CT displaces the bowel loops posteriorly around the spine

MRI: Cyst may have signal intensity ranging from fluid (low on T1W and high on T2W) to fat (high on T1W) depending upon the content of fluid.

Differential Diagnosis

Includes loculated ascites, fluid filled viscus (pseudoascites), ovarian cyst, cystic teratoma and duplication cyst.

Mesenteric and Omental Tumors

Most common neoplasms involving the mesentery are *lymphomas* (usually in the disseminated form) and *metastasis*.

Lymphoma: NHL is more common than Hodgkin's disease. It is usually associated with retroperitoneal lymphadenopathy.

Metastasis may appear on CT as discrete rounded or cake like masses, ill-defined masses or simply as mesenteric fat streakiness.

Primary omental and mesenteric neoplasms are rare and include fibromas, neurofibromas (Figs 11.16A and B), lipomas, lipoblastomas, desmoid, yolk sac tumor.

Fibroma: Is the most common primary mesenteric neoplasm. It appears solid, homogeneous on CT.

Lipomas are well-defined homogeneous mass of fat attenuation (Fig. 11.17).

Lipoblastoma is a heterogeneous mass with soft tissue attenuation areas within a focal fatty mass.

Desmoid tumor occurs typically in post colectomy patients with Gardener syndrome.

Yolk sac tumor is highly malignant. It is the most common gonadal tumor occurring in childhood. Occasionally, however they can arise in mesentery and can appear on CT as well-defined heterogeneous solid mass with low attenuation areas within.

Intraperitoneal teratoma are usually cystic. Identification of multi-tissue origin especially when fat and calcification are seen, can lead to the correct diagnosis.

Cystic mesothelioma is a rare primary neoplasm of peritoneal cavity, seen most commonly in adult females but may occasionally be seen in children. It has a predilection for surface of pelvic viscera.

COLONIC MASSES IN CHILDREN

Colonic masses can also be classified as:
- Congenital
- Inflammatory
- Neoplastic

Congenital

Duplication Cysts[50]

Colonic duplication cysts are much less frequent than in small bowel but if they are large then they can produce mass effect or obstruction of the bowel. Urinary tract obstruction due to pressure on the urinary bladder by rectal duplication cyst has been observed. Ectopic gastric or pancreatic mucosa can cause ulceration, bleeding and perforation. They may be spherical but in about 50 percent of cases it is tubular.

Inflammatory Mass

Appendicular Lump[51]

Appendicitis is reported to be a common cause for abdominal surgery in children in the west. Early diagnosis is important because morbidity increases after appendix perforation. History and examination are often atypical. Up to approximately 25 percent of patients are found to have normal appendix at surgery. Therefore, imaging plays an important role to eliminate negative surgery.

Perforation can lead to generalised peritonitis but a local abscess adjacent to appendix is more likely because perforation is usually contained by the omentum. And in such cases patient may present with lump in RLQ. US is the investigation of choice.

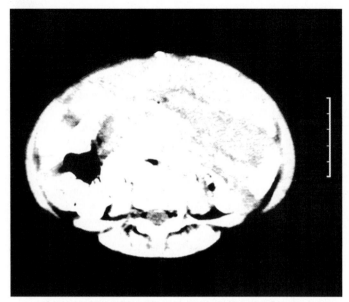

Fig. 11.16A: Mesenteric neurofibroma: CT shows a diffuse relatively homogeneous soft tissue mass in the mesentery

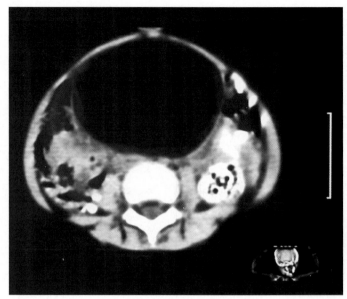

Fig. 11.17: Mesenteric lipoma. On CT a large fat attenuating mesenteric mass is seen

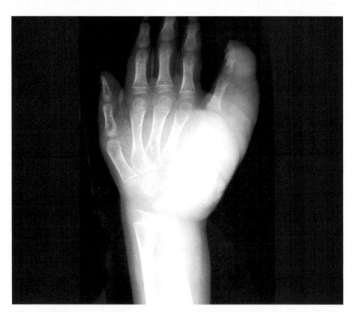

Fig. 11.16B: Mesenteric neurofibroma: Right hand radiograph—a large neurofibromatosis mass on the ulnar side

US: It may show variable findings:

- A mass of mixed echogenicity in RLQ with periappendiceal fluid or intraperitoneal fluid
- Inflamed appendix may be seen as a tubular aperistaltic, noncompressible, blind ending structure with total diameter >6 mm.
- Appendicolith may be seen as an echogenic lesion with an acoustic shadowing (Fig. 11.18A)
- Appendiceal abscess is seen as a hypoechoic mass in the RLQ (Fig. 11.18B) and its extension into the cul-de-sac occurs frequently forming a hypoechoic mass between the bladder and the rectum.

Plain abdominal radiograph: A number of findings may be seen

- Mass effect on the caecum
- Thickened caecal wall
- Air-fluid level in the terminal ileum and caecum.
- Loss of obturator internus fat plane.
- Appendicolith: calcified concretions in the appendix are seen in about 5-10 percent of cases on plain radiograph.

Identification of appendicolith in a child with acute abdominal pain is diagnostic of appendicitis and atleast 50 percent of such patients have perforation, abscess or both.

CT due to its superior soft tissue contrast is more sensitive than US for diagnosis of abscess (Fig. 11.18C).

Neoplasms

Most large bowel tumors in children are benign, i.e. juvenile polyps.[4] Less common causes include hereditary polyposis syndrome and primary colonic malignancy.

Benign Colonic Neoplasms

Isolated juvenile polyp: This is the most common tumor of colon in children between 4-6 years of age. Some consider it inflammatory, others describe them as hamartomatous. These are not true neoplasms. They can be single or multiple and are most commonly (75-85%) located in the rectum or sigmoid region but they can occur anywhere in the colon. They are rarely seen in neonates.

They usually present with bleeding per rectum. Occasionally, there may be anemia, mucoid diarrhea or colocolic intussusception.

Polyposis syndromes: A number of syndromes have been described with multiple colonic polyps (Fig. 11.19). Peutz-Jeghers, Gardner's, Generalized juvenile polyposis syndrome, familial adenomatous colonic polyposis syndrome and Turcot syndrome.

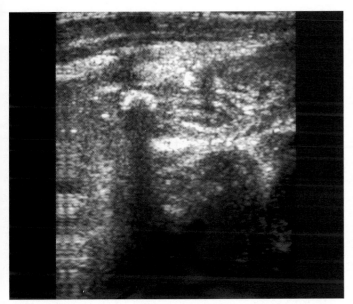

Fig. 11.18A: Acute appendicitis: Longitudinal US in RIF: A dilate, thick walled appendix with an appendicolith producing acoustic shadowing

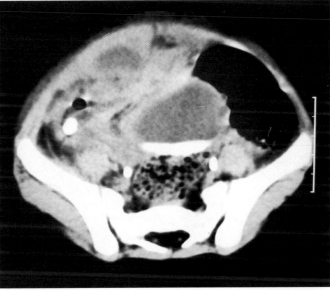

Fig. 11.18C: Acute appendicitis: CECT pelvis: A large appendicular abscess extending to involve the urinary bladder and anterior abdominal walls

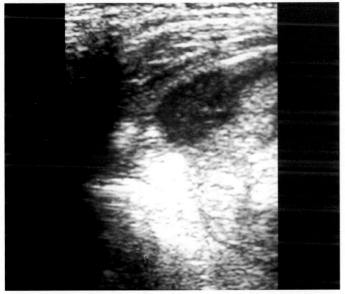

Fig. 11.18B: Acute appendicitis: Transverse US RIF shows a focal hypoechoic mass due to an appendicular abscess

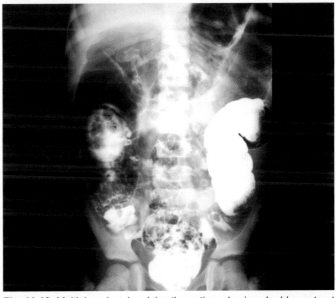

Fig. 11.19: Multiple polyps involving the entire colon in a double contrast barium enema

Malignant Colonic Neoplasm[52,53]

Adenocarcinoma of colon are uncommon in childhood. Most occur in the colon and rectum, usually in the second decade. No sex predilection is observed. In young infants a colonic tumor is more likely to be leiomyoma, leiomyosarcoma and other sarcomas than adenocarcinoma. Predisposing conditions are seen in only about 9-12 percent of cases and includes FAP, Gardner's syndrome, ulcerative colitis, cystic fibrosis.

Clinical features include abdominal pain, nausea, vomiting, diarrhoea, weight loss, GI bleed and obstructive symptoms. In children, the diagnosis of colorectal carcinoma has a much poorer prognosis than in adults for several reasons:

- Because of nonspecific clinical features and a low index of suspicion patients usually present at an advanced stage at the time of diagnosis. About 70 to 90 percent already have local, nodal or metastatic spread at the time of diagnosis compared with 40 percent in adults.
- Aggressive histological subtype: Approximately 50 percent are aggressive mucinous adenocarcinomas as compared to 5 percent in adults.

Imaging: Appearance is similar to that in adults (Figs 11.20 and 11.21).

Plain films are either normal or show features of intestinal obstruction. Mucinous tumors may show areas of punctate calcification at the primary site and also in the metastatic deposits.

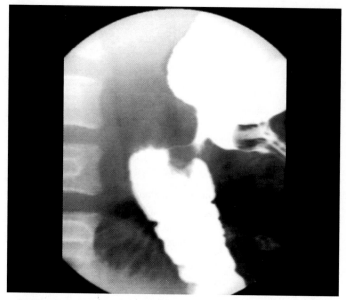

Fig. 11.20A: Adenocarcinoma descending colon: On barium enema short significant narrowing in mid descending colon seen

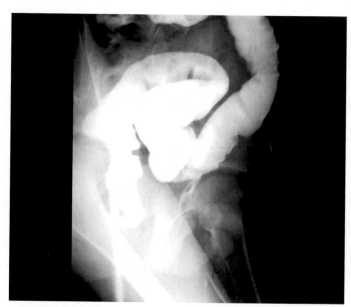

Fig. 11.21A: Carcinoma rectum: Barium enema—marked narrowing and irregularity of the rectum

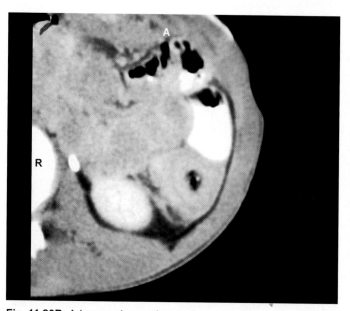

Fig. 11.20B: Adenocarcinoma descending colon: CT at the same level shows concentric wall thickening with luminal narrowing of the affected colon

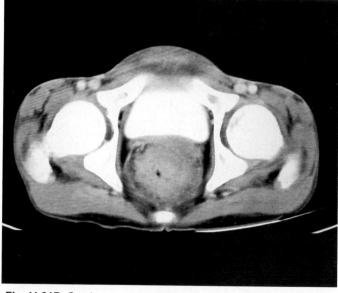

Fig. 11.21B: Carcinoma rectum: CT pelvis shows diffuse thickening of rectal wall with early infiltration of adjacent tissues

Barium enema is used as a screening modality. Intraluminal filling defect or apple core lesion may be seen.

US is not performed for suspected colorectal carcinoma, but when used for evaluation of nonspecific abdominal pain, may demonstrate a mass lesion involving the bowel.

CT is very valuable for diagnosis and staging of disease. The bowel wall thickness, relation of mass to surrounding structures, adenopathy and distant metastasis can be evaluated.

MRI improved soft tissue contrast, but because of expense, low availability, motion artifacts and need for sedation CT is preferred.

GIST: Colonic GIST accounts for only about 5 percent of cases.[27] Features are similar to GIST anywhere in the intestine.[54]

Colon is a much less frequent site for the development of *lymphoma* than the small bowel.

CONCLUSION

- GI masses in children are significantly different when compared with GI masses in adults. In children, primary malignant tumors of GIT hollow viscera are very rare. Masses in intestinal tract are much more likely to be benign developmental lesions like duplication cysts. Benign neoplastic processes are also more common than malignant lesions.

- The ultimate goal of imaging—better patient care—depends on coordinated efforts of pediatric radiologist, pediatrician and pediatric surgeon. The age of patient and the clinical presentation guides the initial imaging technique. Precise diagnostic evaluation allows selection of the proper surgical and medical treatment.

REFERENCES

1. Cairo MS, Grosfeld JL, Weetman RM. Gastric teratoma-unusual cause for bleeding of the upper gastrointestinal tract in the newborn. Pediatrics 1981; 67:721-24.
2. Golden CB, Feusner JH. Malignant abdominal masses in children—Quick guide to evaluation and diagnosis. Pediatr Clin North Am 2002; 49(6):1369-92.
3. Superina RA, Ein SH. Cystic duplications of the esophagus and neuroenteric cysts. J Pediatr Surg 1984; 19:517-30.
4. Parker BR. The abdomen and gastrointestinal tract. In Silverman FN, Kuhn JP (Eds): Caffey's Pediatric X-Ray Diagnosis (9th ed). Mosby, 1993.
5. Gupta AK, Berry M, Mitra DK. Gastric duplication cyst in children-report of two cases. Pediatr Radiol 1994; 24:346-47.
6. Teele RL, Smith EH. Ultrasound in the diagnosis of idiopathic hypertrophic pyloric stenosis. N Engl J Med 1977; 296:1149-50.
7. Hayden CK, Swischuk LE. Ultrasound—The definite imaging modality in pyloric stenosis. Radiographics 1984; 4:517-30.
8. Hallam D, Hansen B, Bodker B, et al. Pyloric size in normal infants and in infants suspected of having hypertrophic pyloric stenosis. Acta Radiol 1995; 36(3):261-64.
9. Neilson D, Hollman AS. The ultrasonic diagnosis of infantile hypertrophic pyloric stenosis: Technique and accuracy. Clin Radiol 1994; 49(4):246-47.
10. Hernanz-Schulman M, Sells LL, Ambrosino MM, et al. Hypertrophic pyloric stenosis in the infant without a palpable olive: Accuracy of sonographic diagnosis. Radiology 1994; 193(3):771-76.
11. Blumhagen JD, Noble HGS. Muscle thickness in hypertrophic pyloric stenosis—Sonographic determination. AJR 1983; 140:221-23.
12. Daniel AB. Pyloric stenosis, hypertrophic. http://www.emedicine.com/ped/topic1103.htm
13. Murphy S, Shaw K, Blanchard H. Report of three gastric tumors in children. J Pediatr Surg 1994; 29(9):1202-24.
14. Mirbagheri SA, Nahidi AR, Mohammod SP. Report of an 8 years old boy presenting with repeated GIT bleeding. http://pearl.sums.ac.ir/AIM/9923/mirbagheri9923.html
15. Mathew M, Gupta A, Narula MK, et al. Gastric teratoma—A report of three cases. Ind J Radiol Imag 2002; 12(4):507-10.
16. Gupta AK, Berry M, Mitra DK. Ossified gastric leiomyoma in a child—A case report. Pediatr Radiol 1995; 25:48-49.
17. Navaro O, Dugougeat F, Daneman A. Sonographic signs that characterize the gastrointestinal origin of abdominal neoplasms in children – 4 case reports. Can Assoc Radiol J 2000; 51(4):250-53.
18. Bluth EI, Merritt CRB, Sullvian MA. Ultrasonic evaluation of the stomach, small bowel and colon. Radiology 1979; 133:677-80.
19. Golden T, Stout AP. Smooth muscle tumours of GIT and retroperitoneal tissue. Surg Gynecol Obstet 1941; 73:784.
20. Thompson WM, Kende AI, Levy AD. Imaging characteristics of gastric lipomas in 16 adults and pediatric patients. AJR 2003; 181:981-85.

21. Dixon WL, Fazzari PJ. Carcinoma of stomach in a child. JAMA 1976; 235:2414-15.
22. Dunnick NR, Harell GS, Parker BR. Multiple "bull's eye" lesions in gastric lymphoma. AJR 1976; 126:965.
23. Ng YY, Healy JC. The radiology of Non-Hodgkin's lymphoma in childhood—A review of 80 cases. Clin Radiol 1994; 49(9):594-600.
24. Kurugoglu S, Mihmanli I, Celkan T, et al. Radiological features in pediatric primary gastric MALT lymphoma and association with Helicobacter Pylori. Pediatr Radiol 2002; 32:82-87.
25. Li P, Wei J, West AB, et al. Epithelial GI stromal tumours of stomach with liver metastases in a 12 years old girl: Aspiration cytology and molecular study. Pediatr Dev Pathol 2003; 6(3):278-79.
26. Oguzkurt P, Akcoren Z, Senocak ME, et al. A huge gastric stromal tumour in a 13 years old girl. Turk J Pediatr 2002; 44(1):65-68.
27. Nguyen VU, Taylor A. Gastric stromal tumours—leiomyoma, leiomyosarcoma. http://www.emedicine.com/radio/topic338.htm
28. Newman B, Girdany BR. Gastric trichobezoars—Sonographic and CT appearance. Pediatr Radiol 1990; 20:526-527.
29. Barr LL, Hyden CK, Stansberry SD, et al. Enteric duplication cysts in childen—Are their ultrasonographic wall characteristics diagnostic? Pediatr Radiol 1990; 20:326-28.
30. Macpherson RI. Gastrointestinal duplications—Clinical, pathologic, etiologic and radiologic considerations. Radiographics 1993; 13:1063-80.
31. Lister J, Rickham PP. Duplication of the alimentary tract. In Rickham PP, Lister J, Irving T (Eds): Neonatal Surgery (2nd ed). London: Butterworth 1990; 474-84.
32. Spottswood SE. Peristalsis in duplication cyst : A new diagnostic sonographic finding. Pediatr Radiol 1994; 24:344-45.
33. Andronikou S, Welman CJ, Kader E. The CT features of abdominal tuberculosis in children. Pediatr Radiol 2002; 32(2):75-81.
34. Denath FM. Abdominal tuberculosis in children—CT findings. Gastrointestinal Radiology 1990; 15(4):303-06.
35. Ozbey H, Tireli GA. Abdominal tuberculosis in children. Eur J Pediatr Surg 2003; 13(2):116-19.
36. Gupta AK, Berry M, Mitra DK. Gastrointestinal smooth muscle tumours in children—Report of three cases. Pediatr Radiol 1994; 24:498-99.
37. Chattopadhyay A, Kumar A, Maruliah M, et al. Duodenojejunal obstruction by a haemangioma. Pediatr Surg Int 2002; 18(5-6):501-02.
38. Vade A, Blane CE. Imaging of Burkitt lymphoma in paediatric patients. Pediatr Radiol 1985; 15:123-26.
39. Sargent MA, Babyn P, Alton DJ. Plain abdominal radiography in suspected intussusception—A reassessment. Pediatr Radiol 1994; 24:17-20.
40. Bowerman RA, Silver TM, Jaffe MH. Real time ultrasound diagnosis of intussusception in children. Radiology 1982; 143:527-29.
41. Harrington L, et al. Ultrasonographic and clinical predictors of intussusception. J of Pediatrics 1998; 132(5):836-39.
42. Stanley A, Logan H, Bate TW, et al. Ultrasound in the diagnosis and exclusion of intussuception. Ir Med J 1997; 90(2):64-65.
43. Intussusception reduction: British Society of Paediatric Radiology draft guidelines for suggested safe practice. http://www.bspr.org.uk/intus.doc
44. Del-Pozo G, et al. Intussuception in children: Current concepts in diagnosis and enema reduction. Radiographics 1999; 19(2):299.
45. Chan KL, Saing H, Peh WC, et al. Childhood intussusception: Ultrasound guide Hartmann's solution hydrostatic reduction or barium enema reduction? J Pediatr Surg 1997; 32(1):3-6.

46. Swischuk LE. The current radiology management of intussusception—A survey and review. Pediatr Radiol 1992; 2:317.

47. Haney PJ, Whitley NO. CT of benign cystic abdominal masses in children. AJR 1984; 142:1279-81.

48. Konen O, Rathaus V, Dlugy E, et al. Childhood abdominal cystic lymphangioma. Pediatr Radiol 2002; 32:88-94.

49. Zarewych ZM, Donnelly LF, Frush DP, et al. Imaging of pediatric mesenteric abnormalities. Pediatr Radiol 1999; 29(9):711-19.

50. Jewell CT, Miller ID, Ehrlich FE. Rectal duplication—An unusual cause for an abdominal mass. Surgery 1973; 74:783-85.

51. Sivit CJ, Newman KD. Appendicitis—Usefulness of ultrasound in diagnosis in a pediatric population. Radiology 1992; 185:549-52.

52. Karnak I. Colorectal cancers in children. J Pediatr Surg 1999; 34(10):1499-1504.

53. Radha Krishnan CN, Bruce J. Colorectal cancers in children without any predisposing factors—A report of eight cases and review of literature. Eur J Pediatr Surg 2003; 13(1):66-68.

54. Karnak I, Kale G, Tanyel FC, et al. Malignant stromal tumour of the colon in an infant: Diagnostic difficulties and differential diagnosis. J Pediatr Surg 2003; 38(2):245-47.

CHAPTER 12

Hepatic and Pancreatic Masses in Children

Akshay Kumar Saxena, Kushaljit Singh Sodhi, Naveen Kalra

Focal hepatic masses in children include benign lesions such as cysts (congenital, i.e. simple or acquired like hydatid cysts), abscesses, granulomas and neoplasms (benign and malignant tumors, primary and metastatic lesions). Malignant neoplasms and abscesses are more common than simple cysts and benign tumors.

Pancreatic tumors are rare in infants and children. They can be cystic or solid, benign or malignant and endocrine or exocrine in origin. Pancreatoblastoma, islet cell tumors and solid and papillary epithelial neoplasms (SPEN) are the most important tumors of childhood. Pseudocysts of pancreas secondary to pancreatitis are more common than cystic tumors of the pancreas.

IMAGING

Ultrasonography (US) and computed tomography (CT) remain the primary imaging modalities for investigating hepatic and pancreatic masses. Majority of the lesions, particularly tumors, require more than one modality to reach at a definitive diagnosis. Ultrasonography is the initial investigation of choice as the location, nature of the lesion (cystic or solid), relationship to adjacent organs, associated lymphadenopathy and invasion of the vascular structures by the mass can all be well seen on US. In children, ultrasonography has the ability to visualize the entire pancreas well because of the relatively large left lobe of liver as an acoustic window during scanning. Color Doppler flow imaging and intra-operative ultrasonography further help in the diagnosis and patient's management.[1]

Once a mass is suspected to be a tumor, dynamic contrast enhanced CT scan should be performed as it is more accurate than US in distinguishing various neoplastic lesions and it has the best capability to assess extrahepatic spread of the disease such as lymphadenopathy and omental or peritoneal spread.[1] However, it is important to note a few technical considerations while performing the CT scan. Many of the patients require sedation for performing a technically satisfactory study. Generally, the sedation is provided by the anesthetists. The radiologist should ensure that the patient undergoes pre-anesthetic check up prior to the date of appointment. In addition, need for keeping the child nil orally on the day of appointment should be carefully impressed upon. Failure to adhere to these precautions may lead to postponement of study. The nil per oral guidelines are less stringent for smaller children and for clear fluids (Table 12.1).[2]

With the advent of multidetector spiral CT, it is now possible to image the abdomen during the arterial and portal venous phases. Lu et al[3] however have advocated that imaging of the pancreas should be done in the 'pancreatic phase' only. This phase occurs in the interval between the arterial and portal venous phase at 40-70 seconds after the bolus injection of contrast at a rate of 3 ml/second. During this phase there is maximum pancreatic parenchymal enhancement with accentuation of the lesion-to-pancreas contrast. The use of this phase alone has the benefit of reducing the radiation exposure to the patient. Single phase evaluation of focal hepatic lesions is also recommended by "Image gently" campaign.[4] Apart from doing the single phase studies, it is important to carefully adjust the KV and mAs according to the weight of the child.[2] This will avoid unnecessary high radiation to these children. Most of the vendors now provide for children specific scanning protocols and radiologists should ensure that technologists are adhering to these protocols.

Magnetic resonance imaging (MRI) is superior to both US and CT in characterizing the lesion and showing its extent, particularly vascular invasion,[5,6] but it is reserved as a problem solving modality because of its inherent limitations namely high cost, lack of easy availability and compulsory sedation in nearly all infants and children which makes its routine use impractical. However due to

Table 12.1: Nil per oral guidelines for CT scan[2]		
Age	*Solids and Milk/Formula*	*Clear liquids*
> 3 years	Stop 6-8 h before sedation	Stop 2-3 h before sedation
6 months 3 years	Stop 6 h before sedation	Stop 2-3 h before sedation
< 6 months	Stop 4-6 h before sedation	Stop 2 h before sedation

the lack of ionizing radiation and multiplanar imaging capabilities, MR and MRCP are especially useful in the pediatric population.

Radionuclide scanning of the liver using ^{99m}Tc-Sulphur colloid has a sensitivity and specificity of 80-85 percent each. It can be supplemented with single photon emission computed tomography (SPECT) which can detect lesions as small as 1 cm diameter (sensitivity and specificity of 90-95% each). Regarding characterization of a known hepatic mass, ^{99m}Tc-labelled red blood cell (RBC) scanning has the greatest utility in diagnosing cavernous hemangiomas by achieving a specificity of nearly 100 percent (barring occasional false positives due to small hepatocellular carcinomas or hypervascular metastasis).[7]

Angiography has limited role except for the vascular road-mapping of tumors when surgery or therapeutic embolization is considered.

Plain radiography is of limited diagnostic value in the evaluation of pediatric masses. Calcification in tumors like hepatoblastoma and pancreatoblastoma may be detected on abdominal radiographs. Pulmonary complications like basal pneumonitis, pleural effusions in hepatic abscesses and pulmonary metastasis may be seen on chest radiographs.

Imaging, usually ultrasonography, may also be required for providing guidance for interventional procedures like fine needle aspiration cytology (FNAC).

HEPATIC MASSES

Malignant Hepatic Tumors

Primary malignant hepatic tumors constitute nearly 1.5 percent of all pediatric tumors and 15 percent of all abdominal masses in children.[8] About 2/3rd of these are malignant, of which hepatoblastoma, hepatocellular carcinoma and rarely sarcomas constitute the majority.[5,9]

HEPATOBLASTOMA

The term hepatoblastoma was coined by Willis in 1962 for hepatic tumors of embryonal origin which were histologically different from hepatocellular carcinoma.[10] Hepatoblastoma is the most frequent malignancy of liver in children and is seen at less than 5 years of age.[2,11] The peak incidence occurs between 18 and 24 months of age. The patient usually presents with an abdominal mass but less frequently anorexia, weight loss, jaundice and pain due to hemorrhage or rupture may be the presenting features. A number of conditions such as Beckwith-Wiedemann syndrome, hemihypertrophy, familial adenomatous polyposis (FAP), Gardner's syndrome, Wilms' tumor, sexual precocity and osteopenia can be associated with hepatoblastoma. Serum alpha-fetoprotein is elevated in about 80 percent of these patients.[9]

Pathologically, hepatoblastoma contains small, primitive, epithelial cells resembling those in fetal liver tissue. When mesenchymal elements like osteoid are also present in addition to epithelial elements, the hepatoblastoma is classified as mixed variant. There is no significant survival difference between the epithelial and mixed forms of hepatoblastoma. Vascular invasion is less frequent compared to hepatocellular carcinoma. Calcification

may be present. The tumor metastasizes most commonly to the lungs followed by lymph nodes, brain, peritoneum and diaphragm.

Several methods are available for staging of hepatoblastoma.[12] The most commonly used is PRETEXT system. This system is predominantly dependent on radiological findings. The liver, in this system, is divided into right anterior (Couniad's segments V and VIII), right posterior (Couniad's segments VI and VII), left medial (Couniad's segments IVa and IVb) and left lateral (Couniad's segments II and III) sections (also called sectors). The caudate lobe and the caudate process, i.e. segments I and IX are currently considered not to have any independent significance in PRETEXT system. The PRETEXT group number reflects the maximum number of contiguous liver sections that are free of tumor (Table 12.2).[12] Extrahepatic spread is classified separately (Table 12.3).[12] In contrast, Children's Oncology Group (widely used in North America) is based on postoperative evaluation (Table 12.4)[12] and, therefore, relies much less on the imaging findings. TNM classification is not widely used for hepatoblastoma.

Table 12.2: PRETEXT staging of hepatic tumors[12]	
PRETEXT-I	One section is involved and three adjoining sections are free
PRETEXT-II	One or two sections are involved, but two adjoining sections are free
PRETEXT-III	Two or three sections are involved and no two adjoining sections are free
PRETEXT-IV	All four sections are involved

Table 12.3: PRETEXT staging of extra hepatic disease[12]	
V +	Involvement of the inferior vena cava and/or all three hepatic veins
P +	Involvement of the main portal vein and/or both left and right branches of the portal vein
E +	Extrahepatic disease in the abdomen
M +	Distant metastases

Table 12.4: Children's oncology group staging of liver cancer[12]	
Stage I	Tumor completely resected
Stage II	Tumor grossly resected with microscopic residual disease
Stage III	Tumor unresectable or resected with gross residual disease
	Nodal involvement
	Tumor spill
	Gross residual intrahepatic disease
Stage IV	Distant Metastases

On imaging, hepatoblastoma is generally seen as a single, well-defined lesion with lobulated outline, mostly located in the right lobe. Less commonly the lesion may involve the left lobe or even be multicentric. On US, the lesion has generally inhomogeneous echotexture, may be hyperechoic[13] with anechoic areas corresponding to necrosis or hemorrhage. Calcifications in the lesion appear as echogenic foci with distal shadowing. A rare cystic form of hepatoblastoma has also been described which is completely anechoic on US but may reveal mural nodule.[11] Hepatoblastoma may also appear as diffuse parenchymal inhomogeneity with multiple cystic lesions.[14] In case of vascular invasion, portal vein may show intraluminal thrombus. On Doppler studies, peak systolic Doppler frequency shifts in the hepatic artery are usually greater than 4 KHz.[9] If available, noncontrast CT (Fig. 12.1A) scan generally reveals hypodense or isodense and calcification may be detected in as many as 50 percent of cases.[15] Calcification is typically coarse and dense in contrast to fine calcification seen in hemangioendothelioma. Other features which differentiate hepatoblastoma from hemangioendothelioma include predominantly hyperechoic pattern, absence of congestive heart failure and markedly elevated level of alpha-fetoproteins in hepatoblastoma. On CECT hepatoblastoma appears as low attenuating mass which may show inhomogeneous enhancement (Fig. 12.1B). In the early phase of dynamic CT, the tumor may

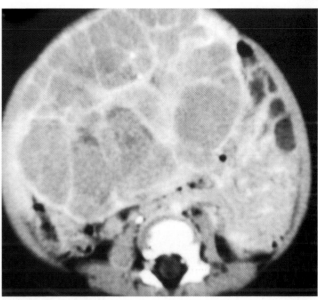

Fig. 12.2: CT in a case of hepatoblastoma shows inhomogeneous enhancement and multiple enhancing septae

appear hyperdense and show rim enhancement indicating increased vascularity. The septations within the tumor are best seen after contrast enhancement (Fig. 12.2).

On MRI, hepatoblastoma appears as low intensity mass on T1WI and increased signal intensity mass on T2WI. Hypointense bands (corresponding to fibrotic areas) may be seen on both T1W and T2W images. Tumor thrombus in the hepatic or portal vein appears as an area of increased signal intensity in the normal flow of vessels. MRI is better than CT and US for demonstration of tumor margins and vascular invasion. However, CT is superior for detecting calcification.

HEPATOCELLULAR CARCINOMA (HCC)

This tumor generally occurs in children older than 5 years. There are two age peaks in childhood, the first is between 2 to 4 years and the second one occurs between 12 to 14 years.[16] Childhood HCC is associated with diseases like glycogen storage disease (Type I), cystinosis, hereditary tyrosinemia, Wilson's disease, alpha 1-antitrypsin deficiency, extrahepatic biliary atresia and giant cell hepatitis. Association with cirrhosis is less common than in adults. Serum alpha-fetoprotein is elevated in 40-50 percent of patients.[6]

HCC can appear as focal, multinodular or diffuse form with variable and non-specific appearances. When solitary, the lesion is common in the right lobe. On sonography, HCC is characterized by variable echogenicity pattern with predominantly hypo-, iso- or hyperechoic echotexture. Calcification may be seen in 10 percent of patients but is less common than in hepatoblastoma. US appearances may be indistinguishable from hepatoblastoma.

On noncontrast CT scan, lesion is of low attenuation and generally reveals inhomogeneous enhancement after contrast. On dynamic CT, majority are hypervascular and may reveal areas of peripheral enhancement in the early vascular phase and later become hypodense to liver parenchyma (Figs 12.3A and B). On MRI, these

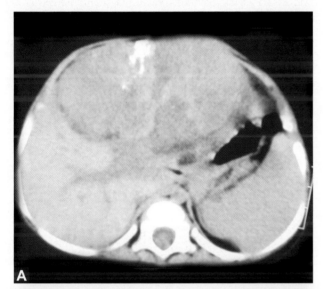

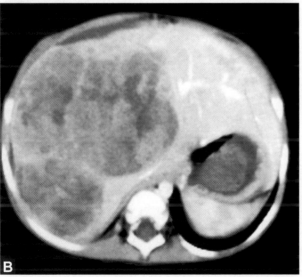

Figs 12.1A and B: (A) NCCT scan in a 14-month-old male patient with hepatoblastoma shows a large well defined hypodense mass replacing the left lobe of liver. Coarse calcification is seen within the mass. (B) CECT in another patient of hepatoblastoma shows heterogeneously enhancing mass lesion in right lobe

tumors are usually hypointense on T1WI and hyperintense on T2WI. The vascular invasion is demonstrated as loss of normal flow void in the vessels.

Fibrolamellar HCC

It is a rare subtype of HCC but it has a better prognosis if resected. This tumor is usually seen in young females (mean age 23 years); but it can occur in children. Alpha-fetoprotein level is usually not elevated.[17] CT reveals a well-defined hypodense mass which shows variable enhancement after contrast injection. A central fibrotic scar and calcification are more commonly seen (30% and 50% of cases respectively)[18] in fibrolamellar subtype of HCC

(Figs 12.4A and B). MRI can be used to distinguish fibrolamellar HCC from focal nodular hyperplasia (FNH). The fibrous central scar of fibrolamellar HCC is hypointense on both T1WI and T2WI. On the other hand, the central scar of FNH is hyperintense on T2WI.[19]

RHABDOMYOSARCOMA

This is the most common tumor of the biliary tree in children and accounts for 0.04 percent of all cancers in children. It occurs at a median age of 3 years and is rare after the first decade.[20] There is a male preponderance. The tumor may arise in the liver, intrahepatic ducts, intrahepatic cyst, gallbladder, cystic duct, extrahepatic duct,

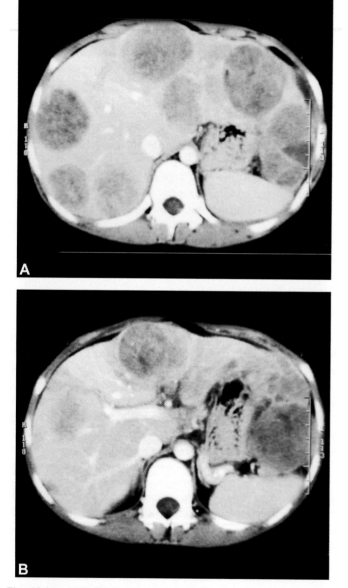

Figs 12.3A and B: CT scan in an 11 year-old male patient with multicentric HCC. There are multiple lesions seen in both lobes of liver which show peripheral enhancement. The left branch of portal vein is not opacified suggestive of invasion

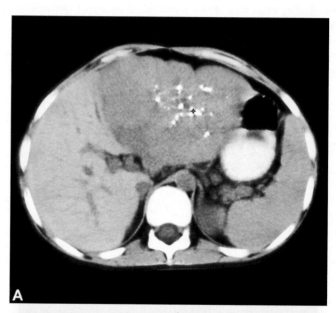

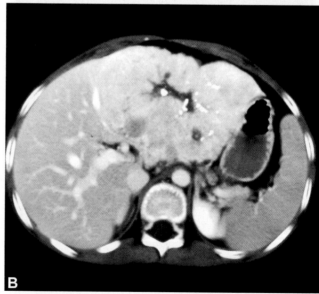

Figs 12.4A and B: CT scan in a 16-years-old female patient with fibrolamellar HCC (A) NCCT shows a well-defined hypodense mass in the left lobe of liver with central calcification and lobulated border. (B) CECT shows inhomogeneous enhancement with central hypodense scar

ampulla or choledochal cyst. Patient usually presents with jaundice and abdominal distention. Ultrasonography (Fig. 12.5A) shows biliary dilatation with a hyperechoic intraductal mass. The portal vein may be displaced but is not thrombosed. Larger lesions have areas of necrosis. CT (Figs 12.5B and C) shows an intraductal mass with or without biliary dilatation. The mass is heterogeneous in attenuation with variable contrast enhancement. On MRI, the mass is of low signal intensity on T1W images and hyperintense on T2W images. MRCP shows dilated ducts and the entire extent of the lesion (Fig. 12.6).

HEPATIC METASTASES

The common primary malignancy to metastasize to liver in children are neuroblastoma, Wilms' tumor, GI tumors, Ewing's sarcoma, rhabdomyosarcoma, lymphomas and leukemias.[2,11] The metastases may be single or multiple (Figs 12.7 and 12.8). These are usually nonspecific lesions appearing hypoechoic on ultrasonography, hypodense on contrast enhance CT scan, hypointense on T1 and hyperintense on T2W MR images. If required, diagnosis can be clinched by fine needle aspiration cytology under sonographic guidance.

Benign Hepatic Neoplasms

These account for one-third of all primary hepatic tumors. Most of these tumors are of vascular origin, viz. infantile hemangioendothelioma and cavernous haemangioma.[9] Less common tumors are mesenchymal hamartoma, focal nodular hyperplasia (FNH) and hepatic adenoma.

INFANTILE HEMANGIOENDOTHELIOMA

Infantile hemangioendothelioma is the commonest benign tumor in children less than one year of age.[2,21] It commonly presents before 6 months of age in more than 85 percent of patients and is more common in females. Hemangioendothelioma may present with high output cardiac failure, asymptomatic hepatomegaly or an abdominal mass. Heart failure occurs in nearly 50% of infants with this tumor.[22] Occasionally, thrombocytopenia due to platelet

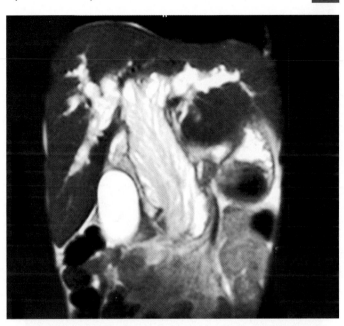

Fig. 12.6: T2W coronal image in a case of biliary rhabdomyosarcoma shows the dilatation of the biliary tree with heterogeneous hyperintensity of the intraductal tumor

sequestration or massive intraperitoneal bleeding and shock due to spontaneous tumor rupture can be the presenting features. Cutaneous hemangiomata are reported in 40 percent of patients.[23] Spontaneous regression has also been described. The clinical as well as radiological features depend on the rate of blood flow and the extent of arteriovenous shunting.

Pathologically, hemangioendothelioma is composed of multiple, round, discrete nodules ranging from 2-15 cm in size. Microscopically, the tumor is quite vascular. There are two histological subtypes.[24] Type 1 consists of variable sized vascular spaces lined by relatively immature plump endothelial cells. Type II has more immature pleomorphic cells with hyperchromatic nuclei and reflects more aggressive form. They may mimic

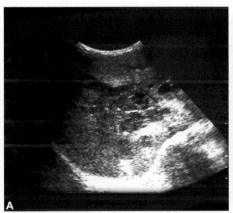
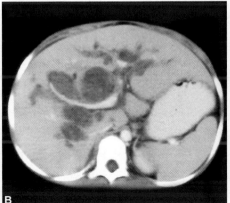
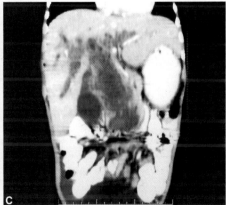

Figs 12.5A to C: An 8-year-old female child with jaundice. (A) Ultrasound scan reveals echogenic soft tissue filling the dilated biliary channels (B) CECT shows biliary radicle dilatation in both lobes of liver with presence of intraluminal heterogeneous attenuation mass. (C) Coronal reconstruction shows the entire extent of the lesion. FNAC revealed biliary rhabdomyosarcoma

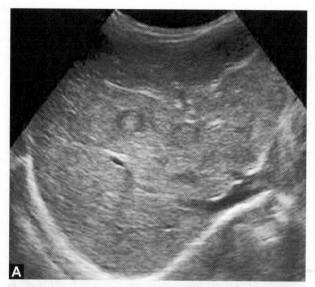

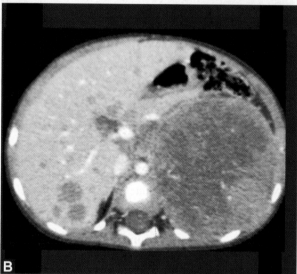

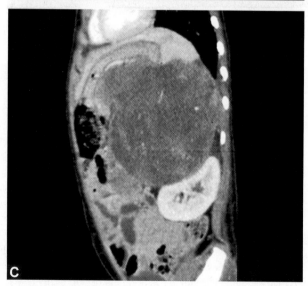

Figs 12.7A to C: (A) Ultrasound reveals multiple target lesions in liver (B) Axial and (C) Reconstructed coronal images of CECT study reveal left adrenal mass with multiple hepatic lesions. FNAC confirmed neuroblastoma

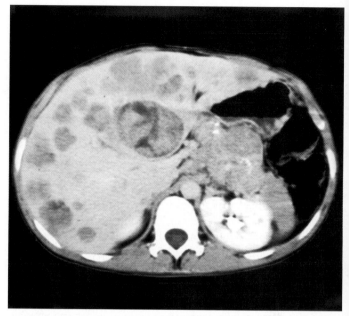

Fig. 12.8: Multiple well-defined hypodense lesions are seen in liver on CECT in a case of pancreatoblastoma metastasizing to liver

hemangioendothelial sarcoma and rare cases of metastasis have also been described.[25] Uncommonly, these tumors may be solitary with a slight predilection for the posterior segment of right lobe.

On sonography the lesion shows multiple well-defined hypoechoic masses throughout the liver (Figs 12.9A and B). Enlargement of the celiac and hepatic arteries along with decreased caliber of the aorta distal to the origin of the celiac artery strongly suggests the diagnosis. Large draining hepatic veins are also seen. Ultrasonography can also be used to monitor the response of hemangioendothelioma to steroid therapy.

On noncontrast CT, these tumors appear as well-defined, homogeneous hypodense masses. Calcification is seen in 40 percent of patients.[16] Early peripheral, nodular enhancement with gradual central filling is seen on dynamic CT scanning similar to hemangioma in adults. Larger lesions usually show incomplete filling with central hypodense areas representing fibrosis and thrombus (Figs 12.9C and D).[26]

When CT or US findings are equivocal, radionuclide or MRI studies can be helpful. Tc-labelled red blood cell scan shows increased activity in the blood pool phase and on delayed scanning. Radionuclide study has nearly 100 percent specificity for the diagnosis and should be used whenever diagnosis is in doubt.[17,27] On MRI, tumor is hypointense on T1WI and hyperintense or heterogeneous on T2WI.

HEMANGIOMA

Hemangiomas may be single or multiple; the latter being associated with hemangiomatosis syndrome of childhood.

Pathologically it is very vascular and shows multiple, dilated, blood filled spaces lined by mature, flat endothelium and separated by fibrous stroma. This lesion does not have any malignant potential.

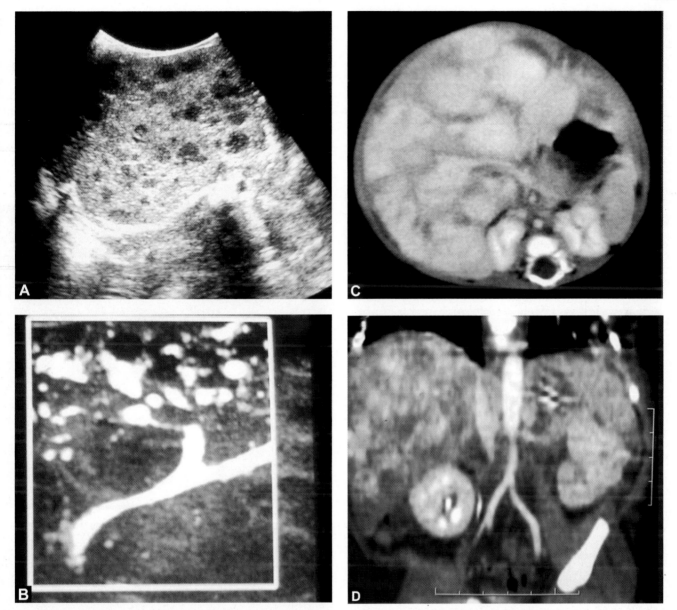

Figs 12.9A to D: Imaging finding in infantile hemangioendothelioma (A) Gray scale ultrasound reveals multiple well defined hypo to anechoic lesions in both lobes of liver. Power Doppler (B) revealed markedly increased vascularity in these lesions *(For color version see Plate 00)*. (C) In another patient axial CECT scan demonstrates multiple enhancing hypervascular lesions diffusedly distributed in both lobes of liver while coronal reformatted image (D) shows sudden change in aortic caliber, distal to celiac artery, which is a characteristic feature of infantile hemangioendothelioma

On sonography, hemangioma is typically small (<3 cm in diameter), homogeneous, well-defined and hyperechoic with distal acoustic enhancement. Larger lesion can be heterogeneous.[28] On noncontrast CT, it is hypo-to isodense and well-defined. On dynamic contrast studies, early, peripheral, dense nodular enhancement with later centripetal fill in is noted (Figs 12.10 A and B). Complete isodense filling occurs in not less than 3 minutes and not more than 30 minutes after injection in 2/3rd of these lesions. When above features can be demonstrated, no further investigation is required. But the lesion can show variable contrast enhancement and variable fill in. In this equivocal state, MRI and scintigraphy are helpful.

On MRI, hemangioma appears hypo-or isointense to liver on T1WI. On T2WI, it shows marked hyperintensity which is maintained even on heavily T2WI.[2] After Gd-DTPA injection, the appearance is similar to CT, i.e. peripheral enhancement with centripetal fill in.

On Tc-labelled red blood cell scanning, it shows increased activity in blood pool phase and on delayed scanning. This study has 100 percent specificity for the diagnosis of hemangioma. For lesion larger than 2 cm, both MRI and ^{99m}Tc RBC imaging have similar accuracy (95%) but for lesion smaller than 2 cm, MRI is more sensitive. However SPECT ^{99m}Tc RBC imaging is more specific than MRI.

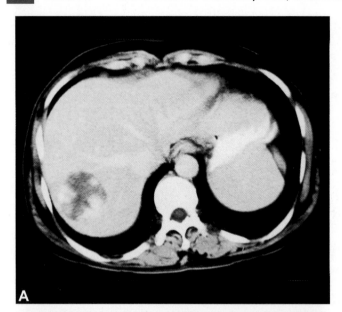

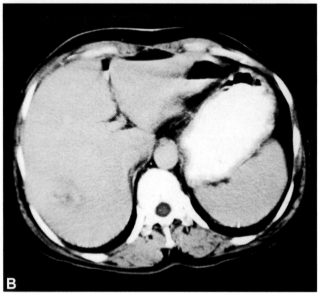

Figs 12.10A and B: (A) Venous phase CECT image in a case of cavenous hemangioma showing dense nodular enhancement in a peripherally located hepatic mass (B) Delayed phase reveals lesion to be almost isodense to liver

Hepatic angiography is rarely required in establishing the diagnosis of hemangioma. Rarely when surgery is contemplated in symptomatic hemangioma, angiography can be helpful in defining the vascular anatomy.

MESENCHYMAL HAMARTOMA

Mesenchymal hamartoma is the second commonest benign hepatic tumor next to vascular lesions.[29] This tumor usually presents as an asymptomatic abdominal mass in children less than 2 years of age and is twice as common in boys than girls. Rarely children may present with cardiac failure due to presence of large shunt in the lesion.

Pathologically, this tumor is seen as a well-circumscribed mass with multiple cystic areas.[29] On sonography,[30] the tumor appears as a well-defined, multilocular mass with anechoic spaces separated by echogenic septae (Figs 12.11A and B). This has been described as 'swiss cheese' appearance.[29] On CT scanning, the tumor is seen as a complex mass containing areas of low attenuation separated by solid septae and stroma which enhance with intravenous contrast administration[31] (Figs 12.12A and B). On MRI, the cystic spaces show high signal on T2WI and low signal on T1WI. The signal intensity however depends on the protein content and presence of hemorrhage within the cysts.

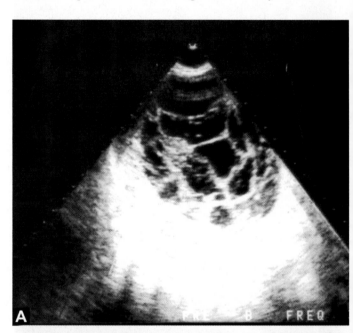

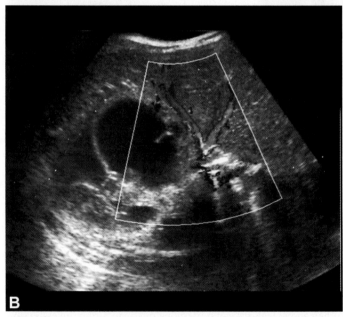

Figs 12.11A and B: (A) US scan in a 7-month-old boy reveals a large multilocular cystic mass with septae in the right lobe of liver in a case of mesenchymal hamartoma (B) Color Doppler reveals absence of intra-lesional blood flow

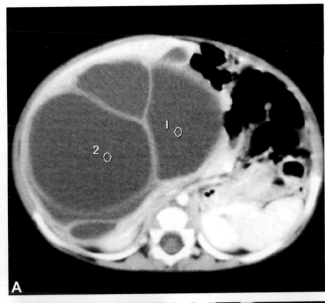

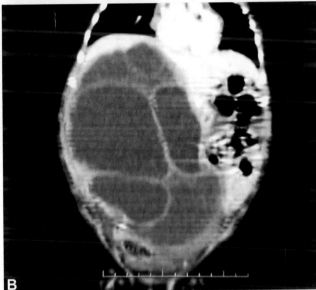

Figs 12.12A and B: CT scan (A) axial and (B) coronal reconstruction in a 7- month-old male patient with mesenchymal hamartoma reveals a multiloculated cystic mass with enhancing septae

FOCAL NONDULAR HYPERPLASIA (FNH) AND HEPATIC ADENOMA

This benign lesion is uncommon and constitutes less than 2 percent of pediatric hepatic tumors.[7] Childhood hepatic adenoma is associated with glycogen storage disease, Fanconi's anemia and galactosemia. Both these tumors are well-circumscribed masses with variable echogenicity and enhancement patterns. However, presence of a central low attenuation scar favors the diagnosis of FNH. When the distinction based on these imaging modalities is uncertain, radionuclide sulphur colloid scintigraphic study is very helpful. As high as 60 percent of FNH accumulate colloid while hepatic adenoma appears as focal defects.[7,9,32] Focal hepatic mass which is seen as hot area on sulphur colloid scan is diagnostic of FNH.

PELIOSIS HEPATIS

This is a rare entity characterized by small blood filled spaces in the liver. It is found in association with type I glycogen storage disease, HIV infection and intake of androgens.[10,16] On US, there are scattered areas of heterogeneous echogenicity of liver along with cystic lesions. CT demonstrates areas of low attenuation which show variable contrast enhancement. MRI shows increased signal intensity on T2WI and variable signal on T1WI depending upon the contents of the cysts.[11]

INFLAMMATORY LESIONS

Pyogenic Hepatic Abscess

These are usually associated with various predisposing conditions like systemic sepsis, appendicitis, inflammatory bowel disease, omphalitis, trauma or chronic granulomatous disease of childhood.[33] In neonates gram-negative, and in older children *Staphylococcus aureus* are the most common organisms. When the abscesses are multiple, they usually are the result of ascending biliary infection. When solitary, right lobe is affected more often. Children often present with fever, upper abdominal pain, tender hepatomegaly and leucocytosis.

The abscesses pass through three stages viz. the stage of suppuration, the stage of liquefaction and the stage of resolution including fibrosis, cystic residual lesion and calcification. These stages influence imaging appearance of the abscesses.

Sonography is the initial and usually the only investigation required in patients suspected to have hepatic abscesses. Abscess may appear anechoic, hypoechoic, hyperechoic or as a complex mass with thick irregular walls and through-transmission (Fig. 12.13). Early lesions tend to be echogenic and ill-defined. If gas is detected it clinches the diagnosis. Occasionally septations, fluid-fluid levels and echogenic debris may be noted.[34]

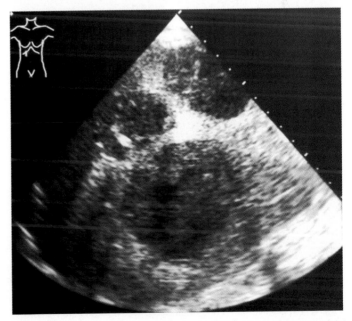

Fig. 12.13: US liver showing multiple pyogenic liver abscesses as multiple hypoechoic lesions with thick irregular wall and coarse internal echoes.

On CT, most abscesses are sharply defined, hypodense masses which may show rim enhancement on contrast administration.[9] Intralesional gas, although highly suggestive of the diagnosis, is seen in only 20 percent of patients. Double-target sign, consisting of a low density central area surrounded by hyperdense zone and then a peripheral hypodense zone may also be noted.

On scintigraphy examination using either Ga-67 or In-111, the lesions are "hot". In-111 scanning provides increased specificity because it is not taken up by benign or malignant lesions. Chest radiographs show elevated hemidiaphragm, pleural effusion, basal atelectasis or infiltrates.

When the diagnosis cannot be established based on clinical or CT findings, percutaneous needle aspiration performed under sonographic or CT guidance can be helpful in diagnosis and also for providing percutaneous aspiration or catheter drainage.[35,36]

Amoebic Hepatic Abscess

It is caused by *E. histolytica* and approximately 3-9 percent of cases of intestinal amoebiasis are complicated by hepatic abscesses. Liver is invaded by one of the three routes viz. (i) portal vein (most common), (ii) lymphatics, or (iii) via direct extension through colonic wall.

Amoebic abscess is most often solitary (85%) and affects the right lobe more (72%) than left lobe (13%). Chest radiograph is abnormal in approximately 50-78 percent of cases which includes elevation of right hemidiaphragm, basal pulmonary infiltrates or pleural effusion. On sulphur colloid scans and gallium scans, the abscess appears as cold center with a hot rim. On ultrasound, the lesion is usually round or oval, hypoechoic mass with homogeneous low level internal echoes and distal acoustic enhancement (Fig. 12.14). Compared to pyogenic abscess, amoebic abscess is more likely to be round or oval in shape (82% vs 60%), sonographically hypoechoic with fine low level echoes (58% vs 36%) and show absence of a definite wall.[37]

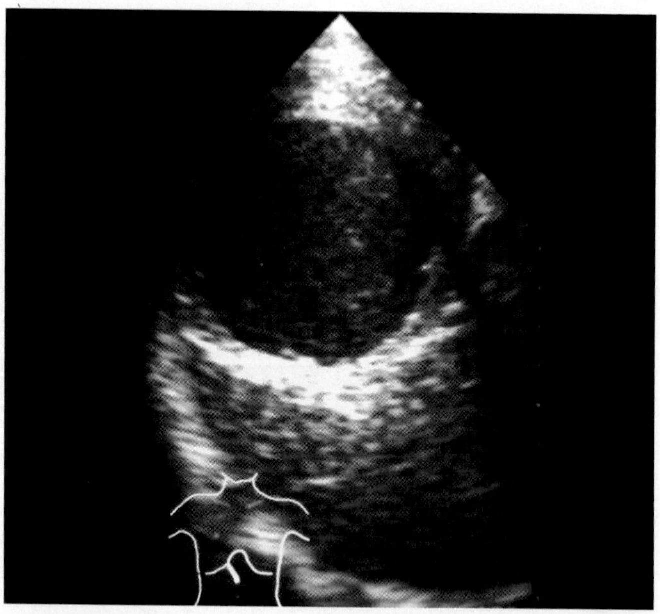

CT appearance of amoebic abscess is variable and nonspecific. Lesion is usually low attenuating (10-20 HU) with an enhancing rim (Fig. 12.15). It may appear uni- or multiocular and may demonstrate nodularity of the margin. On MRI, amoebic abscess appears as a round or oval area showing low signal intensity on T1WI and hyperintensity on T2WI.

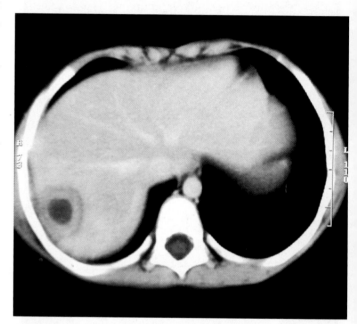

Fig. 12.15: CT scan in a case of liver abscess shows a hypodense lesion with thick wall in the right lobe of liver. A thin rim of perilesional fluid in seen

Fig. 12.14: US liver in a case of amoebic liver abscess shows a well-defined rounded hypoehoic lesion with fine low level internal echoes and an almost imperceptible wall

Fungal Abscess

This is more commonly seen in immunocompromised patients like those receiving chemotherapy, AIDS, lymphoma or acute leukemia. Liver is frequently involved secondary to hematogeneous spread of mycotic infection from other organs, most commonly the lungs. Of the various fungi, candida is the most common agent.[38]

Sonographically four major types are seen (i) "Wheel within a wheel" appearance where a peripheral hypoechoic zone surrounds an inner echogenic wheel which, in turn surrounds a central hypoechoic nidus, (ii) "Bull's eye" lesion where a hyperechoic center is surrounded by hypoechoic rim, (iii) "Uniformly hypoechoic" – the most common appearance (Fig. 12.16) and, (iv) "Echogenic" lesion, caused by scar formation.

On CT scan, most common pattern is multiple, small, rounded lesions of low-attenuation. The lesion may show calcification. It is cold on sulphur colloid and gallium scans. MR shows increased signal intensity on T1WI and STIR (short T1 inversion recovery) sequences.

Granulomatous Lesions

Various granulomatous diseases which may affect liver include tuberculosis, histiocytosis and sarcoidosis.

Echinococcal Disease (Hydatid Cyst)

The disease is worldwide and is most often caused by *Echinococcus granulosus. E. multilocularis* is less common but is more aggressive pathogen and rarely encountered in our country.

Hydatid cyst has three layers. The outer pericyst is formed by the compressed, modified host tissue which is a rigid protective zone. The two inner layers (ectocyst and endocyst) are parasitic in origin. The ectocyst is approximately 1mm thick and may calcify. Innermost germinal layer (endocyst) is the living parasite which produces laminated membrane and scolices. Up to 60 percent of the cysts are multiple.

Plain radiograph shows calcification of the cyst wall in 20-30 percent of cases. Calcification, however, does not indicate death of the parasite.[41] On sulphur colloid scans they are cold and may show a rim of increased activity on gallium scans.

Sonographic appearance depends on the maturity of the cyst. It can be (i) completely anechoic, well encapsulated cyst, (ii) anechoic cyst with hydatid sand, (iii) multiseptated cyst, with daughter cysts and echogenic material within cysts – the characteristic "Water-lily" sign, and (iv) a densely calcified mass. When infected, the hydatid cysts lose their characteristic appearance and are indistinguishable from liver abscess.

On CT (Figs 12.18A to D), hydatid cyst is usually uni- or multilocular, well-defined with either thick or thin wall. Daughter cysts are usually located at the periphery and can be floating freely and altering the patient's position may change the position of these cysts thereby confirming the diagnosis. Curvilinear wall calcification may be seen.

On MR, hydatid cyst has low intensity on T1WI and high signal intensity on T2WI. Pericyst usually has low intensity signal on both TI and T2WI. Calcification is not detected on MR.

Hydatid cyst may rupture into the biliary tree, and pleural, pericardial or the peritoneal cavity, thereby increasing the mortality to 50 percent.[42,43] Presence of undulating membrane on either US or CT suggests contained rupture.

SIMPLE HEPATIC CYST

This arises from bile duct epithelium and is seen in about 5-14 percent of the general population. It is usually asymptomatic and rarely causes pain, biliary obstruction or hepatomegaly.

On sonography (Fig. 12.19), this lesion is usually solitary, well-defined, anechoic and reveals enhanced through transmission. CT features of simple cyst include low attenuating (0-15 HU) lesion with imperceptible or thin smooth walls, homogeneous appearance and total lack of contrast enhancement. On MR, they are sharply demarcated hypointense lesion on T1WI and hyperintense on T2WI.[9]

POLYCYSTIC LIVER DISEASE

This is characterized by multiple liver cysts of varying sizes. Approximately 57-74 percent of patients with adult polycystic kidney disease will show liver cysts. Extent of liver involvement is not proportional to the renal disease. In typical congenital hepatic fibrosis, cysts are not grossly visible. However, in the polycystic variant, numerous large and small cysts coexist with hepatic fibrosis.[44]

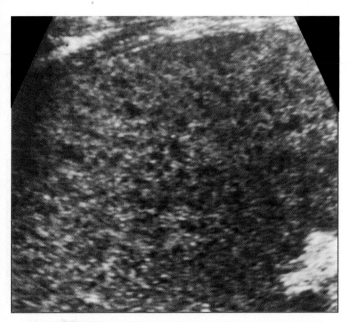

Fig. 12.16: Ultrasound reveals multiple tiny hypoechoic lesions diffusedly scattered in both lobes of liver in a case of candidiasis

Tuberculosis of the liver usually occurs in miliary form with nodules ranging in size from 0.5 to 2 mm which are too small to be seen on US or CT. The commonest finding in such cases is hepatomegaly without focal lesions. A diffusely heterogeneous echotexture on US has also been reported. Macronodular involvement is uncommon[39] and usually manifests as single or multiple focal lesions of varying sizes which are hypoechoic on US and hypodense on CT (Fig. 12.17). These lesions may show peripheral rim enhancement and a central hypodensity due to caseation.[39,40]

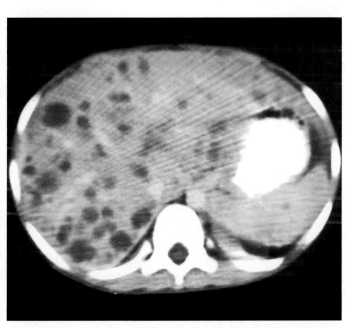

Fig. 12.17: CECT abdomen shows multiple well-defined hypodense lesions in both lobes of liver and spleen. FNAC confirmed tuberculosis

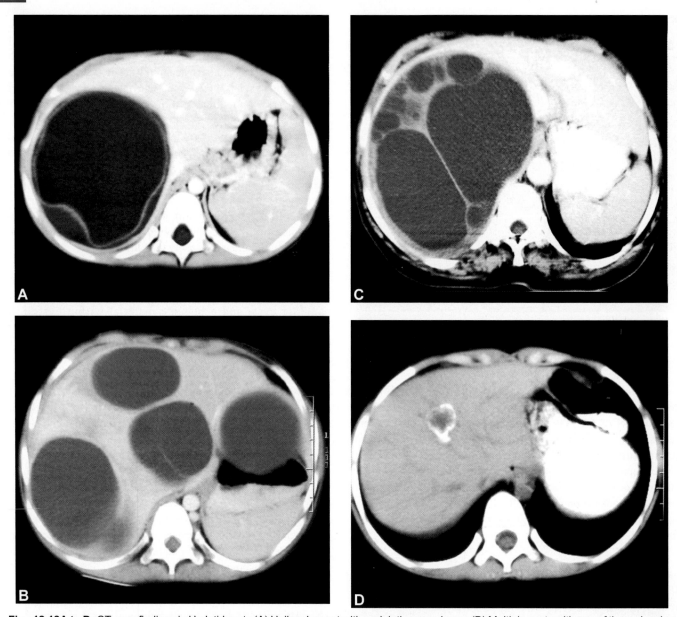

Figs 12.18A to D: CT scan findings in Hydatid cysts (A) Unilocular cyst with undulating membrane (B) Multiple cysts with one of them showing septation (C) Multiseptated cyst in right lobe of liver with multiple peripheral daughter cysts (D) Partially calcified cyst

CAROLI'S DISEASE

This represents type V (Todani) choledochal cyst and is characterized by segmental nonobstructive dilatation of the intrahepatic bile ducts. It is associated with hepatic fibrosis, medullary sponge kidney and infantile polycystic renal disease. Patient presents with abdominal pain secondary to cholangitis or to biliary calculi. US typically shows ectatic ducts surrounding portal vein radicles ('intraluminal portal vein sign').[45] The counterpart of this intraluminal portal vein sign is the 'central dot' sign seen on CT. The common duct and gallbladder are dilated. MRCP is indicated to define the anatomy of the biliary tree in Caroli's disease.

PANCREATIC MASSES

Pancreatoblastoma

The term pancreatoblastoma was first coined by Horie et al for infantile tumors of the pancreas.[46] This tumor is located in the body or tail region of pancreas. According to some authors it is more commonly located in the pancreatic head.[46,47] It usually occurs in newborns and children less than 8 years of age. The mean age at presentation is 6 years. The congenital form is associated with Beckwith-Wiedemann syndrome.[45] Patient presents with an abdominal mass, weight loss, pain, nausea and diarrhea. These tumors secrete alpha-fetoprotein, alpha1-antitrypsin and lactate

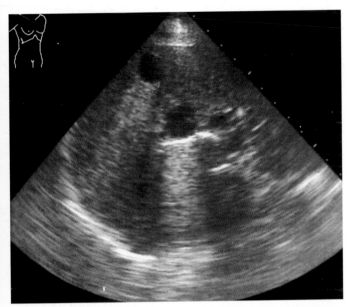

Fig. 12.19: Ultrasound of liver in a 4-year-old child reveals two anechoic lesions with imperceptible wall and distal acoustic enhancement suggestive of simple cysts

dehydrogenase. These tumors are usually large at presentation (7-12 cm) and show areas of necrosis.

Microscopically pancreatoblastoma consists of acinar cells. Small areas of squamous differentiation ('squamoid corpuscles') are typically present. The tumor is well-encapsulated and has a good prognosis after surgery. If metastases are seen at the time of diagnosis, the prognosis is poor.

Barium studies may reveal features of mass effect (Fig. 12.20A). Ultrasound shows a heterogeneous or predominantly hypoechoic mass. Sometimes cystic areas and foci of calcification are seen within the mass (Fig. 12.20B). Even when these tumors are present in the head of pancreas they do not cause biliary obstruction despite their large size (Fig. 12.20C). This is due to the soft and gelatinous consistency of these tumors.[49] The tumor may directly spread into the portal vein.[50] Vascular encasement commonly involves the mesenteric vessels and inferior vena cava. Aortic encasement, however, has not been described.

On CT, the tumor is hypodense and shows mild enhancement. Sometimes it is seen as a multiloculated mass with enhancing septae. Central necrosis may be seen (Figs 12.21A and B). The most common metastases seen in pancreatoblastoma are to the liver. Metastatic spread may also occur to lymph nodes, peritoneal cavity and the lungs. Bony metastases are very rare.

MR shows these tumors as hypointense on T1W images and iso – or hyperintense on T2W images. Contrast enhancement is variable.

Imaging in pancreatoblastoma is required to localize the organ of origin of the mass and to determine the extent of spread. It is important to distinguish pancreatoblastoma from other pediatric masses like neuroblastoma, lymphoma or Wilms' tumor.

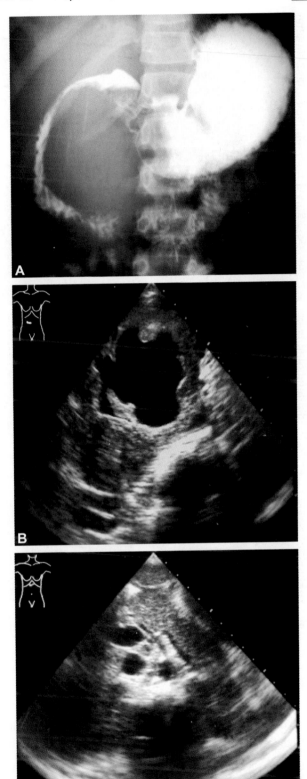

Figs 12.20A to C: A 12- year-old male patient with pancreatoblastoma. (A) Barium meal examination shows widening of the 'C' loop of duodenum with mass effect on the second part of duodenum and gastric antrum. (B) Transverse US images show a large mass in the head of pancreas with central necrotic area (C) The body and tail of pancreas are normal. No ductal dilatation in seen

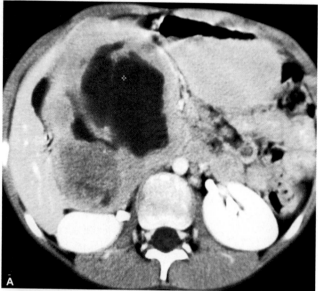

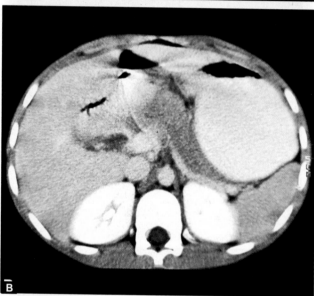

Figs 12.21A and B: (A) CECT in the case of pancreatoblastoma shows a large heterogeneous mass in the head of pancreas with central necrosis (B) There is no dilatation of biliary radicles or pancreatic duct

ISLET CELL TUMORS

Islet cell tumors are rare pancreatic neoplasms that produce and secrete hormones to a variable degree. Insulinoma, glucagonoma, gastrinoma, vasoactive intestinal polypeptide producing tumor and somatostatinoma have been reported in childhood.[11] Insulinomas are the commonest islet cell tumors. The majority of these lesions are solitary (80%) and benign (90%). The usual age of presentation is over 4 years of age although islet cell adenomas have been reported to occur in the neonatal period.

Functional tumors are diagnosed due to the hormonal activity and imaging is needed for preoperative localization. Insulinomas lead to hypoglycemia and the affected children show seizure activity and erratic behavior which is relieved by the administration of glucose. The diagnosis is confirmed by reproducible hypoglycemia in a controlled environment (fasting) and by showing concomitant hyperinsulinaemia. Table 12.5 shows the clinical and laboratory features of patients with functional islet cell tumors.

Nonfunctioning tumors are usually large at time of presentation and contain necrotic and calcified areas. They are easily detected due to the mass effect that they produce.

With the availability of helical CT and MRI, invasive imaging techniques like selective celiac and mesenteric angiography and venography with venous sampling are rarely being used for the diagnosis of islet cell tumors. Selective arteriography is diagnostic in 60 percent to 70 percent of cases while transhepatic portal venous sampling has been reported to have an 86 percent success rate for tumor localization.[51]

Endoscopic ultrasound is an excellent imaging technique with sensitivity and specificity of 93 percent and 95 percent respectively.[52] On US, these tumors are usually seen as well-defined hypoechoic lesions. A hyperechoic rim may sometimes be seen. Isoechoic and hyperechoic lesions have also been described.

On dual phase helical CT, small islet cell tumors are seen as homogeneous hyperattenuating lesions on the arterial as well as portal venous phase. However, these tumors are hypervascular and the attenuation difference between the lesion and the normal pancreatic parenchyma is more in the arterial phase than in the portal venous phase. Nonfunctioning islet cell tumors also have similar characteristics. Larger lesions show heterogeneous enhancement (Figs 12.22A and B). There is no precise data about the sensitivity of biphasic CT for islet cell tumor diagnosis because of the rarity of such studies. The reported sensitivity of CT for localizing functional islet cell tumors is 71 to 82 percent.[53]

Fat suppressed T1WI shows islet cell tumors as low signal intensity lesions compared to the normal pancreas. These lesions are hyperintense on T2WI. Some islet cell tumors may be hypointense on T2WI also due to the presence of fibrous tissue. The sensitivity of MR imaging ranges from 24 to 100 percent.[54] This conflicting data is due to the small reported patient series and the variations in the imaging sequences used.

Table 12.5: Clinical and laboratory features of islet cell tumors		
Functioning islet cell tumor	*Clinical presentation*	*Laboratory findings*
Insulinoma	Hypoglycemic attacks, Atypical seizures	Low fasting plasma glucose, hyperinsulinemia
Gastrinoma	Peptic ulcers, diarrhea, malabsorption	Elevated serum gastrin
Glucagonoma	Necrolytic migratory erythema	Hyperglycemia
VIPoma	Watery diarrhea, flushing	Hypokalemia, achlorhydria, elevated plasma peptide

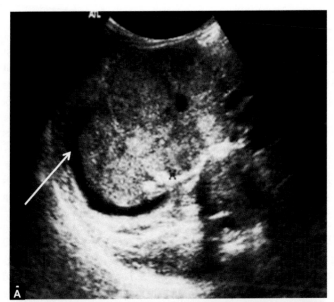

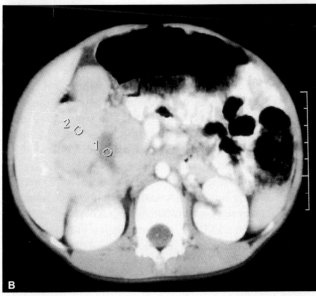

Figs 12.22A and B: An 8-year-old boy with abdominal mass. (A) US reveals a solid mass lesion with duodenum (arrow) draped around it (B) CECT confirms a large heterogeneous mass with central necrosis in the head of pancreas. Histopathological examination of surgical specimen revealed non-functioning neuroendocrine tumor of the pancreas

SOLID AND PAPILLARY EPITHELIAL NEOPLASM (SPEN) (FRANTZ TUMOR)

This tumor was first described by Frantz in 1959. SPEN is an uncommon low grade malignant pancreatic tumor which occurs in young women. The usual age of presentation ranges from 10-74 years with the mean age at diagnosis being 25 years.[55] However it also occurs in the pediatric population .It is common in blacks and East Asian patients.

Patients present with an abdominal mass, pain, nausea and early satiety. The tumor is usually large at presentation and shows areas of necrosis and hemorrhage resulting in cystic cavities. Peripheral calcification is seen in one third of cases.

Microscopically SPEN has characteristic histological features. The solid areas in the lesion are traversed by numerous delicate blood vessels. The disruption of this delicate vascular network leads to intralesional hemorrhage. Acellular spaces form subsequently, which fill with myxoid connective tissue.

On US, the tumor shows variable echotexture. Hyperechoic areas are seen due to hemorrhage. The tumor shows heterogeneous attenuation on CT. On MRI (Figs 12.23A to C), areas of high signal intensity may be seen on T1WI due to presence of hemorrhagic debris within the tumor. A fluid-debris level may be seen on imaging.

SPEN needs to be distinguished from other cystic lesions of the pancreas like microcystic adenoma, mucinous cystadenoma and cystadenocarcinoma, nonfunctioning islet cell tumor and hemorrhagic pseudocysts. Microcystic adenoma is well-circumscribed lesion with microscopic cystic spaces. This lesion is seen in older women and has no malignant potential. Mucinous cystadenoma may have large cystic spaces and shows fluid-debris levels like SPEN. This can be differentiated from SPEN due to the presence of multiple loculi and septations. Mucinous cystadenoma is a premalignant lesion and can transform into cystadenocarcinoma.

MESENCHYMAL TUMORS

These account for 1-2 percent of all pancreatic tumors.[49] These include lymphangioma, lipoma, teratoma, schwannoma and lymphoma. Their exact prevalence in the pediatric population is unknown.

Lymphangioma is a multicystic lesion with cysts of varying sizes separated by thin septa. CT shows a uni- or multilocular cystic mass with enhancing septa. Calcification is rarely seen within the lesion. Pancreatic lymphangioma may be intraglandular or may be connected to the gland by a pedicle. These lymphangiomas are liable to undergo torsion.

Lipoma is seen as homogeneous well-defined nonenhancing lesion with attenuation value of -30 to -120HU.

Pancreatic teratoma originates from pluripotential cells and contains both cystic and solid elements like hair, teeth, cartilage and dermal appendages. On CT, a complex solid cystic mass with calcifications and fatty component is seen.

Pancreas is an unusual site for visceral Schwannomas. In tumors with Antoni type A tissue (organized cellular component), a solid enhancing mass with central necrosis or an in homogeneous hypodense lesion is seen on CT. In tumors with Antoni type B tissue (loose hypocellular component), CT shows a homogeneous fluid attenuation lesion without any significant contrast enhancement.

Less than one percent of non-Hodgkin's lymphoma can be seen in the pancreas. AIDS-related NHL may also involve the pancreas. Pancreatic lymphoma can present as diffuse infiltrating lesion in the pancreas or as focal well-defined mass.

Primary pancreatic sarcoma accounts for 0.6 percent of pancreatic malignancies. CT shows a heterogeneous solid mass with inhomogeneous enhancement.[56] Imaging findings cannot distinguish sarcoma from adenocarcinoma.

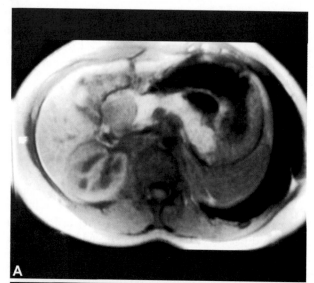

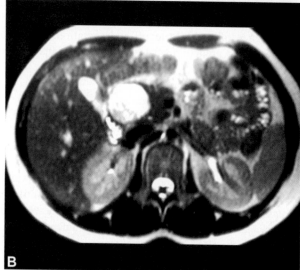

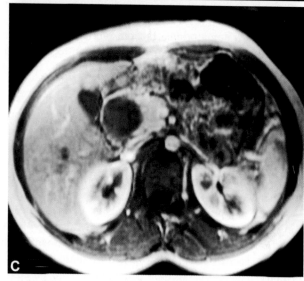

Figs 12.23A to C: Biopsy proven SPEN: (A) Fat saturated T1W and (B) T2W MRI images show the lesion to be hypointense on T1W images and hyperintense on T2W images. The lesion does not show any significant contrast enhancement (C)

PANCREATIC ADENOCARCINOMA

It is the most common pancreatic malignancy occurring in the sixth decade of life but is relatively rare in children. The incidence of pancreatic carcinoma in children is not known. Welch[57] reviewed 38 patients of pancreatic carcinoma in children and found that the age at time of diagnosis ranged from 3 months to 18 years with a mean age of 9.2 years. Abdominal pain and epigastric mass were the common presentations. Unlike in adult patient, jaundice was found to be less common presenting symptom in children.

The imaging features are similar to those seen in adults. Ultrasound shows a poorly defined, homogeneous or inhomogeneous hypoechoic mass in the pancreas. CT assesses the local extension of the tumor and determines the resectability of the lesion.

PSEUDOCYSTS

These are frequent complications of pancreatitis regardless of its etiology. An overall incidence of 10-12 percent has been reported in pancreatitis with a 30 percent incidence in case of traumatic pancreatitis.[58] Thus, pseudocysts occur more often in children with traumatic pancreatitis compared with those with nontraumatic pancreatitis.

Acute pancreatitis is uncommon in childhood. The most common etiology is multisystem disease (Reye's syndrome, sepsis, shock, viral infections, hemolyticuremic syndrome).[59] Other common causes include blunt trauma, congenital anatomic abnormalities, drug toxicity and metabolic diseases. Children with pancreatitis present with abdominal pain, nausea and vomiting.

Ultrasonography is the initial imaging modality for detecting pseudocysts in children with pancreatitis. Pseudocyst is seen as a well-defined anechoic lesion with or without debris. CT is indicated when the pancreas is not well-visualized on ultrasonography. On CT, pseudocyst is seen as a low attenuating lesion with enhancing walls (Figs 12.24A and B). High attenuation in the pseudocyst occurs due to hemorrhage or infection. In case of complicated or recurrent pancreatitis, MRCP is done to evaluate the pancreatic ductal system for congenital ductal anomalies. However for pancreatic duct injury in patients with traumatic pancreatitis, ERCP is required to delineate the site of disruption.

Pancreatic pseudocysts may resolve spontaneously. In the past non-resolving or infected pseudocyst was drained surgically. Percutaneous drainage is an alternative mode of treatment. Its advantages over surgical drainage include early treatment prior to cyst wall maturation and reduction of length and cost of hospital stay.[60]

PANCREATIC TUBERCULOSIS

Abdominal tuberculosis is uncommon in children with a reported incidence of 10 percent under the age of 10 years.[61] Only 1-5 percent of cases of pulmonary tuberculosis are complicated by abdominal tuberculosis. Tuberculosis infrequently involves the pancreas. Pancreatic involvement in children was first reported by Andronikou et al in 2002.[62]

The common presenting features are pain, fever, anorexia and weight loss. Obstructive jaundice, vomiting and anemia are less common symptoms.

modalities can help to reach at a correct preoperative diagnosis in the majority. Awareness of the imaging characteristics, advantages and limitations of different imaging techniques are crucial for diagnosis and management.

REFERENCES

1. Kane RA. Liver imaging update. Seminars in ultrasound, CT and MRI. 1992;13:311-2.
2. Takano H, Smith WL. Gastrointestinal tumors of childhood. Radiol Clin North Am. 1997; 35: 1367-89.
3. Lu DS, Vedantham S, Krasny RM, Kadell B, Berger WL, Reber HA. Two-phase helical CT for pancreatic tumors: Pancreatic versus hepatic phase enhancement of tumor, pancreas, and vascular structures. Radiology 1996;199:697-701.
4. www.imagegently.org last accessed on 15.10.10.
5. Boechat MI, Kangarloo H, Ortega J, et al. Primary liver tumors in children: Comparison of CT and MR imaging. Radiology 1988; 169:727-32.
6. Weinreb JC, Cohen JM, Armstrong E, Smith T. Imaging the pediatric liver: MRI and CT. AJR 1986; 147: 785-90.
7. Drane WE. Nuclear medicine techniques for the liver and biliary system. Update for the 1990s. Radiol Clin North Am. 1991; 29: 1129-50.
8. Weinberg AG, Finegold MJ. Primary hepatic tumors of childhood. Hum Pathol. 1983;14:512-37.
9. Siegel MJ. Pediatric liver and biliary tract. In Margulis, Burhennes, (Eds): Alimentary Tract Radiology 5th edn. Mosby-Year Book Inc., USA, 1994.
10. Willis RA. The pathology of the tumors of children. In Cameron R, Wright GP, (Eds): Pathological Monographs. Oliver and Boyd, London, 1962:57-61.
11. Miller JH, Greenspan BS. Integrated imaging of hepatic tumors in childhood. Part I: Malignant lesions (primary and metastatic). Radiology. 1985; 154: 83-90.
12. Roebuck DJ, Olsen Ø, Pariente D. Radiological staging in children with hepatoblastoma. Pediatr Radiol. 2006; 36: 176-82.
13. Dachman AH, Pakter RL, Ros PR, Fishman EK, Goodman ZD, Lichtenstein JE. Hepatoblastoma: Radiologic-pathologic correlation in 50 cases. Radiology 1987; 164: 15-9.
14. Men S, Hekimoðlu B, Tüzün M, Arda IS, Pinar A. Unusual US and CT findings in hepatoblastoma: A case report. Pediatr Radiol. 1995; 25: 507-8.
15. Amendola MA, Blane CE, Amendola BE, Glazer GM. CT findings in hepatoblastoma. J Comput Assist Tomogr. 1984; 8: 1105-9.
16. Schlesinger AE, Parker BR. Tumors and tumor-like conditions. In Kuhn JP, Slovis TL, Haller JO, (Eds): Caffey's Pediatric Diagnostic imaging. 10th edn. Mosby, USA, 2004: p 1493-1508.
17. Blickman JG , Connolly SA. Pediatric imaging: Liver, biliary tree, and pancreas. In Gazelle GS, Saini S, Mueller PR, (Eds): Hepatobiliary and Pancreatic Radiology, Imaging and Intervention, 1st edn. Thieme, Germany, 1998: p240-70.
18. Brandt DJ, Johnson CD, Stephens DH, Weiland LH. Imaging of fibrolamellar hepatocellular carcinoma. AJR 1988; 151: 295-9.
19. Horton KM, Bluemke DA, Hruban RH, Soyer P, Fishman EK. CT and MR imaging of benign hepatic and biliary tumors. Radiographics. 1999; 19: 431-51.
20. Ruymann FB, Raney RB Jr, Crist WM, Lawrence W Jr, Lindberg RD, Soule EH. Rhabdomyosarcoma of the biliary tree in childhood. A report from the Intergroup Rhabdomyosarcoma Study. Cancer. 1985; 56: 575-81.

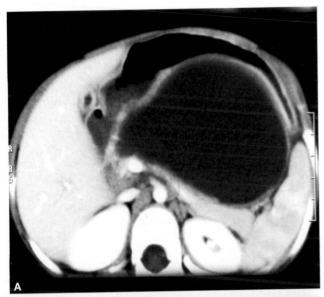

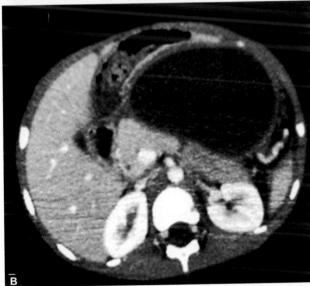

Figs 12.24A and B: (A) CECT in a 3-year-old female patient with pancreatitis and pseudocyst shows a large well-defined fluid attenuation lesion with enhancing wall in the lesser sac. (B) CECT section in another patient with traumatic pancreatitis shows laceration of the pancreas with a fluid collection in the lesser sac

Ultrasound shows an enlarged pancreas with focal hypoechoic lesions especially in the head region. A cystic lesion may sometimes be seen. CT shows multiple hypodense lesions. The imaging findings are nonspecific and may be mimicked by pancreatic carcinoma or focal pancreatitis. Associated ancillary findings such as hypodense peripancreatic or mesenteric lymph nodes, ascites, mural thickening of the ileocaecal region can help in prospectively diagnosing tuberculosis.[63] The diagnosis should however be confirmed on US or CT guided biopsy.

SUMMARY

Hepatic and pancreatic masses in children are a common clinical problem in pediatric population. Judicious use of various imaging

21. Craig JR, Peters RL, Edmondson HA. Tumors of the liver and intrahepatic bile ducts. In Craig JR, Peters RL,Edmondson HA (Eds). Atlas of tumor pathology, fasc 26, ser 2, Wasnigton DC, Armed forces Istitute of Pathology 1989: p 1-280.

22. Smith WL, Franken EA, Mitros FA. Liver tumors in children. Semin Roentgenol 1983; 18: 136-48.

23. Dachman AH, Lichtenstein JE, Friedman AC, Hartman DS. Infantile hemangioendothelioma of the liver: A radiologic-pathologic-clinical correlation. AJR 1983; 140: 1091-6.

24. Dehner LP, Ishak KG. Vascular tumors of the liver in infants and children. A study of 30 cases and review of the literature. Arch Pathol. 1971 ; 92: 101-11.

25. Connolly B. The paediatric liver, biliary tree and spleen. In Grainger RG, Allison DJ, Adam A, Dixon AK, (Eds): *Diagnostic Radiology* 4th edn. Churchill Livingstone, USA, 2001: p 1447-65.

26. Thapa BR, Yaccha S, Narsimharao KL, Gupta HL, Kataryia S, Mehta S. Multinodular infantile hemangioendothelioma of liver. Indian Pediatr. 1988; 25: 199-203.

27. Bar-Sever Z, Horev G, Lubin E, Kornreich L, Naor N, Ziv N, Shimoni A, Grunebaum M. A rare coexistence of a multicentric hepatic hemangioendothelioma with a large brain hemangioma in a preterm infant. Pediatr Radiol. 1994; 24: 141-2.

28. Abramson SJ, Lack EE, Teele RL. Benign vascular tumors of the liver in infants: Sonographic appearance. AJR 1982; 138: 629-32.

29. Ros PR, Goodman ZD, Ishak KG, et al. Mesenchymal hamartoma of the liver: Radiologic-pathologic correlation. Radiology. 1986; 158: 619-24.

30. Narasimharao KL, Narasimhan KL, Katariya S, Suri S, Kaushik S, Mitra SK. Giant hamartoma of liver mimicking malignancy. Postgrad Med J. 1988; 64: 398-400.

31. Stanley P, Hall TR, Woolley MM, Diament MJ, Gilsanz V, Miller JH. Mesenchymal hamartomas of the liver in childhood: Sonographic and CT findings. AJR 1986; 147: 1035-9.

32. Rogers JV, Mack LA, Freeny PC, Johnson ML, Sones PJ. Hepatic focal nodular hyperplasia: Angiography, CT, sonography, and scintigraphy. AJR 1981; 137: 983-90.

33. Chusid MJ. Pyogenic hepatic abscess in infancy and childhood. Pediatrics. 1978; 62: 554-9.

34. Newlin N, Silver TM, Stuck KJ, Sandler MA. Ultrasonic features of pyogenic liver abscesses. Radiology. 1981; 139: 155-9.

35. Towbin RB, Strife JL. Percutaneous aspiration, drainage, and biopsies in children. Radiology. 1985; 157: 81-5.

36. Rajak CL, Gupta S, Jain S, Chawla Y, Gulati M, Suri S. Percutaneous treatment of liver abscesses: Needle aspiration versus catheter drainage. AJR 1998; 170: 1035-9.

37. Ralls PW, Colletti PM, Quinn MF, Halls J. Sonographic findings in hepatic amebic abscess. Radiology. 1982; 145: 123-6.

38. Miller JH, Greenfield LD, Wald BR. Candidiasis of the liver and spleen in childhood. Radiology. 1982; 142: 375-80.

39. Brauner M, Buffard MD, Jeantils V, Legrand I, Gotheil C. Sonography and computed tomography of macroscopic tuberculosis of the liver. J Clin Ultrasound 1989; 17: 563-8.

40. Denton T, Hossain J. A radiological study of abdominal tuberculosis in a Saudi population, with special reference to ultrasound and computed tomography. Clin Radiol. 1993; 47: 409-14.

41. Beggs I. The radiology of hydatid disease. AJR 1985; 145: 639-48.

42. Lewall DB, McCorkell SJ. Rupture of echinococcal cysts: Diagnosis, classification, and clinical implications. AJR 1986; 146: 391-4.

43. Jain R, Sawhney S, Berry M. Hydatid disease: CT demonstration and follow-up of a cystogastric fistula. AJR 1992; 158: 212.

44. Wan SK, Cochlin DL. Sonographic and computed tomographic features of polycystic disease of the liver. Gastrointest Radiol. 1990; 15:310-2.

45. Tomà P, Lucigrai G, Pelizza A. Sonographic patterns of Caroli's disease: Report of 5 new cases. J Clin Ultrasound. 1991; 19:155-61.

46. Horie A, Yano Y, Kotoo Y, Miwa A. Morphogenesis of pancreatoblastoma, infantile carcinoma of the pancreas: Report of two cases. Cancer. 197; 39: 247-54.

47. Willnow U, Willberg B, Schwamborn D, Körholz D, Göbel U. Pancreatoblastoma in children. Case report and review of the literature. Eur J Pediatr Surg. 1996; 6: 369-72.

48. Drut R, Jones MC. Congenital pancreatoblastoma in Beckwith-Wiedemann syndrome: An emerging association. Pediatr Pathol. 1988; 8: 331-9.

49. Klöppel G, Maillet B. Classification and staging of pancreatic nonendocrine tumors. Radiol Clin North Am. 1989; 27: 105-19.

50. Gupta AK, Mitra DK, Berry M, Dinda AK, Bhatnagar V. Sonography and CT of pancreatoblastoma in children. AJR 2000; 174: 1639-41.

51. Grosfeld JL, Vane DW, Rescorla FJ, McGuire W, West KW. Pancreatic tumors in childhood: Analysis of 13 cases. J Pediatr Surg. 1990; 25: 1057-62.

52. Anderson MA, Carpenter S, Thompson NW, Nostrant TT, Elta GH, Scheiman JM. Endoscopic ultrasound is highly accurate and directs management in patients with neuroendocrine tumors of the pancreas. Am J Gastroenterol. 2000; 95: 2271-7.

53. Sheth S, Fishman EK. Imaging of uncommon tumors of the pancreas. Radiol Clin North Am. 2002; 40: 1273-87.

54. Ichikawa T, Peterson MS, Federle MP, Baron RL, Haradome H, Kawamori Y, Nawano S, Araki T. Islet cell tumor of the pancreas: Biphasic CT versus MR imaging in tumor detection. Radiology. 2000; 216: 163-71.

55. Buetow PC, Buck JL, Pantongrag-Brown L, Beck KG, Ros PR, Adair CF. Solid and papillary epithelial neoplasm of the pancreas: Imaging-pathologic correlation on 56 cases. Radiology. 1996 ; 199: 707-11.

56. Ferrozzi F, Zuccoli G, Bova D, Calculli L. Mesenchymal tumors of the pancreas: CT findings. J Comput Assist Tomogr. 2000; 24: 622-7.

57. Welch KJ. The pancreas. In Ravitch MM, Randolph JG, Rowe MI, et al (Eds): Pediatric Surgery 3rd edn. Chicago, IL:Year book, 1984: pp1090-96.

58. Eichelberger MR, Hoelzer DJ, Koop CE. Acute pancreatitis: The difficulties of diagnosis and therapy. J Pediatr Surg. 1982; 17: 244-54.

59. Weizman Z, Durie PR. Acute pancreatitis in childhood. J Pediatr. 1988; 113: 24-9.

60. Amundson GM, Towbin RB, Mueller DL, Seagram CG. Percutaneous transgastric drainage of the lesser sac in children. Pediatr Radiol. 1990; 20: 590-3.

61. Aston NO. Abdominal tuberculosis. World J Surg. 1997; 21: 492-9.

62. Andronikou S, Welman CJ, Kader E. The CT features of abdominal tuberculosis in children. Pediatr Radiol. 2002; 32: 75-81.

63. Takhtani D, Gupta S, Suman K, et al. Radiology of pancreatic tuberculosis: A report of three cases. Am J Gastroenterol. 1996; 91: 1832-4.

CHAPTER 13

Childhood Biliopathies

Veena Chowdhury

Cholestasis is the principal manifestation of hepatobiliary disease and jaundice is the most common clinical problem which necessitates examination of biliary tract in childhood. There are few disorders which can manifest within the first year of life and these present an important challenge because, not only is hepatic structure and function disturbed but also normal development may be retarded or altered by the disease process.

DEFINITION AND PATHOPHYSIOLOGY OF CHOLESTASIS

Cholestasis is defined as a pathological state of reduced bile formation or flow. The clinical state of jaundice occurs in any condition in which substances normally excreted into the bile are retained in varying proportion.[1]

PHYSIOLOGICAL NEONATAL JAUNDICE

Jaundice is the most common problem in the neonatal period, occurring in approximately 60 percent of term infants and 80 percent of preterm infants.[2,3] Metabolism of bilirubin in the neonate is in transition from the fetal stage, when the placenta eliminates bilirubin, to the adult stage, during which bilirubin is excreted from the hepatocytes into the biliary system and then into the gastrointestinal tract. Jaundice occurs when the liver is unable to clear sufficient bilirubin from the plasma. Excessive bilirubin formation or limited uptake and conjugation leads to excess unconjugated bilirubin in the blood. Impaired bile flow and bilirubin excretion result in excess conjugated bilirubin in the blood and urine causing cholestatic jaundice.

During the first 24 hours of life, jaundice may be due to erythroblastosis fetalis, hemorrhage, sepsis and intrauterine infections. Jaundice that appears in the second or third day is usually physiologic but may represent a more severe form of hyper-bilirubinemia of the newborn.[3]

Physiologic jaundice is the most common cause of neonatal jaundice. It has its onset by the third day of life and usually resolves by 7 days of life. The bilirubin levels usually do not exceed 12 mg/dl in full-term infants and 14 mg/dl in preterm infants. The cause of neonatal jaundice should be investigated if:

1. The onset of jaundice is within the first 24 hours of life or if jaundice persists beyond 7 days of life.
2. The bilirubin level is above 12 mg/dl in full-term infants and 14 mg/dl in preterm infants and a direct-reacting bilirubin component exceeds 1 mg/dl at any time.

Breastfed term infants (1 in 200) may have noncholestatic jaundice that persists into the second week of life and if nursing is discontinued, the serum bilirubin falls to normal levels within a few days. This is due to substances in the breast milk of some mothers that impair conjugation of bilirubin.

Nonobstructive jaundice in the neonate and infant is due to sepsis, Rh/ABO incompatibility, red blood cell defects, drug effects, congenital enzyme deficiencies, systemic metabolic disorders, gastrointestinal obstruction and cystic fibrosis.[4,5]

ETIOLOGY OF JAUNDICE IN THE NEONATE AND INFANT

Hepatocellular cholestasis results from impairment of mechanisms of bile formation. The reduction in bile flow with retention of substances normally excreted in the bile is due to an anatomic or functional obstruction in the biliary system resulting in obstructive jaundice. The obstruction may be either at the level of larger extrahepatic bile ducts or at the smaller intrahepatic bile ducts. Major causes of jaundice in neonates are :

Transient Causes
- Hepatic infection
- Sepsis
- Metabolic disease
- Bile plug syndrome
- Adrenal hemorrhage
- Drug related

Persistent Causes
- Neonatal hepatitis
- Biliary atresia
- Choledochal cyst
- Alagille syndrome
- Spontaneous perforation of the common bile duct

Major causes of obstructive jaundice in infancy are:

Common
- Biliary atresia
- Congenital bile duct anomalies (Choledochal cysts)

Uncommon
- Infectious cholangitis
- Primary sclerosing cholangitis
- Langerhans' cell histiocytosis

- Cholelithiasis
- Tumor-Sarcoma botryoides

Biliary atresia accounts for more than 90 percent of cases with obstructive jaundice in infancy.

Other Causes of Cholestasis

Cholestasis may also occur in conditions associated with paucity of ducts. These are:

- Syndromatic paucity: Alagille's syndrome[6]
- Nonsyndromatic ductal paucity

Rare causes of bile duct disease in children are idiopathic congenital stricture of the bile duct, obstruction of bile duct due to pancreatic disease, post-traumatic or spontaneous perforation of the common bile duct, biliary helminthiasis and cystic fibrosis.

DIAGNOSIS OF JAUNDICE IN INFANCY AND CHILDHOOD

The differential diagnosis of cholestasis in neonates and infants is much broader than in children and adults.[7,8] This is because the immature liver is sensitive to injury and the response of immature liver is more limited. The so called "physiologic stasis" results from functional immaturity. The sensitivity of the infant to insults that would not produce cholestasis in the adults, such as gram negative sepsis, heart failure, metabolic disease and exposure to minimally toxic substances alerts the clinician to look beyond the liver for the causes of cholestasis present in the newborn or young infant. A more focussed investigation can be undertaken if these causes are excluded.

The differential diagnosis of hepatobiliary diseases resulting in jaundice in infants is limited, and major concern is to differentiate hepatocellular from obstructive cholestasis because it represents the differential between the disorders of physiology and anatomy or medical versus surgical jaundice. Laboratory tests are often not diagnostic as the biochemical differences between hepatocellular and obstructive cholestasis are few and there is an overlap in values. The diagnosis is usually made with the help of imaging and biopsy.

The imaging modalities routinely used are:

1. Ultrasonography (US)
2. Computed tomography (CT)
3. MRI and MRCP
4. Biliary scintigraphy (^{99m}Tc HIDA scan)
5. Cholangiography—percutaneous transhepatic cholangiography (PTC),
   Endoscopic retrograde cholangiopancreatography (ERCP).

Sonography is the preferred screening method for detection of intrahepatic ductal dilatation and to exclude anatomic anomalies of the extrahepatic biliary system, the most common being choledochal cyst. Sonography may identify other anatomic causes for the patient's jaundice, such as stones or inspissated bile in the bile plug syndrome. Bile plug syndrome is a rare cause of perinantal jaundice of unclear etiology that may be related to total parenteral nutrition or cystic fibrosis in which sludge (echogenic or hypoechoic) in the bile ducts and gallbladder forms plugs and may cause transient gallbladder hydrops and duct dilatation.

Computed tomography can be used to identify associated congenital and acquired abnormalities such as polysplenia and portal hypertension.

Magnetic resonance cholangiopancreatography is an effective noninvasive imaging technique for the evaluation of panreaticobiliary disease in children. [9,10]

Paediatric MR cholangiopancreatography needs to be optimized and tailored to the different body sizes intrinsic to children of various ages. For visualization of small caliber ducts, spatial resolution and SNR needs to be improved. The first step toward such improvement is proper coil selection.[11] Either a phased-array or a surface coil that fits the child well should be used for signal reception. Poor signal in children can be compensated for to some extent by increasing the number of signals averaged to between four and eight. However, this needs to be balanced with the ETL, since increasing the number of signals averaged increases scanning time. Proper slab thickness in 2D FSE and SSFSE imaging is the next step towards obtaining optimal-quality images. Smaller children such as neonates and infants do not need a slab thickness of more than 2 cm. Thin-section (3-5mm) images in the axial and coronal planes, as well as thick slabs in radiating coronal planes, should be acquired. A 3DFSE sequence should be performed whenever breathing is regular. It provides better SNR and spatial resolution than 2D FSE imaging. Moreover, anomalies can be better understood by rotating 3D images. Because neonates and infants usually have irregular breathing with varying respiratory amplitude, 3 D FSE imaging with respiratory triggering may not be possible in many of these patients. SSFSE imaging with varying section thickness can be useful in this situation providing adequate image quality even with free shallow breathing.

Hepatobiliary scintigraphy (^{99m}Tc HIDA scan) **is usually required to differentiate between neonatal hepatitis and biliary atresia.**

Operative cholangiograms are performed to evaluate the intrahepatic and extrahepatic portions of the biliary system as biliary atresia may affect only portions of the biliary tree.

NEONATAL HEPATITIS

Neonatal hepatitis (giant cell neonatal hepatitis) represents a morphologic alteration of the liver that occurs as a nonspecific reaction to various insults. The disease is idiopathic (55%), familial (10%), infectious (20%), and metabolic in 15 percent of cases.[12]

Idiopathic neonatal hepatitis is the most common cause of neonatal cholestasis accounting for one third to two third of cases. The incidence ranges from 1 in 4800 to 1 in 9000 live births. Male preterm infants are more commonly affected.

More than half of neonates with this disorder have jaundice of varying degree within the first week of life, about one-third show failure to thrive and have a fulminant course leading to extensive hepatocellular damage. On clinical examination, hepato-splenomegaly is found and a bleeding diathesis may be present. Laboratory tests reveal abnormal elevation of liver enzyme levels.

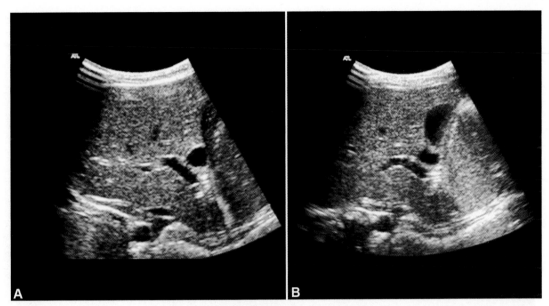

Figs 13.1A and B: Gray scale sonograms of a jaundiced neonate showing increased periportal echogenicity with a normal sized gallbladder – Neonatal hepatitis

Pathology

Liver biopsy is helpful in confirming the diagnosis of idiopathic neonatal hepatitis and in excluding other causes of neonatal cholestasis. Histologic examination demonstrates hepatocellular swelling with marked variation in cell size, portal inflammatory exudate, regeneration and individual cell necrosis, multinucleated giant cells throughout the lobules, and increased extramedullary hematopoiesis.

Imaging Features

Ultrasonography and radionuclide scintigraphy are the most widely used imaging modalities used in this disorder. US findings are, however, nonspecific. The liver may be normal or increased in size with increased periportal echogenicity. Intrahepatic and extrahepatic bile ducts are normal in caliber while the gallbladder may be normal, small, large, or not visualized (Figs 13.1A and B). The normal common bile duct should measure less than 1mm in neonates, less than 2 mm in infants upto 1 year old, less than 4 mm in older children and less than 7 mm in adolescents and adults. In infants the normal gallbladder length is 1.5–3 cm.[13,14] Ikeda et al. have reported that serial ultrasound may be useful in the differentiation of neonatal hepatitis and biliary atresia when the gallbladder is visualized. According to these authors, postprandial gallbladder contraction can be seen in patients with neonatal hepatitis but not in patients with biliary atresia.[15]

A radionuclide hepatobiliary study demonstrates the radiopharmaceutical agent in the bowel, thereby excluding biliary atresia. Nuclear medicine studies of the biliary tree have been the traditional definitive imaging method for the differentiation of biliary atresia from neonatal hepatitis and are typically performed after US. Evaluation of the blood pool and hepatic phases and determination of the presence or absence of radioisotope in the gastrointestinal tract on delayed images are all necessary for the proper investigation of biliary atresia. Patients should be pretreated

with phenobarbital. The oral administration of Phenobarbital for 5 days before the study is said to enhance the biliary excretion of the isotope. If the early scans do not demonstrate isotopic activity in the gastrointestinal tract, delayed scans, up to 24 hours, should be obtained. The presence of radioisotope in the gastrointestinal tract essentially excludes biliary atresia. Scintigraphy has an excellent sensitivity of 96-97% in diffentiating biliary atresia from neonatal hepatitis.[16] Although, most patients with neonatal hepatitis have excretion of the radionuclide into the gut, patients with severe hepatic injury may not have sufficient liver function to excrete detectable amounts of radiotracer into the gastrointestinal tract. Thus, if there is lack of demonstration of the radionuclide in the bowel, the distinction between severe hepatocellular disease and biliary atresia cannot be made with certainty.[17]

On MR imaging, T2 weighted images reveal a collar of high signal intensity surrounding portal vein branches due to periportal edema, however, this finding is nonspecific (Figs 13.2A to E). Overall, if the gallbladder is normal or near normal in size and hepatic bile duct filling occurs, even if it is minimal, the preferred diagnosis should be neonatal hepatitis.

BILIARY ATRESIA (BA)

Extrahepatic biliary atresia (EHBA) accounts for approximately one-third of the cases of neonatal cholestasis, the incidence varying from 1 in 8000 to 1 in 25,000 live births, with females being more commonly affected.[18]

This disorder has a 15 to 30 percent incidence of associated anomalies such as polysplenia, malrotation, trisomy 17-18 and cardiovascular abnormalities, suggesting a congenital etiology.[19] The exact etiology of biliary atresia is unknown, although proposed mechanisms include viral infections, immune-mediated bile duct injury, and autoimmune disease of the biliary tree.[20]

In terms of infection, it is theorized that a viral infection in an infant, first induces a cholangiohepatitis and in response an immune

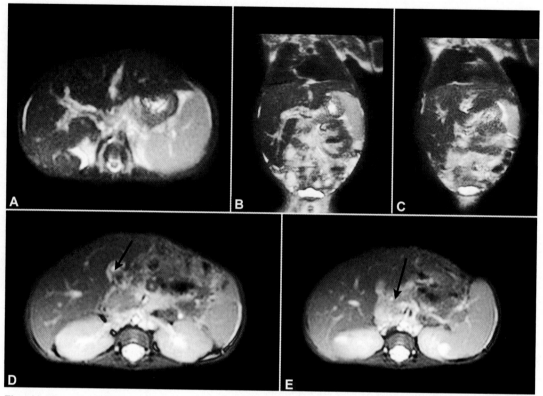

Figs 13.2A to E: HASTE axial (A) HASTE coronal (B,C) revealing a collar of high signal intensity surrounding the portal vein branches due to periportal oedema. TRUFISP axial (D,E) MR images reveal a near normal gallbladder (D) and the intrapancreatic CBD is visualized shown by an arrow (E) Neonatal hepatitis

response is invoked. This entails the production of α-fetoprotein, an immune response regulator that attempts to control the disease process. Characteristically, it is elevated in infants with neonatal hepatitis but not in infants with biliary atresia. This is of considerable importance because it has also been demonstrated that those patients with elevated α-fetoprotein generally do not go on to develop biliary atresia, while those with low levels do. This would suggest that some infants are able to control the initial viral infection better than others and that those who are not able to, develop biliary atresia. Based on this concept, different degrees of biliary duct obliteration will be seen, infants with reasonably well-preserved ducts, infants with ducts that appear hypoplastic and are visible only on microscopic examination and infants with no remaining bile ducts at all and finally a few with cystic transformation of the intrahepatic bile ducts. Thus, main interlobar ducts are present in their entire course in the early stages of the disease, but they diminish in number and size with time (The "disappearing bile duct syndrome").

Pathology

In the first month of life histologic findings in the liver may be indistinguishable from those of neonatal hepatitis, and the two diseases may, in fact be different final processes of a single initial disease state.

Liver biopsy after the first month of life will help differentiate the two diseases. While biliary atresia shows many of the same histologic features as neonatal hepatitis, proliferation of bile ducts in all the portal tracts is an additional cardinal feature.

Based on the predominant site of atresia the following classification of anatomical variants has been evolved:[21,22]

Type I	Obliteration of the common bile duct but proximal ducts are patent.
Type II	Common hepatic duct is obliterated but dilated bile ducts are found at porta hepatitis.
Type IIA	Both cystic and common bile duct are patent.
Type IIB	Obliteration of both cystic and common bile duct.
Type III	No patent hepatic or hilar ducts.

If untreated, the vast majority of cases of EHBA progress to irreversible biliary cirrhosis and death. Because the treatment for biliary atresia and neonatal hepatitis are very different (surgical in the former and medical in the latter), definitive diagnosis is mandatory. Diagnostic imaging tests with or without liver biopsy are utilized to help facilitate a rapid diagnosis because the likelihood of re-establishing bile flow after Kasai hepatoportoenterostomy is greater if the procedure is performed within the first 2 months after birth.[22,23]

Imaging Features

Ultrasonography

A spectrum of changes may be seen sonographically in cases of biliary atresia, depending on the type and severity. Both the liver

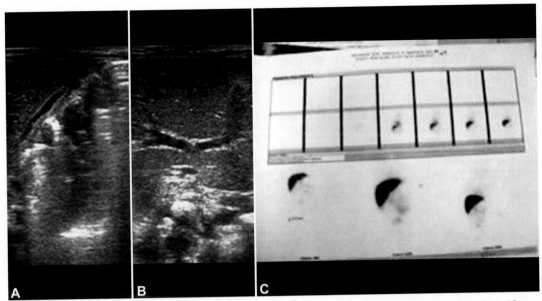

Figs 13.3A to C: Sonography reveals an atretic gallbladder. The length of the gallbladder is less than 19 mm with an irregular wall and an indistinct mucosal lining (A) Bile duct is not identified anterior to the portal vein (B) HIDA scan reveals no bowel opacification (C) Biliary atresia (*For color version see plate 1*)

size and the echogenicity of hepatic parenchyma, may be normal or increased. There may be decreased visualization of the peripheral portal venous vasculature, indicative of fibrosis.[24]

Gallbladder Length and Gallbladder Contraction

On US, an atretic gallbladder that appears small, has an irregular contour and lacks echogenic mucosal lining is the characteristic imaging finding of biliary atresia (Figs 13.3A to C). A combination of three gallbladder features i.e. (i) The length of the gallbladder less than 19 mm, (ii) an irregular wall (iii) indistinct mucosal lining – the so called "gallbladder ghost triad" is diagnostic of biliary atresia.[25] Gallbladder contraction is evaluated by calculating the contraction index (CI) as follows:[26]

$$CI (\%) = \frac{\text{fasting volume-postprandial volume} \times 100}{\text{Fasting volume}}$$

The volume of the gallbladder is calculated as $0.52 \times$ width $\times$ width $\times$ length. A normal contraction index has been reported to be 86% ± 18% (mean ± SD) in a 6 week old infant and 67% ± 42% in a four months old infant. If the contraction index was less than mean ± SD, the gallbladder was described as uncontracted. An uncontracted gallbladder is more suggestive of biliary atresia than of neonatal hepatitis or other causes of infantile cholestasis.[26]

Although, the finding of a normal sized gallbladder usually implies neonatal hepatitis, it may also be seen when the atretic common bile duct is distal to the insertion of the cystic duct. About 10 percent of infants with biliary atresia are found to have a normal gallbladder with a diameter greater than 1.5 cm. Change in gallbladder size after a milk feeding suggests patency of the common hepatic and common bile ducts and is seen only with neonatal hepatitis.

Biliary Atresia Splenic Malformation Syndrome

This syndrome has been reported by Davenport et al.[27] Biliary atresia can be associated with polysplenia, situs inversus, an interrupted inferior vena cava and other cardiovascular anomalies. Furthermore, infants with BA have a degree of hepatic fibrosis or cirrhosis and the majority have some evidence of portal hypertension as early as 8 weeks. Biliary atresia is associated with polysplenia in 10-12 percent of cases. The abdomen should be examined for signs of end-stage liver disease including ascites, hepatofugal flow in the portal and splenic veins and collateral venous channels.

Triangular Cord Sign

Several investigators have recently reported the importance of assessing for the presence or absence of an echogenic triangular cord seen just cranial to the bifurcation of the portal vein on US. This echogenic region corresponds to fibrous tissue found adjacent to the portal vein bifurcation in cases of biliary biliary atresia (Fig. 13.4). In their series of 61 infants with neonatal cholestasis, Park et al found that US had a diagnostic accuracy of 95 percent, a sensitivity of 85 percent, and a specificity of 100 percent when using the presence of the triangular cord sign to identify infants with biliary atresia.[28,29,30]

Objective Criteria of Triangular Cord Sign in Biliary Atresia on US

Biliary atresia is characterized by fibrous obliteration of the extrahepatic bile duct with fibrous ductal remnant in the porta hepatis. The hepatic ducts transform into a fibrous ductal remnant that is usually anterior and slightly cranial to the hepatic artery and the portal vein. The fibrous ductal remnant takes the same

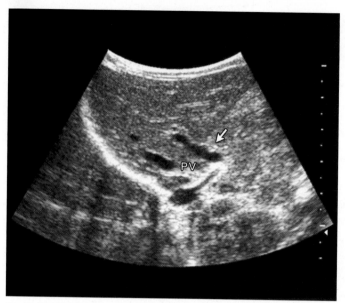

Fig. 13.4: US of a neonate with biliary atresia showing an echogenic triangular cord anterior to the portal vein - "Triangular cord" sign.

course as the common hepatic duct and smoothly tapers proximally along both sides of the intrahepatic ducts. Thus, the location of the fibrous ductal remnant in the porta hepatis should be the same as that of the common hepatic duct. The original definition of the TC sign was based on the idea that this fibrous ductal remnant could

be seen as a thick tubular or triangular echogenic density along the anterior aspect of the portal vein.

The normal possible structures positioned along the anterior aspect of the portal vein, include the anterior wall of the right portal vein, the anterior wall of the right hepatic artery and the common hepatic duct. Lee et al, therefore, took the thickness of the echogenic anterior wall of the right portal vein which they called as EARPV.[31] The triangular cord sign was defined as thickness of the EARPV of more than 4 mm on a longitudinal scan. They stated that the triangular echogenic density was hard to measure exactly on a transverse scan because of errors related to its tapering structure into the liver. Also, the fibrous ductal remnant may not be in the pattern of a triangular, cone-shaped fibrous mass. Other patterns of the fibrous ductal remnant do not appear as triangular echogenic density on a transverse scan, hence they used a longitudinal scan rather than a transverse scan for measurement. These authors, thus proposed that the TC sign be defined as a thickness of the EARPV or the echogenic anterior wall of the right portal vein of more than 4 mm on a longitudinal scan as an objective criterion of diagnosing biliary atresia (Figs 13.5A to C). The use of this criterion for the diagnosis of biliary atresia resulted in a sensitivity of 80%, specificity of 98%, a positive predictive value of 94%, a negative predictive value of 94% and an accuracy of 94%.[31]

Color Doppler US in Biliary Atresia

The triangular cord sign cannot always be found in every patient. The detection of this sign is largely operator dependent. This sign

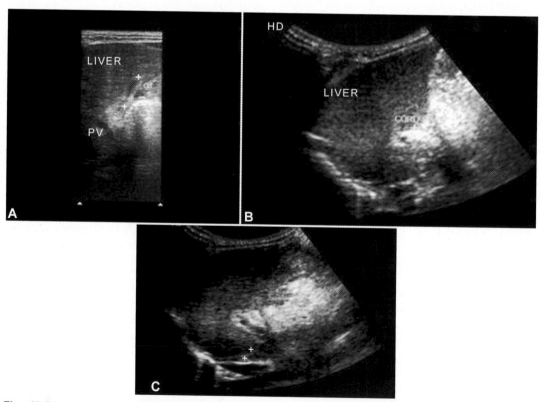

Figs 13.5A to C: Sonography images revealing an atretic gallbladder (A). Scans revealing an echogenic area anterior to the portal vein. The thickness of the EARPV or the echogenic anterior wall of the right portal vein is seen to measure more than 4 mm (B,C) Biliary atresia

enlargement and the branches of the intrahepatic peripheral hepatic artery manifested with irregular contrs suggestive of peripheral occlusion.[32] It has been stated that enlargement may be a compensatory change to improve the blood supply for the biliary trees or a secondary change of liver cirrhosis or a vascular malformation (Figs 13.6A and B). Enlargement of the hepatic artery diameter (> 1.5 mm at the level of the proximal right hepatic artery) or a value of 0.45 for the hepatic artery diameter to portal vien diameter ratio is highly suggestive of biliary atresia.[33] Color Doppler US can also be used to detect hepatic subcapsular flow in patients with biliary atresia. Uflaker and Pariente reported the presence of angiographically demonstrable perivascular arterial tufts in the periphery of the hepatic arterial circulations in patients with biliary atresia and suggested that these findings may be useful in the diagnosis.[34] Hepatic subcapsular flow has been reported to have sensitivity, specificity, positive and negative predictive values of 100%, 86%, 88% and 100% respectively for the diagnosis of biliary atresia.[34]

Hepatobiliary scintigraphy definitively excludes biliary atresia if gut excretion of radiotracer is observed. But this test demonstrates poor accuracy (56%) and specificity (35%), with a sensitivity of 96 percent[28] (Fig. 13.7).

More recently, investigators have evaluated the ability of MRI and MR cholangiography to diagnose biliary atresia. Jaw et al found that the common hepatic ducts and common bile duct could be readily visualized in control subjects and infants with neonatal hepatitis, whereas infants with surgically confirmed biliary atresia failed to demonstrate a visible common bile or hepatic duct on MRCP.[35] In their study, Giubaud et al found that failure to visualize the extrahepatic bile ducts on MRCP and presence of high signal intensity periportal thickening has a strong association with the presence of biliary atresia.[36,37]

Contrast Enhanced MR Cholangiography for Evaluation of Biliary Atresia

Mangafodipir trisodium (Mn-DPDP) is a non radioisotopic liver specific contrast medium that is taken up mainly by the liver cells and excreted into the biliary system. The active ingredient in Mn-DPDP is manganese dipryidoxyl diphosphate, a metal chelate of manganese that is essentially a paramagnetic T1 enhancer.[38] After intravenous administration, a proportion of manganese is slowly released from the chelate and binds to the blood/protein and the main uptake of manganese occurs in the liver. Enhancement of the liver parenchyma peaks after 5-10 minutes and plateaus over several hours.[39] Most of the manganese is then eliminated through the biliary route with about 20% excreted in the urine. Precontrast images are compared with the post contrast and contrast material filling of the gallbladder, extrahepatic bile duct, duodenum or small bowel loops is observed. Contrast enhanced MR cholangiography can also yield functional information similar to that obtained with hepatic scintigraphy, anatomic information similar to that yielded by conventional contrast-enhanced cholangiography and cross-sectional information similar to that obtained at computed tomography and US. Thus, a prominent gallbladder and extrahepatic bile duct filling, together with duodenal excretion of

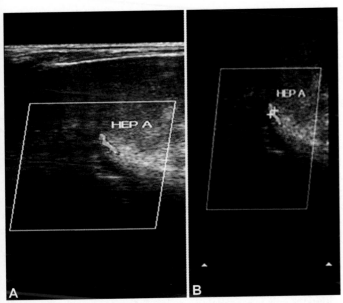

Figs 13.6A and B: Color Doppler showing color fill in of the hepatic artery which is enlarged. The diameter of the artery >1.5 mm – Biliary atresia (*For color version see plate 1*)

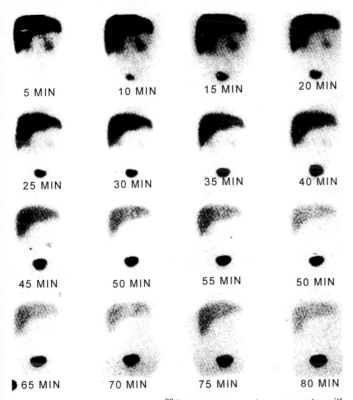

Fig. 13.7: Scintigraphy using [99m] TC IDA scan in a neonate with cholestasis shows good hepatocyte extraction of the radiotracer but no bowel opacification due to biliary atresia

can also be masked in the presence of diffuse periportal echogenicity due to nonspecific inflammation or cirrhosis. A few authors have described enlargement of the hepatic artery as a useful sign in the diagnosis of biliary atresia. In an angiographic study of biliary atresia, all patients with biliary atresia had hepatic artery

Mn-DPDP within 1 hour are definite exclusion criteria of biliary atresia.

Kasai Operation

In the Kasai operation, the porta hepatis is dissected and a loop of small intestine is brought up and anastomosed to the exposed draining biliary radicles.[40] This bowel loop, if it is fluid filled, may be seen in the region of the porta hepatis on postoperative US scans. Biliary scintigraphy can be used to evaluate the patency of the portoenterostomy. Isotopic activity should appear in the bowel by 1 hour after administration. Patients may develop ascending cholangitis with cystic dilatation of the intrahepatic bile ducts and subsequent "bile lakes" secondary to stasis.[41] These accumulations of bile are easily seen on US, CT and magnetic resonance imaging (MRI) and can be drained percutaneously with variable results. Though the operation is successful in more than 50% of patients when performed under the age of 2-3 months, but, because of progressive obliteration of the bile ducts, survival rates drop rapidly when surgery is performed after this age. At times, even with good short-term to mid-term results, cholangitis, cirrhosis and portal hypertension may develop. These patients ultimately need to undergo liver transplantation.

HEPATOBILIARY CYSTIC MALFORMATIONS

Choledochal Cyst

Choledochal cysts are uncommon anomalies of the biliary system with dilatation of the extrahepatic and/or intrahepatic bile ducts. Their incidence in Western countries is approximately 1 in 15,000 live births.[42] About 60 percent of cases are diagnosed before the age of 10, with about 20 percent of patients remaining asymptomatic until adulthood and 75 percent occur in females. Choledochal cysts are generally considered congenital in origin, since they are seen even in foetuses and neonates.

Etiopathogenesis

Yotsuyanagi theorized that unequal proliferation of epithelial cells occurred within the primitive solid bile ducts, with cyst formation occurring at these more "active" locations on subsequent recanalization. Alonso-Lej postulated that cystic dilatation was a result of a primary weakness in the bile duct wall. Subsequently, Babbitt (1969) theorized that an anomalous insertion of the common bile duct into the pancreatic duct with a long common channel caused chronic reflux of digestive pancreatic enzymes into the biliary tree, leading to inflammation, dilation, and scarring. This theory of choledochal cyst development is currently the most popular and is supported by the occurrence of an anomalous pancreaticobiliary junction in 10.5 to 58 percent of cases.[43]

The following classification system to describe the various types of choledochal cysts was initially developed by Alonso-Lej et al[44] and subsequently revised by Todani et al:[45]

Type IA – Cystic choledochal dilatation
Type IB – Focal segmental dilatation
Type IC – Fusiform choledochal dilatation

Type II – Eccentric dilatation of CBD referred to as choledochal diverticulum
Type III – Focal dilatation of the intraduodenal portion of CBD - choledochocele
Type IVA – Intrahepatic and extrahepatic cysts
Type IVB – Multiple extrahepatic cysts (may overlap with Type I)
Type V – Single or multiple dilatation of the intrahepatic ducts (Caroli's disease).

Choledochal cysts may manifest clinically with the classic triad of jaundice, abdominal pain and palpable mass. They may be discovered during prenatal sonography. Laboratory abnormalities are often consistent with obstructive jaundice. Surgical resection is the treatment of choice for choledochal cysts to avoid the potential complications of cholelithiasis, choledocholithiasis, cystolithiasis, cholangitis, cirrhosis, pancreatitis, portal hypertension, cyst rupture with bile peritonitis and malignant degeneration with development of cholangiocarcinoma. Malignancy arising within the cyst is reported to occur in 2.5 to 15 percent of cases.[46]

Hepatobiliary anomalies associated with choledochal cysts include single or multiple intrahepatic and extrahepatic biliary duct strictures, pancreatic duct strictures, ectopic pancreas, malrotation, double common bile duct, double gallbladder, gallbladder atresia, congenital hepatic fibrosis and sclerosing cholangitis.

Anomalous Junction of the Pancreaticobiliary Duct (AJPB)

In general, the main pancreatic duct and the common bile duct open into the second part of the duodenum separately or by a common channel. A common channel is present in 60-80% of people and 20-40% of the population have separate openings for the two ducts.[47] The length of the normal common channel ranges from 1 to 12 mm, with a mean of 4.5 mm.[48] AJPB is defined as the presence of a common channel longer than 15 mm with or without dilatation of the common channel (>5 mm). Many patients with AJPB have associated choledochal cysts. The pathogenesis of choledochal cyst is complex. Babbitt et al. proposed that AJPB predisposes to the reflux of pancreatic juice into the bile duct because pressure is higher in the pancreatic duct. High amylase levels in the bile aspirated from choldedochal cysts confirm the presence of reflux and this finding supports this theory. However, AJPB is not associated with all cases of choledochal cyst. Wiedmeyer et al. identified ectasia of the common channel, larger than 5mm in diameter, in addition to a long common channel as important radiographic findings in the diagnosis of choledochal cyst.[49]

AJPB was classified according to the system of Kimura et al.as type BP when the common bile duct joins the pancreatic duct at a right angle and as type PB when the pancreatic duct joins the common bile duct at an acute angle.[50] Komi proposed a new classification of AJPB into types I, II, and III. Type I, or type BP, is divided further into type Ia or Ib according to whether the common channel is or is not dilated.[51] The normal caliber of the common channel is 3-5 mm. Similarly, type II is divided into type

IIa or IIb. Type III is subclassified as types IIIa, IIIb, and IIIc, which is equivalent to Warshaw's types of pancreas divisum with biliary dilatation. Recently, Guelrud et al. added a Y type AJPB to describe a long common channel without common bile duct dilatation.[52]

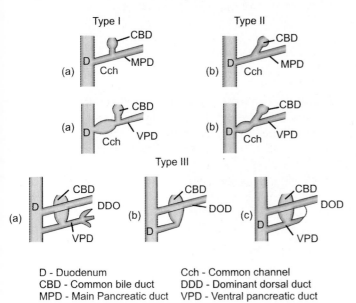

Type I

(a)

Type II

(b)

(a)

(b)

Type III

(a) (b) (c)

D - Duodenum
CBD - Common bile duct
MPD - Main Pancreatic duct

Cch - Common channel
DDD - Dominant dorsal duct
VPD - Ventral pancreatic duct

The most common complications of choledochal cyst is ascending cholongitis. Eventually, cirrhosis of the liver can occur with subsequent portal hypertension. Spontaneous cyst rupture has also been reported. There is a 20 fold increased incidence of carcinoma of the biliary tree in a patient with choledochal cyst. The risk is low in the first decade of life but increases with advancing age. AJPB has also been implicated as a cause of bile duct and gallbladder carcinoma and pancreatitis. Carcinoma is a recognized complication of choledochal cyst, with a reported frequency of 3-28%. There is a 12 to 16 times higher incidence of carcinoma in choledochal cyst, and the risk is especially high in patients with cystolithiasis.[53] Bile duct carcinoma appears to be related to long standing ulceration and inflammation and the formation of carcinogens in the bile. Cystolithiasis and cholelithiasis reflect the effects of prolonged stasis and infection. It has been postulated that, in AJPB, pancreatic juice refluxes freely into the biliary tree, leading to chronic inflammation and metaplasia. When pancreatic juice mixes with bile, lysolecithin and phospholipase A2 are produced, which may also be irritants. In patients with choledochal cyst, irritation occurs in the cyst rather than in the gallbladder, so there is a high incidence of choledochus carcinoma.[54] The incidence of carcinoma of the gallbladder is 73% in patients with AJPB without a choledochal cyst and only 10% in patients with AJPB with a choledochal cyst. AJPB not only predisposes to biliary tract anomalies but also causes pancreatic duct abnormalities. Guelrud et al. found that dysfunction of the sphincter of Oddi associated with AJPB is responsible for episodes of recurrent pancreatitis.[52] They associated AJPB with 28% of patients with recurrent pancreatitis. The combination of AJPB and choledochal cyst is responsible for protein plugs and pancreatolithiasis. Kaneko et al. proposed that increased mucin

production from the bile duct caused by pancreatico biliary maljunction is responsible for protein plug formation.[55] These protein plugs are usually seen in the common channel but may be seen distal to the common channel as reported by Yamataka et al.[56] Pancreatolithiasis in patients with choledochal cyst ranges from 0.2% to 33%, as noted by various investigators.[55,56]

Imaging Features

On plain radiograph a soft tissue mass may be appreciated in the right upper quadrant adjacent to the liver. The cyst wall rarely demonstrates calcification, but opaque calculi may be visible.

An upper GI series demonstrates anterior displacement of the first and second portions of duodenum and gastric antrum, widening of the duodenal sweep. On barium enema, there is inferior displacement of the hepatic flexure.

Choledochal cysts of types I, II or III are detected at sonography as anechoic or hypoechoic cystic lesions in the region of the porta hepatis ventral to the portal vein with communication to the biliary tree (Figs 13.8A to C). The gallbladder is seen separate from the cystic lesion. The rapid, almost focal transition between a grossly dilated and nondilated biliary system is further indication of the presence of a choledochal cyst. US is the recommended initial imaging study in the newborn infant with persistent jaundice in whom the differential diagnostic consideration include choledochal cyst, biliary atresia, neonatal hepatitis etc. Choledochal cyst and biliary atresia might occur together in neonates[57] (Fig. 13.9). Depending on the type of choledochal cyst, other intrahepatic cysts may or may not be demonstrated. The pancreas and pancreatic duct should be examined for evidence of pancreatitis or ductal dilatation.

Hepatobiliary scintigraphy confirms excretion of radiotracer into the choledochal cyst, but yields limited anatomic delineation and is insufficient for determining cyst type or planning surgical reconstruction. At times the choledochal cyst does not fill with the radionuclide and the diagnosis can be missed.

CT is helpful in demonstrating the size and extent of both extrahepatic and intrahepatic choledochal cysts. It can globally delineate the relationship of the cystic mass to adjacent intraperitoneal and extraperitoneal structures, allowing a thorough evaluation of the abdominal cavity and retroperitoneum. Mural irregularities or focal nodularity within the choledochal cyst, suggesting malignant changes, may be identified by CT and US.

On MRI, long T1 and T2 relaxation times characteristic of fluid can confirm the cystic nature of the lesion when US yields inconclusive results because of internal echoes within the cyst (Figs 13.10A and B), (Figs 13.11A to E). MRI can also yield detailed information on surrounding abdominal anatomy.

For preoperative planning, MR cholangiopancreatography (MRCP) may be performed (Figs 13.12A to D). MRCP is a noninvasive procedure and provides the best available projection image for revealing the extent of choledochal cyst in children and adults (Figs 13.13A and B). Thin slice and thick slab MR images enable visualization of the accessory pancreatic duct and the common channel. The global quality of images obtained with single-slab images is better than that of maximum-intensity-

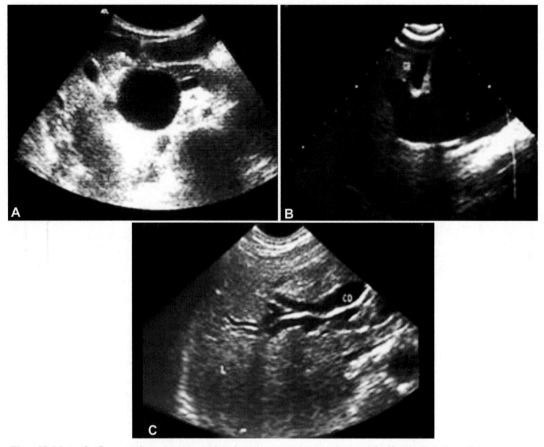

Figs 13.8A to C: Gray scale sonograms showing segmental, saccular and fusiform dilatation of the common bile dutc – Types IA, IB and IC choledochal cysts respectively

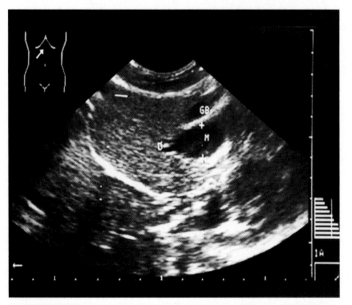

Fig. 13.9: Sonogram showing a diffuse increase in liver echogenicity with saccular dilatation of distal CBD – biliary atresia with associated choledochal cyst

projection images in adults with suspected biliary or pancreatic abnormalities (Figs 13.14A and B), (Fig.13.15). In a study by Chan et al, anomalous pancreaticobiliary ductal union was not visualized on MRCP using a two-dimensional turbo spin-echo sequence with the MIP technique. However, in pediatric patients, MRCP with a half-Fourier acquisition of a single shot fast spin-echo or a turbo spin-echo sequence might increase the sensitivity of anomalous pancreaticobiliary ductal union detection.[48,49] The main drawback of using MRCP for the determination of anomalous pancreaticobiliary ductal union seems to be that large choledochal cysts obscure the common channel. ERCP is regarded as the most definitive and reliable diagnostic method of revealing choledochal cysts and anomalous pancreaticobiliary ductal union[50] (Figs 13.16A and B).

Surgeons need an exact anatomic map of the pancreaticobiliary ductal union because it is essential that the choledochal cyst be completely resected without pancreatic ductal injury. Surgical excision with Roux-en-Y anastomosis gives excellent results and reduces bile stasis, risk of cholangitis and malignancy. When the anatomy is more complicated, a simple drainage is carried out but these patients have risk of recurrent cholangitis, lithiasis, pancreatitis and cancer (Figs 13.17A and B), (Figs 13.18A to C) and (Figs 13.19A and B).

The differential diagnosis of choledochal cyst includes several other cystic lesions including hepatic cyst, enteric duplication cyst, pancreatic pseudocyst, hepatic artery aneurysm and spontaneous perforation of the common bile duct. Use of careful 2D imaging combined with CDFI can readily differentiate these conditions.

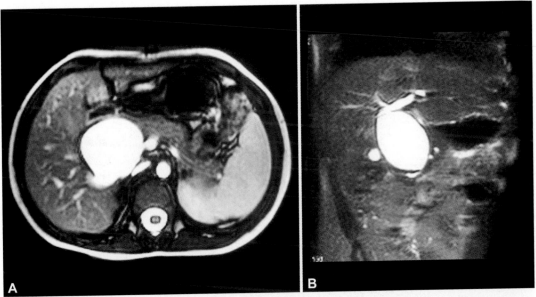

Figs 13.10A and B: True FISP axial and HASTE coronal MR images showing a cystically dilated common bile duct due to Type I choledochal cyst

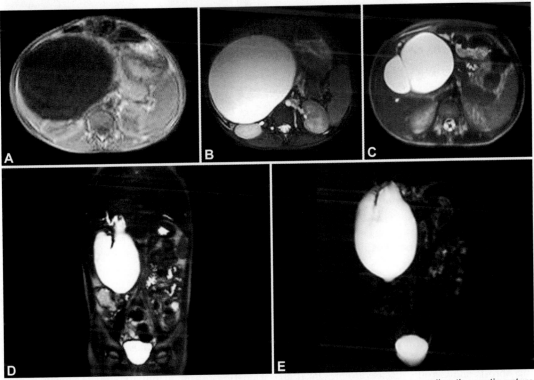

Figs 13.11A to E: Axial, T$_1$ W (A). Axial T$_2$ W (B,C) and HASTE coronal (D) images revealing the cystic nature of the choledochal cyst seen as hypointense signal on T$_1$ and hyperintense on T$_2$ W MR images. A small septation is seen within the cyst. RARE sequence showing the cyst to a saccular dilatation of the common bile duct Type I A choledochal cyst

CAROLI'S DISEASE

Caroli's disease is Type IV (Alonson-Lej) or type V (Todani) Choledochal cyst.

Caroli's disease or communicating cavernous ectasia of the intrahepatic bile ducts is a rare congenital disorder with segmental, saccular dilatation of the intrahepatic bile ducts. Although,

congenital cystic dilation of the intrahepatic bile ducts was first described by Vachell and Stevens in 1906, Caroli first clearly defined this disease entity in 1958.[61]

It is an autosomal recessive disorder and is among the ductal plate malformations that occur at different levels in the developing biliary tree. The disease results from the arrest of or a derangement

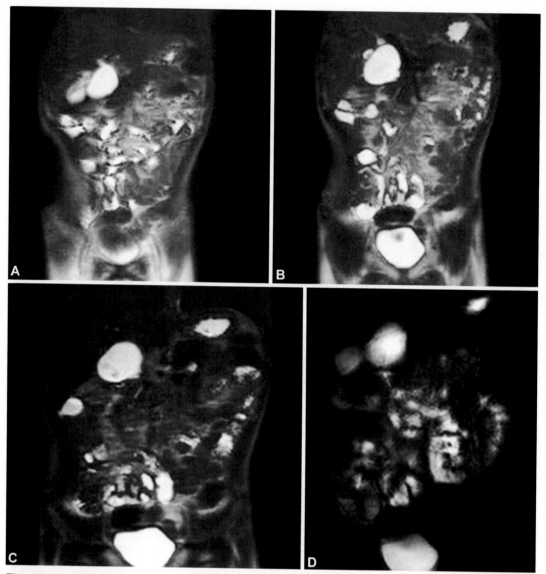

Figs 13.12A to D: HASTE coronal (A to C) and RARE sequence (D) MR images showing a focal segmental dilatation of the common bile duct. The normal caliber duct proximal and distal to the dilatation is visualized – Type IB choledochal cyst

in the normal embryologic remodeling of ducts and causes varying degrees of destructive inflammation and segmental dilatation. When the large intrahepatic bile ducts are affected, the result is Caroli's disease. Abnormal development of the small interlobular bile ducts results in congenital hepatic fibrosis. Features of both congenital hepatic fibrosis and Caroli's disease are present if all levels of the biliary tree are involved and this condition has been termed "Caroli's syndrome". Two primary types of the disease have been identified:

1. Non-hereditary form (Type I), also known as the "sporadic pure type" is often limited to one hepatic lobe (usually the left lobe). Multifocal saccular dilatations of segmental bile ducts are frequently accompanied with calculi formation and recurrent bacterial cholangitis.
2. Hereditary form (Type II) involves the entire liver. The bile duct dilatation is usually less prominent than in Type I, and the

patients present with abnormalities related to hepatic fibrosis and portal hypertension.

Associated conditions, including choledochal cysts and cystic lesions of the kidney known as autosomal— recessive polycystic kidney disease (ARPKD) occur mainly in the hereditary form.[62] Hepatic fibrosis, medullary sponge kidney, nephronophthisis are other associated conditions.

Although, the Todani classification of choledochal cysts includes Caroli's disease as a type V choledochal cyst, the current understanding of the pathogenesis of Caroli's disease makes it unlikely that these entities are related. The cause of Caroli's disease is unknown. Postulated mechanisms include occlusion of the hepatic artery in the neonatal period with associated ischaemia of the bile ducts. Abnormal growth rate of the biliary epithelium and lack of the normal involution of the ductal plates surrounding the portal tracts, leads to biliary cysts surrounding the portal tracts.

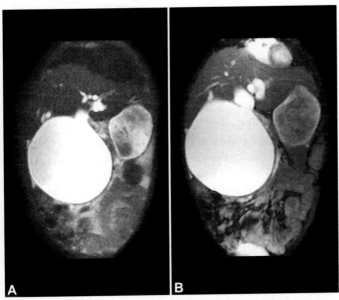

Figs 13.13A and B: HASTE coronal MR images revealing a large eccentric dilatation of the CBD seen as a large outpouching from the CBD – Type II choledochal cyst/choledochal diverticulum

Caroli's disease has an autosomal recessive inheritance and is often associated with renal disorders whereas choledochal cysts are congenital and not associated with renal disorders.[63]

Caroli's disease typically develops during childhood or early adulthood with recurrent episodes of right upper quadrant or epigastric pain, fever, and sometimes jaundice (typical triad).

Liver function tests may be normal or demonstrate mild elevations in serum alkaline phosphatase and transaminase levels.

Complications of the "simple form" of Caroli's disease include cholelithiasis, choledocholithiasis, intrahepatic calculi, intrahepatic abscesses, subphrenic abscesses, and cholangiocarcinomas.

Bloustein reported a 7 percent incidence of malignancy in Caroli's disease.[64] Portal hypertension, although less common, does occur with the fibroangioadenomatous form of Caroli's disease and the patient may have episodes of hematemesis secondary to variceal bleeding.

Pathology

Pathologically, two forms of the disease have been recognized:
1. The "simple" form, which is more common, is characterized by dilatation of the intrahepatic bile ducts and is most often manifested as repeated episodes of ascending cholangitis.
2. The "fibroangioadenomatic" form is characterized by congenital hepatic fibrosis, portal hypertension and bleeding esophageal varices.[63]

Imaging Features

The spectrum of radiologic appearances of Caroli's disease ranges from segmental to diffuse biliary dilatation, from saccular to fusiform dilatation, and from isolated intrahepatic involvement to intra- and extrahepatic involvement.[65-67]

Plain films occasionally show gallstones, intrahepatic calculi, or medullary nephrocalcinosis. Excretory urography may demonstrate the renal tubular ectasia of medullary sponge kidney or the corticomedullary cystic changes of renal cystic disease.

US demonstrates sonolucent intrahepatic tubular structures converging on the porta hepatis, representing the grossly dilated intrahepatic biliary tree. The dilated ducts may give the appearance of surrounding the portal vein radicles ("the intra aluminal portal vein sign") Toma et al believed this sign to be pathognomonic Caroli's disease.[68] On color Doppler they show lack of color fill-in *the dilated ducts and colour flow can be seen in portal vein branches*. It is important to demonstrate a communication between these multiple dilated structures in order to distinguish Caroli's

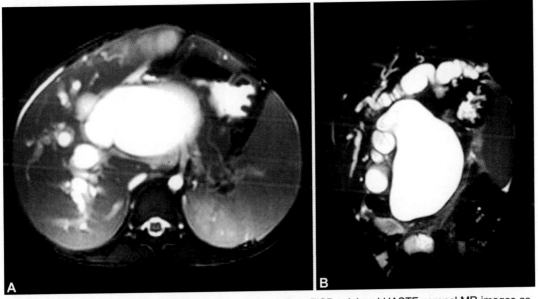

Figs 13.14A and B: Type IVA choledochal cyst seen on True FISP axial and HASTE coronal MR images as cystically dilated intra and extrahepatic bile ducts

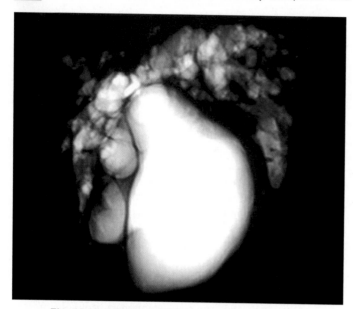

Fig. 13.15: SSFSE (RARE) image showing Type IVA choledochal cyst

disease from polycystic liver disease or multiple hepatic abscesses. Additional, findings include intrahepatic calculi, bulbar protrusions into the ductal lumina, bridge formation across dilated ductal lumina, and portal radicles surrounded by dilated bile ducts ("central dot" sign).

Intrahepatic dilatation of the bile ducts with multiple cysts can also be seen in Byler's disease but the large cysts do not communicate with the biliary system. Renal sonography may show medullary cysts, loss of corticomedullary differentiation, or increased medullary or parenchymal echogenicity.[65]

CT depicts low-density, irregular, dilated cystic structures communicating with the biliary tree[66] (Figs 13.20A and B). CT is an excellent modality to show the extent of the disease especially the intrahepatic ductal ectasia. A central dot may be seen that corresponds to the intraluminal portal vein seen sonographically. These will enhance on administration of contrast. If the ducts are only minimally dilated the connections will be better seen on CT than US[69] (Figs 13.21A and B), (Figs 13.22A to C) and (Fig. 13.23).

CT cholangiography has also been described as a noninvasive method of confirming the biliary nature of the disease process.

Hepatic scintigraphy may show multiple filling defects if the ducts are sufficiently dilated. Biliary imaging with, ^{99}Tc iminodiacetic acid compounds show focal defects during the hepatic phase that gradually increases in activity as the radiopharmaceutical collects in the dilated ducts while the remainder of the liver shows decreased activity with time. Radiotracer activity in the gastrointestinal tract will be seen but is frequently delayed because of the stasis.[70]

The cholangiographic features of Caroli's disease are well established as saccular or fusiform dilatation of the intrahepatic bile ducts, irregular bile duct walls, strictures, and stones. Segmental ductal dilatation is more common (82%) than diffuse ductal dilatation with alternating areas of stricture and dilation. The presence of diffuse fusiform dilatation of the extrahepatic duct measuring 3 cm or less in diameter combined with the characteristic intrahepatic ductal findings may be helpful in differentiating patients with Caroli's disease from patients with choledochal cyst and intrahepatic biliary dilatation.

• Direct bile duct opacification by ERCP or PTC is the most sensitive method for investigating bile duct abnormalities, and, more specifically, for demonstrating communications between cystic dilatations and bile ducts, however, both techniques are invasive and carry a risk of complications including sepsis and bleeding.[65]

Advantages of MRCP consist of depiction of the entire biliary tree in a noninvasive fashion and a spatial resolution as high as

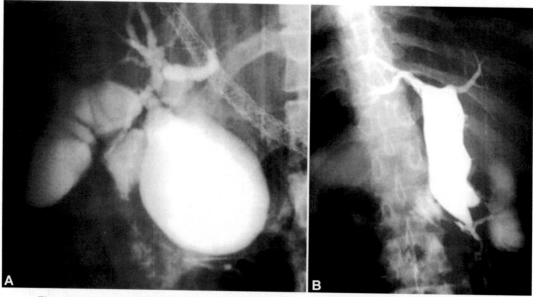

Figs 13.16A and B: ERCP images illustrating saccular and fusiform dilatation of common duct with nondilated intrahepatic biliary radicles – Type I choledochal cysts

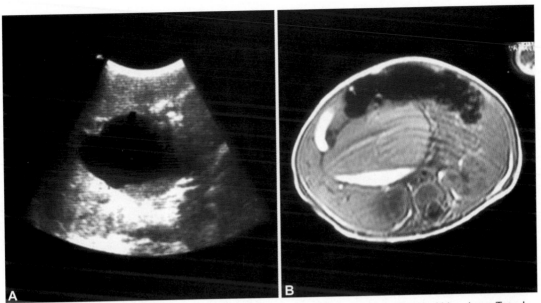

Figs 13.17A and B: US(A) and T1W axial (B) MR image showing fluid–sludge level within a huge Type I choledochal cyst

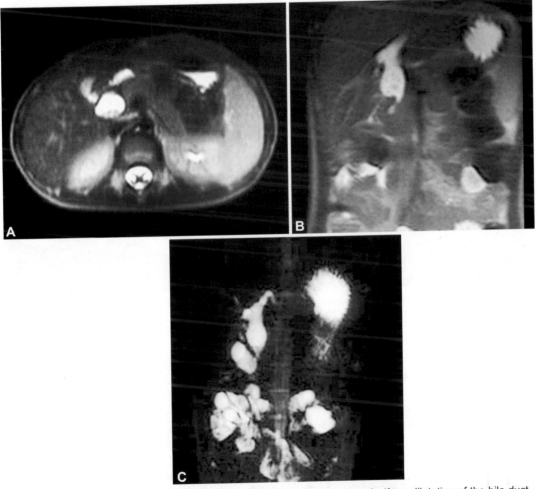

Figs 13.18A to C: HASTE axial (A) and coronal (B) MR images reveal a fusiform dilatation of the bile duct. Multiple hypointense foci suggestive of calculi seen within – Type IC choledochal cyst with calculi

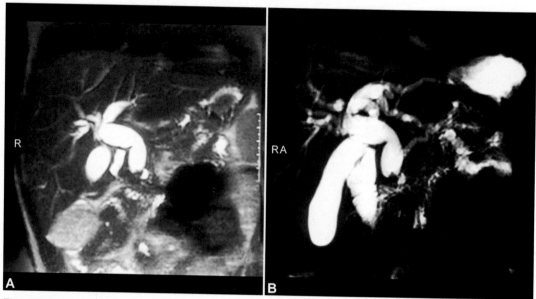

Figs 13.19A and B: HASTE coronal and SSFSE MR images illustrate fusiform dilatation of common duct with an irregular polypoid filling defect at its lower end – Malignant transformation in a Type I choledochal cyst

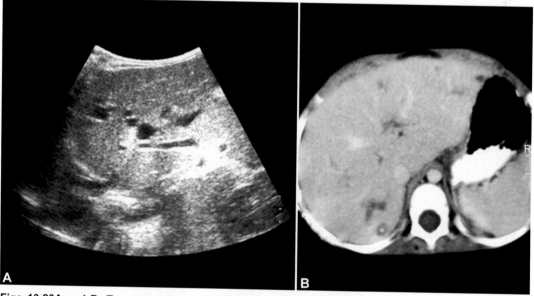

Figs 13.20A and B: Transverse sonogram(A) showing multiple intrahepatic cysts communicating with the biliary tree. CECT (B) in another patient showing segmental intrahepatic duct dilatation with the "central dot" sign – Caroli's disease

1.5 mm.[67] Guy et al (2002) reported three main patterns of Caroli's disease using an MR imaging protocol which included MRCP and a dynamic contrast-enhanced study.[71]

i. The first pattern was characterized by multiple cystic ectasias connected with fusiform dilatations of the intrahepatic bile ducts throughout the liver. On gadolinium-enhanced scans, the 'dot sign' was seen as a tiny dot or an internal septum showing strong contrast enhancement due to a portal radicle surrounded by a dilated bile duct.

ii. The second pattern was characterized by isolated fusiform dilatation of the intrahepatic bile ducts.

iii. The third pattern was characterized by a monoliform dilatation of the left intrahepatic bile ducts with hepatic cystic lesions.

MRCP may be useful in the evaluation of a suspected malignancy. The modality has the added benefit of revealing both intraluminal and extraluminal disease and has recently been reported as an aid in the diagnosis of malignancy in Caroli's disease.

The differential diagnosis of Caroli's disease includes primary sclerosing cholangitis, recurrent pyogenic cholangitis, polycystic liver disease, a choledochal cyst, biliary papillomatosis, and (occasionally) obstructive biliary dilatation.[63]

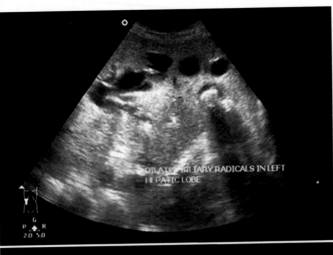

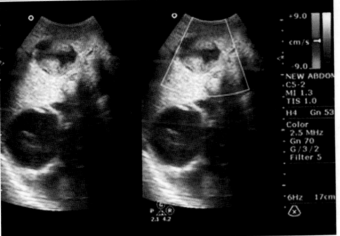

Fig. 13.21: Ultrasound images in an adolescent male showing multiple saccular areas of biliary dilatation within the liver parenchyma. Echogenic foci with distal acoustic shadowing seen in one of the cysts s/o intraductal calculi. One of the larger cysts shows presence of soft tissue along the walls (*For color version see plate 2*)

Congenital Hepatic Fibrosis

Congenital hepatic fibrosis, with or without associated biliary duct ectasia, is an autosomal recessive inherited abnormality. The associated renal abnormalities are infantile and adult polycystic disease, renal dysplasia, and medullary cystic disease.[72] Those patients who present as newborns or infants do so because of the severity of their renal disease which usually dictates their course and prognosis. Those patients who present later in childhood or in adulthood have less renal involvement and frequently come to attention because of hepatomegaly or portal hypertension.

US characteristics of congenital hepatic fibrosis described by Alvarez et al is a large liver with or without splenomegaly depending on the presence or absence of portal hypertension.[72] The hepatic echogenicity is homogeneously or heterogeneously increased. With associated Caroli's disease there will be intrahepatic biliary duct ectasia and dilatation of the gallbladder. If portal hypertension is present, its characteristic imaging findings will be seen.[73] Associated renal lesions can also be identified and should always be sought. CT does not have a routine role in this disease but may be performed if complications are suspected or in

the evaluation of patients with portal hypertension.[74] MR angiography can demonstrate vascular sequelae of portal hypertension and MR cholangiopancreatography may reveal biliary cysts or intra- or extrahepatic biliary duct dilatation or ectasia.[75]

PRIMARY SCLEROSING CHOLANGITIS (PSC)

Primary sclerosing cholangitis (PSC) is an uncommon, progressive idiopathic chronic cholestatic disorder characterized by inflammation of bile ducts leading to their fibrosis and destruction. It can involve both intrahepatic and extrahepatic ducts, gallbladder and small bile ducts down to the interlobular ducts in any combination. There may be focal or diffuse liver involvement.

Pathology

Pathologically, the extrahepatic ducts are thickened with small lumen, described as cord-like or ropelike ducts and the intrahepatic ducts are almost always affected. Histologically, the constellation of reduced numbers of small bile ducts, surrounded by cuff of fibrous tissue, ductular proliferation, copper deposition, and piecemeal necrosis is very suggestive of PSC.

- PSC is an uncommon condition in infants and children. It can present either alone or in association with ulcerative colitis, histiocytosis X and immune deficiency. In children many cases are idiopathic with a subset of it presenting in the neonatal period.[76] The neonatal form presents with jaundice within the first two weeks of age which resolves by one year. These children develop cirrhosis between 1 and 10 years of age.

No definite test is available for the diagnosis of primary sclerosing cholangitis and diagnosis is based on the combination of biochemical, histological and imaging data.

Radiological visualization of biliary tree is essential for its diagnosis and cholangiographic techniques are the gold standard.

Imaging Features

On sonography, extensive thickening of intrahepatic and extrahepatic ducts is depicted as brightly echogenic tissue surrounding the portal venules and common duct. Intraluminal debris consisting of non-shadowing, mobile echogenic particles may be present, consistent with pus, biliary sludge or desquamated bile duct epithelium. Irregular, multisegmental intrahepatic biliary dilatation on sonography can suggest PSC (Figs 13.24A and B).

CT may show a spectrum of findings including intrahepatic duct pruning, beading, and skip dilatation. Most commonly, multifocal discontinuous areas of minimal intrahepatic biliary dilatation without a mass are seen (Figs 13.24C and D). As benign reactive lymphadenopathy may occur in PSC, it should not be taken as a strong indicator of malignancy without other supportive signs.

Cholangiography is the gold standard for diagnosis of PSC and ERCP is preferable to PTC for demonstrating the intrahepatic and extrahepatic ductal narrowing and dilatations with "skip" lesions.

Magnetic resonance imaging has been used to evaluate children with sclerosing cholangitis and has demonstrated peripheral wedge shaped areas of high signal in association with dilated bile duct.[10]

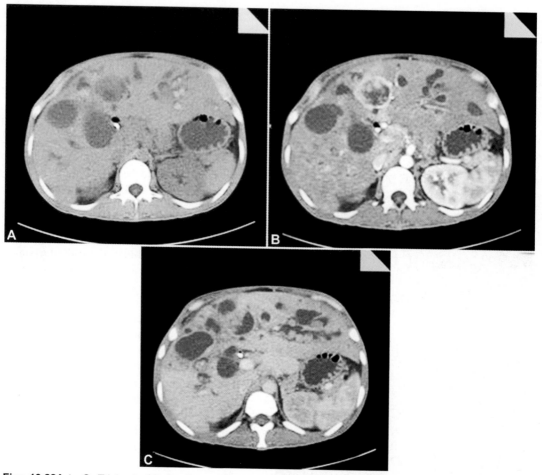

Figs 13.22A to C: Triphasic CT showing multiple saccular dilatations of the biliary tree (A). Hepatic arterial phase showing intense enhancement of the polypoidal mass (B) and a washout is seen in the portal venous phase (C). The intraluminal portal vein sign is well seen on the portal venous phase – Caroli's disease with a mitotic polypoidal mass

The biliary tree is markedly irregular with areas of stricture and focal dilatation proximal to the stricture (Figs 13.25A to C).

The prognosis of PSC in children is variable and hepatocellular carcinoma, as a complication of PSC seen in adults, has not been reported in children.[77]

CYSTIC FIBROSIS

Symptomatic liver disease is seen in 2-18 percent patients of cystic fibrosis and can be the presenting feature of this disorder.[78] Rarely the patient may present in the neonatal period with cholestatic jaundice. Focal or multilobular biliary cirrhosis can be attributed to intrahepatic bile plugging causing ductular obstruction, with common and intrahepatic bile duct strictures.

Initially the liver function tests may be normal but later there is mild to moderate elevation of liver enzymes and as the disease advances, conjugated bilirubin levels are also elevated.

Imaging Features

Sonography and CT can demonstrate intrahepatic ductal dilatation which is often focal or multifocal with intraductal echogenic foci with or without shadowing due to inspissated bile and stones (Fig. 13.26).

Hepatobiliary scintigraphy shows intraparenchymal and intrahepatic ductal retention of activity with delayed clearance of isotope and a nonvisualized or poorly visualized gallbladder.

Cholangiography reveals features similar to PSC including variable dilatation, narrowing and beading of the intrahepatic ducts with occasional strictures of the common bile duct.[78]

DESTRUCTIVE CHOLANGITIS ASSOCIATED WITH LANGERHANS' CELL HISTIOCYTOSIS

Some infants develop an acute hepatitis like picture while others develop severe progressive cholestasis with duct lesions.[79]

Pathology

There is marked destruction of intrahepatic bile ducts and their walls show intense necrosis, inflammation and fibrosis. Periductal bile lakes are seen due to extrusion of bile into the surrounding parenchyma.

Imaging Features

Cholangiography shows "puff of smoke" appearance in the parenchyma around major bile ducts due to the leakage of bile and contrast.

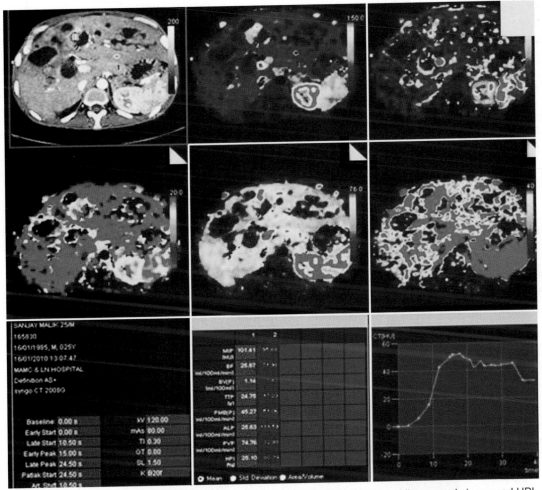

Fig. 13.23: Perfusion study with ROI placed over the intraductal lesion and normal liver reveals increased HPI values 80.79% for the lesion. Higher BF BV PMB HPI are observed. Biopsy revealed it to be a intraductal cholangiocarcinoma (*For color version see plate 2*)

BILE DUCT PAUCITY

Bile duct paucity is present when histologic examination demonstrates that the ratio of intralobular ducts to portal tracts is less than 0.9.[80] Disorders with bile duct paucity have been divided into two major groups: non-syndromic and syndromic bile duct paucity (SBDP), or Alagille's syndrome.

Non-syndromic bile duct paucity refers to many conditions associated with bile duct paucity including idiopathic, metabolic (a-IAT deficiency, hypopituitarism, cystic fibrosis), infectious (rubella, congenital syphilis, CMV, hepatitis B), immunologic, chromosomal (Down's syndrome) and miscellaneous disorders (Zellweger's syndrome, Ivemark's syndrome).[81]

- Alagille's syndrome (SBDP, Watson-Alagille syndrome, arteriohepatic dysplasia) is recognized as an important and relatively common cause of neonatal jaundice and cholestasis in older children with an estimated incidence of 1 in 100,000 births. The syndrome, which is inherited in an autosomal dominant pattern, is characterized by a typical facies, hepatic abnormalities, cardiovascular abnormalities, musculoskeletal, vertebral, ocular and genitourinary abnormalities, marked mental retardation, and growth failure.[6] The abnormal facies include a large forehead, small pointed chin, hypertelorism and a poorly developed nasal bridge. Ocular abnormalities are most typically posterior embryotoxon and pigmentary retinopathy. The cardiovascular abnormalities include pulmonary artery hypoplasia or stenosis.

Imaging Features

On US, the liver shows increased echogenicity and may demonstrate evidence of regenerating cirrhotic nodules. In addition, US helps to exclude any surgically correctable cause of jaundice. There is progressive decrease in ducts after three months of age and extrahepatic ducts are narrowed or hypoplastic. Presence of a patent biliary tract on HIDA distinguishes bile duct paucity from biliary atresia.

SPONTANEOUS PERFORATION OF CBD

Perforation usually occurs at the junction of the cystic and common hepatic duct and rarely it occurs in the common hepatic or common bile duct or the gallbladder. The etiology is uncertain but several

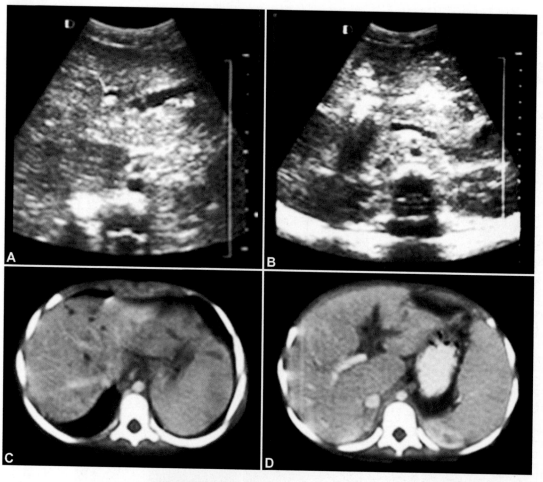

Figs 13.24A to D: (A and B) Transverse sonograms of liver showing irregular intrahepatic biliary dilatation with shadowing and nonshadowing intraluminal echogenic debris – primary sclerosing cholangitis. (C and D) CECT scans of the same patient show tubular structures in left lobe with "skip" areas of biliary dilatation

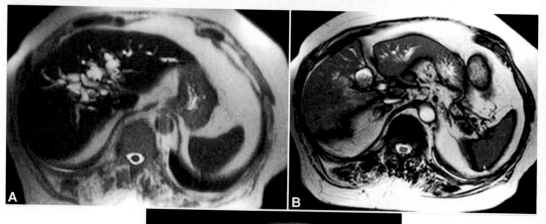

Figs 13.25A to C: HASTE axial (A,C) TRUFISP axial (B) MR images revealing irregular multisegmental intrahepatic biliary dilatation with evidence of pruning and skip dilatation. Intraluminal debris is seen as a hypointense material filling the common duct and the biliary radicles—primary sclerosing cholangitis

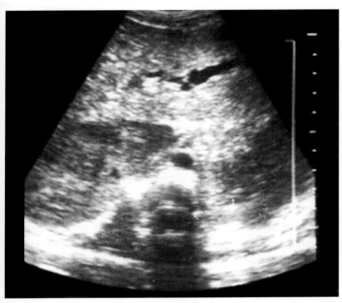

Fig. 13.26: US of a child with cystic fibrosis reveals irregular left hepatic duct dilatation with nonshadowing intraluminal echogenic foci

causes have been postulated including developmental weakness of the bile duct wall, wall weakness resulting from the reflux of pancreatic secretions, calculi or inspissated bile.

It is seen in infants within the first three months of life who present with jaundice and ascites. The liver function tests are essentially normal.

Diagnosis is established based on clinical, sonographic and scintigraphic findings.

Imaging Features

Sonography reveals normal ducts with fluid in the peritoneal cavity. The fluid may be septated and is located in subhepatic region.

Hepatobiliary scintigraphy depicts the leak.

INSPISSATED BILE SYNDROME (IBS)

IBS is an uncommon cause of jaundice in neonates. Sludge may be seen within the gallbladder as low-level echoes without distal shadowing. It may also be seen within the biliary ducts associated with partial or complete ductal obstruction. IBS may be associated with massive hemolysis (Rh incompatibility), hemorrhage (intraabdominal, intracranial or retroperitoneal), and increased enterohepatic circulation in various intestinal diseases (Hirschsprung disease, intestinal atresias and stenoses).[82]

JAUNDICE IN OLDER CHILDREN

The causes of jaundice in older children can be divided into primary diseases of the hepatocytes and obstructive causes.

Hepatocellular Causes

Hepatocellular disease can be subdivided into hepatitis (both acute and chronic) and metabolic.

HEPATITIS

Acute hepatitis may be caused by infection, toxic agents or drugs.

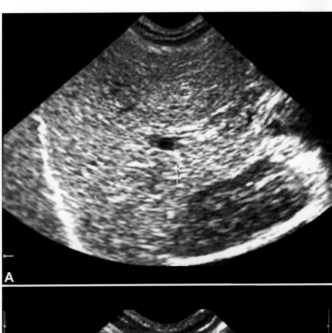

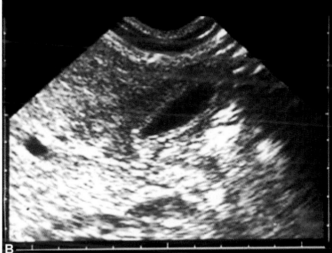

Figs 13.27A and B: Gray scale sonograms of a child with acute hepatitis reveal hepatomegaly with bright portal radicles (A) and a diffusely thickened gallbladder wall (B)

Imaging Features

On US, the liver size may be normal or enlarged with diffuse decrease in parenchymal echogenicity and brightly echogenic portal venous walls due to edema in the hepatocytes. The gallbladder wall may be diffusely thickened with intraluminal sludge[83] (Figs 13.27A and B).

CHRONIC ACTIVE HEPATITIS

Imaging Features

Sonograms generally show increased hepatic parenchymal echogenicity with a coarsened echotexture and decreased visualization of the peripheral portal venous vasculature (Fig. 13.28).

On T2W MR images of patients with acute or chronic active hepatitis, a periportal cuff of high signal intensity can often be seen, corresponding to inflammation. However, this finding is

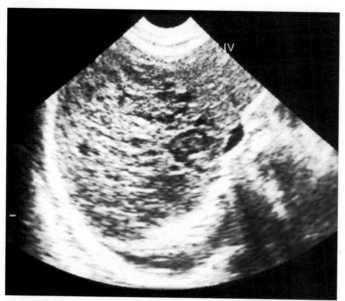

Fig. 13.28: US in a case of chronic active hepatitis shows coarsened liver echotexture with multiple ill-defined hypoechoic nodules

non-specific. In some patients with focal inflammatory changes or fibrosis, diffuse or regional high signal intensity can be identified on T2W images. Enlarged periportal lymph nodes are common in patients with hepatitis.[84]

METABOLIC

Metabolic causes of jaundice include Wilson's disease, cystic fibrosis, glycogen storage disease, tyrosinuria and α1-AT deficiency. The sonographic findings are nonspecific with the liver often appearing hyperechoic with decreased visualization of the peripheral portal venous vasculature. Liver biopsy may be necessary to confirm the diagnosis.

CIRRHOSIS

Cirrhosis is rare in neonates but may occur in older children as a cause of jaundice. Various etiological factors that cause childhood cirrhosis include chronic hepatitis, congenital hepatic fibrosis, biliary atresia, cystic fibrosis, metabolic disease, Budd-Chiari syndrome and total parenteral nutrition.

Duplex and color Doppler evaluation of biliary vessels is important in pediatric patients with chronic liver disease to establish whether the flow is hepatopedal or hepatofugal; presence of varices and collateral venous channels, evidence of spontaneous portosystemic shunts, if "portalization" of the hepatic veins is evident and if satisfactory flow is seen in the hepatic artery and IVC [85] (Figs 13.29A and B).

Portal Hypertensive Biliopathy

It is a rare cause of childhood cholestasis. Portal hypertensive biliopathy (PHB) is defined as abnormal biliary changes that take place most likely secondary to extrahepatic portal vein obstruction (EHPVO) with portal hypertension.[86] This condition may be asymptomatic or could lead to a cholestatic state which is rare in children. The term "portal biliopathy" actually describes an intra- or extrahepatic biliary stricture in patients with portal cavernoma.[87] Portal cavernomas are usually associated with portal hypertension, which frequently causes bleeding from esophageal or gastric varices. Cavernomatous transformation of the portal vein may also lead to biliary obstruction (Figs 13.30A and B). In fact, portal cavernous transformation gives rise to many dilated pericholedochal and periportal collaterals that bypass the portal

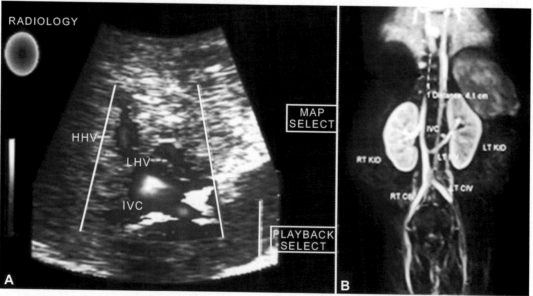

Figs 13.29A and B: (A) Doppler image of a child with Budd-Chiari syndrome showing attenuated hepatic veins and intrahepatic IVC. MIP MR venogram (B) of the same patient well depicts the long segment of IVC attenuation

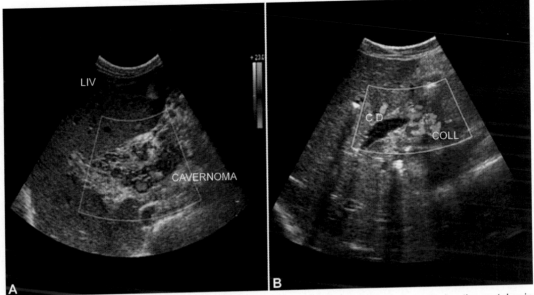

Figs 13.30A and B: Doppler images revealing multiple anechoic tubular structures replacing the portal vein with color fill in s/o portal cavernoma formation. There is extrinsic compression with resultant dilatation of the common bile duct – portal hypertensive biliopathy (*For color version see plate 3*)

vein obstruction. Extrinsic compression of the common duct by dilated venous collaterals together with pericholedochal fibrosis from the inflammatory process causing portal thrombosis may lead to biliary stricture and dilatation of the proximal biliary tree.[88] This condition sometimes causes the formation of secondary biliary stones and cholangitis. There are 2 types of clinical features in portal biliopathy: (i) those related to chronic cholestasis, probably explained by strictures caused by either compression of the biliary lumen by enlarged collaterals or by ischemia and (ii) those related to biliary stones, which are probably responsible for biliary pain and cholangitis.

The diagnosis of PB is mostly made by ERCP. The typical changes are irregularities in the CBD and hepatic ducts (smooth tapering strictures) and localized saccular dilatations. Filling defects suggestive of CBD stones may be seen. Abdominal ultrasound provides additional information regarding the presence of gallbladder varices (tortuous vessels in and around the gallbladder) and is helpful to provide the complete spectrum of PB.

Chandra et al have graded the severity of biliopathy changes as follows:[89]
- Type I—Involvement of extrahepatic bile duct
- Type II—Involvement of intrahepatic bile duct
- Type IIIa—Involvement of extrahepatic bile duct and unilateral intrahepatic bile duct (left or right)
- Type IIIb—Involvement of extrahepatic bile duct and bilateral intrahepatic bile duct.

Treatment is focussed on the management of portal hypertension and relief of obstructive jaundice due to the portal cavernoma is managed endoscopically. Stenting with or without balloon dilatation of CBD is recommended and the stent needs to be replaced regularly. Portosystemic shunt surgery can be done in cases which cannot be managed endoscopically.

BILIARY TRACT NEOPLASMS

Embryonal Rhabdomyosarcoma (Sarcoma Botryoides)

Sarcoma botryoides is a variant of embryonal rhabdomyosarcoma that arises in proximity to the mucosal surface of a hollow viscus or body cavity. After choledochal cyst, sarcoma botryoides is the most common cause of obstructive jaundice in children post infancy.[90,91] Average age at onset is four years with a 2:1 female preponderance. Children present with malaise, fever, jaundice and death is usually from local invasion of contiguous structures.

Pathology

Biliary sarcoma botryoides usually grows from or along the wall of the common bile duct beneath the lining mucosa, with polypoid projections into the lumen. The projecting polyps often undergo hemorrhage and necrosis and are covered by biliary epithelium overlying a dense zone of neoplastic cells (cambium layer) resembling rhabdomyoblasts.[90]

Imaging Features

Sonography and CT show intrahepatic duct dilatation and a soft tissue mass in the region of the common bile duct or porta hepatis. MRCP and direct cholangiography reveal grapelike intraluminal filling defects, usually in extrahepatic ducts, that obstruct the duct only after the tumor has reached a considerable size. Ducts proximal to the obstruction are usually not as dilated as ducts containing the tumor.[91]

DISEASES OF THE GALLBLADDER

Cholelithiasis

Cholelithiasis is uncommon in otherwise healthy children but certain conditions are associated with increased risk of cholelithiasis.

Pathogenesis of Gallstones in Infancy and Childhood

Pigmented gallstones predominate in infants and children. Cholecystitis occurs in premature infants on prolonged parenteral nutrition, following bouts of sepsis, repeated blood transfusions and use of diuretics. An enlarged distended gallbladder filled with sludge may develop before the evolution of cholelithiasis.

Chronic hemolytic disorders are also associated with gallstones. Thirty to sixty percent of patients with sickle cell disease develop pigment stones. Older children and adolescents without an identifiable cause of cholelithiasis are more likely to be obese females.

Other predisposing causes include pancreatic abnormalities and intestinal problems that interfere with the normal enterohepatic circulation such as inflammatory bowel disease, cystic fibrosis and the short gut syndrome. Cystic fibrosis can also produce cholelithiasis.

Imaging Features

Ultrasonography is the most sensitive, specific and the only imaging technique required for demonstrating gallstones and any associated dilatation of the intrahepatic or extrahepatic bile ducts[92,93] (Figs 13.31 and 13.32).

Acute Acalculus Cholecystitis and Acute Hydrops of the Gallbladder

Acute acalculus cholecystitis is an acute inflammation of the gallbladder without gallstones which is associated with infection or systemic illness. Infections due to streptococcal group, gram-negative organisms including *Salmonella, Shigella, E.coli* and parasitic infestation with ascariasis or giardia lamblia may be the cause of acute acalculus cholecystitis. Systemic vasculitis from periarteritis nodosa and Kawasaki disease are more often associated with acute hydrops of the gallbladder. Sometimes congenital narrowing or inflammation of the cystic duct or compression by lymph nodes may be the cause of acalculus cholecystitis. The diagnosis is based on the clinical findings of right upper quadrant or epigastric pain, nausea, vomiting, fever and jaundice. An enlarged gallbladder may be palpable. Laboratory investigations reveal elevated alkaline phosphatase and bilirubin with leukocytosis.

- Sonography reveals a distended gallbladder without calculi. The gallbladder appears biconvex on longitudinal scan instead of its normal ovoid shape. The gallbladder wall is edematous and measures more than 3 mm. US findings in cholecystitis include thickened gallbladder wall, distention of the gallbladder, pericholeycytic fluid, biliary sludge gallbladder wall edema, irregularity of the gallbladder wall (may suggest

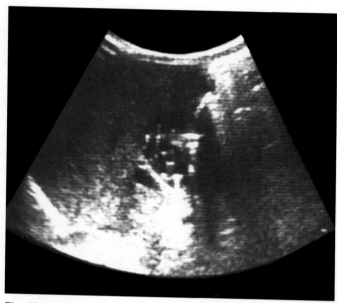

Fig. 13.31: US showing multiple echogenic foci within the gallbladder lumen causing distal shadowing – gallstones in a neonate

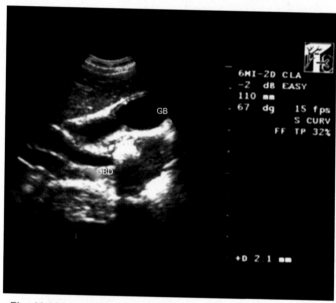

Fig. 13.32: Gray scale sonogram of a nine-year old child showing choledocholithiasis with proximal CBD dilatation

gangrene) and echogenic nonshadowing foci in gallbladder wall (may suggest emphysematous change).[94]

Serial imaging of the gallbladder is useful in following the course of the illness.[95]

To conclude hepatobiliary cholestasis in childhood is both a diagnostic and therapeutic challenge. New diagnostic tools, experience in endoscopy, better imaging and understanding of the molecular mechanisms underlying childhood cholestasis have contributed to an early diagnosis with improved management and better outcome for these children. A multimodality imaging approach is required for the diagnosis of obstructive biliopathies.[96]

REFERENCES

1. Elias E, Boyer JL. Mechanims of intrahepatic cholestasis. In Popper H, Schaffer F (Eds): Progress in Liver Diseases. New York: Crune and Stratton 1979; 4:457-70.

2. Maisels MG. Neonatal jaundice. In Avery GB (Ed): Neonatology, Pathophysiology and Management of the Newborn. Philadelphia: JB Lippincott, 1987.

3. Kliegman RM, Behrman RE. Jaundice and hyperbilirubinaemia in the newborn. In Behrman RE, Vaughan VC III (Eds): Nelson Textbook of Pediatrics (13th edn). Philadelphia: WB Saunders, 1987.

4. Ferry GD, Selbi ML, Udall J, et al. Guide to early diagnosis of biliary obstruction in infancy. Clin Pediatrics 1985; 24:305-11.

5. Markle BM, Potter BM, Majd M. The jaundiced infant and child. Semin Ultrasound 1980; 1:123-33.

6. Alagille D, Estrada A, Hadchovel M. Syndromatic paucity of interlobular bile ducts (Allagille syndrome or arteriohepatic dysplasia); Review of 80 cases. J Pediatrics 1987; 110:195-200.

7. Balistreri WF. Neonatal cholestasis. J Pediatrics 1985;106:171-84.

8. Fitzgerald JF. Cholestatic disorders of infancy. Pediatric Clinics of North America 1988; 35:357-73.

9. Delaney L, Applegate KE, Karmazyn B, Akisik MF, Jennigs SR. MR Chalongiopancreatography in children: feasibility, safety an initial experience. Paediatr Radiol 2008; 38:64-75.

10. Tipnis NA, Dua KS, Werlin SA. A retrospective assessment of magnetic resonance chalongiopancreatography in children. J Paediat Gastroentrol 2008; 46:59-64.

11. Chavhan GB, Babyn PS, Manson D, Vidarsson L. Paediatric MR Cholangiopancreatography: Principles, Technique and Clinical Applications. Radiographics 2008; 28:1951-62.

12. Moyer MS, Balisteri WF. Prolonged neonatal obstructive jaundice. In Walker WA, Durie PR, Hamilton JR, et al (Eds): Pediaric Gastrointestinal Disease. Philadelphia: BC Decker, 1991.

13. Carroll BA, Oppenheimer DA, Muller HH. High frequency real time ultrasound of the neonatal biliary system. Radiology 1982; 145:437-40.

14. McGahan JP, Phillips HE, Cox KL. Sonography of the normal pediatric gallbladder and the biliary tract. Radiology 1982; 144:873-75.

15. Ikeda S, Sera Y, Akagi M. Serial ultrasonic examination to differentiate biliary atresia from neonatal hepatitis – special reference to changes in size of the gallbladder. Eur J. Paedtr 1989; 148:396.

16. Nadel HR. Hepatobilary scintigraphy in children. Seminar Nucl. Med 1996; 26:25-42.

17. Majd M. Nuclear Medicine. In Franken EA Jr, Smith WL (Eds): Gastrontestinal Imaging in Pediatrics. (2nd edn). New York: Harper and Row 1982; 530-79.

18. Lilly JR. Biliary atresia: The jaundiced infant. In Welch KJ, Randolph JG, Ravitch MM (Eds): Pediatric Surgery Chicago: Year Book,l 1985.

19. Abramson SJ, Berdon WE, Altman RP, et al. Biliary atresia and non-cardiac polysplenia syndrome: US and surgical considerations. Radiology 1987; 163:377-9.

20. Sokol RJ, Mack C. Etiopathogenesis of biliary atresia. Semin Liv Dis 2001; 21:517-24.

21. Miyano T, Fujimoto T, Ohya T. Current concept of treatment of biliary atresia. World Journal Surgery 1993; 17:332-36.

22. Kasai M. Treatment of biliary atresia with special reference to hepatic portoenterostomy and its modifications. Prog Pediatric Surgery 1974; 6:5.

23. Balisterie WF, Grand R, Hoofnagal JH, et al. Biliary atresia: Current concepts and research directions. Hepatology 1996; 23:1682-92.

24. Kirks DR, Coleman RE, Filson HC, et al. An imaging approach to persistent neonatal jaundice. AJR 1984; 142:461-5.

25. Tan Kendrick AP, Phua OB, Ooi Bc, Tan CE. Biliary atresia making the diagnosis by gallbladder ghost triad. Paedr. Radiol 2003; 33:311-15.

26. Kanegawa K, Akasaka Y, et al. Sonographic diagnosis of biliary atresia in pediatric patients using the "Triangular Cord" Sign Versus gallbladder Length and Contraction. AJR 2003; 181:1387-90.

27. Davenport M, Savage M, Mowat AP, Howard ER. The biliary atresia splenic malformation syndrome. Surgery 1993; 113:662-8.

28. Park WH, Choi SO, Lee HJ, et al. A new diagnostic approach to biliary atresia with emphasis on the ultrasonographic triangular cord sign: Comparison of ultrasonography, hepatobiliary scintigraphy and liver needle biopsy on the evaluation of infantile cholestasis. J Pediatric Surgery 1997; 32:1555-9.

29. Kotb MA, Kotb A, Sheba MF, et al. Evaluation of the triangular cord sign in the diagnosis of biliary atresia. Pediatrics 2001; 108:416-20.

30. Brun P, Gauthier F, Bouchar D, et al. Ultrasound findings in biliary atresia in children. Ann Radiol 1985; 28:259.

31. Lee HJ, Lee SM, Park WH, Choi SO: Objective criteria of Triangular cord sign in biliary atresia on US scans. Radiology 2003; 229:395-400.

32. dos Santos JL, da Silveira TR, da Silva VD, Cerski CT, Wagner MB. Medial thickening of hepatic artery branches in biliary atresia: A morphometric study. J Paed. Surg 2005; 40:637-42.

33. Kim WS, Cheon JE, Youn BJ, et al. Hepatic arterial diameter measured with US: Adjunct for US diagnosis of biliary atresia. Radiology 2007; 245:549-55.

34. Uflacker R, Pariente DM. Angiographic findings in biliay atresia. Cardiovasc Intervent Radiol 2004; 27:486-90.

35. Jaw TS, Kuo YT, Liu GC, et al. MR cholangriography in the evaluation of neonatal cholestasis. Radiology 1999; 212:249-56.

36. Arcement CM, Meza MP, Arunmanla S, et al. MRCP in the evaluation of pancreatobiliary disease in children. Pediatr Radiol 2001; 31:92-7.

37. Giubaud L, Lachaud A, Touraine R, et al. MR cholangiography in neonates and infants: Feasibility and preliminary applications. AJR 1998; 170:27-31.

38. Mitchell DG, Alam F. Mangafodipir trisodium: Effects on T1 and T2 weighted MR cholangiography. J Magn Reson Imaging 1999; 9:366-368.

39. Ryeom HK, Choe BH, et al. Biliary atresia: Feasibility of Mangagfodipir Trisodium Enhanced MR cholangiography for Evaluation. Radiology 2005; 235:250-8.

40. Kasai M, Kimura S, Asakura Y, et al. Surgical treatment of biliary atresia.J Pediatr Surg 1968; 3:665.

41. Takahashi A. Tsuchida Y, Suzuki N, et al. Incidence of intrahepatic biliary cysts in biliary atresia after hepatis portoenterostomy and histopathologic findings in the liver and porta hepatic at diagnosis. J Paediatr Surg 1999; 34:1364.

42. Sela-Herman S, Scharschmidt BF. Choledochal cyst, a disease for all ages. Lancet 1996; 347:779.

43. Babbitt DP. Congenital choledochal cyst: New etiologic concept based on anomalous relationships of common bile duct and pancreatic bulb. Ann Radiol 1969; 12:231-40.

44. Alonso-Lej F, Rever Jr WB, Pessagno DJ. Congenital choledochal cysts, with a report of 2, and an analysis of 94 cases. Surg Gynecol Obstet 1959; 108:1-30.

45. Todani T, Watanabe Y, Narusue M, et al. Congenital bile duct cysts. Am J Surg 1977; 134:263-69.

46. Todani T, Tabuchi K, Watanabi Y, et al. Carcinoma arising in the walls of congenital bile duct cysts. Cancer 1979; 44:1134-41.

47. DiMagno EP, Shorter RG, Taylor WG, Go LW. Relationship between pancreaticobiliary ductal anatomy and parenchymal histology. Cancer 1982; 49:361-8.

48. Misra SP, Gulati P, Thorat VK, et al. Pancreaticobiliary ductal union in biliary diseases. An endoscopic retrograde cholangiopancreaticographic study. Gastroenterology 1989; 96:907-12.

49. Wiedmeyer DA, Stewart ET, Dodds WJ, et al. Choledochal cyst: findings on cholangio pancreatigraphy with emphasis on ectasia of the common channel. AJR 1989; 153:969-72.

50. Kimura K, Ohto M, Saisho H, et al. Association of gallbladder carcinoma and anomalous pancreaticobiliary duct union. Gastroenterology 1985; 89:1258-65.

51. Komi N. New classification of anomalous arrangement of the pancreaticobiliary ductal (APBD) in choledochal cyst: A proposal of new Komi classification of APBD. J Jpn Pancr Soci 1991; 6:234-43.

52. Guelrud M, Morera C, Rodrigues H, et al. Sphincler of Oddi dysfunction in children with recurrent pancreatitis and anomalous pancreaticobiliary union: An etiologic concept. Gastrointest Endoscopy 1999; 50:194-9.

53. Voyles CR, Smajda C, Shands WC, et al. Carcinoma in choledochal cysts. Arch Surg 1983; 118;969.

54. Nagi B, Kochhar R, Bhasin D, Singh K. Endoscopic retrograde cholangiopancreatography in the evaluation of anomalous junction of the pancreaticobiliary duct and related disorders. Abdom Imaging 2003; 28:847-52.

55. Kaneko K, Ando M, Ito T, et al. Protein plug causes symptoms in patients with choledochal cysts. Am J Gastroenterol 1997; 92:1018-21.

56. Yamtaka A, Segawa O, Kobayashi H, et al. Intraoperative pancreatoscopy for pancreatic stone debris distal to the common channel in choledochal cysts. J Paed. Surg 2000; 35:1-4.

57. Torrisi JM, Haller JO, Velcek FT. Cloledochal cyst and biliary atresia in the neonate: Imaging findings in five cases. AJR 1990; 155:1273-6.

58. Chan Y, Yeung C, Fork T, et al. Magnetic resonance cholangiography: feasibility and application in the pediatric population. Pediatr Radiol 1998; 28:307-11.

59. Dinsmore JE, Murphy JJ, Jamieson D. MRCP evaluation of choledochal cysts. J Pediatric Surgery 2001; 36:829-30.

60. Lamb WWN, Lamb TPW, Saing H, et al. MR cholangiography and CT cholangiography of pediatric patients with choledochal cysts. AJR 1999; 173:401-05.

61. Caroli J, Soupault R, Kossakowsky J, et al. La Dilatation Polycystique congenitale des voies biliairis intrahepatiques. Semin Hop Paris 1958; 14:128-35.

62. Lonergan GJ, Rice RR, Suarez ES. Autosomal recessive polycystic kidney disease: Radiologic-pathologic correlation. Radiographics 2000; 20:837-55.

63. Levy AD, Rohrmann CA, Murakata LA, et al. Caroli's disease: Radiologic spectrum with pathologic correlation. AJR 2002; 179:1053-57.

64. Bloustein PA. Association of carcinoma with congenital cystic conditions of the liver and bile ducts. Am J Gastroenterol 1977; 67:40-6.

65. Miller WJ, Sechtin AG, Campbell WL. Imaging findings in Caroli's disease. AJR 1995; 165:333-7.

66. Choi BI, Yeon KM, Kim SH, et al. Caroli disease: Central dot sign in CT. Radiology 1990; 174:161-3.

67. Pavone P, Laghi A, Basso N, et al. Caroli's disease: Evaluation with MRCP. Abdom Imaging 1996; 21:117-9.

68. Toma P, Lucigraj G, Pelizza A. Sonographic patterns of Caroli's disease report of 5 new cases. J Clin Ultrasound 1999; 19:155.

69. Sood GK, Mahaptra JR, Khurana, et al. Caroli disease : Computed tomographic diagnosis. Gastrointest Radiol 1991; 16:243.

70. Sty JR, Hubbard AM, Starshak RJ. Radionuclide hepatobiliary imaging in congenital tract ectasia (Caroli disease) Paed Radiol 1982; 12:111.

71. Guy F, Cognet F, Dranssart M, et al. Caroli's disease: magnetic resonance imaging features. Am Radiol 2002; 12:2730-6.

72. Alvarez A, Bernard O, Brunelle F, et al. Congenital hepatic fibrosis in children. J Paediatr 1981; 99:370.

73. Premkumar A, Berdon WE, Levy J, et al. The emergence of hepatic fibrosis and portal hypertension in infants and children with autosomal recessive polycystic kidney disease: initial and follow up sonographic findings. Paedtr Radiol 1988; 18:123.

74. Summerfield JA, Nagaguchi Y, Sherlock S, et al. Hepatobiliary fibropolycystic diseases clinical and histological review of 51 patients. J Hepatol 1986; 2:141.

75. Brancatelli G, Federle MP, et al. Fibropolycystic liver disease: CT and MR Imaging findings. Radiographics 2005; 25:659-70.

76. Debray D, Pariente D, Uryoas E. Sclerosing cholangitis in children. J Pediatrics 1994; 124:49.

77. Sisto A, Feldman P, Garel L. Primary sclerosing cholangitis in children: Study of five cases and review of the literature. Pediatrics 1987; 80:918-23.

78. Oppenheimer EH, Esterly JR. Hepatic changes in young infants with cystic fibrosis. Possible relation to focal biliary cirrhosis. J Pediatrics 1975; 86:683.

79. Leblanc A, Hadchouel M, Jehan P. Obstructive jaundice in children with Histiocytosis X. Gastroenterology 1981; 80:143.

80. Piccoli DA, Witzleben CL. Disorders of intrahepatic bile ducts. In Walker WA, Hamilton JR, Walker-Smith JA, et al (Eds): Pediatric Gastrointestinal Disease, Philadelphia: BC Decker, 1991.

81. Altman RP. Personal communication, 1992.

82. Pfeiffer WR, Robbinson LH, Balsara VJ. Sonographic features of bile plug syndrome. J Ultrasound Med 1986; 5:161-63.

83. Kurtz AB, Rubin CS, Cooper HS, et al. Ultrasound findings in hepatitis. Radiology 1980; 136:717-23.

84. Donnelly LF, Bisset GS III. Pediatric hepatic imaging. Radiol Clin North Am 1998; 36:413-27.

85. Subramanyam BR, Balthazar EY, Horri SC, et al. Sonography of portosystemic venous collaterals in portal hypertension. Radilogy 1983; 146:161-6.

86. Matary WZ, Roberts EA, Kim P, et al. Portal hypertensive biliopathy: A rare cause of childhood cholestasis. Eur J Padiatr 2008; 167:1339-42.

87. Perego P, Cozzi G, Bertolini A. Portal bioliopathy. Surgical Endoscopy. 2002 (online publication).

88. Malkan GH, Bathia SJ, Bashir K. Cholangiopathy associated with portal hypertension.Gastroint Endos 1999; 49:344-8.

89. Chandra R, Kapoor D, Tharakan A, et al. Portal biliopathy.J Gastro Hepatol 2001; 16:1086-92.

90. Orloff MJ, Charters AC. Tumours of the gallbladder and bile ducts. In Bockus HL (Ed): Gastroenterology. Philadelphia: WB Saunders, 1976.

91. Davis GL, Kissane JM, Ishak KG. Embryonal rhabdomyosarcoma (Sarcoma botryoides) of the biliary tree: A report of five cases and review of the literature. Lancet 1969; 24:333-42.

92. Debray D, Pariente D, Gauthier F. Cholelithiasis in infancy: A study of 40 cases. J Pediatrics 1993; 122:385-91.

93. Greenberg M, Kangarloo H, Cochran ST, et al. The ultrasonographic diagnosis of cholecystitis and cholelithiasis in children. Radiology 1980; 137:745-49.

94. Coughlin JR, Mann DA. Detection of acute cholecystitis in children. J Can Assoc Radiol 1990; 41:213.

95. Gubernick JA, Rosenberg HK, Kessler A, et al. US approach to jaundice in infants and children. Radiographics 2000; 20:173-95.

96. Mortele KJ, Rocha TC, et al. Multimodality Imaging of pancreatic and biliary congenital anomalies. Radiographics 2006; 26:715-31.

CHAPTER **14**

Congenital Anomalies of the Urinary Tract

Smriti Hari, Arun Kumar Gupta

INTRODUCTION

Anomalies of the urogenital tract are among the most common organ system anomalies found in the neonate. With use of real-time ultrasound (US) as a screening test in healthy infants, Steinhardt et al found that 3.2 percent of infants had an abnormality of the genitourinary tract and one-half of these patients required surgical intervention.[1] Prompt and accurate imaging analysis of these anomalies is important so that correctible abnormalities can be treated in a timely manner. Correct diagnosis can also help in genetic workup that may aid in future pregnancy planning.

Imaging Modalities

Diagnostic imaging of pediatric urologic disorders is continuously changing as technological advances are made. Although, the backbone of pediatric urologic imaging has been US, voiding cystourethrography (VCUG), and radionuclide scintigraphy, newer and advanced modalities are increasingly becoming important. The small physical habitus of infants and children and absence of abdominal fat make US an ideal imaging method for providing excellent anatomic images of the urinary system. US has replaced intravenous urography (IVU) as the initial examination, and the results of US usually determine what further examination is required. The role of IVU is to answer specific questions (e.g. to show the calyceal anatomy which may be helpful in establishing the cause of a small kidney), and to differentiate some unusual causes of ureteral obstruction (ureteral valve, ureteral polyp, retrocaval ureter) from the usual pelviureteric junction (PUJ) obstruction.[2] VCUG is essential for the evaluation of the anatomy and abnormalities of the bladder and urethra. Diuretic renography is used to differentiate obstructive from nonobstructive hydronephrosis or hydroureter. It is performed by the intravenous injection of a radiopharmaceutical Tc-diethylene triamine pentaacetic acid (DTPA) or Tc-mercaptoacetyl glycyl3 (MAG3) that is extracted rapidly from the bloodstream and excreted by the kidney. US is the preferred modality when anatomic detail is required, whereas diuretic renography is better for quantitative functional information, such as differential renal function.

Antenatal Sonography

It is estimated that a structural fetal anomaly is detected by antenatal sonography in 1 percent of all screened pregnancies.

Of these anomalies, a fifth are believed to be manifestations of genitourinary origin, second only to those found within the central nervous system.[3] Fetal sonography allows for early detection of renal lesions, especially those characterized by hydronephrosis. Because it has been shown that renal growth and development are affected adversely by prenatal urinary tract obstruction, antenatal hydronephrosis has become a common indication for postnatal renal and bladder sonography. Once postnatal hydronephrosis or hydroureteronephrosis is detected, the radiologic workup should include evaluation for vesicoureteral reflux (VUR) and posterior urethral valve (PUV), evaluation of individual renal function, and determination of whether the lesion is obstructive or nonobstructive. The most common causes of nonobstructive hydronephrosis are VUR and nonobstructive primary megaureter; "prune-belly syndrome" is a much less common cause. Obstructive causes include PUJ obstruction, ureterovesical junction (UVJ) obstruction, ureteral ectopia with or without ureterocele, and PUV (in boys).[4]

Magnetic Resonance Urography (MRU)

MRU has become a useful adjuvant in evaluating urogenital anomalies when the results of conventional imaging modalities are inconclusive.[5] MRU is a powerful examination that has the distinct advantage of providing both anatomic and functional information in one examination. MRU allows a one-stop-shop evaluation of the renal parenchyma, collecting system, vasculature, bladder, and surrounding structures. MRU has intrinsic high soft tissue contrast resolution and multiplanar 3D reconstruction capabilities, without the use of radiation. Additionally, MRU allows quantification of numerous renal functional parameters including transit times, an index of glomerular filtration rate (GFR), and differential renal functions. A comprehensive MRU protocol is a 2-part imaging technique composed of precontrast sequences (static MRU) and postcontrast sequences (dynamic or excretory MRU).

Static MRU (Precontrast Imaging)

Static MRU uses heavily T2-weighted fluid-sensitive sequences in which urine-containing structures are bright. These T2-weighted images serve to delineate the anatomy of the renal collecting systems and ureters. 3D respiratory triggered T2 sequences can be reconstructed to create maximum intensity

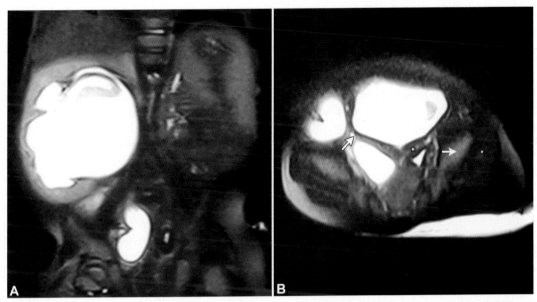

Figs 14.1A and B: MR Urogram: (A) Coronal HASTE image shows gross right hydroureteronephrosis and empty left renal fossa in a one year old child, (B) Axial HASTE image demonstrates the dysplastic, small left pelvic kidney (star) and the right lower ureteric stricture (arrow), the cause of proximal gross hydroureteronephrosis

projections (MIPs) and volume rendered images of the entire collecting system. Additional, high-quality axial T2 sequences are also obtained to provide a high-resolution view of the renal parenchyma. MRU has been shown to be superior to US both in the detection of occult upper pole moieties and in demonstrating ureteral ectopy.[6] In this instance, excretory function of the kidney is not a limiting factor in diagnosing an ectopic ureter because the static-fluid MRU images are sufficient. This is also true for the detection of dysplastic ectopic kidneys that are very difficult to see with other imaging modalities (Figs 14.1A and B). MRU can also clarify the anatomy and complications related to complex urinary tract anomalies, such as crossed fused renal ectopia and horseshoe kidney.

Dynamic MR Urography (Postcontrast Imaging)

Dynamic MRU not only provides anatomic information including that of the vascular system, it also offers functional information, which is in many ways analogous to a nuclear medicine study. Intravenous gadolinium is administered and sequential 3D dynamic sequences of the whole urinary tract are acquired. These images can be presented as a MIP and a cine loop. The former provides morphologic information. The dynamic sequences are the basis of the functional calculation, assess renal perfusion, evaluate renal transit and excretion, and allow generation of signal intensity versus time curves. MRU has been shown to be superior to renal scintigraphy in many regards.[7] MRU has superior contrast and temporal and spatial resolution, and MRU has been shown to be superior to renal scintigraphy in many regards.[10] MRU has superior contrast and temporal and spatial resolution, and can provide precise anatomic information, which radionuclide studies cannot. MRU has also been shown to be superior to renal scintigraphy in distinguishing between pyelonephritis and scar.[8]

Limitations

Although MRU is a powerful study with numerous advantages, few limitations do exist. MRU can have relatively long imaging times and is sensitive to motion artifact, which necessitates sedation for young children. An important limitation of the dynamic postcontrast part of the MRU is that it can be contraindicated in patients with moderate renal insufficiency. As stated, excretory MRU involves the administration of intravenous gadolinium and requires excretion into the collecting systems. Although, it was previously thought that gadolinium could be safely administered in patients with renal insufficiency/failure in an effort to avoid iodinated contrast material, relatively recent reports have linked the disorder nephrogenic systemic fibrosis (NSF) to gadolinium administration.[9] New recommendations are to make every effort to avoid administering gadolinium-based contrast material in patients with moderate-to-severe renal insufficiency (GFR <30 ml/min).

Voiding Urosonography (VUS)

VUS is a relatively new modality in the detection of VUR in children. Although, VCUG and radionuclide cystography are currently the two methods most commonly used to evaluate for VUR, recent developments of commercially available echoenhancing agents have significantly improved the sonographic detection of fluid movement within the urinary tract. The most commonly used echoenhancing agent is Levovist (Bayer-Schering, Berlin, Germany). This introduces stabilized microbubbles, which allow improved visualization of fluid movement. More recently, a newer-generation US contrast agent, namely SonoVue (Bracco, Milan, Italy), is starting to be used. These US contrast agents have made VUS a reliable alternative to VCUG and radionuclide cystography with the distinct advantage of avoiding ionizing radiation and, at the same time, increasing the detection rate of VUR. Overall, the VUS examination consists of scanning the patient before, during, and after the intravesical administration of US contrast agent, as well as during voiding. The kidneys, ureter, and bladder are then imaged to assess for possible VUR, which is diagnosed by the presence of echogenic microbubbles in either the ureters or the renal pelves. VUS can be used in workup of urinary tract infections, follow-up of known VUR, and in the evaluation of reflux in renal transplant patients.

CT Angiography (CTA) and CT Urography (CTU)

State-of-the-art CT technology offers two advanced imaging protocols for pediatric urological applications: CTA and CTU. Among many technical factors, CTA and CTU require precise synchronization between contrast medium delivery and the scan acquisition. For CTA, synchronization is to the arterial or venous phase, whereas for CTU, synchronization is to the delayed excretory renal phase. Although inherently dependent on radiation and iodinated contrast medium, CTA and CTU can be performed safely in pediatric patients using low radiation and contrast medium dose strategies. Current state-of-the-art scanners offer 64- to 320-channel multidetector-row CT (MDCT) technology. Both isotropic (0.50–0.75 mm thick images) and high-resolution (1.25–1.50 mm thick images) datasets can be generated. In most instances, however, a high-resolution acquisition provides sufficient detail for accurate CTA and CTU diagnoses. In selecting this mode, patients are exposed to less radiation, as MDCT collimation will not be submillimeter. Additional, strategies and acquisition parameters to control radiation exposure include restricting coverage to the anatomy of interest and using the lowest possible voltage (kVp) and amperage (mA). Coverage, voltage, and amperage all have direct relationships with the amount of patient radiation exposure. Voltage options include 80, 100, 120, and 140 kVp; 80 kVp is recommended until 50 kg, 100 kVp from 50 to 90 kg, and 120 kVp greater than 90 kg. Amperage is typically prescribed using an automated dose algorithm, which delivers a variable range of amperage over the length of the coverage, based on prescan determined body density and a targeted threshold value for acceptable noise. Using a 64-channel MDCT scanner for abdominal CTA and abdominopelvic CTU in neonates to adolescent patients, average radiation exposures are approximately 1 to 2 mSv with scan times of 1.5 to 4.0 seconds.[10] This radiation dose is equivalent to that of approximately 50 to 100 chest radiographs. As with 3D MRI-MRA and 3D US, CTA, and CTU, datasets are transferred to a workstation for real-time display and review using a combination of multiplanar and curved planar reconstructions, 3D volume rendering, and maximum intensity projections. Pediatric CTA and CTU are considered only after US and MRI have been exhausted or when CT is considered superior for clinical imaging objectives. Emphasizing the advantages of CT, appropriate primary indications for CTA or CTU include the presence of metallic hardware and implantable devices; the requirement for higher spatial resolution; and the need for rapid scan time, such as in emergent imaging or in the high-risk

sedation/ anesthesia patient. Once there is a decision to proceed forward with CT, the pediatric urology patient should be screened to confirm normal renal function and an absence of contrast allergies. CTA applications for the pediatric urology patient include evaluation of suspected or known renovascular hypertension, crossing renal hilar vessels (in the setting of PUJ obstruction), renal aneurysms, small-vessel vasculitis, renal venous occlusive disease (i.e. tumour invasion), vascular malformations (in the setting of hematuria), and traumatic renovascular injury. Additional, indications include preoperative vascular mapping (i.e. before resection of vascular renal and adrenal tumors) and if involved with hemodialysis access care, assessment of upper or lower extremity dysfunctional grafts and fistulas. Diagnostic quality pediatric renal CT arteriograms are motion free, achieving robust enhancement of extraparenchymal renal arteries through to at least the third to fourth order intraparenchymal segments. CTU applications include the evaluation of suspected or known congenital anomalies, obstructive uropathy, trauma, reflux nephropathy, and papillary necrosis. Acquisitions may be performed as a single dedicated urographic 8 to 10 minutes delay acquisition or as a second series following a routine CT or CTA acquisition. Diagnostic quality CT urograms, achieve dense enhancement of the upper and lower collecting systems and the bladder, while maintaining enhancement in the renal parenchyma. As with MRU or conventional IVU, evaluation addresses the number, caliber, contour, course, and patency of native and anomalous upper and lower collecting systems.

The Neonatal Kidney

The normal US appearance of the neonatal kidney (Fig. 14.2) is markedly different from that of an older child or an adult, i.e. the

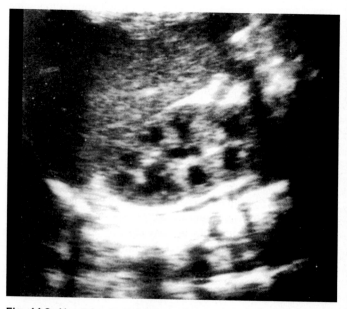

Fig. 14.2: Normal neonatal kidney. The cortex is relatively thin and echogenic, the medullary pyramids appear large and relatively hypoechoic and minimal sinus structures are seen

cortex is thinner and more reflective than the liver, the pyramids are large and relatively hypoechoic compared with the cortex, the capsule is not well-defined and the sinus fat is much less noticeable.[11] The age of transition from the neonatal to an adult pattern is very variable and may occur at 2 to 3 months after birth, but can persist for up to 6 months of age.

The large pyramids have been mistaken for renal cysts. The important diagnostic features of the neonatal renal medulla are the pyramids with their regular triangular shape, with the base on the cortex and the highly reflective foci of the arcuate vessels on the triangular base. The infant kidney is often lobulated in outline because of residual fetal lobulations, and this should not be mistaken for scarring.

Dynamic radionuclide scans are generally best obtained after 4 weeks of age when some renal maturity has occurred. The neonatal DTPA scan is characterized by poor visualization of the kidneys. Relatively poor function as seen on nuclear scanning does not imply irreversible damage, and no long-term management decisions should be taken on the basis of these results; rather the scan should be repeated either when the infant is older (around 3 months) or following a drainage procedure.[12]

IVU requiring administration of an osmotically active contrast medium may be detrimental to the immature kidney of a neonate; it may also aggravate renal vein thrombosis or medullary necrosis. Even in normal neonates, an IVU may fail to outline the kidneys, especially in the first 48 hours of life. These considerations suggest that there is generally no place for an IVU in the first 2-3 days of life. US is the imaging modality of choice for the kidneys in the first week of life. If an IVU is undertaken, delayed images at 6, 12 and 18 hours may be necessary to visualize the kidneys. IVU should be done with a non-ionic contrast medium at a concentration of 30 percent iodine up to a maximum dose of 3 ml per kg.

Embryologic Development of the Urinary Tract

The following brief review of the embryologic development of the urinary tract is very helpful in understanding these congenital genitourinary malformations. The renal parenchyma is derived from the primitive metanephros, which arises from mesenchymal tissue in the presacral area.[13] This primitive tissue is referred to as the nephrogenic blastema. As the primitive metanephros migrates upwards and matures, it takes the form of normal kidney. A specific rotation also occurs so that whereas the renal pelvis originally points anteriorly, a gradual inward and medial turning takes place. Any arrest along this line results in an abnormal orientation of the kidney and some degree of malrotation.

The ureteric bud develops as an outpouching from the metanephric or Wolffian duct at a site near the cloaca. It soon separates from the Wolffian duct and opens into the portion of the cloaca destined to become the urinary bladder. Then the ureteric bud grows upwards and eventually meets the primitive renal parenchymal tissue. At its upper end it forms the renal pelvis and then divides to form the calyces and the collecting tubules. The cloaca forms the larger portion of the bladder and urethra.

The Wolffian duct descends and forms the epididymis, ejaculatory duct and vas deferens in the male. In the female, the Wolffian duct disappears and the Mullerian ducts give rise to the female internal genitalia.

ABNORMALITIES OF KIDNEY

Renal Agenesis

Renal agenesis, the complete congenital absence of renal tissue results from the failure of the ipsilateral ureteric bud to contact the nephrogenic blastema. The ipsilateral ureter and renal artery are absent. There is ipsilateral absence of the trigone and ureteral orifice of the bladder when evaluated by cystoscopy.

Bilateral renal agenesis is the most severe anomaly of the genitourinary system and occurs in 1 to 3 per 10,000 live births. It is noted predominantly in males and is incompatible with life. On prenatal US, severe oligohydramnios, absence of fetal bladder and both kidneys are highly suggestive of bilateral renal agenesis. Early neonatal death is usually because of pulmonary hypoplasia resulting from a lack of transmitted pulsations from amniotic fluid necessary for tracheobronchial tree development. Affected fetuses develop a Potter facies (flattened nose, recession of chin, epicanthic folds, low set ears and hypertelorism) as well as brachycephaly and clubfoot as a result of markedly restricted space for growth.

Unilateral agenesis occurs in about 1 in 1000 of the general population, predominantly in males and on the left side. Sonographically, fetuses with unilateral renal agenesis have a normal amount of amniotic fluid and a readily visualized urinary bladder. The contralateral kidney may be large secondary to compensatory hypertrophy. The most common associated genitourinary anomalies include uterovaginal atresia (or duplication) in females and absent seminal vesicle or seminal vesicle cyst in males.[14]

A number of syndromes are associated with unilateral renal agenesis, such as the VACTERL association, Fanconi pancytopenia, Kallman syndrome, and Fraser syndrome. Abnormalities of the remaining kidney have been described in up to 90 percent of patients. The most common abnormality is VUR followed by renal ectopia and malrotation, PUJ obstruction and multicystic dysplasia.

Imaging Features

In clinical practice it is quite difficult to be certain that one is dealing with true unilateral agenesis since a very small non-functioning kidney may be either ectopic or located medially in the renal bed overlying the transverse processes of the lumbar vertebra. A combination of US and ^{99m}tc dimercaptosuccinic acid (DMSA) scan is needed to make the diagnosis. US might show that a non-excreting kidney on scintigraphy is actually present but abnormal. Conversely, scintigraphy might reveal a small unilateral dysplastic/hypoplastic kidney that was difficult to be evaluated on US, but which is nonetheless present and retains some function. If the US and nuclear studies fail to show a small kidney, then contrast enhanced CT should be done before RGP.

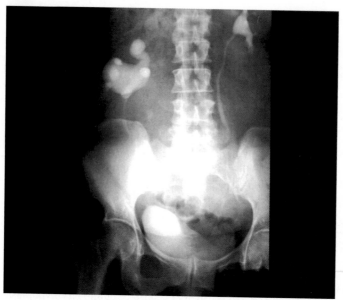

Fig. 14.3: Rotational anomaly of the kidney: IVU showing right caudal ectopia with a rotational anomaly. Note that the calyces are facing medially while the pelvis is facing laterally

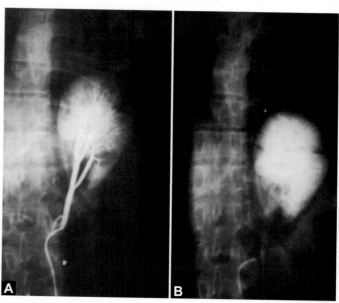

Figs 14.4A and B: Thoracic kidney: Conventional angiogram showing intrathoracic left kidney being supplied by an abnormally long renal artery

RGP can exclude renal agenesis if it shows pelvicalyceal system and ureter on the suspected side.

Rotational Anomalies

As the kidney ascends in fetal life from its origin in the pelvis to its final position opposite the second lumbar vertebra, it undergoes a 90° inward rotation along its longitudinal axis so that finally the renal hilum is directed medially and slightly forward. Any anomaly in this process, results in deficient, excessive, or reversed rotation. In incomplete rotation, or nonrotation, the hilum continues to face anteriorly, the calices project out from either side of the pelvis on a standard frontal radiograph, and the proximal ureter is displaced laterally. In excessive rotation, the normal inward rotation is prolonged beyond 90° so that the hilum faces posteriorly or posteromedially and the renal vessels lie posterior to the kidney. In reversed rotation, the kidney rotates outward with the renal hilum facing laterally, the proximal ureter is displaced laterally, and the renal vessels lie anterior to the kidney (Fig. 14.3). Non-rotation and incomplete rotations are most common rotational anomalies. They may be unilateral or bilateral and often accompany ectopia or fusion anomalies. In an IVU, oblique views are of great help in establishing that the malrotated kidney is otherwise normal.[15]

Anomalies of Renal Position

Normally, the kidneys are located opposite 1st-3rd lumbar vertebrae. Anomalies of renal position range from minor degrees of unilateral malposition to totally abnormal positioning of both kidneys. The clinical significance of this finding lies in the fact that these ectopic kidneys are more susceptible to trauma, iatrogenic injury, obstruction, calculi, reflux and infection. There is a high incidence of aberrant and multiple renal arteries and veins.

Ipsilateral/Uncrossed Ectopia

In this anomaly, the ectopic kidney is on the same side as the vesical opening of its ureter. It can be further divided into cranial or caudal ectopias according to whether they are above or below the normal position. In cranial renal ectopia, the affected kidney, usually the left, is within the lower thorax posteriorly, either below a localized diaphragmatic eventration or within a diaphragmatic hernia (intrathoracic kidney).[16] In caudal renal ectopia the abnormal kidney lies below normal position; it may be abdominal (above iliac crest, below L3), iliac (iliac fossa) or pelvic (true pelvis).

Imaging Features

Chest X-ray shows a thoracic kidney as a well-defined, posteroinferior mediastinal mass. IVU confirms the thoracic location of the kidney. CT may show the diaphragmatic defect through which the kidney passes and the adrenal gland is seen lying above, behind or below the kidney. Blood supply is from an elongated renal artery from aorta at normal level (Figs 14.4A and B), or occasionally from an accessory renal artery from thoracic aorta. In cases of caudal renal ectopia, renal outline is not visible in expected position on an abdominal X-ray. Bowel gas can be seen to occupy the renal fossa; typically the hepatic and splenic flexures are repositioned. IVU shows the malrotated, ectopic kidney with a bizarre pattern of calyces draining into the bladder via a short ureter. Tightly coned views can miss early nephrogram as the ectopic kidney may not be included in the field of view. Fluoroscopic spot views may be required to delineate the course of ureters. Adrenal gland remains in normal location; appears linear on CT and the colonic flexures, spleen and tail of pancreas are seen occupying the empty renal fossa. CT can easily distinguish the ectopic kidney from various abdominal and pelvic masses (Fig. 14.5A). Delayed imaging is helpful in hydronephrosis

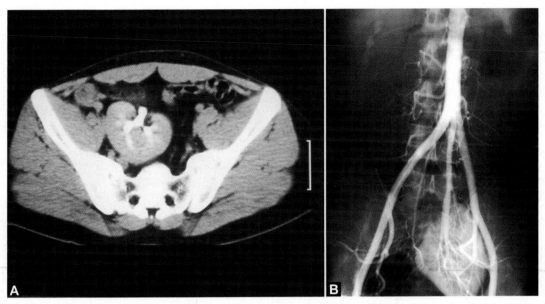

Figs 14.5A and B: Pelvic kidney: (A) Contrast enhanced CT axial image showing ectopic right kidney lying in the right iliac fossa, (B) Aortogram showing an ectopic left pelvic kidney drawing its blood supply from the aortic bifurcation

and to delineate distal ureters. CT angiography can be used for mapping of renal vasculature. Renal arteries are seen to arise lower than normal and may be multiple. When the kidney is pelvic, the arterial supply usually arises from the aortic bifurcation (Fig. 14.5B). These aberrant arteries may cross and obstruct the ureter. It is important to recognize these vessels prior to aortic surgery as they may be inadvertently injured. DMSA scan detects ectopic kidney by outlining the kidney shape. A ptotic kidney has to be differentiated from a caudal renal ectopia. In ptosis of kidney the renal artery arises from normal site and the ureter is redundant.[17]

Crossed Renal Ectopia

In crossed renal ectopia the kidney is located in opposite side of midline from its ureteral orifice. It may occur with fusion (most common), without fusion (15%), or in a solitary kidney (least common).[18] In fused crossed ectopia (unilateral fused kidney), the kidney crosses the midline to the opposite side of the body and fuses with the kidney on that side. Crossed, fused renal ectopia is more common in males and on the right side. The anomalous kidney usually lies below the orthotopic kidney, and the fusion is between the lower pole of the orthotopic kidney and the upper pole of the ectopic kidney. Malrotation, particularly in the ectopic kidney, is the rule. Occasionally, the pelvis of the lower, ectopic kidney faces laterally (sigmoid or S-shaped kidney) or is horizontal (L-shaped kidney). In rare cases, the two fused kidneys are at the same level and are fused completely (unilateral lump kidney). Instances of bilateral crossed renal ectopia and of crossed ectopia of a solitary kidney have been reported.[19] The importance of these conditions is that it may present as an abdominal mass or as an obstructive uropathy with PUJ obstruction. There is an increased incidence of VUR into the crossed kidney.

Imaging Features

The US reveals an unusually large kidney on the affected side with an absent kidney on the opposite side. If the kidneys are not fused, they may be seen to move separately from each other during respiration. In cases of fused ectopia, the renal sinuses lie in different planes, run in different directions and the fused kidneys are inseparable. The diagnosis of renal ectopia is generally established from the IVU or CT. IVU delineates the morphology of the crossed kidneys and shows the insertion of ureter into the trigone on the side of origin (Fig. 14.6). CT with

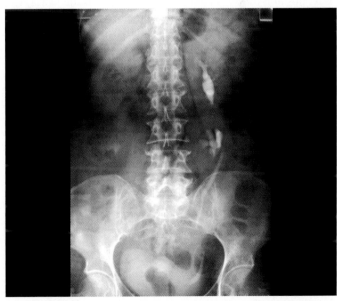

Fig. 14.6: Crossed fused ectopia. IVU showing the right kidney crossing over and fusing with the lower pole of left kidney

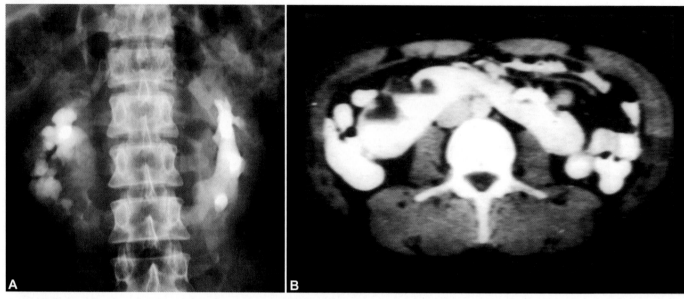

Figs 14.7A and B: Horseshoe kidney: (A) IVU shows the typical U-shape of the horseshoe kidney. The calyces are pointing medially and the pelvis faces laterally, (B) CECT showing a horseshoe kidney with hydronephrosis on the right side and an isthmus of functioning renal parenchyma

thin slices is helpful in showing the degree of separation of the kidneys. CT angiography can show the anomalous vascular supply arising from the vessels in the vicinity.

Horseshoe Kidney

The horseshoe kidney is the most frequent renal fusion anomaly, occurring in 1 in 400 people. It is characterized by fusion of the lower poles across the midline. The kidney is lower in position than a normal kidney and lies anterior to the aorta and inferior vena cava. The horseshoe kidney's polar fusion results in an isthmus of tissue (parenchymal or fibrous) between the two. The usual position of the isthmus is at the junction of the aorta with the inferior mesenteric artery. The isthmus prevents normal renal rotation. The ureters exit the anteriorly positioned renal pelves to descend inferiorly. Most (90%) cases are asymptomatic. Horseshoe kidneys are at greater risk than normal kidneys for PUJ obstruction as well as VUR, infection, urolithiasis and malignancy. Carcinoma of the renal pelvis and Wilms' tumor are more likely to occur in the horseshoe kidney.[20] The abnormal position also leaves the kidney more susceptible to trauma. Many anomalies are associated with horseshoe kidney. Urinary tract anomalies include PUJ obstruction, duplicated collecting systems, ureterocele, megaureter, and renal dysplasia. Horseshoe kidney may be associated with Turner's syndrome, trisomy 18, Fanconi's anemia, and Laurence-Moon-Biedl syndrome, or as a part of VACTERL association.

Imaging Features

On X-ray the lower poles of the kidneys are seen to lie too close to the spine and sometimes the isthmus may be seen. US shows the curved configuration of the horseshoe kidney with elongated, poorly defined lower poles.[21] IVU reveals that the nephrogram is U-shaped and the lower calyces descend towards the midline near the isthmus, resulting in the "hand-holding calyces" appearance

(Fig. 14.7A). The lower calyces are often medial to the ureter on the same side. As each ureter crosses the isthmus, it curves laterally and then assumes a normal medial course giving rise to the "flower-vase" appearance. The renal pelvis is usually large and extrarenal with an abnormally high insertion of the ureter. PUJ (more common) or UVJ obstruction may lead to delayed clearing of the contrast. VCUG often demonstrates VUR. CT is especially useful in showing the degree and site of fusion, and whether the isthmus is composed of functioning renal parenchyma or of fibrous tissue (Fig. 14.7B). Renal parenchymal changes (scarring, cystic disease) and collecting system abnormalities (duplex system, hydronephrosis, calculi) are also picked up on CT.[22] Angiographic images show renal arterial supply from aorta, common iliac, internal iliac, external iliac or inferior mesenteric arteries.

Ureteropelvic Duplication (Duplex Kidney)

A duplex kidney shows two separate pelvicaliceal systems. The two draining ureters may join before emptying into the bladder (partial duplication/bifid ureters) or insert separately into the bladder (complete duplication). 85 percent of completely duplicated ureters follow the Weigert-Meyer rule according to which the upper ureter inserts into the bladder in a position more inferior and medial to the orifice of the lower moiety ureter. In these cases, the ectopic ureter draining the upper pole moiety frequently ends in a ureterocele and is obstructed, whereas reflux typically occurs into the lower moiety. The duplication process may involve the entire urinary tract: from the renal parenchyma to urethra.

Imaging Features

The US diagnosis of a duplex kidney is usually straightforward, the calyces forming two distinct echo complexes with intervening renal parenchyma. Separate renal pelves are often visible along

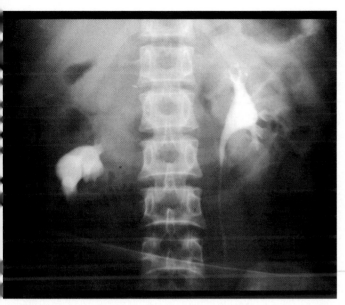

Fig. 14.8: Duplex right kidney. IVU shows that the upper moiety is non-functioning and displaces the lower pelvicaliceal system downwards, producing the "drooping lily sign"

with separate proximal ureters. Distal nondilated ureters are more difficult to image because of bowel gas. One should carefully look for associated ureterocele and assess for the presence and location of ureteral jets in the bladder. Concomitant genital anomalies, especially uterine should also be looked for.

On IVU or CT Urography, duplex kidney is well seen with double ureters leading to two jets of contrast. There is poor or no excretion by the upper pole moiety. Nonfilling of the obstructed upper pole moiety results in the downward displacement of the lower pole calyces, called the "drooping lily" sign (Fig. 14.8). Lower pole may also show calyceal clubbing with thinning and scarring of overlying renal parenchyma. VCUG demonstrates reflux into the lower pole ureter and the frequently present ureterocele at the distal end of upper pole ureter. Saddle reflux or yo-yo reflux is unique to partial duplications which have a single distal ureter. It refers to the refluxed contrast first entering one moiety, draining and then entering the other moiety of the duplicated pelvicaliceal system. Occasionally, nuclear scan is the first to suggest a renal duplication. Renal scan is helpful in estimating differential function, drainage and scarring. MR urography is often the best modality when an ectopic ureter can not be shown by any other imaging modality.[23] Coronal thick slab sequences are most useful in this regard.

Renal Hypoplasia

In simple renal hypoplasia, also called miniature or dwarf kidney, the affected kidney is significantly smaller than normal, but is otherwise well formed both grossly and histologically, and functions normally in proportion to its mass. The main renal artery and its branches are uniformly small. On IVU, it is small, usually excretes contrast material well, smooth in outline, has normal appearance but has fewer than normal (less than 7) calyces, and a normal ureter. The opposite kidney is usually large owing to

compensatory hypertrophy. It does not affect total kidney function unless the opposite kidney is diseased or absent, but rarely it may cause severe hypertension in the neonate.[24]

Cystic Renal Dysplasia

Renal dysplasia is a congenital renal parenchymal malformation in which abnormal nephrons and mesenchymal stroma are found in absence of either neoplasm or infection. It occurs in 2 to 4 in every 1,000 births. Cystic renal dysplasia has been classified into 4 types.[25] Type I is infantile or Autosomal Recessive Polycystic Kidney Disease (ARPKD); II, Multicystic Dysplastic Kidney Disease (MDK); III, Autosomal Dominant (Adult Type) Polycystic Kidney Disease (ADPKD); and IV, cystic renal dysplasia due to early urinary tract obstruction (at any level).

Autosomal Recessive Polycystic Kidney Disease (ARPKD)

ARPKD is a single gene disorder characterized by bilateral, symmetrical renal cystic disease involving distal convoluting tubules and collecting ducts. There is 25 percent likelihood of recurrence in a future pregnancy. Pathologically, there is saccular dilatation of renal collecting tubules noted as hundreds of tiny 1-2 mm cysts on gross examination. In ARPKD the liver is always involved by hepatic cysts, bile duct ectasia and periportal fibrosis. Clinically, it is characterized by a variable mixture of renal failure and portal hypertension. ARPKD is divided into four categories: Perinatal, neonatal, infantile and juvenile, depending upon the age at the time of presentation. It is generally accepted that the abnormality is expressed within a spectrum that varies from predominant renal and minimal hepatic involvement in the infant, to predominant hepatic and minimal renal involvement in the late childhood.[26]

Imaging Features

Plain radiograph shows bilateral large flank masses (enlarged kidneys) that displace the bowel gas centrally. Dilated renal collecting tubules are, too small to be imaged on US as separate cysts and because of the numerous acoustic interfaces provided by the cyst walls the kidney appears solid and homogeneously hyperechoic (Fig. 14.9A). The size of kidneys is 2-4 standard deviations more than the mean size, in majority of patients. The enlarged kidneys maintain their reniform shape and show absent or poor corticomedullary differentiation. Dilated renal collecting tubules are seen radially arranged from the hilum to the periphery in two-third patients when high frequency linear transducer is used.[27] Cysts are only occasionally visible and they are small (0.5 to 1 cm). A characteristic perirenal halo may be seen, representing the peripherally compressed hypoechic normal cortex around the hyperechoic medulla. Tiny, punctuate, echogenic foci develop with time due to calcium deposition and correlate with renal failure. These foci do not show posterior acoustic shadowing, but may cause ring-down artifacts.

IVU is seldom performed today. Decreased renal function leads to poor visualization of the pelvicaliceal system. Classic urographic appearance, best seen on delayed films taken 6-24

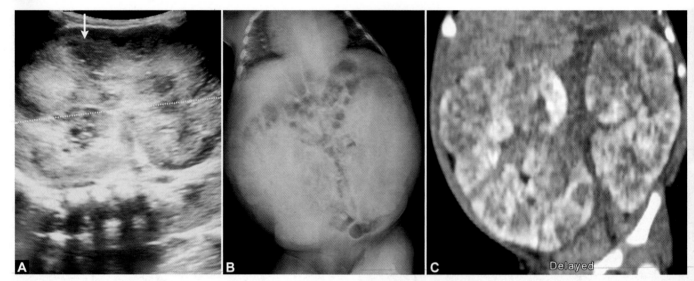

Figs 14.9A to C: Autosomal Recessive Polycystic Kidney: (A) US shows markedly enlarged, homogeneously hyperechoic, kidney with absent corticomedullary differentiation. A characteristic perirenal halo is also seen (arrow), representing the peripherally compressed hypoechoic normal cortex around the hyperechoic medulla, (B) Radiograph taken postcontrast enhanced CT shows classic persistence of contrast in the dilated tubules leading to a streaked nephrogram, (C) Contrast enhanced CT shows bilateral symmetrically enlarged kidneys showing a prolonged striated nephrogram, due to trapping of contrast in the medulla

hours after the administration of IV contrast medium, was persistence of contrast in the dilated tubules leading to a streaked nephrogram (Fig. 14.9B).

CT shows bilateral symmetrically enlarged kidneys with multiple punctuate calcific foci. Contrast enhanced CT shows a prolonged striated nephrogram (Fig. 14.9C), due to trapping of contrast in the medulla. There is minimal excretion of contrast and the bladder is typically empty or small. Few small cysts (2 cm) may be identifiable within the kidneys.

Nuclear scan shows loss of kidney outline with patchy, tracer uptake with focal defects throughout the renal parenchyma.

Antenatal US diagnosis of ARPKD can be made when oligohydramnios with markedly enlarged, echogenic kidneys is noted. In general, earlier the diagnosis is made, worse is the prognosis. These infants are at risk for pulmonary hypoplasia and often die in the neonatal period due to pulmonary complications.

Multicystic Dysplastic Kidney (MDK)

MDK is the second most common abdominal mass in a neonate after hydronephrosis, with an incidence of 1 in 4300 live births. The affected kidney is non-functioning, replaced by numerous cysts and dysplastic tissue. It varies in size from 10-15 cm to only 1-2 cm. Classically, two forms are recognized on imaging;

- *Pelvi-infundibular* MDK, the more common type results from atresia of renal pelvis and proximal ureter in early fetal life. The cysts represent the dilated calyces.
- *Hydronephrotic* MDK, the less frequent type results from atresia of the proximal segment of the ureter (sometimes the entire ureter). In this form cysts represent the entire pelvicaliceal system.

The abnormality is usually unilateral with a normal contralateral kidney allowing for a good prognosis. Bilateral

disease, including bilateral MDK (19%) or MDK with contralateral kidney agenesis (11%), is lethal. There is a 3 to 5 percent familial recurrence of the disease suggesting a genetic influence.[28] The importance of recognizing MDK lies in the knowledge that, approximately 30-50 percent of affected patients have contralateral renal abnormalities including vesicoureteral reflux, PUJ obstruction, and ureterovesical junction obstruction.[29] Postnatally, the natural history of MDK is one of progressive involution of the cystic spaces within the first two years of life.

Imaging Features

MDK is often discovered on routine prenatal US or during an US investigation of a flank mass in the neonate.[30] The findings include the presence of variably-sized cysts separated by echogenic areas throughout the kidney. Outer contour is often lobulated with outer cyst walls forming the margins of the mass. There is no demonstrable communication between these cysts, and no normal renal parenchyma is seen (Fig. 14.10). The kidney may lose its reniform contour. Microscopically, connective tissue, thick walled cysts, small groups of tubules and poorly formed glomeruli are seen between cysts. Color Doppler shows minimal flow in the parenchyma and the central hilar vessels tend to be small. In the majority of cases US allows a definitive diagnosis to be made, however in a small percentage of cases in the neonate it may be difficult to distinguish between a multicystic dysplastic kidney and a large PUJ obstruction. In the multicystic kidney there is usually one 'cyst' which is larger than the others and lies laterally, whereas in PUJ obstruction the dilated renal pelvis is centrally located and the peripheral calyces are seen to extend from it (Figs 14.11A and B). The kidney maintains a reniform shape and its parenchyma surrounds the dilated calyces. In such situations dynamic nuclear imaging may be useful since the

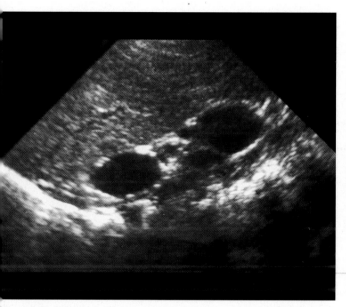

Fig. 14.10: Multicystic Dysplastic Kidney US shows variably-sized cysts separated by echogenic areas throughout the kidney. There is no demonstrable communication between these cysts, and no normal renal parenchyma is seen

demonstration of function indicates PUJ obstruction. In MDK, initial blood flow images show perfusion but sequential images demonstrate lack of any excretory function. CECT also shows multiple low attenuation cysts (debris may lead to higher attenuation in some cysts) replacing normal renal parenchyma. There is minimal or no contrast enhancement and no excretion on delayed images.

Autosomal Dominant (Adult Type) Polycystic Kidney Disease (ADPKD)

ADPKD is a hereditary disease characterized by the presence of multiple bilateral renal macrocysts. There is cystic involvement of liver (50%), pancreas (9%), spleen, brain, ovaries or testes (1%). It has autosomal dominant inheritance with a high degree of penetrance. This disorder most frequently manifests after the third decade of life but now is frequently being diagnosed in infants and children. Children with ADPKD may have hypertension, proteinuria or hyperlipidemia. ADPKD is rarely seen in utero because less than 5 percent of nephrons are cystic antenatally.

Imaging Features

Renal cysts are rarely seen in normal children; hence, when imaged, although at times part of some syndromes, one must consider the possibility of ADPKD. Analysis of the US or medical history of older family members can help make the diagnosis. Cysts are readily seen in the affected adults, with a reported US sensitivity of 100 percent in those more than 30 years of age. Renal contor is typically normal early in life, becoming bosselated as more cysts develop.[31] Renal size and echotexture is normal in young patients, aside from the few small cysts.

IVU shows mildly to markedly enlarged kidneys. Dystrophic calcification of cyst walls and renal calculi are typically only seen

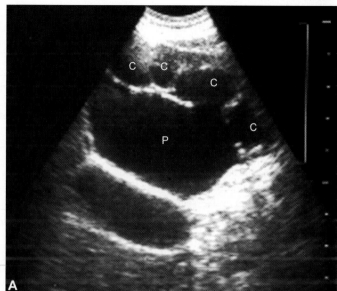

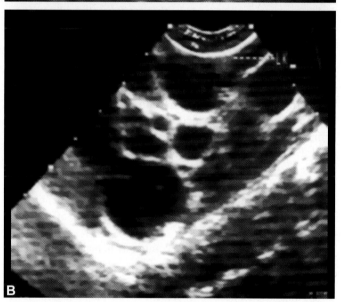

Figs 14.11A and B: (A) PUJ obstruction: Longitudinal US scan of the kidney showing a central distended pelvis (P) and communicating dilated calyces (c), (B) Multicystic dysplastic kidney: The kidney is replaced by multiple simple appearing cysts, which are not connected to each other, the largest ones are peripherally situated

in adult patients. Smoothly marginated rounded, radiolucent defects may be seen in the nephrographic phase, leading to a "Swiss-cheese" pattern. The pelvicaliceal system is splayed around the renal cysts.

Contrast enhanced CT can readily show the nonenhancing hypodense cysts with intervening normally enhancing renal parenchyma and the associated cysts in the liver, pancreas or spleen. Cysts complicated by hemorrhage appear hyperdense (60-90 HU) and may be associated with perinephric hematoma due to rupture. Cyst wall calcification and secondary calculi are easily identified. Infected cysts are hypodense with thick walls showing variable contrast enhancement. Adjacent renal fascia is also thickened with stranding of the perinephric fat. MRI is useful in equivocal cases as it can reliably demonstrate hemorrhage within the cysts as T1 hyperintensity, fluid-fluid levels or T2 hypointense hemosiderin deposition.

PUJ Obstruction

Idiopathic obstruction at the PUJ is a major cause of obstructive uropathy at all ages and is the most common cause of neonatal hydronephrosis.[32] The etiology of obstruction is varied and in more than half the cases obstruction is functional rather than anatomical. Histologically, the PUJ shows a deficiency of muscle fibers with an increase in collagen tissue. This results in an impaired transmission of the peristaltic waves and urine from the renal pelvis to the ureter (segmental dysfunction, adynamic segment).[33] Obstruction may also be due to an intrinsic stenosis of the PUJ, an infolding of the local mucosa and musculature or local kink and angulation of the ureter associated with adhesions and overlying fibrous bands. An aberrant renal artery to the lower pole of the kidney crossing the PUJ is seen in about one-third of patients.[34]

PUJ obstruction may occur in a duplex system where it almost always affects the lower moiety. Malrotated, horseshoe and ectopic kidneys are prone to PUJ obstruction, mainly due to aberrant and multiple arterial vasculature. PUJ obstruction has also been reported to be associated with primary megaureter and VUR. In unilateral PUJ obstruction, the opposite kidney is sometimes absent, duplicated or cystic dysplastic. There is a definite relationship between fetal urinary obstruction and cystic renal dysplasia. The location and timing of obstruction *in utero* appear to determine whether dysplasia, cystic dysplasia or ordinary hydronephrosis will result.[35] Whatever the cause, the renal pelvis and calyces fail to empty leading to various degrees of dilatation with corresponding degree of atrophy of the renal parenchyma.

PUJ obstruction occurs more commonly in males than females and the left side is more commonly affected. There can be bilateral involvement in 10-30 percent of patients. Newborns and infants (if not diagnosed antenatally) present with a palpable abdominal lump. Older children may present with intermittent abdominal pain with vomiting, hematuria or urinary tract infection.

Imaging Features

In infants with known or suspected hydronephrosis from a prenatal US, a re-evaluation by abdominal US should be done soon after birth followed by a diuretic DTPA nuclear scan and, if still indicated, by a conventional urogram. In other patients, both infants and older children, the diagnosis is often suggested on sonography. On US, the hydronephrotic kidney is often enlarged and contains a central cystic structure, representing the renal pelvis, around which and communicating with it are multiple cystic areas corresponding to the dilated calyces. US can also evaluate the degree of cortical atrophy. As the ureter is not dilated, it is not visualized.

Duplex Doppler can be used to differentiate obstructive from non-obstructive dilatation of the renal collecting system. A resistive index (RI) of more than 0.7 in the peripheral intrarenal

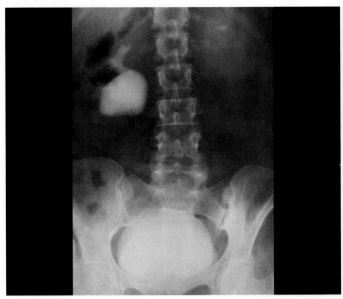

Fig. 14.12: PUJ obstruction. IVU showing dilatation of right renal pelvis out of proportion to the calyces, with abrupt narrowing at the junction of pelvis with ureter

arteries indicates obstructive dilatation. However, the RI value is age-dependent and in children less than 4 years of age the RI is normally greater than 0.7. In these cases the RI of the affected system can be compared with the opposite side.[36] Measurements of the resting RI and after a diuretic challenge, i.e. 10 minutes following intravenous frusemide, can give better results in the pediatric population. The post-frusemide study shows an increase in RI in both the obstructed and non-obstructed kidneys, but the obstructed kidney shows a significant increase of greater than 0.1.[37]

On IVU, the classical PUJ obstruction presents with delayed opacification of the collecting system, marked pyelocaliectasis, narrowing at PUJ, incomplete visualization of a normal sized ureter, and retention of contrast material in the collecting system on delayed films (Fig. 14.12). In severe cases the nephrographic phase of the urogram may show an opaque rim of functioning parenchyma of variable thickness peripherally with multiple centrally placed round radiolucencies representing dilated calyces (rim sign).[38] Contrast in the compressed and realigned or dilated collecting tubules of Bellini may be visible in the early phase of the study as dense curved bands (calyceal crescents)[39] or as a row of dense dots located around the outer border of the calyces. The markedly dilated pelvis and calyces fill only on delayed films and absence of function is uncommon.

The urographic appearance of PUJ obstruction varies depending upon the cause. Obstructing vessels may produce a linear or band like oblique crossing defect in the proximal ureter.[40] Both intrinsic stenosis and functional obstruction cause a focal, smooth narrowing. In most PUJ obstructions the extrarenal pelvis enlarges out of proportion to the degree of caliectasis. Rarely, PUJ obstruction occurs with an intrarenal pelvis, in which case caliectasis may be in proportion with or relatively more severe than the pyelectasis.

Diuresis renography can help in two circumstances: (i) to confirm that a prominent renal pelvis is not obstructed and (ii) to bring out a suspected intermittent PUJ obstruction. It is an adjunct to the basic IVU. Furosemide, 0.5 mg/kg is injected intravenously, 15-20 minutes after the injection of contrast. Films are taken at 5, 10 and 15 minutes after the diuretic injection. In non-obstructive PUJ, all contrast material should clear by 10 minutes. Delayed clearance, appearance of pyelocaliectasis and/or flank pain is the classic signs of a flow related PUJ obstruction.[41]

Radionuclide studies give the best objective assessment of renal function. Diuresis renography effectively separates obstructive from non-obstructive dilatation in many patients and can also localize the probable site of obstruction. Even in patients with equivocal test results, serial renograms are useful to assess whether urine transport is stable or deteriorating.

VCUG is done in infants with PUJ obstruction to exclude coincidental reflux.[42] Older children need VCUG only if a dilated ureter has been demonstrated on IVU or US or if urinary infection is present.

CT is needed in very few circumstances. CT is the best method for assessing isthmus anatomy when PUJ obstruction involves a horseshoe kidney. It may also be used to determine the level of obstruction in non-functioning kidneys. Hydronephrosis without ureterectasis places the obstruction near or at the PUJ.

The Prominent Normal Extrarenal Pelvis

Rounded extrarenal pelvis is seen in approximately 10 percent of normal individuals. It tends to be flabby, distensible, often narrow or closed at outlet and may appear turgid during some phases of IVU (Fig. 14.13). The features which caution against diagnosing this as PUJ obstruction are: The absence of symptoms, prompt appearance of contrast material in the calyces, normal sized calyces with sharp fornices and prompt drainage on films made with the patient prone/erect.

Postoperative Evaluation

Postsurgical edema at the anastomosis frequently causes partial obstruction in the early postoperative period and gradual resolution takes place over days to weeks. Routine imaging studies during this interval are likely to be confusing and misleading.

Serial diuretic radionuclide renography is probably the most informative way to monitor urodynamics postsurgically as long as renal function is satisfactory. Improvement in function and/or drainage has been shown by renography in approximately 90 percent of patients.[43]

IVU or renography should be done 3 to 6 months postoperatively. Following successful PUJ repair the contour of the renal pelvis will be altered according to the type of surgery performed. Reduction in size of the renal pelvis reflects the extent of the plastic repair and is not, *per se*, an indication that obstruction is gone.

Improvement in the emptying rate should result in earlier appearance of contrast material in the upper ureter compared with preoperative studies. Although, drainage may still be delayed in

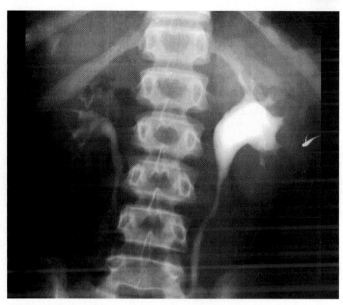

Fig. 14.13: Left extrarenal pelvis without obstruction. Though the pelvis appears distended it tapers smoothly into the ureter with no evidence of hold up of contrast

comparison with the normal, contralateral kidney, this should not be taken as evidence for persistent obstruction. Calyces that were minimally dilated preoperatively may return completely to normal after surgery, but if moderate or severe caliectasis was well established, little or no change is common. Maximum improvement is attained by 6 months. Increased caliectasis or further delay in appearance of contrast material in the ureter at 6 months always indicates a poor clinical result.

In view of the unpredictability of pyelocaliectasis following PUJ repair, US has limited usefulness for postsurgical evaluation. Moreover, different states of hydration and bladder filling affect the caliber of the collecting system and make interpretation difficult. A decrease in both renal size and pelvic dilatation has been observed by US immediately following PUJ surgery in uncomplicated cases. The comparison of renal RI as measured by duplex Doppler in pre- and post-pyeloplasty cases can be used as an index to assess the postsurgical status.

ANOMALIES OF THE URETER

Ectopic Ureter

An ectopic ureter is one that does not insert at its normal position at the superolateral aspect of the bladder trigone. Intravesical ectopia is not so common and is manifested by the ureter opening either lateral or caudal to the normal opening.

Extravesical ectopia is more common and also more clinically important. It is more common in girls than in boys and is associated with a duplicated system in at least 85 percent of cases. It is the upper pole ureter that opens ectopically. In girls the ectopic ureter may open in the urethra, vestibule or vagina and a common presenting feature is continuous leakage of urine with a normal voiding pattern. In boys, the anomalous ureter may insert in the prostatic urethra, near the bladder neck or sometimes in the genital ducts. Urinary incontinence is not a problem with boys

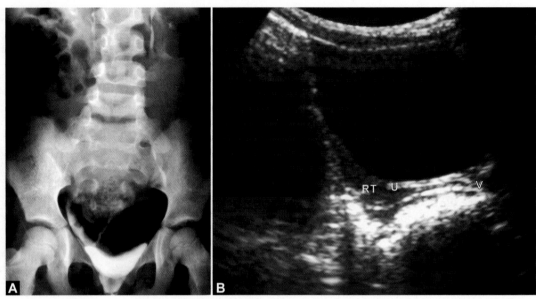

Figs 14.14A and B: Ectopic ureter: (A). Delayed IVU fim showing the low-lying ectopic insertion of the right ureter into the vagina which has been opacified by contrast, (B) US showing mildly dilated right ureter draining into the vagina in a 6-year-old girl with complaints of continuous dribbling of urine

since the ectopic opening is above the strongly developed external sphincter but urinary tract infection is a common clinical manifestation.

Imaging Features

The renal parenchyma drained by the ectopic ureter is often dysplastic and its function is usually decreased or absent. The corresponding pelvicalyceal system and ureter draining ectopically may be visualized on delayed films of an IVU (Fig. 14.14 A). A non-functioning second system can be suspected when the visualized pelvicalyceal system is displaced downward and laterally. When the aberrant ureter empties in the urethra, reflux into the ectopic ureter is occasionally demonstrated in the voiding study. In girls, a vaginogram may show reflux in the affected ureter if this terminates in the vagina. US is helpful if the anomalous ureter is dilated, in which case it can be followed down to and beyond the bladder (Fig. 14.14B). Renal scan can demonstrate function not apparent in the urogram. Recently, MR urography has proved capable of displaying dilated collecting systems, ectopic ureters, and ureteroceles. It has an advantage over US and IVU in that it is capable of demonstrating ectopic extravesical ureteric insertions, thereby providing a global view of the malformation.

Ureterocele

Ureterocele is a cystic dilatation of the intravesical segment of the ureter projecting into the lumen of the bladder. It is of two types—Simple ureterocele and Ectopic ureterocele.

Simple Ureterocele

In simple ureterocele, stenosis of the distal end of the normally positioned ureteral orifice leads to ballooning of the segment immediately above it, forming the ureterocele which presents as a rounded cystic mass. It is more commonly bilateral and is seen in non-duplicated systems. Complications include stone formation and urinary tract infection.

Imaging Features

A simple ureterocele may be demonstrated on US, VCUG or IVU. The ureterocele is located at the lateral angle of the trigone, and is entirely within the bladder. The findings on excretory urography are characteristic. In the early films, the ureterocele is seen as a round, radiolucent defect at the trigone. As contrast collects within the bladder and in the ureterocele a radiolucent halo representing the nonopacified wall of the ureterocele is seen. This is the well known "Cobra head" appearance (Fig. 14.15). On US, ureterocele may be seen as a cystic mass projecting into the lumen of the bladder. On real time US scanning the ureterocele may show distension and collapse with ureteric peristalsis (Figs 14.16A and B). On VCUG the negative defect of the ureterocele is best seen during early filling of the bladder before the contrast becomes too dense and before the intravesical pressure compresses the ureterocele.

Ectopic Ureterocele

Ectopic ureterocele is more common than the simple type and is unilateral in 90 percent of patients. It differs from simple ureterocele in several respects.[44]

- Ectopic ureterocele commonly occurs in a duplicated system and is almost always connected with the upper moiety ureter.
- The ureter connected with the ureterocele enters the bladder wall at the normal site, descends towards the bladder neck submucosally, passes through the internal urethral sphincter and terminates ectopically in the proximal urethra. In contrast to the simple ureterocele in which the cyst is formed by herniation of distal end of the ureter, the ectopic ureterocele

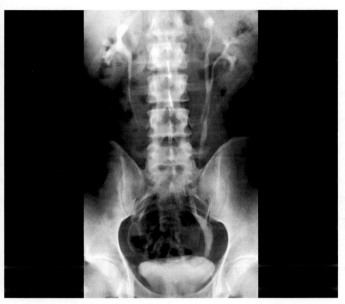

Fig. 14.15: Simple Ureterocele. IVU showing duplex left kidney. The ureter draining the lower moiety inserts into the lateral trigone of the bladder ending into a ureterocele. A radiolucent halo representing the nonopacified wall of the ureterocele is seen producing the "Cobra head" appearance

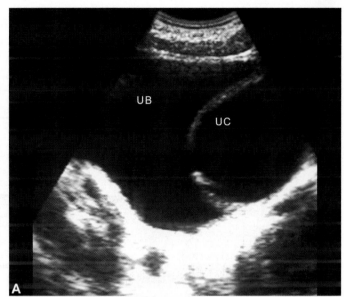

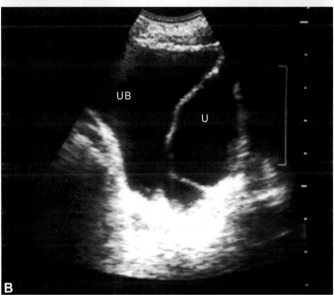

Figs 14.16A and B: Ectopic ureterocele: (A) US shows the ureterocele as an intravesical cyst attached to the posterolateral wall of the bladder (cyst within a cyst appearance) (B) Dynamic scanning shows a collapsing ureterocele

represents the dilatation and protrusion of the entire submucosal segment of the ureter into the lumen of the bladder and at the bladder neck.

- Ectopic ureterocele has a broad base and is usually larger than the simple intravesical type. It is located more inferiorly in the bladder and extends to the bladder neck area or urethra. The ureter connected with ureterocele is often dilated and tortuous.

Imaging Features

US is the single, most important investigation to diagnose ectopic ureterocele. It shows not only the ureterocele but also the upper pole collecting system of a duplex kidney which is typically dilated and is continuous with the dilated tortuous ureter entering the ureterocele (The upper pole kidney may not be seen on IVU). The ureterocele is seen as an intravesical cystic lesion of variable size attached to the posterolateral wall of the urinary bladder (cyst within cyst).

Renal scintigraphy has an important role in evaluation of functional status of kidneys in these patients.

On IVU the ectopic ureter and its insertion point may be visualized, although IVU is now performed less frequently because the dilated upper pole often shows reduced function and is rarely opacified. The visualized pelvicalyceal system of the lower moiety is displaced downwards and laterally by the dilated non-visualized upper moiety. Ureterocele is usually seen as a rounded and eccentric filling defect at the base of the urinary bladder (Fig. 14.17). The outline of the ureterocele is usually clearly defined by the contrast material except for its lower margin which is confluent with the bladder base and bladder neck. This is in contrast to the simple ureterocele which is intravesical and therefore completely outlined.

Primary Megaureter

Primary megaureter, is an uncommon, non-hereditary lesion caused by an adynamic distal segment that prevents normal, caudal progression of ureteral peristalsis.

The diagnosis of primary megaureter is usually made from the IVU. Typically the dilated ureter tapers smoothly but abruptly just above the ureterovesical junction. The terminal aperistaltic segment varies between 0.5 to 4 cm in length. Mild forms are common, resulting only in fusiform dilatation of the lower ureter. Even when the entire ureter is affected, the lower third shows greatest dilatation.

At its extreme, primary megaureter causes severe obstructive hydronephrosis with parenchymal thinning and loss of renal

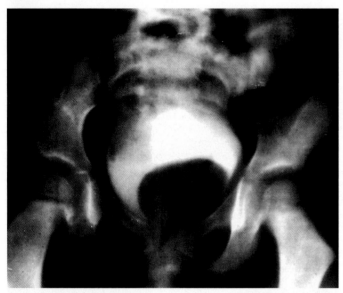

Fig. 14.17: Ectopic ureterocele. Contrast filled bladder on an IVU shows the ureterocele as a well defined eccentrically placed filling defect confluent with the bladder base

function. In bilateral cases, dilatation is often asymmetrical. Calculi may form or trap proximal to the adynamic segment and often remain long enough to become very large (Figs 14.18A and B).

Real time US shows ureterectasis, disproportionately greater dilatation of the lower ureter, hyperperistalsis with to and fro movement of urine, and the relatively narrowed adynamic distal segment.

VCUG should always be performed to make sure VUR is not the major cause of a wide ureter. Although, the strict definition of primary megaureter excludes patients with reflux, ipsilateral reflux has been seen in a significant number of children with otherwise classical findings of primary megaureter. Clues to the diagnosis of primary megaureter being primary rather than secondary to reflux are:

- The distal ureteral segment is normal in caliber
- The opacity of refluxed contrast material in the ureter and collecting system is less than that in the bladder, indicating dilution by stagnant urine trapped above the aperistaltic segment, and
- There is delayed drainage of contrast-laden urine back into the bladder.[45]

ANOMALIES OF THE URINARY BLADDER

Agenesis

Agenesis of the bladder is a rare anomaly that is more commonly seen in females. When seen, it is mostly part of a complex anomaly in a stillborn fetus. On antenatal US, bladder absence may be simulated by recent emptying, requiring follow-up imaging. An axial US image of the umbilical arteries as they course lateral to the bladder can help point out where the bladder should be imaged in the fetus.

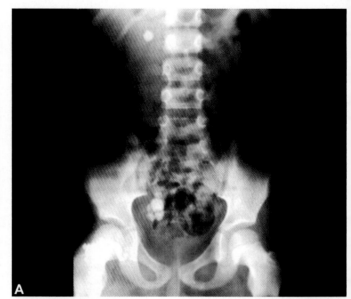

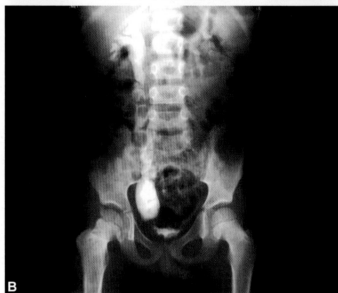

Figs 14.18A and B: Calculi complicating primary obstructive megaureter. (A) Plain radiograph of the pelvis shows large, faceted stones in the right hemipelvis, and a single right renal calculus. (B) IVU shows grossly dilated juxtavesical segment of the primary megaureter in which the faceted stones are located

Complete Duplication

Complete duplication of the urinary bladder and related anomalies are also extremely rare.[46] Two bladders lie side by side separated by peritoneal fold. Each bladder has a separate urethra (Fig. 14.19). Bladder may be compartmentalized into two parts by a septum in the sagittal or coronal plane. The complete septum results in a ureter draining into the closed portion resulting in a dysplastic or nonfunctional kidney. IVU shows one kidney with an associated hemibladder.

Bladder Exstrophy

Exstrophy of the bladder (Fig. 14.20) occurs as a result of defect in the formation of anterior abdominal wall. Exstrophy is the most

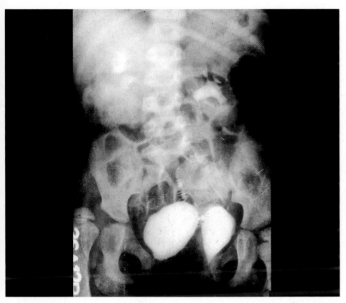

Fig. 14.19: Bladder duplication. IVU showing duplication of the urinary bladder in the sagittal plane

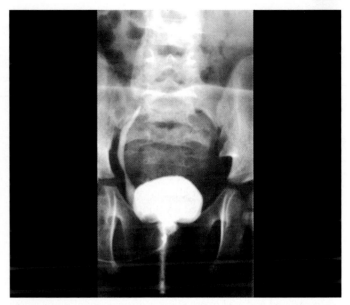

Fig. 14.20: Exstrophy of the bladder: (Postoperative patient). Evidence of diastasis of symphysis pubis with reconstructed bladder seen. Also bilateral VUR seen

common anomaly of the urinary bladder.[47] In its most severe manifestation, the rectus abdominus muscle is widely separated and bladder lies open and everted on the anterior abdominal wall. The bladder mucosa is continuous with the skin. The exposed transitional cell mucosa often undergoes metaplasia, creating an increased risk for adenocarcinoma of the bladder. With an associated epispadias the urethral mucosa covers the dorsum of a short penis and the urethra opens on the dorsal surface of the penis. Plain radiograph of abdomen and pelvis demonstrates diastasis of the symphysis pubis. On intravenous urography there is a wide lateral curve of the pelvic portion of the distal ureters, which then turn slightly medially and upwards and pass through the bladder wall in a perpendicular direction.

Bladder Diverticulae

Congenital bladder diverticulae occur almost exclusively in boys. Most bladder diverticulae are localized outpouchings of the bladder mucosa between fibers of the detrussor muscles (pseudo-diverticulae) resulting from a congenital or acquired defect in the bladder wall. Bladder diverticulae may be primary (idiopathic), secondary or iatrogenic (postoperative).

Primary or idiopathic diverticulae are the most common, occur anywhere but most frequently in the trigonal areas. A common type of bladder diverticulum, referred to as paraureteral diverticulum or "Hutch diverticulum", is located laterally and cephalad to the ureteral orifice (Fig. 14.21). Associated VUR is present in about half of the patients. This is because the presence of the diverticulum alters the normal slanted insertion of the ureter into the bladder. A large diverticulum may cause bladder outlet obstruction. Bladder diverticulae may be seen in several syndromes, e.g. Cutix Laxa, Ehlers-Danlos syndrome, Fetal alcohol syndrome. In male infants, bladder diverticulum must be distinguished from bilateral protrusion of the urinary bladder into

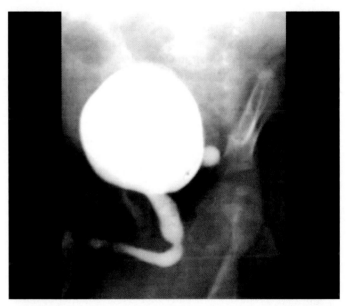

Fig. 14.21: Hutch diverticulum: MCU showing a paraureteric (Hutch) diverticulum

the inguinal rings anteriorly. These outpouchings also called "bladder ears" are transient and disappear with growth. Lateral VCUG usually helps differentiate between the two conditions.

Secondary diverticulae develop as a result of chronically increased intravesical pressure and are seen mostly in patients with posterior urethral valves or other causes of severe lower urinary tract obstruction and in patients with neurogenic bladder disease.

Iatrogenic diverticulae are most often seen in the anterior wall of the bladder at the site of previous vesicostomy or suprapubic drainage catheter and at VUJ following ureteral reimplantation.

Bladder diverticulae are best imaged by contrast cystography, US and CT. The appearance of diverticulae varies with location, size and pressure effect due to adjacent structures and the presence of complicating stone or tumor. A wide neck diverticulum fills and empties readily with the bladder, if the neck of diverticulum is narrow with poor emptying, the diverticulum may be better appreciated on post void film.

Neurogenic Bladder

In contrast to adult patient in whom neurogenic bladder is most often due to an acquired, usually traumatic spinal cord lesion, the vast majority of children affected with this disorder have a myelomeningocele or a related myelodysplastic anomaly (occult spinal dysraphism, sacral agenesis).

Myelomeningocele can occur at any level of the spine but is most often located in the lumbosacral area. The radiographs of the affected area show widening of the neural canal, defective posterior neural arches, absence of the posterior spinous processes, and widened interpedicular distance involving several segments, with elongated and flattened or defective pedicles.

Occult myelodysplasia is a group of congenital anomalies of the spinal cord in which the overlying skin is intact although cutaneous stigmata of the disorder may be present such as local hair overgrowth, hyperpigmentation, hemangioma, a skin dimple, or an ill-defined soft tissue mass due to a lipoma. These anomalies include tethered cord, diastematomyelia, intraspinal lipoma, dermoid cyst, and hamartoma. Radiographs of the spine may show osseous changes similar to those seen in myelomeningocele, and sometimes scoliosis or broad vertebral bodies.

Children with this disorder commonly have inappropriate detrusor muscle contraction and external sphincter relaxation, resulting in uncontrolled voiding pattern with incomplete bladder emptying.[48] Initially, the upper tracts are normal but due to poor bladder emptying secondary changes of reflux and infection result.

Complete evaluation of patients suspected of having neurogenic bladder requires VCUG for assessment of lower urinary tract, US and one of the functional studies of IVU or scintigraphy for upper tract. However, for the diagnosis of primary cause, examination with plain radiographs and MRI is essential.

On VCUG, bladder is usually elongated, pointing upwards (Christmas tree shape) with varying degrees of trabeculation and sacculation (Fig. 14.22). Rarely bladder may be large, smooth, atonic type. During voiding, bladder neck and proximal posterior urethra are dilated forming a funnel shape with the point of the funnel directed caudally at mid posterior urethra level. Distal urinary stream is usually poor with significant post void residual urine. Associated VUR is common. Urodynamic techniques have assumed a major role in the evaluation of neurogenic bladder and contributed significantly to the management.

Megacystis

Megacystis is a descriptive term for a large, smooth walled bladder. It may be a normal variation or a congenital anomaly of little clinical significance. A large smooth walled bladder is a

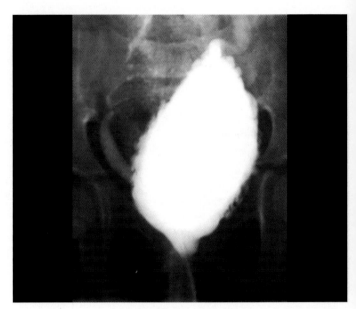

Fig. 14.22: Neurogenic bladder: Bladder is elongated upwards with trabeculations and sacculations

common finding in Prune Belly syndrome. It may be seen in patients with excessive urine formation, e.g. Diabetes insipidus. Uncommonly it may be seen in neurogenic disease.

Prune Belly Syndrome

Prune belly syndrome is a rare congenital syndrome usually affecting the males. The term prune belly refers to a lax, wrinkled abdominal wall, which is frequently associated with other anomalies.[49] The syndrome comprises of deficiency of abdominal muscles, undescended testis and urinary tract anomalies. On voiding cystourethrography, bladder is enlarged and elongated but lacks trabeculations and dilated high placed posterior urethra is a characteristic finding (Fig. 14.23). Upper tract findings include renal dysmorphism or marked hydroureteronephrosis. Non-functioning kidney may also be seen.

Urachal Anomalies

In early fetal life the bladder extends to the umbilicus where it is in continuity with the allantois. As the fetus grows the cephalad part of bladder narrows to form a channel, the urachus, which obliterates into a fibrous cord called the medial umbilical ligament. Failure of the urachus to regress may result in one of the following 4 types of congenital anomalies:[50]

Types of Anomalies

- Patent urachus
- Urachal cyst
- Urachal sinus
- Urachal diverticulum

Patent urachus: The failure of the entire course of the urachus to close results in an open channel between the bladder and the umbilicus. A patent urachus is diagnosed in a newborn when urine is seen leaking from the umbilicus.

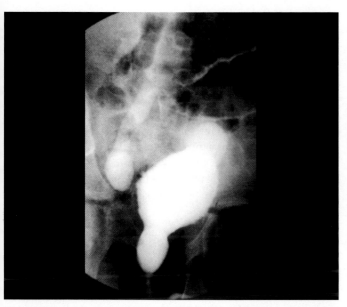

Fig. 14.23: Prune belly syndrome. VCUG showing enlarged and elongated bladder that lacks trabeculations, dilated high placed posterior urethra and dilated right ureter

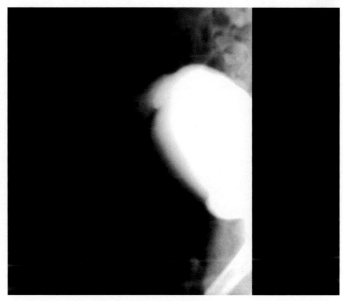

Fig. 14.24: Urachal diverticulum: Blind ending dilated urachus seen at the anterior superior aspect of the bladder

Urachal cyst: It results from obliteration of both the umbilical and the vesical ends of the urachal lumen with an intervening portion remaining patent and fluid filled. Generally, it occurs in that part of the urachus which is closer to the bladder. It usually remains clinically obscure till complicated by either infection or rarely a tumor.

Urachal sinus: Urachal sinus is a blind ending dilatation of the urachus at the umbilical end.

Urachal diverticulum: Urachal diverticulum is a blind ending dilatation of the urachus at the anterosuperior aspect of the bladder as a result of failure of closure of the urachus at the bladder end (Fig. 14.24).

The diagnosis of patent urachus can be made either by catheterization of the bladder through the umbilicus or by VCUG with films taken in lateral projection. Diagnosis of urachal sinus is made by catheterization and opacification of the umbilical fistula. Urachal diverticulum is demonstrated by VCUG with films in lateral projection. Diagnosis of urachal cysts is more difficult. The cystogram may show only an extrinsic compression on the dome of the bladder in the mid line or slightly to one side. US, CT or MRI may demonstrate the lesion better.

ABNORMALITIES OF THE URETHRA

Posterior Urethral Valve

Posterior urethral valve is the most common congenital obstructive lesion of the urethra and the most important cause of end stage renal disease in boys. Three types of posterior urethral valves (PUV) have been recognized based on urethroscopic findings.[51]

Type I: Two fibroepithelial valve like folds originate from the lower pole of the verumontanum and course obliquely to the most distal portion of the prostatic urethra. The two folds fuse anteriorly,

leaving a cleft as the only passage for urine. This is the most common form of PUV.

Type II: PUV related to superior urethral crest and its fins, is believed to be very rare or non-existent.

Type III: This type of PUV is also relatively less common as compared to Type I. In patients with this type of valve a transverse membrane is seen in the posterior urethra just below the verumontanum sometimes near the urogenital diaphragm.

Imaging Features

VCUG is the gold standard for imaging PUV. On voiding films, the posterior urethra is markedly dilated and elongated down to the level of PUV. The transition between the dilated posterior and anterior normal urethra is abrupt with a thin stream (Fig. 14.25). The valves may be seen as two radiolucent lines. A posterior indentation or posterior lip is often present at the level of bladder neck due to bladder neck hypertrophy. Reflux of contrast into the prostatic or ejaculatory ducts may occur and a prominent utricle may be seen. Classic PUV is not visible on a retrograde urethrogram since the valves are displaced and flattened against the urethral wall by the retrograde flow of contrast.

Secondary, obstructive changes of varying severity develop in the bladder, ureters and kidneys. The bladder becomes hypertrophied and trabeculated and develops saccules and diverticulae. In approximately 50 percent of patients VUR may be present.[52] The ureters are often dilated, elongated and tortuous, along with hydronephrosis. Associated renal dysplasia of varying degree is common and the affected kidney may be small.

Apart from VCUG, US is a valuable modality for evaluation of PUV. US evaluates size of the kidneys, thickness of renal parenchyma, degree of hydronephrosis, dilatation of the ureters, and bladder wall thickness. Mid line sagittal scans of the base of the bladder through suprapubic approach or through perineum

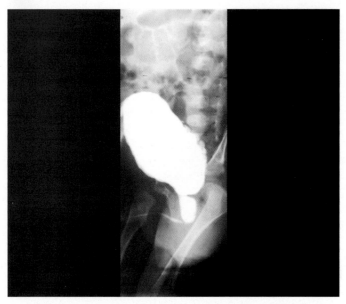

Fig. 14.25: Posterior urethral valve: MCU showing markedly dilated posterior urethra and thin stream of contrast in anterior urethra. Bladder shows back pressure changes of multiple saccules and diverticulae

may show dilatation of the proximal posterior urethra.[53] Evaluation of kidneys may be carried out by nuclear scan.

The newborns with PUV and severe degree of obstructive changes may be associated with Potter facies and pulmonary hypoplasia. Abdominal distension and palpable abdominal masses due to an enlarged bladder and kidneys may be noted. A localized perirenal urinoma or urinary ascites due to a rent in the caliceal fornix or in the bladder may also contribute to the abdominal enlargement. The prenatal US may reveal bilateral hydronephrosis, hydroureters, a thickened bladder wall and a dilated posterior urethra in sagittal scans (Keyhole sign).[54] Fetal MRI is the best imaging test for antenatal diagnosis in late gestation when ossifying pelvic bones interfere with the visualization of bladder outlet on sonography.

Posterior Urethral Polyp

This is a relatively uncommon lesion of the male posterior urethra and is usually diagnosed in children between 3 to 6 years of age but may be seen even in infants or adults. The lesion is also called congenital polyp of the verumontanum which consists of an elongated, freely mobile polypoid mass on a long stalk originating from the verumontanum. It is a benign hamartomatous lesion. The symptoms are those of intermittent urethral obstruction. On VCUG urethral polyp is seen as a rounded/oval filling defect in the distal posterior urethra. At the end of voiding the polyp is displaced upwards at the level of bladder outlet.[55]

Prostatic Utricle and Mullerian Duct Cyst

Prostatic utricle is a small diverticulum of the prostatic urethra located in verumontanum between the two openings of the ejaculatory ducts and extends backwards and slightly upwards for a short distance within the medial lobe of the prostate. The utricle is occasionally seen on routine VCUG as a tiny diverticulum

of few millimeters length. Large size prostatic utricle occasionally may be seen in normal males and in other conditions, e.g. Male hypospadias, Prune Belly syndrome and anorectal anomalies.

Mullerian duct cyst or cyst of the prostatic utricle is a cystic dilatation of an obstructed utricle occurring in patients with otherwise normal lower urinary tract. The obstruction could be due to congenital valves, mucosal folds, or local infection. The cysts vary in size from a few cm in diameter to a large pelvic mass, displacing the bladder upwards and forwards and sometimes obstructing the urethra. Stones may form in these cysts. The cysts may communicate with urethra by a minute tract. The cystic nature and location of the pelvic mass is readily determined by US, CT or MRI.

Cowper's Duct Cyst

Cowper's glands are paired structures located on either side of the membranous urethra within the urogenital diaphragm. Their ducts are directed forward through the bulb of the corpus spongiosum to end in the ventral aspect of the bulbar urethra. The ducts and the glands may sometimes be opacified during VCUG. Abnormalities of the Cowper's duct are uncommon. Syringoceles or cystic dilatation occurs most commonly in infants and young children secondary to narrowing of the duct orifice. Clinical findings include recurrent urinary tract infection and obstructive voiding symptoms. Rarely Cowper's duct cyst appears as a perineal mass. The dilated duct is seen on VCUG as a filling defect on the ventral surface of the bulbar urethra. Reflux of contrast material into a patulous or perforated syringocele opacifies the dilated duct.

Male Hypospadias/Epispadias

Hypospadias is a condition in which the urethral meatus opens on the ventral surface of the penis at a point proximal to the glans. In epispadias, in contradistinction, the urethral orifice is located on the dorsal aspect of the penis. Epispadias is usually seen in association with various forms of exstrophy. Epispadias in female is associated with a short patulous urethra, widely separated labia and a bifid clitoris. In either, hypospadias or epispadias, VCUG demonstrates a foreshortened urethra.

Anterior Urethral Diverticulum and Anterior Urethral Valve

Anterior urethral diverticulum, although uncommon, is the second most common cause of congenital urethral obstruction in boys. Anterior urethral diverticulum is a saccular outpouching of the ventral aspect of the anterior urethra commonly near penoscrotal junction. The diverticulum has a well defined valve like anterior lip and a less well defined posterior lip. The diverticulum fills during voiding, thereby narrowing and obstructing the true urethra. Complications resulting from the presence of diverticulum are incomplete bladder emptying and infection. On VCUG, the typical saccular diverticulum of the anterior urethra fills with contrast material and appears as an oval shaped structure on the ventral aspect of anterior urethra (Fig. 14.26). At times RGU may be required to demonstrate the neck of the diverticulum.

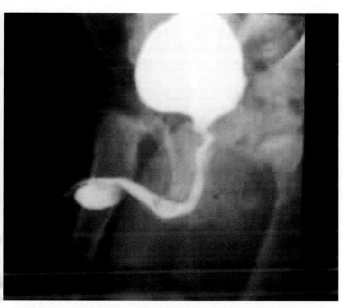

Fig. 14.26: Anterior urethral diverticulum: A large diverticulum is seen on the ventral aspect of the anterior urethra

Anterior urethral valve is a semilunar fold similar to anterior lip of a urethral diverticulum with absence of posterior lip. 40 percent of the anterior urethral valves are located in the bulbar urethra, 30 percent at the penoscrotal junction, and 30 percent in the pendulous urethra. VCUG is the diagnostic modality of choice for anterior urethral valves. Typically, the urethra appears dilated proximal to the valve and narrowed distal to it. A valve may appear as a linear filling defect along the ventral wall, or it may be indicated by an abrupt change in the caliber of the dilated urethra.

Urethral Duplication

Urethral duplication may be complete or incomplete and may take several forms. Two separate structures may originate from the bladder and persist with separate external drainage; a common urethra may originate from the bladder and duplicate distally; or a duplicated origin may unite distally into a single external orifice.[56] According, to the location of the accessory urethral opening on the dorsal or ventral aspect of the penis, urethral duplications are divided into epispadiac (more common) and hypospadiac types. The diagnosis is made by VCUG or catheterization and opacification of both the urethras.

Megalourethra

Megalourethra is a rare anomaly in which abnormal development of the corpus spongiosum and corpus cavernosum results in congenital dilatation of penile urethra without obstruction. On VCUG the penile urethra is seen markedly dilated and fusiform, with tapering both distally and proximally into a relatively normal urethra. Sometimes, the anomaly affects a small portion of the urethra. The anomaly may occur as an isolated lesion but is seen more commonly in prune belly syndrome.

Scaphoid megalourethra is more common than fusiform type. It consists of a localized saccular dilatation of the penile urethra caused by a localized absence of the corpus spongiosum. During voiding the affected part of urethra balloons markedly causing a large smooth bulge on the ventral surface of the urethra assuming a scaphoid configuration.[57]

Congenital Meatal Stenosis

Congenital meatal stenosis is a pin point narrowing of the urethral orifice and is seen in patients with hypospadias. Acquired meatal stenosis is more common than congenital stenosis. VCUG demonstrates dilatation of the urethra proximal to a narrowed meatal orifice. Radiologic evaluation of meatal stenosis, however, is usually not required.

REFERENCES

1. Steinhardt JM, Kuhn LP, Eisenberg B. Ultrasound screening of healthy infants for urinary tract abnormalities. Pediatrics 1988; 82:609-12.
2. Kraus SJ. Genitourinary Imaging in Children in Pediatric Urology. Pediatr Clin North Am 2001; 48:1381-424.
3. Johnson CE, Elder JS, Judge NE, et al. The accuracy of antenatal ultrasonography in identifying renal abnormalities. Am J Dis Child 1992; 146(10):1181-4.
4. Harvie S, McLeod L, Acott P, Walsh E, Abdolell M, Macken MB. Abnormal antenatal sonogram: An indicator of disease severity in children with posterior urethral valves. Can Assoc Radiol J 2009; 60(4):185-9.
5. Payabvash S, Kajbafzadeh AM, Saeedi P, Sadeghi Z, Elmi A, Mehdizadeh M. Application of magnetic resonance urography in diagnosis of congenital urogenital anomalies in children. Pediatr Surg Int 2008; 24(9):979-86.
6. Staatz G, Rohrmann D, Nolte-Ernsting CC, et al. Magnetic resonance urography in children: Evaluation of suspected ureteral ectopia in duplex systems. J Urol 2001; 166:2346-50.
7. Perez-Brayfield MR, Kirsch AJ, Jones RA, et al. A prospective study comparing ultrasound, nuclear scintigraphy and dynamic contrast enhanced magnetic resonance imaging in the evaluation of hydronephrosis. J Urol 2003; 170:1330-4.
8. Grattan-Smith JD, Jones RA. MR urography in children. Pediatr Radiol 2006; 36: 1119-32.
9. Grobner T. Gadolinium—a specific trigger for the development of nephrogenic fibrosing dermopathy and nephrogenic systemic fibrosis? Nephrol Dial Transplant 2006; 21:1104-8.
10. Brody AS, Frush DP, Huda W, et al. Radiation risk to children from computed tomography. Pediatrics 2007; 120:677-82.
11. Han BK, Babcock DS. Sonographic measurements and appearances of normal kidneys in children. AJR 1985; 145:611-16.
12. De Brugn R, Gordon I, Mc Hugh K: Pediatric Uroradiology. In Grainger RG, Allison D (Eds): Diagnostic Radiology: A Textbook of Medical Imaging. New York: Churchill Livingstone 2001; 1717-64.
13. Sadler TW (Ed). Langman's Medical Embryology, edn, 9. Philadelphia, PA, Lippincott Williams and Wilkins, 2004.
14. Trigaux JP, Van Beers B, Delchambre F. Male genital tract malformations associated with ipsilateral renal agenesis: Sonographic findings: J Clin Ultrasound 1991; 19:3-10.
15. Shalaby-Rana E, Lowe LH, Blask AN, et al. Imaging in pediatric urology. Pediatr Clin North Am 1997; 44:1065-89.
16. Jefferson KP, et al. Thoracic kidney; a rare form of renal ectopia. J Urol 2001; 165(2):502.
17. Pennington DJ, Zerin JM. Imaging of the urinary tract in children. Pediatr Ann 1999; 28:678-86.

18. Glodny B, Petersen J, Hofmann KJ, Schenk C, Herwig R, Trieb T, Koppelstaetter C, Steingruber I, Rehder P. Kidney fusion anomalies revisited: Clinical and radiological analysis of 209 cases of crossed fused ectopia and horseshoe kidney. BJU Int 2009; 103(2):224-35.

19. Gu LL, et al. Crossed solitary renal ectopia. Urology 1991; 38(6): 556-8.

20. Begin LR, Guy L, Jacobson SA, et al. Renal carcinoid and horseshoe kidney: A frequent association of the two rare entities– a case report and review of the literature. J Surg Oncol 1998; 68:113-9.

21. Strauss S. Sonographic features of horseshoe kidney: J ultrasound Med 2000; 19(1):27-31.

22. Pozniak MA, Nakada SY. Three-dimensional computed tomographic angiography of a horseshoe kidney with ureteropelvic junction obstruction. Urology 1997; 49(2):267-8.

23. El-Nahas AR, Abou El-Ghar ME, Refae HF, Gad HM, El-Diasty TA. Magnetic resonance imaging in the evaluation of pelvi-ureteric junction obstruction: An all-in-one approach. BJU Int 2007; 99(3):641-5.

24. Tokunaka S, Osanai H, Hashimoto H, et al. Severe hypertension in infant with unilateral hypoplastic kidney. Urology 1987; 29:618-20.

25. Osathanondh V, Potter EL. Pathogenesis of polycystic kidneys. Survey of results of microdissection. Arch Pathol 1964; 77:510-2.

26. Turkbey B, Ocak I, Daryanani K, Font-Montgomery E, Lukose L, Bryant J, Tuchman M, Mohan P, Heller T, Gahl WA, Choyke PL, Gunay-Aygun M. Autosomal recessive polycystic kidney disease and congenital hepatic fibrosis (ARPKD/CHF). Pediatr Radiol 2009; 39(2):100-11.

27. Traubici J, Daneman A. High-resolution renal sonography in children with autosomal recessive polycystic kidney disease. AJR Am J Roentgenol 2005; 184(5):1630-3.

28. Srivastava T, Garola RE, Hellerstein S. Autosomal dominant inheritance of multicystic dysplastic kidney. Pediatr Nephrol 1999; 13(6):481-3.

29. Kaneyama K, Yamataka A, Satake S, Yanai T, Lane GJ, Kaneko K, Yamashiro Y, Miyano T. Associated urologic anomalies in children with solitary kidney. J Pediatr Surg 2004; 39(1):85-7.

30. Eckoldt F, Woderich R, Smith RD, Heling KS. Antenatal diagnostic aspects of unilateral multicystic kidney dysplasia—sensitivity, specificity, predictive values, differential diagnoses, associated malformations and consequences. Fetal Diagn Ther 2004; 19(2):163-9.

31. Avni FE, Guissard G, Hall M, Janssen F, DeMaertelaer V, Rypens F. Hereditary polycystic kidney diseases in children: Changing sonographic patterns through childhood. Pediatr Radiol 2002; 32(3):169-74.

32. Talner LB. "Specific causes of obstruction". In Pollack HM (Ed): Clinical Urography. Philadelphia: WB Saunders Co 1990; 2:1629-751.

33. Park JM, Bloom DA. The pathophysiology of UPJ obstruction. Current concepts. Urol Clin North Am 1998; 25(2):161-9.

34. Khaira HS, Platt JF, Cohan RH, Wolf JS, Faerber GJ. Helical computed tomography for identification of crossing vessels in ureteropelvic junction obstruction-comparison with operative findings. Urology 2003; 62(1):35-9.

35. Beck AD. The effect of intrauterine urinary obstruction upon the development of fetal kidney. J Urol 1971; 105:784.

36. Platt JF, Rubin JM, Ellis JH, et al. Duplex Doppler US of the kidney-differentiation of obstructive from non-obstructive dilatation. Radiology 1989; 171:515-17.

37. Malleck R, Bankiee AA, Hainz E, et al. Distinction between obstructive and non-obstructive hydronephrosis: Value of diuresis duplex Doppler sonography. AJR 1996; 166:113.

38. Ramsey PG. Opacification of the renal parenchyma in obstruction and reflux. Paediatr Radiol 1976; 4:226.

39. Dunbar JS Nogardy MB. The calyceal crescent—a roentgenographic sign of obstructive hydronephrosis. AJR 1970; 110:520.

40. Stephens FD. Ureterovascular hydronephrosis and the "aberrant" renal vessels. J Urol 1982; 128:984.

41. Whitfield HN, Britton KE, Hendry WF, et al. Furosemide intravenous urography in the diagnosis of PUJ obstruction. Br J Urol 1985; 57:351.

42. Lebowitz RL, Blickman JG. The coexistence of ureteropelvic junction obstruction and reflux. AJR 1983; 140:231.

43. Lupton EW, Testa HJ, Lawsan RS, et al. Diuresis renography and the results of pyelplasty for idopathic hydronephrosis. Br J Urol 1979; 51:449.

44. Nussbaum AR, Dort JP, Jeffs RD, et al. Ectopic ureter and uterocoele: Their varied radiographic manifestations. Radiology 1986; 159:227-35.

45. Blickman JG, Lebowitz RL. The coexistence of primary megaureter and reflux. AJR 1984; 143:1053.

46. Dunetz GN, Bauer SB. Complete duplication of bladder and urethra. Urology 1985; 25:179-82.

47. Cohen HL, Kravets F, Zucconi W, Ratani R, Shah S, Dougherty D. Congenital abnormalities of the genitourinary system. Semin Roentgenol 2004; 39(2):282-303.

48. Bauer SB. Neurogenic bladder dysfunction. Paed Cli North America 1987; 34:1121-40.

49. Jennings RW. Prune Belly syndrome. Semin Paed Surg 2000; 9:115-20.

50. Suita S, Nagasaki A. Urachal remnants. Semin Paediat Surg 1996; 5:107-15.

51. Wendelin SH. The urinary bladder. In Davidson AJ, Hartman DS (Eds): Radiology of the Kidney and Urinary Tract Philadelphia: WB Saunders Co 1994; 607-48.

52. Chatterjee SK, Banerjee S, Basak D, et al. Posterior urethral valves: The scenario in a developing center. Paed Surg Int 2001; 17:2-7.

53. Cohen HL, Susman M, Haller JO, et al. Posterior urethral valve: Transperineal US for imaging and diagnosis in male infants. Radiology 1994; 192:261-4.

54. Eckoldt F, Heling KS, Woderich R, Wolke S. Posterior urethral valves: Prenatal diagnostic signs and outcome. Urol Int 2004; 73(4):296-301.

55. Silverman FN, Kuhn JP. Abnormalities of the lower urinary tract. Caffey's Paediatric X-ray Diagnosis: An Integrated Imaging Approach (9th ed). Mosby 1993; 1278-98.

56. Effman EL, Lebowitz RL, Colodny AH. Duplication of urethra. Radiology 1976; 119:179-85.

57. Kester RR, Woopan UM, Ohm HK. Congenital megalourethra. J Urol 1990; 4:1213-5.

CHAPTER 15

Urinary Tract Infections (including VUR and Neurogenic Bladder)

Kushaljit Singh Sodhi, Akshay Kumar Saxena

Urinary tract infection (UTI) is a common febrile illness in children. Although, most of these children recover with an excellent prognosis, a minority will still have long-term complications and sequelae, such as hypertension, chronic renal insufficiency, and end-stage renal failure. These potential complications are the basis for rapid appropriate investigations, prompt treatment, and subsequent customized follow-up of UTI in children.[1,2] Interventions, such as follow-up imaging, antibiotic prophylaxis, and surgical correction, are thought to reduce the incidence of the long-term complications.[3-5]

The urine culture is a critical component of the workup for a presumed UTI. The culture identifies the organism causing the infection and helps guide treatment with right antibiotics. The traditional definition for a clinically significant UTI is more than 100,000 cfu/mL.[3,4] However, lower numbers can also constitute a UTI because of additional factors (e.g. hydrational dilution and frequent voiding).[3,4]

Incidence

It has been estimated that 7 percent of girls and 2 percent of boys have a UTI prior to 6 years of age.[3,6] During the first year of life more boys than girls are diagnosed with a UTI, with uncircumcized boys having a 10-fold greater risk than those circumcized.[3,6] This trend reverses after the first year of life, with more girls than boys being diagnosed with a UTI.

Of children who have UTI, between 25 and 40 percent are found to have vesicoureteral reflux (VUR).[5,7] Of children who have febrile UTI, 50-91 percent are found to have defects on renal cortical scintigraphy, indicating acute pyelonephritis (APN).[5,8] However, when VUR is present, renal cortical abnormalities are shown by scintigraphy in 79-86 percent of the kidneys.[8]

Although, these statistics show that VUR is a precipitating factor in APN, studies[5,9] have also found that 61 percent of kidneys with evidence of APN on scintigraphy did not have VUR, and 53 percent of refluxing kidneys did not have any defect on scintigraphy to suggest APN. Therefore, VUR and APN frequently also occur independently of one another.[9,10]

Of children with APN diagnosed by scintigraphy, 38-57 percent will develop permanent renal scarring.[5,11,12] A recent study by Oh et al[13] found a correlation between the severity VUR grade and frequency of APN on renal scintigraphy; however, the likelihood of APN becoming permanent renal scarring was independent of the VUR grade.

Radiological Modalities for Imaging of UTI

Imaging may entail renal ultrasound (US) for the detection of congenital abnormalities, obstruction, and scarring; micturating cystourethrography (MCU) for the identification of vesicoureteric reflux; and ^{99m}Tc-labeled dimer captosuccinic acid (DMSA) renal scintigraphy for the determination of scarring. Depending on the clinical scenario, one or more of these examinations may be performed after a child's first episode of UTI; indeed, in many cases, all three investigations are performed.[1]

Role of Ultrasound in First Time UTI

Ultrasound has always been a part of the routine evaluation of first time UTI because it is very useful in depicting structural abnormalities such as asymmetric renal size, hydronephrosis, and duplex kidneys. Ultrasound is a noninvasive study which requires no sedation or ionizing radiation.

However, due to its low yield for additional clinical information, its role has been questioned in many recent articles. Zamir et al[14] found that ultrasound failed to alter clinical management in any of 255 first uncomplicated UTI patients. Many other studies raise concern that routine ultrasound for UTI may not be justifiable, given its somewhat negligible effect on patient management.

On the contrary, in a more recent study, Huang et al[15] found ultrasound abnormalities in 112 (28.7%) of 390 children with UTI residing in a country in which antenatal ultrasound is routinely performed. The abnormalities detected included asymmetric renal size, intermittent hydronephrosis, and duplicated collecting system. The presence of these findings correlated to a higher prevalence and grade of VUR. The authors concluded that routine ultrasound for UTI is worth performing.

Vesicoureteral Reflux

Vesicoureteral reflux (VUR) refers to the retrograde passage of urine from the bladder into the ureter and often to the calices. VUR can occur due to one of the following causes:[16,17]

- Abnormality of ureterovesical junction (UVJ).
- Marginally competent UVJ becoming incompetent due to urinary tract infection.
- Lateral ureteral ectopia.
- Abnormal bladder wall, e.g. Prune belly syndrome.
- Bladder outlet obstruction and neurogenic bladder.
- Reflux following interference of UVJ (iatrogenic).

As it is generally believed that VUR correlates to risk of renal scar development, pediatric patients with UTI undergo various imaging tests to detect vesicoureteral reflux.

Pathophysiology of VUR and Pyelonephritis

The distal most part of ureter traverses obliquely through the bladder wall into the ureteral orifice. Over a period of time, as the bladder distends with urine, increasing compression of the intramural and submucosal segment of ureter prevents retrograde flow of urine into the distal most ureter. However, the effectiveness of this particular valvular function is dependent on the length of the distal ureteral segment that lies within the bladder wall: a shorter intramural–submucosal segment increases the likelihood of VUR.[5] The normal length of the intramural–submucosal segment varies with age in children, is reported to range from 7 to 12 mm.[18] The objective of ureteral reimplantation surgery for VUR is to construct a more oblique ureteral course through the bladder wall, thus lengthening the intramural–submucosal segment.[5]

Pyelonephritis on the other hand, is usually caused by ascending bacterial infection in the urinary tract. VUR and urinary stasis predispose urine in the renal pelvis to infection. Bacteria are thus able to enter the renal parenchyma, leading to inflammation and edema. Subsequently, the parenchymal microvasculature becomes compressed, which can lead to ischemia, microabscess formation, and necrosis.[5] If the renal parenchyma is unable to recover from these injuries, permanent renal scarring with loss of parenchymal volume and function can also result. Renal cortical scintigraphy with ^{99m}Tc-dimercaptosuccinic acid (DMSA) is considered to be the imaging technique of choice to detect acute pyelonephritis and renal scarring because of its high sensitivity,[5,19] both entities appear as photopenic defects on DMSA scans, and the radiologist/nuclear physician has to rely on the clinical time course to distinguish between the two entities.

Imaging Findings in Acute Pyelonephritis

Urographic (Intravenous Urography-(IVU)) findings consist of diffuse renal enlargement, decreased patchy or striated nephrogram, delayed calyceal opacification and attenuation or effacement of the PCS. Renal US may be entirely normal or may show generalized or patchy decrease (rarely increase) in parenchymal echogenicity with decreased vascularity (Fig. 15.1). US is mainly performed for detection of associated abnormalities, e.g. calculi, obstructive uropathy or nephrocalcinosis.[20]

Renal cortical scintigraphy with ^{99m}Tc glucoheptonate (GH) or DMSA with a sensitivity of 91 percent and specificity of 99.9 percent, is the imaging procedure of choice for acute pyelonephritis.[21] Cortical scintigraphy demonstrates a pattern of

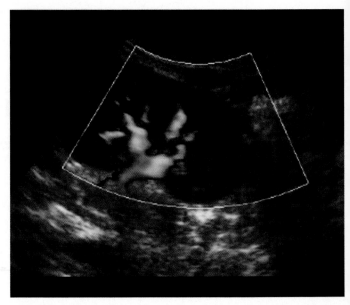

Fig. 15.1: Power Doppler ultrasound of kidney reveals a well defined area of altered echogenicity at lower pole, which demonstrates decreased flow and perfusion, corresponding to acute pyelonephritis (*For color version see plate 3*)

focally reduced or absent cortical accumulation of the radiopharmaceutical with no evidence of volume loss; the defects may be solitary, multiple, or involve the entire kidney giving rise to a mottled tracer distribution (Figs 15.2 and 15.3). On contrast-enhanced computed tomography (CECT) and contrast-enhanced magnetic resonance (CEMR), the affected kidney may show a striated nephrogram with multiple, poorly enhancing wedge shaped (rarely round and irregular) areas fanning out from the calyces, and reaching upto the cortex of the kidney (Fig. 15.4).

All children with acute pyelonephritis require US and DMSA scans in the acute phase; if the US is normal but the isotope scan is abnormal, follow-up scanning 3-6 months later is suggested, to detect whether the kidney has healed or scarred.[20,22]

Acute Focal Bacterial Nephritis

In this form of acute pyelonephritis, which is also called acute lobar nephronia, the inflammatory process is localized or segmental, often affecting a renal pole or one moiety of a duplex kidney. On renal ultrasound, the swollen part of the kidney appears as a hypoechoic poorly marginated mass with low-level echoes scattered throughout. Acute infection produces wedge-shaped areas with decreased perfusion on Doppler US.[23]

These are better shown with power Doppler.[20] However, Power Doppler US is not as sensitive for pyelonephritis as renal scintigraphy performed with DMSA. CECT shows poor and mottled enhancement of the area sometimes associated with wedge-shaped hypodense zones. In general, the renal mass is not sharply defined from rest of the kidney and lacks a well defined wall in contrast with a renal abscess which shows a relatively well defined wall which enhances on CECT. A decreased uptake of the tracer is seen on nuclear scintigraphy. IVU shows

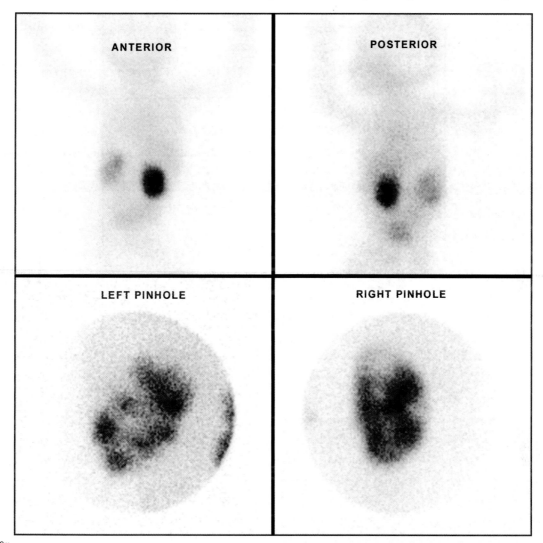

Fig. 15.2: ^{99m}Tc DMSA scan showing multiple photopenic areas in both kidneys, suggestive of pyelonephritis (*For color version see plate 4*)

localized enlargement of part of the kidney with focally reduced nephrographic density and is non-specific for pyelonephritis.

Grading of VUR

The accepted technique for reporting and grading VUR is the International Reflux Study Committee's classification for radiographic grades of reflux, which was suggested as a system to provide standardization of reporting technique.[24] The classification is shown below and should be used in radiology reports wherever possible so that effective communication between clinicians and radiologists takes place.

Grade I: Reflux to the ureter but not to the kidney.

Grade II: Reflux to the ureter, pelvis and calyces without dilatation.

Grade III: Reflux to the calyces with mild dilatation or tortuosity of the ureter, mild dilatation of renal pelvis and calyces, with normal or slightly blunted calyceal fornices.

Grade IV: Reflux into moderately dilated ureter and pelvicalyceal system with blunting of the fornices but preservation of papillary indentation.

Grade V: Reflux into grossly dilated ureter and pelvicalyceal system with loss of papillary indentation.

Imaging of VUR

1. Micturating cystourethrogram (MCU)
2. Radionuclide cystography (RNC)
3. Voiding urosonography (VUS)
4. MRI

Micturating Cystourethrogram (MCU)

Micturating cystourethrogram (MCU), also known as voiding cystourethrogram (VCUG) is one of the most commonly performed fluoroscopic investigations in pediatric radiology departments.[25] It is currently the investigation of choice for delineating the anatomy and determining the function of the lower urogenital tract.[25] It is the primary diagnostic procedure for evaluation of VUR in children. MCU should be used to document the presence of VUR and to determine the grade of reflux and whether reflux occurs during micturation or during bladder filling (Figs 15.5 and 15.6).

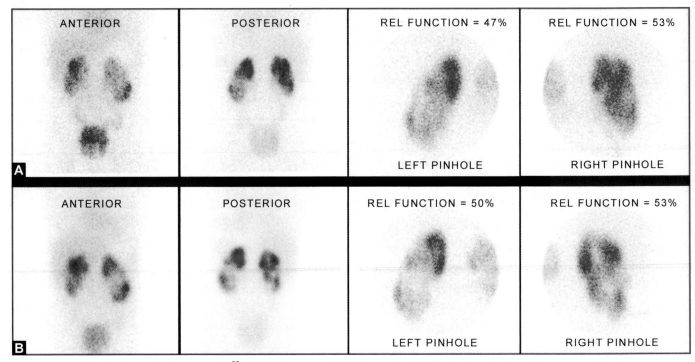

Figs 15.3A and B: Consecutive ⁹⁹ᵐTc DMSA scans in 2008 (A) and 2010 (B) showing persistent photopenic defects in both kidney cortices, indicative of renal scarring (*For color version see plate 4*)

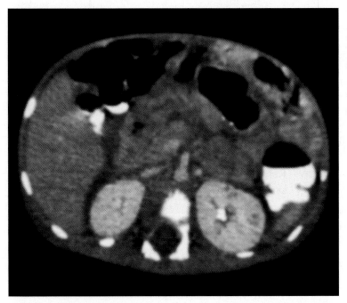

Fig. 15.4: CECT abdomen demonstrates well defined poorly enhancing areas of acute pyelonephritis in left kidney

A proper technique is essential for performing MCU. Catheterization should be performed using strict aseptic technique and contrast medium should be instilled via the gravity drip method and not by hand injection. This prevents the introduction of contrast medium under pressure and is less likely to cause transmucosal contrast medium absorption and consequent contrast reactions.[26]

Recommended views for MCU study[25] are:
1. Early filling view of bladder.
2. Full bladder view. The expected bladder capacity (in milliliters) for children less than 2 years of age is calculated using the formula (age+2)×30.[25,27]
3. Voiding urethra view. This should be obtained by turning boys in the right or left anterior oblique position. For girls supine position is obtained.
4. Renal view following voiding. To determine if any contrast medium has reached the kidneys (reflux).
5. Bladder view following voiding. This assesses the degree of bladder emptying. The majority of children under 1 year of age do not empty their bladder completely during a VCUG,[28] but a complete bladder emptying episode does help, exclude bladder neuropathy.

The last three images should be repeated as part of a cyclical voiding study.

Practice and Concept of Cyclical Voiding

It has been recommended that in order to increase the diagnostic yield of VUR in MCU examinations, cyclical voiding is required. Obtaining a second voiding cycle has been shown to increase the detection of VUR significantly.[25,29,30] The increased detection rate using cyclical voiding can be as high as 19.5 percent.[29] Grade 5 reflux has been detected on a second repeat cycle, where no VUR was seen on the first void.[29] Second-cycle voids can also increase the grade of reflux that was detected on the first void.[29,30] This is most important when grade 1 reflux is upgraded to grade 2 or above, since many clinicians will not treat grade 1 reflux alone.

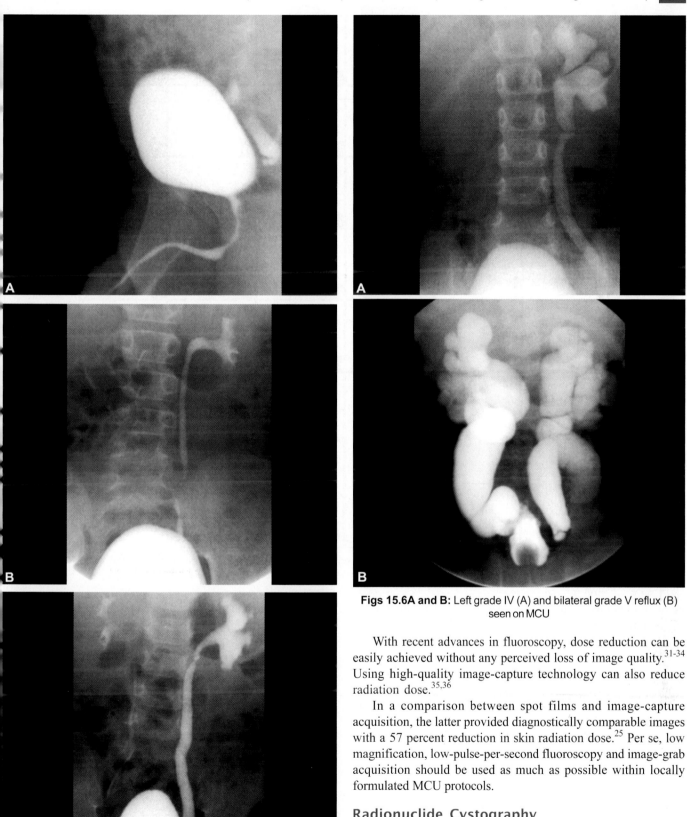

Figs 15.6A and B: Left grade IV (A) and bilateral grade V reflux (B) seen on MCU

Figs 15.5A to C: Grade I-III Vesico-ureteral reflux. MCU reveals left sided grade I reflux (A), grade II reflux (B) and grade III reflux (C)

With recent advances in fluoroscopy, dose reduction can be easily achieved without any perceived loss of image quality.[31-34] Using high-quality image-capture technology can also reduce radiation dose.[35,36]

In a comparison between spot films and image-capture acquisition, the latter provided diagnostically comparable images with a 57 percent reduction in skin radiation dose.[25] Per se, low magnification, low-pulse-per-second fluoroscopy and image-grab acquisition should be used as much as possible within locally formulated MCU protocols.

Radionuclide Cystography

Reflux can also be graded, with radionuclide cystography (Fig. 15.7). There are two types of radionuclide cystography: Direct and Indirect.

Indirect radionuclide cystography is performed by IV injection of a radiopharmaceutical such as [99m]Tc

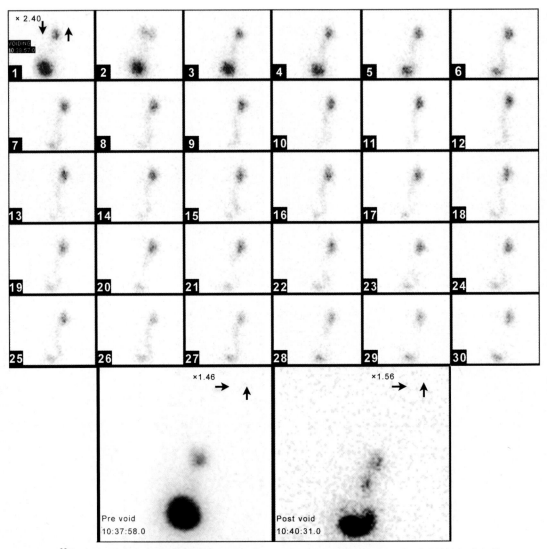

Fig. 15.7: ^{99m}Tc sulphur colloid DRCG: Retrograde movement of tracer is seen from the right kidney into the upper ureter, indicative of high grade right sided VU reflux (*For color version see plate 5*)

mercaptoacetyltriglycine (^{99m}Tc-MAG3) or ^{99m}Tc-diethylene-triaminepentaacetic acid (^{99m}Tc-DTPA) followed by dynamic imaging of the kidneys.[5] A time–activity curve will show a sudden rise in activity in the renal pelvis when VUR occurs. The main advantage of indirect RNC is that bladder catheterization is not required, although an IV catheter is needed.

The reported sensitivity of indirect RNC, is less than direct RNC, and ranges between 22 percent and 51 percent.[5,37] If indirect RNC is to be performed, it should be restricted to patients in whom bladder catheterization is impossible. To maximize sensitivity, patients should be toilet-trained.

The radionuclide cystogram has traditionally had approximately 1/100th of the radiation exposure of a standard MCU.[3] Further, because imaging is continuous with a direct radionuclide cystogram (versus intermittent with fluoroscopy), it seems to be more sensitive in determining reflux than a traditional contrast VCUG.[3,38,39] Fluoroscopic MCU is more accurate at grading reflux, however, and can show spinal abnormalities,

bladder and urethral anatomy, periureteral diverticula, and other upper tract detail that cannot be identified with radionuclide cystography.[3,4]

The commonly accepted practice is to perform MCU as the initial test for the presence and severity of VUR as well as any anatomic abnormalities. RNC is typically used at follow-up to determine if VUR subsequently persists or resolves, especially after antireflux surgery and in girls with first-time UTI because urethral pathology is far less common in girls or when there is a low clinical suspicion of VUR.[40] The sensitivity of RNC has been found to be equal to or slightly higher than that of MCU.[38,41,42] Some studies have found that VCUG is more likely to miss reflux due to its noncontinuous imaging and that RNC is more likely to miss grade I reflux because of its poor anatomic detail.[39,42]

The gonadal radiation dose in RNC has been reported in the range of 10–20 µGy.[5,43] A tailored, low-dose fluoroscopy technique using "last–frame grabber" technology can potentially result in a VCUG gonadal dose as low as 17–52 µGy.[5,44] As stated above, the use of modern variable-rate pulsed fluoroscopy reduces effective radiation dose by eightfold compared with older continuous fluoroscopy machines; however, the effective dose of VCUG performed with this technique is still ten-fold higher than that received during RNC.[45]

To summarize, nuclear cystography has an advantage due to the lower radiation dosage, which makes it an excellent tool for screening female patients and for follow-up of patients of both sexes. The disadvantages are difficulty in recognizing important anatomical details, i.e, associated bladder disease, e.g. bladder diverticula and male urethra.

Ultrasound in VUR

Echoenhanced cystosonography has now emerged as a promising new method for detecting and grading VUR without exposing patients to ionizing radiation.

Recent studies[46] have shown that ureteral dilatation has the best diagnostic accuracy for the ultrasound based diagnosis of both all-grade and high-grade VUR (compared with pelvic dilatation, renal length, urinary tract dilatation, and corticomedulary differentiation) with 73 percent sensitivity and 88 percent specificity for the detection of high grade VUR.

In voiding urosonography (VUS) intravesical administration of US contrast agent (USCA) is performed for the diagnosis of vesicoureteric reflux (VUR).[47] Many institutions now recognize VUS as a practical, safe, radiation-free modality with comparable or higher sensitivity than direct radionuclide cystography (DRNC) and voiding cystourethrography (VCUG), respectively.

The basic procedural steps of VUS are:
1. US of the kidneys and bladder.
2. Bladder catheterization and intravesical administration of normal saline and USCA.
3. Repeat scan of the bladder and kidneys during and after bladder filling and finally all through voiding.[47,48]

Reflux is ranked in grades 1–5 similar to that for VCUG. The most commonly used USCAs are first generation ultrasound contrast agent, Levovist (Bayer-Schering Pharma, Berlin, Germany) and second generation ultrasound contrast agent SonoVue (Bracco, Milan, Italy).[47,48] Harmonic Imaging (HI) improves the detection of microbubbles and increases the sensitivity of VUS.[47]

Micturating Cystourethrogram versus Voiding Urosonography

The largest comparative study between VCUG and VUS with the intravesical administration of the second generation USCA SonoVue, published to date, is by Papadopoulou et al.[49] It comprises a total of 228 children, 123 boys and 105 girls, 6 days to 13 years old, with a total of 463 pelvi-ureteral-units (PUUs). SonoVue was administered at a dose of 1 ml/bladder filling. In 161 (35%), PUUs reflux was detected by one or both methods. In 90 (56%), PUUs reflux was detected only by VUS and in 14 (9%), PUUs only by VCUG. This implies a 47 percent higher reflux detection rate for SonoVue-enhanced VUS compared to VCUG,

which is almost 1.5-times higher than the highest reported rate for Levovist-enhanced VUS.[48] Concordance of VUS and VCUG was 78 percent. More importantly refluxes missed by VCUG were of higher grades (2 grade 1, 65 grade II, 19 grade III, 4 grade IV) compared to those missed by VUS (8 grade I, 5 grade II, 1 grade III). When VCUG was used as the reference method, the sensitivity of VUS was 80 percent. When all refluxing PUUs in either method were considered as true positive, sensitivity of VUS and VCUG was 92 and 64 percent, respectively. These results emphasize that as VUS with a second generation USCA is a safe modality with a much higher sensitivity, it has the potential to become the study of choice in future.

Eva K et al[50] also evaluated the sensitivity of VUS using a second generation ultrasound (US) contrast agent and compared it with standard fluoroscopic voiding cystourethrography (VCUG) in a study group comprising 183 children. VUR was detected in 140 out of 366 cases (38%); in 89 (24.3%) by both methods, in 37 (10.1%) by VUS only, and in 14 (3.8%) by VCUG only. Although, there was considerable agreement in the diagnosis of VUR by VUS and VCUG ($\kappa = 0.68$, standard error [κ] = 0.04), the difference in the detection rate of reflux between VUS and VCUG was significant ($p < 0.00001$). Their findings also suggest that contrast enhanced harmonic VUS using a second generation contrast agent is superior to VCUG in the detection and grading of VUR, and it should be the method of choice in UTI.

Most of the publications on VUS are from Europe.[47,48] Limited availability of these contrast agents, however limits its wider use. However, this is a very promising investigation and has the potential to change the conventional management algorithm of VUR.

Role of MRI in UTI Imaging

Although, MR urography has yielded very promising results in obstructive uropathy, its role in MR cystography is yet to be established. Few recently published articles on direct and indirect MR cystography techniques have shown technical feasibility details,[51,52] however, there have been no studies comparing it with VCUG.

MRI with its great anatomical detail can help in detection of pyelonephritis and scarring. Many studies have established superior or atleast similar sensitivity of MRI to DMSA scintigraphy, in acute pyelonephritis and scarring. It also offers additional advantage of being a radiation free modality and provides structural detail even in children with poor renal function.

Guidelines for Imaging in UTI: From History to Current Perspective

First set of guidelines were published by Royal college of physicians (RCP) in 1991 for imaging of UTI in children.[53,54] It was recommended that every child between 0 and 7 years of age with first UTI should have an ultrasound and DMSA scan. Children who are in first year of life should also have a Micturating Cystourography (MCU). These guidelines obviously led to huge burden on radiology departments.

Subsequent to this, practice parameters were established by the American Academy of Pediatrics (AAP) in 1999,which guided physicians in the evaluation of UTI in infants and children.[55,56] Their recommendations for imaging workup were broad, advocating ultrasound and voiding cystourethrography (VCUG) or radionuclide cystography (RNC) in all infants and young children (< 2 years old) with UTI. The American Academy of Family Physicians suggested performing DMSA scanning after treatment of UTI to evaluate for permanent renal scarring.[56] This imaging algorithm and its variants have been described as the "bottom-up" approach because the initial diagnostic concern is detection of VUR. Once VUR is diagnosed, the patient is presumed to be at increased risk for renal scarring, and DMSA scanning is performed several months later to detect any permanent renal scarring.

Since, the 1999 recommendations, physician's experience in managing pediatric UTI and published scientific data has expanded. As a result, there has been a gradual drift away from the AAP guidelines, resulting in several imaging algorithms that can differ among various physicians, practice groups, cities, countries, and continents. One recent survey by Shah et al[57] showed only a 61 percent adherence rate to the AAP imaging guidelines.

Another evolution in practice guidelines is now seen in the 2007 European Society of Pediatric Radiology recommendations.[58] This algorithm advocates ultrasound examination of all pediatric UTI patients, and if the ultrasound is normal and there is clinical suspicion for APN, early DMSA scanning is performed at the time of the acute infection. If the DMSA scan shows evidence of APN, then VCUG or RNC is performed later to evaluate for VUR.[5] Normal findings on DMSA scanning obviate subsequent VCUG or RNC.[59,60]

This reversal in the sequence of DMSA scanning and cystography has been referred to as the "top-down" approach by Lim et al because the initial diagnostic concern is now that of APN, not VUR.[5] The rationale behind most of these recent guidelines is that only 47 percent of VUR is severe enough to cause APN.[5,9] Therefore, it may not be worthwhile to diagnose and treat all cases of mild VUR. Conversely, 61 percent of APN occurs in children who do not have reflux;[5,9] using the presence of VUR as the criterion to decide which patients will undergo continued follow-up results in great potential to underdiagnose APN in children without reflux.

To prevent serious long-term sequelae such as hypertension and renal failure, it is now believed that the critical clinical goal is the early recognition of infants and children who are at risk of permanent renal scarring. Detection of APN using DMSA renal scintigraphy may be a more sensitive and appropriate screening tool than VCUG or RNC to determine who is at risk for renal scarring.[5]

DMSA for Renal Scar: When is the best time to scan?

There is no consensus amongst the physicians and radiologists on what is the best time to perform DMSA scan for renal scarring.It is vital as the affected patients would need appropriate urinanalysis,interval renal imaging, hypertensive check ups and follow-ups. In their consensus report, Piepsz et al[61] found that there is no consensus: 42 percent of experts perform DMSA scanning at 3 months, 33 percent at 6 months, and 15 percent at 12 months after the acute UTI. Agras et al.,[62] have demonstrated in a group of 37 children with DMSA scintigraphic defects, 13 (38.2%) had persistent defects at 6 months but only six (17.6%) showed defects at 12 months after acute UTI. This study suggests a high rate of continuing resolution of pyelonephritis even beyond 6 months after infection and that a 12–month time interval is more reliable for determining the presence of permanent renal scarring.

Treatment Guidelines for Reflux

The significance of reflux deals with the issue of recurrent pyelonephritis and potentially renal scarring. A common dilemma has been the decision to treat or not to treat a particular child. Traditional therapy has included long-term prophylactic antibiotic treatment, to prevent infections alongside observation, in anticipation of the child outgrowing the reflux.[3]

High spontaneous resolution rates have been obtained, especially for lower grades of reflux, but admittedly with the cost of long-term use of antimicrobials and repeated imaging with MCUs. Surgical intervention has traditionally been reserved for those children who have noncompliance with medical therapy, or nonresolution of VUR, febrile breakthrough UTIs, and progression of renal scarring, after prolonged follow-up.[3]

Bauer et al in their review article on UTI,[3] have described results of a recent metaanalysis of ten trials, involving 964 children, which compared long-term antibiotics and surgical correction of VUR with antibiotics (seven trials); antibiotics with no treatment (one trial);and different materials for endoscopic correction of VUR (two trials). Risk of UTI by 1 to 2 and 5 years was not significantly different between surgical and medical groups. Surgical treatment did result in a 60 percent reduction in febrile UTI by 5 years but no concomitant significant reduction in risk of new or progressive renal damage at 5 years.

American Urological Association has convened the Pediatric Vesicoureteral Reflux Guidelines Panel to make a set of guidelines to determine when to treat reflux medically versus surgically.[63] As is evident from the recommendations, surgery is recommended for higher grades of reflux. Different surgical treatment options are available to these children. The standard surgical care has always been open surgical repair (e.g. ureteral reimplantation). After various attempts made to minimize the morbidity, extravesical approach has been proposed. Success rates for surgical techniques are 98 percent for curing reflux. These surgical developments, combined with a new general tendency to avoid overuse of antibiotics, have resulted in a drift toward earlier surgery. This has been emphasized even more by the use of laparoscopic techniques in many centers.[64] In endoscopic treatment of reflux, however, success rates of 70-90 percent for curing reflux have been reported and VCUGs remain essential for endoscopic treatment. It is important to remember that not all VUR

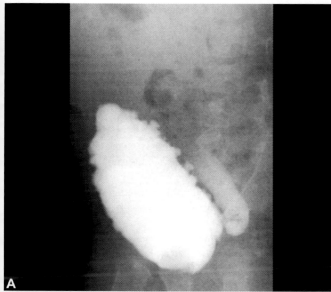

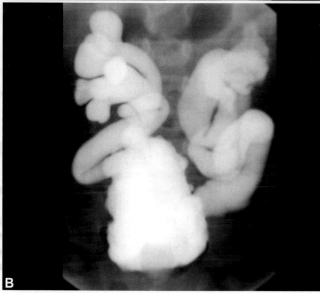

Figs 15.8A and B: Neurogenic bladder: MCU shows an elongated bladder with trabeculations and sacculations with grade I VUR (A) MCU in another patient showing neurogenic bladder with grade V VUR (B)

needs intervention, and treatment does not always prevent complications.[65]

Neurogenic Bladder

In contrast to adult patient in whom neurogenic bladder is most often due to an acquired, usually traumatic spinal cord lesion, the vast majority of children affected with this disorder have a myelomeningocele or a related myelodysplastic anomaly (occult spinal dysraphism, sacral agenesis).

Myelomeningocele can occur at any level of the spine but is most often located in the lumbosacral area. The radiographs of the affected area show widening of the neural canal, defective posterior neural arches, absence of the posterior spinous processes, and widened interpedicular distance involving several segments, with elongated and flattened or defective pedicles.[16]

Occult myelodysplasia is a group of congenital anomalies of the spinal cord in which the overlying skin is intact although cutaneous stigmata of the disorder may be present such as, local hair overgrowth, hyperpigmentation, hemangioma, a skin dimple, or an ill-defined soft tissue mass due to a lipoma. These anomalies include tethered cord, diastematomyelia, intraspinal lipoma, dermoid cyst, and hamartoma. Radiographs of the spine may show osseous changes similar to those seen in myelomeningocele, and sometimes scoliosis or broad vertebral bodies.

Children with this disorder commonly have inappropriate detrusor muscle contraction and external sphincter relaxation, resulting in uncontrolled voiding pattern with incomplete bladder emptying.[16,66] Initially, the upper tracts are normal but due to poor bladder emptying secondary changes of reflux and infection result.

Complete evaluation of patients suspected of having neurogenic bladder requires MCU for assessment of lower urinary tract, US and one of the functional studies of IVU or scintigraphy for upper tract. However, for the diagnosis of primary cause, examination with plain radiographs and MRI is essential. In case of nonavailability of MRI, myelography with nonionic contrast followed by CT is mandatory.

On MCU, bladder is usually elongated, pointing upwards (Christmas tree shape) with varying degrees of trabeculation and sacculation (Figs 15.8A and B). Rarely bladder may be large, smooth, atonic type. During voiding, bladder neck and proximal posterior urethra are dilated forming a funnel shape with the point of the funnel directed caudally at midposterior urethra level. Distal urinary stream is usually poor with significant post void residual urine. Associated vesicoureteral reflux is common.[16] Urodynamic techniques have assumed a major role in the evaluation of neurogenic bladder and contributed significantly to the management.

Acknowledgments

We wish to thank Dr Anish Bhattacharya, Associate Professor, and Dr B.R. Mittal, Prof and Head, Department of Nuclear medicine, for their kind help and support in providing images of ^{99m}Tc DMSA scans and ^{99m}Tc sulphur colloid DRCG scans.

REFERENCES

1. Luk WH, Woo YH, San Au-Yeung AW and Chan JCS . Imaging in Pediatric Urinary Tract Infection: A 9-Year Local Experience. AJR 2009; 192:1253-60.
2. Larcombe J. Urinary tract infection in children: Clinical evidence. BMJ 1999; 319:1173-5.
3. Bauer R, Kogan BA. New Developments in the Diagnosis and Management of Pediatric UTIs. Urol Clin N Am 2008; 35:47-58.
4. Linda S. Urinary tract infections in infants and children. In: Walsh P, (Ed). 8th edn. Campbell's urology, vol. 3. Baltimore (MD): Saunders 2002; p. 1846-84.
5. Lim R .Vesicoureteral Reflux and Urinary Tract Infection: Evolving Practices and Current Controversies in Pediatric Imaging. AJR 2009; 192:1197-208.
6. Marild S, Jodal U. Incidence rate of first-time symptomatic urinary tract infection in children under 6 years of age. Acta Pediatr 1998; 87:549–52.

7. Cleper R, Krause I, Eisenstein B, Davidovits M. Prevalence of vesicoureteral reflux in neonatal urinary tract infection. Clin Pediatr (Phila) 2004; 43:619-25.

8. Rushton HG, Majd M. Dimercaptosuccinic acid renal scintigraphy for the evaluation of pyelonephritis and scarring: A review of experimental and clinical studies. J Urol 1992; 148:1726-32.

9. Ditchfield MR, De Campo JF, Cook DJ, et al. Vesicoureteral reflux: An accurate predictor of acute pyelonephritis in childhood urinary tract infection? Radiology 1994; 190:413-5.

10. Sastre JB, Aparicio AR, Cotallo GD, Colomer BF, Hernandez MC. Urinary tract infection in the newborn: Clinical and radio imaging studies. Pediatr Nephrol 2007; 22:1735-41.

11. Lin KY, Chiu NT, Chen MJ, et al. Acute pyelonephritis and sequelae of renal scar in pediatric first febrile urinary tract infection. Pediatr Nephrol 2003; 18:362-5.

12. Zaki M, Badawi M, Al Mutari G, Ramadan D, Adul Rahman M. Acute pyelonephritis and renal scarring in Kuwaiti children: A follow-up study using ^{99m}Tc DMSA renal scintigraphy. Pediatr Nephrol 2005; 20:1116-9.

13. Oh MM, Jin MH, Bae JH, Park HS, Lee JG. Moon du G. The role of vesicoureteral reflux in acute renal cortical scintigraphic lesion and ultimate scar formation. J Urol 2008; 180:2167-70.

14. Zamir G, Sakran W, Horowitz Y, Koren A, Miron D. Urinary tract infection: Is there a need for routine renal ultrasonography? Arch Dis Child 2004; 89:466-8.

15. Huang HP, Lai YC, Tsai IJ, Chen SY, Tsau YK. Renal ultrasonography should be done routinely in children with first urinary tract infections. Urology 2008; 71:439-43.

16. Vashist S. Radiology of lower Urinary tract; In Diagnostic Radiology. Pediatric Imaging 2nd edn, Jaypee Brothers 2004; 11:208-22.

17. Alon U, Berant M, Pery M. Intravenous pyelography in children with urinary tract infection and vesicoureteral reflux. Pediatrics 1989; 83:332-7.

18. Cussen LJ. Dimensions of the normal ureter in infancy and childhood. Invest Urol 1967; 5:164-78.

19. Ataei N, Madani A, Habibi R, Khorasani M. Evaluation of acute pyelonephritis with DMSA scans in children presenting after the age of 5 years. Pediatr Nephrol 2005; 20:1439-44.

20. Sandhu MS, Lal A. Pediatric Kidney: Medical Conditions. Radiology of lower Urinary tract;9; 160-181 in Diagnostic Radiology. Pediatric Imaging 2nd edn, Jaypee Brothers, 2004.

21. Jakobson B, Soderlungh S, Berg U. Diagnostic significance of ^{99m}Tc-DMSA scintigraphy in urinary tract infection. Arch Dis Child 1992; 67:1338-42.

22. Lebowitz RL, Mandell J. Urinary tract infection in children: Putting radiology in its place. Radiology 1987; 165:1-9.

23. Dubbins PA. The kidney. In Allen PL, Dubbins PA, Pozniak MA and McDicken WN (Eds): Clinical Doppler ultrasound. New York. Churchil livingstone 2000; 169-90.

24. International Reflux Study Committee (1981): Medical versus surgical treatment of primary vesicoureteral reflux: A prospective international reflux study in children. J Urol 1981; 125:277-83.

25. Agrawalla S, Pearce R, Goodman TR. How to perform the perfect voiding cystourethrogram. Pediatr Radiol 2004; 34:114-9.

26. Weese DL, Greenberg HM, Zimmern PE. Contrast media reactions during voiding cystourethrography or retrograde pyelography. Urology 1993; 41:81-3.

27. Kaefer M, Zurakowski D, Bauer SB, et al. Estimating normal bladder capacity in children. J Urol 1997; 158:2261-4.

28. Sillen U. Bladder function in healthy neonates and its development during infancy. Urology 2001; 166:2376-81.

29. Papadopoulou F, Efremidis SC, Economou A, et al. Cyclic voiding cystourethrography: Is vesicoureteral reflux missed with standard voiding cystourethrography? Eur Radiol 2002; 12:666-70.

30. Paltiel HJ, Rupich RC, Kiruluta HC. Enhanced detection of vesicoureteral reflux in infants and children with use of cyclic voiding cystourethrography. Radiology 1992; 184:753-5.

31. Boland GW, Murphy B, Arellano R, et al. Dose reduction in Gastrointestinal and genitourinary fluoroscopy: Use of grid-controlled pulsed fluoroscopy. AJR Am J Roentgenol 2000; 175:1453-7.

32. Hernandez RJ, Goodsitt MM. Reduction of radiation dose in pediatric patients using pulsed fluoroscopy. AJR Am J Roentgenol 1996; 167:1247-53.

33. Lederman HM, Khademian ZP, Felice M, et al. Dose reduction fluoroscopy in pediatrics. Pediatr Radiol 2002; 32:844-8.

34. Brown PH, Silberberg PJ, Thomas RD, et al. A multihospital survey of radiation exposure and image quality in pediatric fluoroscopy. Pediatr Radiol 2000; 30:236-42.

35. Bazopoulos EV, Prassopoulos PK, Damilakis JE, et al. A comparison between digital fluoroscopic hard copies and 105 mm spot films in evaluating vesicoureteric reflux in children. Pediatr Radiol 1998; 28:162-6.

36. Diamond DA, Kleinman PK, Spevak M, et al. The tailored low dose fluoroscopic voiding cystogram for familial reflux screening. J Urol 1996; 155:681-2.

37. De Sadeleer C, De Boe V, Keuppens F, Desprechins B, Verboven M, Piepsz A. How good is technetium-99m mercaptoacetyltriglycine indirect cystography? Eur J Nucl Med 1994; 21:223-7.

38. Unver T, Alpay H, Biyikli NK, Ones T. Comparison of direct radionuclide cystography and voiding cystourethrography in detecting vesicoureteral reflux. Pediatr Int 2006; 48:287-91.

39. McLaren CJ, Simpson ET. Direct comparison of radiology and nuclear medicine cystograms in young infants with vesico-ureteric reflux. BJU Int 2001; 87:93-7.

40. Lebowitz RL. The detection and characterization of vesicoureteral reflux in the child. J Urol 1992; 148:1640-2.

41. Sukan A, Bayazit AK, Kibar M, et al. Comparison of direct radionuclide cystography and voiding direct cystography in the detection of vesicoureteral reflux. Ann Nucl Med 2003; 17:549-53.

42. Saraga M, Stanicic A, Markovic V. The role of direct radionuclide cystography in evaluation of vesicoureteral reflux. Scand J Urol Nephrol 1996; 30:367-71.

43. Van den Abbeele AD, Treves ST, Lebowitz RL, et al. Vesicoureteral reflux in asymptomatic siblings of patients with known reflux: Radionuclide cystography. Pediatrics 1987; 79:147-53.

44. Kleinman PK, Diamond DA, Karellas A, Spevak MR, Nimkin K, Belanger P. Tailored low-dose fluoroscopic voiding cystourethrography for the reevaluation of vesicoureteral reflux in girls. AJR 1994; 162:1151-4; discussion 1155-6.

45. Ward VL, Strauss KJ, Barnewolt CE, et al. Pediatric radiation exposure and effective dose reduction during voiding cystourethrography. Radiology 2008; 249:1002-9.

46. Leroy S, Vantalon S, Larakeb A, Ducou-Le-Pointe H and Bensman A. Vesicoutertral reflux in children with urinary tarct infection: Comparison of Diagnostic Accuracy of Renal US criteria. Radiology 2010; 255:890-8.

47. Darge K. Voiding urosonography with US contrast agent for the diagnosis of vesicoureteric reflux in children: An update Pediatr Radiol 2010; 40:956-62.

48. Darge K. Voiding urosonography with ultrasound contrast agents for the diagnosis of vesicoureteric reflux in children. Pediatr Radiol 2008; 38:40-53.

49. Papadopoulou F, Anthopoulou A, Siomou E, et al. Harmonic voiding urosonography with a second generation contrast agent for the diagnosis of vesicoureteral reflux. Pediatr Radiol 2009; 39:239-44.

50. Éva K, Nyitrai A,Várkonyi I, et al. Voiding urosonography with second generation contrast agent versus voiding cystourethrography. Pediatr Nephrol 2010; 25:2289-93.

51. Teh HS, Gan JS, Ng FC. Magnetic resonance cystography: Novel imaging technique for evaluation of vesicoureteral reflux. Urology 2005; 65:793-4.

52. Takazakura R, Johnin K, Furukawa A, et al. Magnetic resonance voiding cystourethrography for vesicoureteral reflux. J Magn Reson Imaging 2007; 25:170-4.

53. [No authors listed]. Guidelines for the management of acute urinary tract infection in childhood. Report of a Working Group of the Research Unit, Royal College of Physicians. J R Coll Physicians Lond 1991; 25:36-42.

54. Biassoni L, Chippington S. Imaging in Urinary tract Infections: Current Strategies and New Trends. Seminars in Nucl Medicine 2008; 38:56-66.

55. [No authors listed]. Practice parameter: The diagnosis, treatment, and evaluation of the initial urinary tract infection in febrile infants and young children. American Academy of Pediatrics. Committee on Quality Improvement. Subcommittee on Urinary Tract Infection. Pediatrics 1999; 103:843-52.

56. Ross JH, Kay R. Pediatric urinary tract infection and reflux. Am Fam Physician 1999; 59:1472-8, 1485-6.

57. Shah L, Mandlik N, Kumar P, Andaya S, Patamasucon P. Adherence to AAP practice guidelines for urinary tract infections at our teaching institution. Clin Pediatr (Phila) 2008; 47:861-4.

58. Riccabona M, Avni FE, Blickman JG, et al. Imaging recommendations in pediatric uroradiology: Minutes of the ESPR workgroup session on urinary tract infection, fetal hydronephrosis,urinary tract ultrasonography and voiding cystourethrography. Barcelona, Spain, June 2007. Pediatr Radiol 2008; 38:138-45.

59. Preda I, Jodal U, Sixt R, Stokland E, Hansson S. Normal dimercapto-succinic acid scintigraphy makes voiding cystourethrography unnecessary after urinary tract infection. J Pediatr 2007; 151:581-4.

60. Tseng MH, Lin WJ, Lo WT, Wang SR, Chu ML, Wang CC. Does a normal DMSA obviate the performance of voiding cystourethro-graphy in evaluation of young children after their first urinary tract infection? J Pediatr 2007; 150:96-9.

61. Piepsz A, Blaufox MD, Gordon I, et al. Consensus on renal cortical scintigraphy in children with urinary tract infection: Scientific Committee of Radionuclides in Nephrourology. Semin Nucl Med 1999; 29:160-74.

62. Agras K, Ortapamuk H, Naldoken S, Tuncel A, Atan A. Resolution of cortical lesions on serial renal scans in children with acute pyelonephritis. Pediatr Radiol 2007; 37:153-8.

63. Elder JS, Peters CA, Arant B Jr, et al. Pediatric vesicoureteral reflux guidelines panel summary reporton the management of primary vesicoureteral reflux in children. J Urol 1997; 157:1846-51.

64. Yeung CK, Sihoe JD, Tam YH, et al. Laparoscopic excision of prostatic utricles in children. BJU Int 2001; 87:505-8.

65. Lorenzo AJ, Khoury AE. Endoscopic treatment of reflux: Management pros and cons. Curr Opin Urol 2006; 16:299-304.

66. Bauer SB. Neurogenic Bladder dysfunction. Paed Cli North America 1987; 34:1121-40.

CHAPTER 16

Renal and Retroperitoneal Masses

Anju Garg

The retroperitoneum is a potential space that extends along the posterior most aspect of the abdominal cavity from the level of the diaphragm to the pelvic brim. Masses in this space can arise from the kidneys, adrenal glands, lymph nodes, lymphatic channels, sympathetic ganglia or other neural tissue and iliopsoas muscle. As symptoms of retroperitoneal disease are non-specific and physical examination is difficult, retroperitoneal masses grow quite large before they are detected.

IMAGING

The multitude of diagnostic imaging modalities available for evaluation of abdominal masses in infants and children requires a logical and analytical approach to avoid unnecessary expense, radiation and potential morbidity. Ultrasound (US) is the most frequently selected first imaging modality on the basis of availability, ease of performance (as there is no need for intravenous contrast or patient sedation), low cost and absence of radiation exposure. The highest possible frequency probes should be used to maximize resolution. Color Doppler enables characterization of tumor vascularization and assessment of vascular invasion. US has a high diagnostic efficacy for common pediatric abdominal masses and in many cases it may give a complete diagnosis obviating the need for any further investigation. If the US examination is technically limited because of excessive bowel gas or body habitus, or if the mass is incompletely evaluated by US or thought to be neoplastic, computed tomography or magnetic resonance imaging can be done. In the case of a suspected neoplasm, these modalities further refine the differential diagnosis, define the local and regional extent of the mass and detect metastases.

Computed tomography (CT) is an extremely accurate and fast imaging modality, displaying high quality cross sectional images. Multidetector CT allows excellent reconstructions in planes other than the original scanning plane. Isotropic multiplanar reconstructions (MPRs) of thin overlapping slices in the coronal and sagittal plane provide excellent delineation of the location and extent of retroperitoneal masses. The use of pre- and post-contrast scanning should be minimized in children; the use of oral contrast is helpful in distinguishing bowel from nodal disease. Short sedation may be required, especially in younger children. A relative disadvantage of CT is the radiation exposure. Chest CT may be required in cases of suspected neoplasms to evaluate presence of lung metastases.

The advantages of *magnetic resonance imaging (MRI)* include its unique ability to directly acquire multiplanar images, superior contrast resolution and lack of ionising radiation. Its major disadvantages are cost, limited availability and need for sedation. Faster scanners and newer imaging sequences currently allow accurate lesion characterisation in a reasonably short scanning time. Typical sequences used are pre-contrast T1- and T2-weighted gradient echo sequences and post contrast fat suppressed T1-weighted images. Images should be obtained in at least two orthogonal planes to permit direct evaluation of extent of retroperitoneal disease.

Conventional abdominal radiographs infrequently provide a definite diagnosis for a suspected abdominal mass but can suggest a mimicking process such as constipation and fecal retention or a distended urinary bladder. The nature of an abdominal mass can sometimes be inferred on abdominal radiographs by the presence or absence of calcification in the mass and the location of the mass as indicated by the pattern of bowel displacement and other signs of mass effect.

With the availability of cross-sectional imaging modalities like US, CT and MRI, *intravenous urography* has a very limited role to play in the evaluation of suspected cases of retroperitoneal or even renal masses as it provides only indirect evidence of the mass.

The first step in evaluating these masses is to decide whether the mass is located in the retroperitoneal space. Anterior displacement of retroperitoneal organs and major abdominal vessels strongly suggest that the mass arises in the retroperitoneum. After confirming the retroperitoneal location, the next step is to decide whether it is arising from a retroperitoneal organ or is a primary retroperitoneal tumor arising outside the major retroperitoneal organs. Certain radiologic signs have been described to determine the origin of a mass.[1] When a tumor arises from an organ, the organ appears to be embedded in the tumor. This is called the *positive embedded organ sign*. When a tumor compresses an adjacent pliable organ (such as the hollow viscera or IVC), it deforms the organ into a crescent shape. This is the *negative embedded organ sign* and is seen in primary retroperitoneal tumors. When the edge of an adjacent organ is distorted into a "beak", it indicates that the tumor probably arises from the organ. This is called the *"positive beak sign"*. On the other hand, when an adjacent organ has rounded edges, it indicates that the retroperitoneal mass does not arise from that organ, this finding is called a *negative beak sign* (Figs 16.1A to D). When a

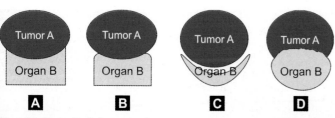

Figs 16.1A to D: Schematic diagram showing possible relationships of retroperitoneal masses to retroperitoneal organs.[1] (A and B) Beak sign. Drawings illustrate the positive beak sign (A), in which Tumor A arises from Organ B, and the negative beak sign (B), in which Tumor A does not arise from Organ B. (C and D) Embedded organ sign. Drawings illustrate the negative embedded organ sign (C), in which Tumor A simply compresses Organ B, and the positive embedded organ sign (D), in which Tumor A arises from Organ B so that the organ appears to be embedded in the tumor.

Table 16.1: Most common age at presentation for renal neoplasms[3]

Renal neoplasm (Prevalence)	Age range	Peak age
Wilms' tumor (80%)		
Unilateral form	1–11 y	3½ y
Bilateral form	2 mo–2 y	15 mo
Nephroblastomatosis	Any age	6–18 mo
Mesoblastic nephroma (3%)	0–1 y	1–3 mo
Clear cell sarcoma (4-5%)	1–4 y	2 y
Rhabdoid tumor (2%)	6 mo–9 y	6–12 mo
Miscellaneous tumors (7%)		
Renal cell carcinoma	6 mo–60 y	10–20 y*
Multilocular cystic renal tumor	3 mo–4 y	1–2 y
(Cystic nephroma)		
Angiomyolipoma	6–41 y	10 y†
Ossifying renal tumor of infancy	6 d–14 mo	1–3 mo
Metanephric adenoma	15 mo–83 y	None
Renal medullary carcinoma	10–39 y	20 y
Lymphoma		
Hodgkin	>10 y	Late teens
Non-Hodgkin	Any age child	<10 y

*von Hippel–Lindau syndrome, †Tuberous sclerosis, neurofibromatosis, von Hippel–Lindau syndrome

large mass arises from a small organ, the organ sometimes becomes undetectable – the *phantom (invisible) organ sign*.

RENAL MASSES

Renal masses can be congenital, infective, inflammatory or neoplastic in nature. Non-neoplastic masses have been discussed elsewhere in the book and this chapter will deal with the renal neoplasms in children.

An abdominal mass in a child in the first year of life is usually of renal origin. Benign renal masses (mainly developmental, only 20% being true neoplasms)[2] predominate in early infancy, but beyond the first year of life and during the first decade, primary tumors of the kidney become more common. The various pediatric renal neoplasms, their frequency and age of presentation are given in Table 16.1.[3]

WILMS' TUMOR (NEPHROBLASTOMA)

Wilms' tumor was first described by a German surgeon named Max Wilms in 1899. It is the commonest renal malignancy in childhood accounting for 80-90 percent of pediatric renal tumors and 12 percent of childhood cancers. It is rare during the first year of life and is commonly seen between 1-5 years of age with a peak at 3 years.[4] Occasionally Wilms' tumor has been described in teenagers and adults.

Etiopathogenesis

Wilms' tumors can arise sporadically, can develop in association with genetic syndromes, or can be familial. Upto 12 percent of children with Wilms' tumor have associated congenital anomalies. The incidence of co-existent genitourinary anomalies– cryptorchidism, hypospadias, ambiguous genitalia, horseshoe kidney – is the highest (5%) followed by hemihypertrophy (2.5%), and aniridia (1%). Thirty-three percent of children with sporadic aniridia develop Wilms' tumor and these tumors are frequently bilateral. Certain syndromes have a predisposition to Wilms' tumor. These include the Beckwith-Wiedeman syndrome (macroglossia, exomphalos, gigantism), Denys-Drash (pseudohermaphroditism, glomerulonephritis), Sotos (cerebral gigantism), Bloom (immunodeficiency and facial telangiectasia) and Perlman syndromes.[2] Wilms' tumor has also been reported in children with neurofibromatosis, with imperforate anus and rectourethral fistula.

Two loci on chromosome 11 have been implicated in the genesis of a minority of Wilms' tumors. Locus 11p13 is known as the WT1 gene, and locus 11p15 is known as the WT2 gene. An abnormal WT1 gene is present in patients with WAGR syndrome (Wilms' tumor, aniridia, genitourinary abnormalities, mental retardation) or Drash syndrome; an abnormal WT2 gene is present in patients with Beckwith-Wiedeman syndrome or hemihypertrophy. However, the genetics of Wilms' tumor appear to be multifactorial, and abnormalities at other sites, including chromosomes 1, 12, and 8, are also recognized. Familial Wilms' tumor is rare, occurring in approximately 1 percent of cases, and is not associated with mutations in chromosome 11.[5]

Clinical Features

Most children present with a painless abdominal mass often discovered accidentally by the parents or by the physician on a routine examination. The mass is hard rather than firm, non-tender and commonly unilateral. Wilms' tumor can be bilateral in 4–13 percent of children of which two-thirds are synchronous and one-third metachronous.[6] Bilateral tumors occur earlier, have a higher incidence of associated congenital anomalies and a higher incidence of nephroblastomatosis than seen in unilateral tumors.[7]

If the tumor ruptures or if hemorrhage occurs, there may be rapid enlargement of the mass with development of acute symptoms. Fever, leucocytosis, malaise, anorexia and gross or microscopic hematuria may occur. Hypertension can occur due to disruption of blood flow to and from the kidney, compression of renal tissues by tumor or rarely production of renin by the tumor itself.[8] Rarely, some tumors may become hormonally active and can cause Cushing's syndrome or hypoglycemia.

Table 16.2: Staging system for National Wilms' tumor study[10]

Stage I:	The tumor is limited to the kidney and is excised completely.
Stage II:	The tumor extends beyond the kidney but is excised completely. Capsular penetration, renal vein involvement, and renal sinus involvement may also be found. No residual tumor apparent at or beyond margins of excision.
Stage III:	Residual intra-abdominal tumor (nonhematogenous) exists after the completion of surgery. Lymph node findings are positive, or peritoneal implants are found. Tumor extends beyond surgical margins either microscopically or macroscopically.
Stage IV:	Hematogenous or lymph node metastasis has occurred outside the abdomen or pelvis.
Stage V:	Synchronous bilateral involvement has occurred. Each side is assigned a stage from I to III, and histology is based on biopsy findings.

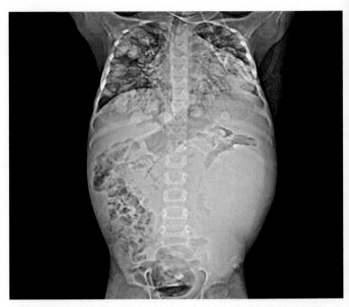

Fig. 16.2: Plain radiograph of the chest and abdomen shows evidence of a soft tissue mass in the left lumbar and iliac fossa with displaced bowel loops. Multiple rounded opacities seen scattered through both lung fields - pulmonary metastasis.

Pathology

Wilms' tumor is characterized by an abnormal proliferation of the metanephric blastema cells, which are believed to be primitive embryologic cells of the kidney. The gross appearance of a Wilms' tumor is that of a large, bulky, solid mass with a well defined pseudocapsule of compressed renal parenchyma that separates it from the rest of the kidney, with distortion of the renal parenchyma and collecting system. The tumor typically spreads by direct extension and displaces adjacent structures but does not usually encase or elevate the aorta. Foci of hemorrhage, necrosis and cyst formation are commonly found, specially if the tumor is large or has previously been treated with radiation or chemotherapy. There may be vascular invasion of the renal vein and inferior vena cava with occasional extension into the right atrium. Metastases are most commonly found in the lungs (85% of cases), liver, and regional lymph nodes.

Histologically, the classic Wilms' tumor is "triphasic": it contains epithelial (tubular, glomerular), blastemal (small round cells), and stromal (spindle, myxoid) cell lines. Not all tumors however, contain all cell lines and the proportion as well of degree of differentiation of cell lines is highly variable from one tumor to the next.[9] Apart from the predominant cell lines, the prognosis of children with Wilms' tumor is heavily dependant on the presence of anaplasia. Its presence has been found to be more significant than tumor staging when assigning prognosis. A 'favorable' histology lacks anaplastic changes, whereas one with "unfavorable" histology demonstrates extreme nuclear and mitotic atypia characteristic of anaplasia. Approximately 90 percent of Wilms' tumors are of 'favorable" histology.

Staging

The current staging according to the North American National Wilms' Tumor Study Group (NWTSG) is based on surgical, pathological and radiological findings and is given in Table 16.2.[10]

Imaging

Plain abdominal radiographs show evidence of a large flank mass. Calcification is seen in less than 10 percent of cases.[2] *Chest radiographs* are routinely done in all cases to look for evidence of lung metastases which indicate advanced stage disease (Fig. 16.2).

On *US* the tumor is visualized as a predominantly solid, slightly hyperechoic mass causing gross renal enlargement. A clear margination of the tumor from the rest of the kidney is often possible due to the pseudocapsule which may be hypo- or hyperechoic (Figs 16.3A and B). Normal native renal tissue can be difficult to detect and is typically stretched at the periphery of the lesion. It may show hydronephrotic changes. Cystic areas are often seen within the mass which correlate with presence of hemorrhage or cystic degeneration. Invasion of the IVC and extension into the right atrium can be readily detected on US (Fig. 16.4). Intrahepatic IVC can be assessed relatively easily but differentiation of invasion from displacement and compression may be difficult. A clue to the presence of obstruction is the dilatation of the hepatic veins. Doppler can also confirm the presence of a thrombus and show its extent. Thrombus confined to the renal vein is less easy to detect because of distortion. US is excellent for detecting the tumor itself and its vascular extension but is limited in its ability to assess extracapsular extension of tumor, lymph node involvement and small contralateral tumors.

Abdominal *CT scan* is more sensitive than ultrasound in identifying tumor extent, nodal, liver and contralateral kidney involvement.[11] CT has the advantage of detecting the precursor condition, nephroblastomatosis.[12] On CT, Wilms' tumor is seen as a large, well defined mass of heterogeneous attenuation, which enhances to a lesser degree than the normal renal parenchyma. The normal renal parenchyma can be seen stretched and splayed at the periphery of the mass - the "positive beak sign". Areas of low attenuation coincide with tumor necrosis and/or fat deposition. Calcification may be seen in a few cases (Figs 16.3C, 16.5

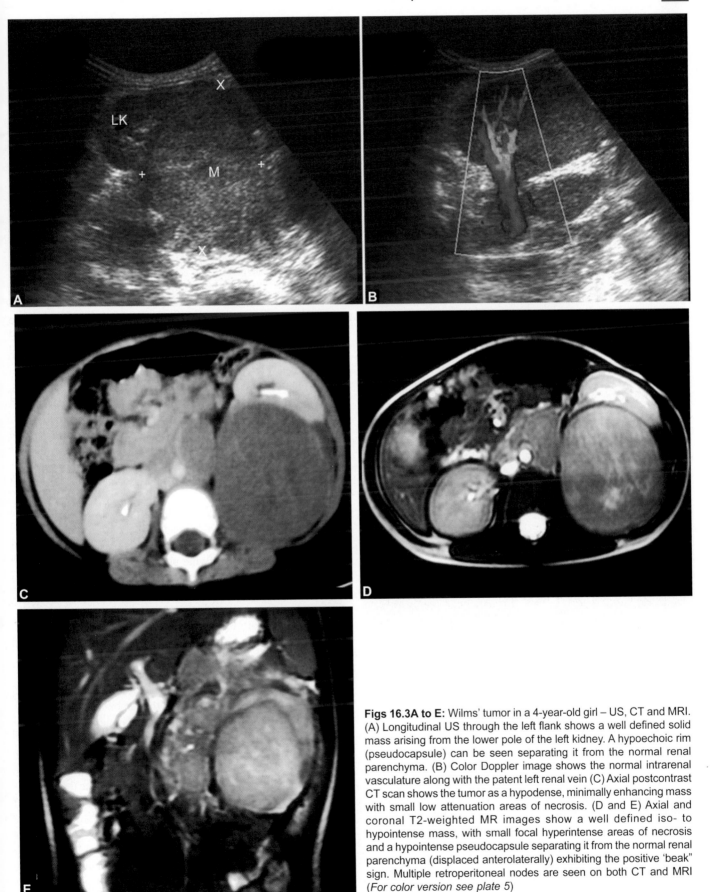

Figs 16.3A to E: Wilms' tumor in a 4-year-old girl – US, CT and MRI. (A) Longitudinal US through the left flank shows a well defined solid mass arising from the lower pole of the left kidney. A hypoechoic rim (pseudocapsule) can be seen separating it from the normal renal parenchyma. (B) Color Doppler image shows the normal intrarenal vasculature along with the patent left renal vein (C) Axial postcontrast CT scan shows the tumor as a hypodense, minimally enhancing mass with small low attenuation areas of necrosis. (D and E) Axial and coronal T2-weighted MR images show a well defined iso- to hypointense mass, with small focal hyperintense areas of necrosis and a hypointense pseudocapsule separating it from the normal renal parenchyma (displaced anterolaterally) exhibiting the positive 'beak" sign. Multiple retroperitoneal nodes are seen on both CT and MRI (*For color version see plate 5*)

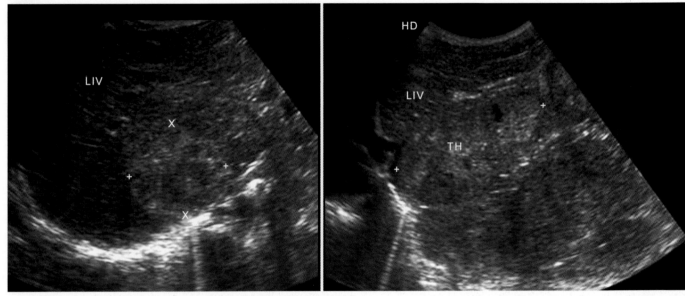

Fig. 16.4: Transverse and longitudinal US image in a case of Wilms' tumor showing an isoechoic thrombus (TH) filling the IVC

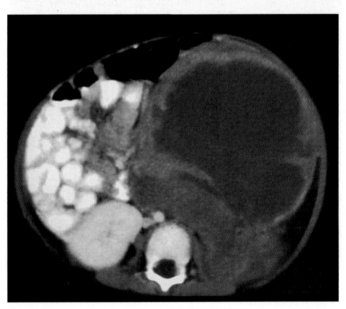

Fig. 16.5: Cystic Wilm's tumor. Contrast enhanced axial CT shows a Wilms' tumor of the left kidney with a large cystic component within. The tumor mass extends across the midline, displacing the aorta and IVC to the right, but not elevating or encasing these vessels (unlike neuroblastoma).

and 16.6A and B). Capsular invasion may be suggested by a pattern of exophytic growth and contour irregularity. Contrast enhanced CT scan allows evaluation of the renal veins and inferior vena cava for tumor thrombus though sensitivity is less than sonography (Fig. 16.6C).[13] CT scan may identify regional adenopathy, although it cannot differentiate tumor replacement from reactive adenopathy. Nodal involvement differentiates between stage II & III, but neither CT nor surgical exploration is accurate and its distinction remains histological at present. Peritoneal, omental and mesenteric involvement of Wilms' tumor can be depicted accurately by CT.

On *MR imaging* the tumor appears as a well defined mass with signal intensity similar to that of the spleen and slightly lower than that of the normal renal cortex on T1W images. On T2W images, the tumor appears isointense to normal renal cortex. Areas of high signal intensity correspond to the presence of hemorrhage or necrosis. The pseudocapsule is seen as a hypointense rim surrounding the tumor on both T1 and T2 pulse sequences (Figs 16.3D and E). On contrast administration the tumor enhances heterogeneously and characteristically less than the normal renal parenchyma.

MR imaging can accurately assess tumor size, gross composition, and regional spread, although, as with all other imaging modalities, it cannot define subtle capsular invasion.[2] It can also accurately identify the presence of liver metastases and caval thrombus. Advantages over US and CT scan include the use of specific flow sequences in the search for tumor thrombus and multiplanar imaging in evaluating caval displacement by tumor.

With the diagnostic information provided by US, CT/MRI, the role of intravenous urography (IVU) has significantly reduced in the present day imaging work-up of Wilms' tumor. On IVU, both frontal and lateral views are required for a proper 3-dimensional concept of the mass. The appearance of the tumor on the IVU depends on the location of the tumor within the kidney. An intrarenal mass can be seen to cause splaying and distortion of the calyces. Tumors in the upper pole and posterior location cause more calyceal distortion than lower pole or anterior tumors, which can readily grow exophytically. A centrally located tumor may cause a hydronephrotic appearance associated with calyceal distortion.

Chest CT and pulmonary metastases: The role of CT scan of the chest in the evaluation and subsequent management of pulmonary lesions found only on CT is controversial and its prognostic importance is equivocal.[14,15] Chest CT, currently required by the NWTSG-5 imaging protocol, is a highly sensitive technique in the evaluation of parenchymal lung disease and enables

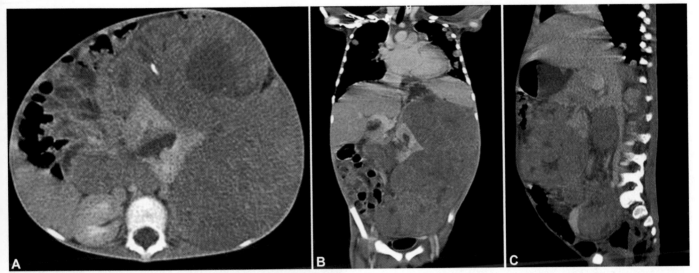

Figs 16.6A to C: MDCT of a large left Wilms' tumor. (A and B) Axial CT and coronal MPR shows a large heterogenous left renal mass with areas of low attenuation due to necrosis. Small focus of calcification is also seen. Residual renal parenchyma is displaced anteromedially by the mass and shows the positive "embedded organ" sign. The mass enhances less than the normal renal parenchyma. Note the ill defined nodular hypoattenuating area anterior to the right kidney, aorta and IVC representing adenopathy. Vessels are not encased or elevated. Multiple metastases can be seen in the lung fields. (C) Parasagittal MPR image shows the entire IVC which is compressed by the mass but there is no invasion or thrombus formation

the identification of lesions not visible on chest radiographs. It is also more sensitive in the detection of calcified nodules. Controversy arises in staging the disease when chest CT identifies lesions (CT-only lesions) not seen on chest radiographs. The results of many studies have shown that treating according to chest CT findings does not change the final outcome of children with Wilms' tumor.[14] Also, it has been shown that CT-only lesions are not invariably tumor, demonstrating the need for histopathological confirmation.[16]

Differential Diagnosis

The most important differential diagnosis of a Wilms' tumor is *neuroblastoma*. Although Wilms' tumor characteristically arises from the kidney whereas a neuroblastoma displaces the kidney, differentiation may be difficult in the presence of a large exophytic Wilms' tumor or with renal invasion of neuroblastoma. Features favoring Wilms' tumor are non-homogeneous internal structure of tumor with hemorrhage and necrosis, round or oval shape with regular margins and absence of calcification. Classical features of an abdominal neuroblastoma are ill-defined margins, tumor calcifications, tumor extension across midline, displacement and encasement of vascular structures. Encasement of aorta, paravertebral extension and invasion of spinal canal, if seen, are highly predictive of neuroblastoma whereas tumor invasion of IVC suggests Wilms' tumor.

Other differentials are mesoblastic nephroma (seen in children younger than 6 months), renal cell carcinoma (peak age 10-20 years), clear cell sarcoma and rhabdoid tumor of the kidney.

Treatment and Prognosis

The treatment strategy of Wilms' tumors has become a model for the successful multidisciplinary approach to pediatric solid tumors.

North American practice is initial surgical removal of the tumor followed by adjuvant chemotherapy dictated by the staging found at surgery. European oncologists favor initial chemotherapy (after biopsy confirmation in the UK) with later resection. The optimal surgery includes a transperitoneal approach with biopsy of adjacent regional lymph nodes, whether enlarged or not. Nephrectomy is usually carried out except in the setting of bilateral Wilms' tumors where partial nephrectomies, when possible, are indicated to preserve as much normal kidney tissue with the hope of avoiding or delaying the subsequent onset of chronic renal failure. The prognosis for Wilms' tumor patients is excellent and there is little evidence to suggest that the overall relapse-free survival is adversely affected by either approach. The 4-year overall survival rate, and presumed cure, ranges between 86 percent and 96 percent for stages I–III disease, is up to 83 percent for stage IV and 70 percent for stage V disease. Patients with the much less common diffuse anaplastic Wilms' tumors have a much poorer outcome, however. Their 4-year survival figures are 45 percent for stage III and only 7 percent for stage IV disease.[17]

Follow-up and Screening

Follow-up care after treatment must be long (if possible, lifelong) because Wilms' tumor may recur after several years. Most relapses occur within the chest and abdomen, and 94 percent of relapses occur within the first 2 years following diagnosis. Follow-up consists of chest radiography, abdominal ultrasonography and CT scan or MRI every 3 months for the first 2 years, every 6 months for another 2 years, and once every 2 years thereafter.[2]

Screening for Wilms' tumor in patients with associated syndromes should begin at 6 months of age with initial computed tomography (CT) followed by serial ultrasonography (US) every 3 months up to 7 years of age. After the age of 7 years, screening can be discontinued because the risk of developing Wilms' tumor decreases significantly.[6,18]

NEPHROBLASTOMATOSIS

The nephrons of the kidney develop from the metanephric blastema. This development is normally complete by the 36th week of intrauterine life. The term "nephrogenic rests" implies persistence of the metanephric blastema beyond 36 weeks of gestation. Nephroblastomatosis is the presence of multiple nephrogenic rests. These abnormal foci of persistent nephrogenic cells are regarded as precursor lesions and have the potential for malignant transformation into Wilms' tumor. They are found incidentally in 1 percent of infants. It is currently believed that nephrogenic rests give rise to approximately 30–40 percent of unilateral Wilms' tumors,[6] and they are found in up to 99 percent of bilateral Wilms' tumors.[19]

Pathology

Nephrogenic rests are classified histologically as *dormant, sclerosing, hyperplastic*, or *neoplastic*. Dormant and sclerosing rests are usually microscopic and not considered to have malignant potential. *Hyperplastic* and *neoplastic* rests are grossly visible as small nodules surrounded by normal parenchyma. Nephrogenic rests can also be classified into *perilobar* and *intralobar* on the basis of location and the syndromes with which they are associated. Perilobar rests lie in the peripheral cortex or columns of Bertin. They are associated with Beckwith-Wiedemann syndrome and hemihypertrophy, Perlman syndrome, and trisomy 18. Malignant degeneration into Wilms' tumor is most common in patients with Beckwith-Wiedemann syndrome and hemihypertrophy, occurring in 3 percent of cases.[6] Intralobar rests are considerably less common than the perilobar type but have a higher association with Wilms' tumor development. These rests are found in 78 percent of patients with Drash syndrome and nearly 100 percent of patients with sporadic aniridia and are also seen in patients with WAGR syndrome.

Imaging Features

Nephroblastomatosis may either be *diffuse* or *multifocal*. In the more common *multifocal* type, the nephrogenic rests resemble normal renal cortex on all modalities and can be scattered throughout the kidneys; US shows large, irregularly lobulated kidneys with hypoechoic to isoechoic homogeneous mass like regions within the renal parenchyma. These masses are often asymmetric and peripheral and the corticomedullary differentiation is poor. They are better defined on contrast enhanced CT and MRI as focal non enhancing masses (Fig. 16.7).[20] In general, these nodules appear fairly homogeneous in contrast to a Wilms' tumor which is always heterogeneous in appearance.

The *diffuse* form typically manifests as reniform enlargement with a thick hypoechoic rim on US. This abnormal tissue surrounds the renal periphery and compresses the centrally located residual parenchyma. At CT, the peripheral rim of nephroblastomatosis is homogenously hypodense and non-enhancing, and causes distortion of the pelvicalyceal system. The remaining functional

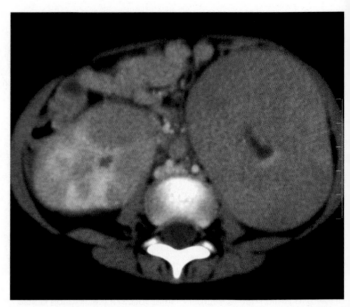

Fig. 16.7: Nephroblastomatosis in a 1 year old child. Contrast enhanced axial CT scan shows large non-enhancing hypodense masses in both the kidneys, larger on the left. Histological examination showed Wilms' tumor on the left

parenchyma may characteristically exhibit a pattern resembling stag's antlers. On MRI, the nephroblastomatosis is homogeneously hypointense on T1W images and varies from iso- to hyperintensity on T2W images. It is best seen after contrast administration becoming sharply demarcated from the highly enhancing normal renal parenchyma.

MRI may be able to distinguish a sclerotic from a hyperplastic nephrogenic rest.[21] Sclerotic rests are thought to be in a regressive phase and to thus lack the potential to develop into a Wilms' tumor. Sclerotic rests typically appear dark on T2-weighted images, whilst hyperplastic rests are usually hyperintense, similar to Wilms' tumor. In the setting of bilateral nephroblastomatosis or bilateral Wilms' tumors on treatment, it is thought that hypointense lesions on T2-weighted images (sclerotic rests) may simply be observed, whereas hyperintense lesions may require further chemotherapy or local resection.[21] CT is unable to make this distinction.

The *differential diagnosis* of nephroblastomatosis includes renal lymphoma, leukemia or even polycystic kidneys.

MESOBLASTIC NEPHROMA (BOLANDE'S TUMOR)

Mesoblastic nephroma is the most common solid renal tumor identified in the first 3-6 months of life. It is a non-familial, benign tumor arising from the renal connective tissue. Originally thought to represent congenital Wilms' tumor, it was first described as a separate entity by Bolande et al in 1967.[22]

Clinical Presentation

A large, palpable abdominal mass in a neonate is the most common presentation. The peak age at presentation is approximately 3 months. Additional signs and symptoms include hematuria, hypertension, vomiting, and hypercalcemia, seen in a minority of cases. Increased renin levels are often present. Some cases are

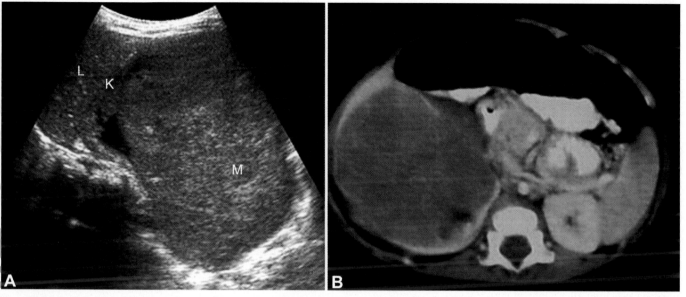

Figs 16.8A and B: Mesoblastic nephroma (A). Longitudinal US and (B) Contrast enhanced axial CT in a 6-month-old infant with a palpable abdominal mass shows a large, central, solid homogeneous mass arising from the right kidney. The enhancing normal renal tissue is seen along the periphery in B. (M = mass, K = hydronephrotic kidney, L = liver)

detected at prenatal sonography and may be associated with polyhydramnios, hydrops, and premature delivery.

Pathology

Grossly, mesoblastic nephroma has a yellow, homogeneous, rubbery appearance likened to a *uterine leiomyoma* with no capsule and poorly defined margins. Unlike Wilms tumor, foci of hemorrhage and necrosis are uncommon in this entity. The tumor has 2 morphologic variants – namely, the classic and cellular type. Microscopically, the classic type shows sheets of benign connective tissue and mature spindle cells arranged in bundles and fascicles with entrapped dysplastic tubules and glomeruli. The cellular variant is highly cellular, with immature mesenchymal cells and a high number of active mitotic figures, but no significant pleomorphism. Tumor *necrosis* and hemorrhage are more frequently seen with the cellular variant. These tend to have a poorer prognosis and are mainly seen in infants and children older than 3 months.[20]

Imaging

On US imaging, a mesoblastic nephroma appears typically as a well defined, solid, homogeneous lesion (Fig. 16.8A). There may be some heterogeneity due to hypoechoic areas of hemorrhage or necrosis. A distinctive "ring sign" may be seen in typical intrarenal CMN, This vascular ring sign, as described by Chan et al,[23] is an anechoic or hypoechoic vascular ring surrounding the tumor on ultrasound and is considered a feature of the typical or nonaggressive mesoblastic nephroma. On color Doppler examination, this vascular ring demonstrates significant vascularity, and on spectral Doppler examination, it demonstrates both arterial and venous waveforms.

CT and MRI demonstrate the presence of a large solid, mostly homogeneous intrarenal mass typically involving the renal sinus. On contrast administration the tumor shows no or minimal enhancement (Fig. 16.8B). Entrapment of urine or collecting system may lead to the excretion of contrast material within the mass. Areas of necrosis may be seen with the aggressive variant. On MRI the mass shows intermediate signal intensity, similar to the renal cortex and the skeletal muscle on the T1- and increased signal on the T2-weighted images. The benign or the classic mesoblastic nephroma may demonstrate a peripheral, markedly enhancing ring on the postcontrast T1-weighted images, corresponding to the vascular ring seen on US.

On prenatal sonography a mesoblastic nephroma may be first diagnosed when the detailed fetal anomaly scan is performed at 18-20 weeks' gestation, as a unilateral, solid paravertebral mass with low level echoes. Differentiation between a solid and a cystic mass can easily be made on ultrasound to differentiate between a mass and hydronephrosis. Associated polyhydramnios is common and is thought to occur due to increased renal blood flow and impaired renal concentrating ability leading to fetal polyuria and subsequent polyhydramnios. If the mass is very large, it may be difficult to determine the organ of origin in some cases. Fetal MRI may be helpful in determining the organ of origin.

Differential Diagnosis

Imaging cannot definitively differentiate a mesoblastic nephroma from a congenital Wilms' tumor. Histologic examination is the only definitive test. The younger age of presentation, lack of well defined margins, absence of tumor capsule, and central intrarenal location with involvement of renal sinus favor the diagnosis of mesoblastic nephroma. Other differential diagnoses include multicystic dysplastic kidney and congenital adrenal neuroblastoma.

Treatment and Prognosis

Mesoblastic nephroma generally exhibits benign behavior and is successfully treated with nephrectomy alone. Rarely, the lesion may recur locally if incompletely resected or metastasize to the lungs, brain, or bones. Therefore, it is currently recommended that patients be closely followed-up for 1 year after surgical resection.[3] The prognosis is best if the tumor is diagnosed and resected before 6 months of age.

CLEAR CELL SARCOMA

Clear cell sarcoma of the kidney once thought to be a variant of Wilms' tumor, accounts for 4–5 percent of primary renal tumors in childhood.[2] The peak incidence is at 1–4 years of age, and a male predominance has been reported.[3] It has a nonspecific presentation, most often manifesting as an abdominal mass. The tumor is characterized by its aggressive behavior and is associated with a higher rate of relapse and mortality than Wilms' tumor. It may metastasize to the bones, lymph nodes, brain, liver, and lungs; in some cases long after nephrectomy.

Pathology

At gross analysis, the tumor is soft and well circumscribed. At histologic analysis, small cells with inconspicuous nucleoli and ill-defined cell membranes and a prominent capillary network commonly characterize this tumor. However, there is a spectrum of appearances, in which only 20 percent have clear cells.[3]

Imaging

Imaging studies do not allow differentiation of clear cell sarcoma from Wilms' tumor. A sharply demarcated solid intrarenal mass without intravascular extension is seen on all modalities. Bone metastases may be osteolytic, osteoblastic or mixed. The discovery of a metastatic lesion in the skeleton in a child with a presumed diagnosis of Wilms' tumor should suggest that the tumor is likely to be a clear cell sarcoma. Once diagnosed, a 99mTc-MDP bone scintigraphy is indicated for staging purposes.

Treatment consists of nephrectomy and chemotherapy with current survival rates of 60-70 percent.[3] The most common site of recurrence is bone and current recommendations of the NWTSG-5 include periodic screening with bone scintigraphy and skeletal survey.

RHABDOID TUMOR

Rhabdoid tumor of the kidney (RTK) is a rare, highly aggressive malignancy of early childhood comprising 2 percent of all pediatric renal malignancies.[3] It was formerly considered a Wilms' tumor variant with unfavorable histology, but is now recognized as a separate entity. Rhabdoid tumor is seen early in life: 80 percent of cases occur in patients less than 2 years and 60 percent before 1 year of age. The median age at presentation is 11 months with a slight male predominance.[24]

Clinical Presentation

Most patients present with advanced stage disease and symptoms maybe referable to metastatic disease. Concomitant brain tumor or other soft tissue tumors are distinctive features of this entity.

Pathology

The macroscopic appearance of rhabdoid tumor is nonspecific. It arises centrally (unlike Wilms' tumor) and has an infiltrative growth pattern. Local invasion of renal parenchyma and renal vein are common. Distant metastases to the lung and liver are also common and association with synchronous and metachronous brain metastases is a distinctive feature. Association with synchronous primary brain tumors has been reported in 10-15 percent of patients. Primitive neuroectodermal tumor, ependymoma, and cerebellar and brainstem astrocytoma have all been documented.[24] Soft tissue and thymic tumors may also occur in association with malignant rhabdoid tumor.

At histologic analysis, the tumor is characterized by monomorphic cells with prominent eosinophilic nucleoli and characteristic filamentous intracytoplasmic inclusions.[25] Some areas of the tumor may superficially resemble the blastemal pattern of Wilms' tumor.

Imaging

In most instances, RTK cannot be differentiated from Wilms' tumor based on imaging alone. US, CT and MRI show a large heterogenous mass, characteristically involving the renal hilum with associated vascular invasion. If present, a number of features may suggest the diagnosis of RTK: subcapsular fluid collections, tumor lobules separated by dark areas of necrosis or hemorrhage, and linear calcifications outlining tumor lobules.[26] Vascular and local invasion is common. Radiological investigation should also include cross-sectional imaging for the common sites of metastases (lung, liver, brain), bone scintigraphy and skeletal survey (bone metastases).

Treatment and Prognosis

Of all the pediatric renal tumors, the prognosis of children with RTK is the poorest. Despite aggressive surgery and chemotherapy, RTK has the poorest prognosis amongst all pediatric renal tumors. There is a high rate of local tumor recurrence following surgical resection. Survival is poor, with an 18-month survival rate of only 20 percent.[26]

RENAL CELL CARCINOMA

Renal cell carcinoma (RCC) is primarily a tumor of the adult population and less than 2 percent of all cases occur in the pediatric age range. The mean age of presentation is 9 years. Although Wilms' tumor is much more common than any other malignancy in the first decade of life, Wilms' tumor and RCC have an almost equal incidence in the second decade.[27]

Renal cell carcinoma is associated with von Hippel–Lindau syndrome, in which the tumors tend to be multiple and manifest at a younger age. This syndrome must be ruled out in pediatric patients diagnosed with renal cell carcinoma, especially when the tumor is bilateral.[27]

Clinical Presentation

Clinical manifestations are similar to those in adults. Gross painless hematuria, flank pain, and a palpable mass are the most common presenting symptoms. Hematuria is more frequent in patients with renal cell carcinoma than in patients with Wilms' tumor.

Pathology

The tumor forms an infiltrative solid mass with variable necrosis, hemorrhage, calcification, and cystic degeneration. There is distortion of the normal renal architecture and formation of a pseudocapsule. The tumor invades locally with spread to adjacent retroperitoneal lymph nodes. Metastases to the lungs, bones, liver, or brain are found in 20 percent of patients at diagnosis. Compared with Wilms' tumor, renal cell carcinoma is more likely to manifest bilaterally and more likely to metastasize to bone.[2]

Imaging

RCC and Wilms' tumor may be indistinguishable based on imaging features alone. RCC tends to be smaller and exhibits calcifications more frequently (25% of RCC versus 9% of Wilms' tumor).[6] On CT and MRI, RCC appears as a heterogeneous intrarenal mass, due to the presence of necrosis and/or hemorrhage. Ring like calcifications may be present. On contrast administration, the mass shows little or no enhancement.

MULTILOCULAR CYSTIC RENAL TUMOR

The term multilocular cystic renal tumor (MCRT) refers to two distinct entities: cystic nephroma (CN) and cystic partially differentiated nephroblastoma (CPDN). Both are benign renal tumors that have well defined margins and consist entirely of cystic lesions with multiple thin walled septations. In CN, the septa are composed entirely of differentiated tissues. If immature or blastemal cells are present in the septa, the lesion is termed CPDN.[20]

Multilocular cystic renal tumors have a biphasic age and sex distribution - two-thirds occur in a predominately male pediatric population between 3 months and 2-years-old; approximately one-third occur in a mostly female population, with a peak in the 5th and 6th decades of life.[28] There is no association with cysts in other organs and only sporadic association with other congenital anomalies.

Clinical Presentation

Presenting symptoms vary with patient age. Children typically present with a painless, progressively enlarging, palpable abdominal or flank mass that has a variable growth rate and may be discovered incidentally. Adults can present with a variety of nonspecific signs and symptoms, including abdominal and flank pain, urinary tract infection, and hypertension.[28]

Pathology

CN and CPDN are indistinguishable from each other on gross examination and consist of a well defined multiloculated mass of non communicating cysts that is surrounded by a thick fibrous capsule and compressed renal parenchyma. The mass is typically large and commonly arises from the lower pole of the kidney. Calcification is rare. Necrosis and hemorrhage are uncommon but

are usually seen in association with herniation of the tumor into the renal pelvis or ureter, which damages the thin layer of transitional epithelium.[28]

At microscopic examination, however, CN is clearly distinct from CPDN. In CN, the septa consist of fibrous tissue, which may contain well-differentiated epithelial cells. The presence of poorly differentiated tissues or blastemal cells in the septa characterize CPDN. It is essential to distinguish between cystic nephroma and CPDN because the blastemal component theoretically portends the risk of Wilms' tumor development.

Imaging

Abdominal radiography may demonstrate a soft-tissue mass. Curvilinear and peripheral calcification may be seen, although it is uncommon. On US, CT and MRI, a MCRT typically appears as an intrarenal multicystic mass with no solid or nodular elements (Figs 16.9A and B). The loculi can range in size from microscopic to 4 cm in diameter and very small loculi may mimic solid components because of their innumerable, closely packed acoustic interfaces.[29,30] On CT the cystic spaces have an attenuation value similar to or slightly greater than water. On MR T1-weighted images the cyst contents show variable signal intensities, depending on the concentration of old hemorrhage or protein and a high signal intensity on T2-weighted images. Septal enhancement is seen on contrast administration on both CT and MRI. Associated urinary tract obstruction may be evident.

Differential Diagnosis

The main differential diagnosis is cystic Wilms' tumor. Identification of solid nodular elements in the septa should suggest the diagnosis of WT and not MCRT. Other lesions that may mimic MCRT include multicystic dysplastic kidney, cellular variety of mesoblastic nephroma, clear cell carcinoma and renal cell carcinoma.[20]

Treatment and Follow-up

Because neither the clinical nor the imaging features of MCRT can predict its histologic characteristics, surgery—either nephrectomy or nephron-sparing surgery—is required for both diagnosis and treatment.[29] If pathologic analysis proves that the tumor is a CPDN, regular noninvasive monitoring is suggested because the presence of blastemal cells in the septa of a CPDN implies the potential for more aggressive behavior, despite the usually benign course of the tumor.

ANGIOMYOLIPOMA

Angiomyolipomas (AML) are benign hamartomatous masses in the kidney containing fat, smooth muscle and blood vessels in varying proportions. Upto 80 percent of all patients with tuberous sclerosis (both adults and children) have angiomyolipomas.[2] When associated with tuberous sclerosis, these tumors are more likely to be multifocal, bilateral and of greater size. Association with neurofibromatosis and von Hippel-Lindau syndrome has also been described.

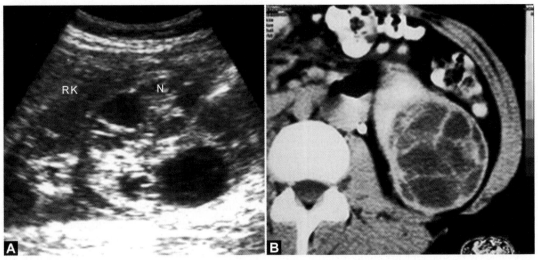

Figs 16.9A and B: Multilocular cystic nephroma. (A) Longitudinal US and (B) Contrast enhanced axial CT demonstrate an intrarenal sharply circumscribed, multiloculated mass with enhancing septae on CECT

Clinical Presentation

Most commonly AMLs are found incidentally in asymptomatic children. Clinical symptoms are related to the occurrence of tumor bleeding which correlates with the size of tumor. AMLs smaller than 4 cm are usually asymptomatic. Those larger than 4 cm are more likely to bleed spontaneously and manifest clinically as pain and hematuria or even severe life threatening hemorrhage.[2,31]

Pathology

On gross examination, angiomyolipoma appears as an intrarenal mass, varying in diameter from 3 - 20 cm. It is well demarcated from surrounding compressed renal parenchyma but it has no capsule. Rarely it may behave aggressively and invade the collecting system, renal vein, IVC and retroperitoneal lymph nodes. Microscopically, a mixture of lipomatous tissue, blood vessels and smooth muscle characterizes angiomyolipoma.

Imaging

Imaging studies are diagnostic if a characteristic fatty component is identified. On US, AML is seen as a heterogeneous mass, predominantly echogenic, without through transmission (Fig. 16.10A). CT is the most reliable imaging modality and shows the presence of a renal mass with significant fat attenuation within it (Figs 16.10B and C). However, in the case of small lesions thin sections and single voxel measurements may be needed to confirm the diagnosis.[32] MRI can also detect fat within an AML which gives high signal intensity signal on both T1- and T2-weighted images. The signal intensity decreases on out of phase T1W and fat suppressed pulse sequences. Angiography which may be performed for embolization of a focal lesion prior to surgery, shows a hypervascular lesion with tortuous, somewhat aneurysmal arteries, venous puddling, but no vascular encasement or arteriovenous shunting.[33]

Screening, Follow-up and Treatment

Conservative management is recommended for patients with known masses smaller than 4 cm. In children with tuberous sclerosis, it is expected that by 10 years of age, 80 percent will have developed angiomyolipomas if monitored. The intensity of monitoring varies between centres. Serial US examinations every 2-3 years before 10 years of age and every 8-12 months thereafter are recommended, with the aim of identifying and monitoring growing lesions.[3] Lesions that have bled or lesions larger than 4 cm may require renal-sparing surgery or selective transcatheter embolization in an attempt to spare as much renal parenchyma as possible.[2]

OSSIFYING RENAL TUMOR OF INFANCY

Ossifying renal tumor of infancy is a rare benign renal mass and is reported only in young children ranging from 6 days to 14 months. Boys are more commonly affected than girls.[34,35] The tumor is relatively small (2-3 cm) and resembles renal calculi, except that it is attached to the renal parenchyma. The mass is centrally located at or near the renal papilla from where it extends in a polypoid fashion into the collecting system. Microscopically, ossifying tumors are composed of an osteoid core, osteoblasts and proliferating spindle cells.

Imaging

The renal outline is usually maintained; however, filling defects with partial obstruction of the collecting system are often seen. Because of its location within the collecting system and its characteristic ossification, ossifying renal tumor of infancy may mimic a staghorn calculus, which would be exceedingly rare in the age group in which this lesion occurs. At US, the mass is echogenic with shadowing, and hydronephrosis may be present. CT shows a well defined mass, often calcified, with poor enhancement.[3]

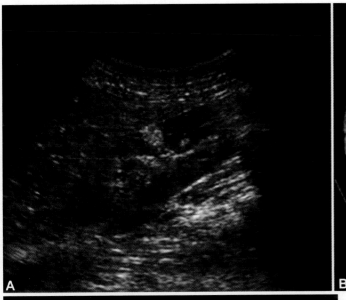

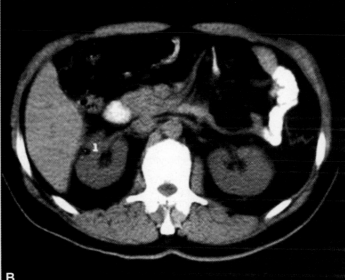

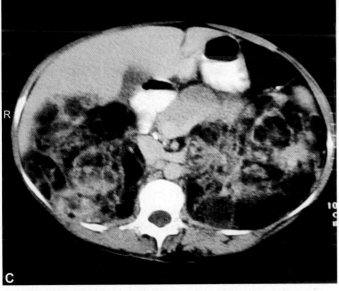

Figs 16.10A to C: Angiomyolipoma. (A) Longitudinal US of the right kidney shows a small well defined hyperechoic mass in peripheral cortex. (B) Contrast enhanced axial CT shows fatty attenuation (-50 HU) in the mass. (C) Contrast enhanced CT shows large hetrogeneous masses in both kidneys with multiple fat density areas in a child with tuberous sclerosis

METANEPHRIC ADENOMA (NEPHROGENIC ADENOFIBROMA, EMBRYONAL ADENOMA)

Metanephric adenoma is a benign renal tumor that can occur at any age and has been reported in patients as young as 15 months and as old as 83 years. It is more common in female patients.[3] Presenting features include pain, hypertension, hematoma, a flank mass, hypercalcemia, and polycythemia.

Imaging

At US, the mass is well defined and solid. It can be hypoechoic or hyperechoic or even cystic with a mural nodule. Doppler evaluation shows the lesion to be hypovascular. CT shows an iso- to hyperattenuating mass which enhances less than normal renal parenchyma. Small calcifications may be present.[36]

LYMPHOMA

Lymphoma either involves the kidney secondarily from direct retroperitoneal extension or by hematogenous metastases. In children, non-Hodgkin lymphoma—especially Burkitt lymphoma—is more likely to involve the kidney. As many as 62 percent of patients with lymphoma have renal involvement at autopsy although only 3–8 percent of these patients demonstrate renal involvement at CT.[3,37] The existence of primary renal lymphoma without evidence of systemic disease is still debatable.

Clinical Presentation

Lymphomatous involvement of the kidney typically does not produce symptoms until late in the disease. Flank or abdominal pain, hematuria, anemia, weight loss, and a palpable mass are the most common clinical findings. Hypertension is rare.[3]

Imaging

Imaging findings are variable and include solitary or multiple renal masses or nodules, diffuse infiltration, direct invasion from contiguous retroperitoneal extension, and least commonly isolated perinephric disease. The most common radiologic pattern is

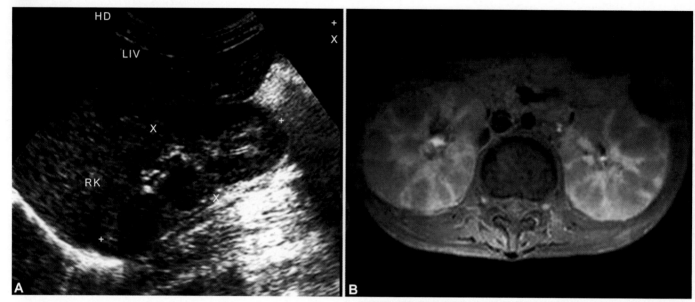

Figs 16.11A and B: (A) Renal lymphoma. Longitudinal US through the kidney shows multiple focal hypoechoic masses in the kidney. (B) Renal Leukemia. Post-contrast T1-weighted axial image shows leukemic infiltration of the kidneys in a 12-year-old boy as multiple non enhancing nodular lesions in the renal parenchyma. This appearance is indistinguishable from that of lymphoma.

multiple parenchymal masses or nodules that occasionally distort the renal contour and displace the collecting system. Lymphomatous masses have a nonspecific CT appearance. They are usually homogeneous, hypodense on non-enhanced and contrast-enhanced images, and may mimic multiple renal cysts. At US, they are hypoechoic and may demonstrate increased through transmission (Fig. 16.11A). On MRI, lymphomatous nodules exhibit signal intensity slightly higher than that of muscle on T1- and higher than fat on T2-weighted images.

Diffuse infiltration of the kidney may result in reniform enlargement. Retroperitoneal disease occasionally leads to vascular and ureteric encasement. Perinephric involvement can arise from retroperitoneal disease (most commonly) or transcapsular spread of parenchymal involvement. The CT findings of perinephric disease are variable and include small curvilinear areas of high attenuation, soft-tissue attenuation nodules, thickening of the Gerota fascia, or a mass contiguous with retroperitoneal disease.

LEUKEMIA

Renal involvement by leukemia is rare at presentation but may occur at relapse. Renal involvement generally occurs along with involvement of other extramedullary sites such as mediastinum, liver, pancreas, lymph nodes, etc. Renal symptoms such as hypertension or renal failure are rare. Leukemic infiltration of the kidneys most commonly causes bilateral, diffuse renal enlargement with distortion of the calyceal system. solitary or multiple focal nodular deposits may be seen in the renal parenchyma. On imaging, the kidneys are enlarged but maintain their shape. There is loss of corticomedullary differentiation on US with a heterogeneous echotexture. CT and MRI show the same findings, i.e. bilaterally enlarged kidneys with loss of corticomedullary differentiation,

altered parenchymal attenuation and decreased cortical enhancement.[2] Nodular deposits are seen as hypoechoic on US which are non enhancing on CT and MRI (Fig. 16.11B). The differential diagnosis includes nephroblastomatosis, lymphomatous deposits and simple cysts.

PRIMARY NEUROGENIC TUMORS OF THE KIDNEY

Primitive Neuroectodermal Tumor (PNET)

PNETs are rare malignant lesions most commonly occurring in the chest and extremities but have been reported to occur in the kidney. At histological examination, the tumor features small round cells and areas of extensive necrosis. On imaging, these lesions resemble Wilms' tumors. A large heterogeneous mass with areas of necrosis and minimal or no enhancement are found. Calcifications may be present.[20]

Neuroblastoma

Primary renal neuroblastomas have been reported but are rare. Imaging appearances resemble those of Wilms' tumor. Secondary renal involvement from contiguous adrenal and retroperitoneal neuroblastoma is more common and an incidence of 20 percent of cases has been reported.[38] Renal invasion occurs more frequently in undifferentiated histology and high stage (3 or 4) tumors. Extension may occur by tumor spread along vessels or by direct infiltration of the renal capsule, specially the upper pole contiguous with the adrenal gland.

Other rare primary tumors of the kidney are *renal medullary carcinoma,[3] metanephric stromal tumor and hemangiopericytoma* or *reninoma.[2] Metastases* to the kidney are extremely rare in children. Osteosarcoma metastases have been reported.[39]

CYSTIC DISEASES OF THE KIDNEY

Although simple cysts of the kidneys are more common in adults, they are more frequent in childhood than was previously appreciated and may even be seen *in utero*. The routine use of US nowadays and its high sensitivity in the diagnosis of cystic lesions, account for the increased number of cysts reported.

It is believed that if a cyst is small, asymptomatic and meets all the standard US criteria for a simple cyst (no internal echoes or septations, good through transmission, smooth wall) then no further evaluation is required. Follow-up sonography is recommended to detect changes in the size or appearance of the cyst that might indicate the need for surgical treatment. If a cyst is symptomatic (producing hypertension or dangerously attenuating the overlying cortex), surgery may be indicated despite a benign appearance at US.

If a cystic lesion fails to meet the criteria for a simple renal cyst, then additional imaging studies, e.g. CT or MRI, are indicated, to exclude developmental lesions (e.g. multicystic dysplastic kidney) or cystic neoplasms (cystic Wilms' tumor, clear cell sarcoma and multilocular cystic renal tumor).

ADRENAL MASSES

Adrenal masses in children may be due to neoplasms, hemorrhage, abscess and cysts. Neoplasms of the adrenal gland may arise from the medulla or the cortex. Medullary neoplasms are of neural crest origin and so may arise not only from the adrenal medulla but also from the sympathetic chain and include neuroblastoma, ganglioneuroblastoma, ganglioneuroma and pheochromocytoma. Adrenal cortical neoplasms are the carcinoma and adenoma. Rarely other neoplasms like smooth muscle tumors can occur in children.

NEUROBLASTOMA

Neuroblastoma (NBL) is by far the most frequent adrenal neoplasm, being the third most common pediatric malignancy, after leukemia and central nervous system tumors.[40] It is also the most common malignancy encountered in the first month of life. The median age of diagnosis is 2 years and 90 percent of the diagnoses are made in children under the age of 5 years.[41] The tumor is congenital and cases have been identified on in utero ultrasound examination. There is a genetic predisposition to neuroblastoma and the tumor has occurred in siblings and in identical twins.[42]

Site

Neuroblastomas arise from primordial neural crest cells, which are the precursors of the sympathetic nervous system. As a result they can be found anywhere along the sympathetic chain or in the adrenal medulla. Two thirds of NBLs are located in the abdomen and of these approximately two-thirds arise in the adrenal gland and the rest from the retropritoneal sympathetic ganglia, followed by the posterior mediastinum (20%).[43] Less common sites are the pelvis (2–3%) and the neck (1–5%). Occasionally, in the presence of metastatic disease, no definite primary tumor can be found.

Clinical Features

NBL has overall a wide spectrum of clinical symptoms which depend on the site, extent and the biological features of the primary tumor, and the presence of distant metastatic disease. The majority of children with NBL present with a palpable abdominal mass. This may be an incidental finding in an otherwise healthy child or in a child clearly unwell with lethargy, anemia, weight loss and failure to thrive from widespread dissemination of tumor. In half of the patients with intraspinal tumor extension, peripheral neurologic deficits and neurological symptoms from compression of the nerve roots or the cord may be present.[42] Metastatic involvement of the periorbital bones and soft tissues results in ecchymosed orbital proptosis, which is also described as "raccoon eyes" and may be misinterpreted as non-accidental injury. Compression of the optic nerves by metastases may cause blindness. Massive hepatic metastases can cause increased intra-abdominal pressure and death from respiratory insufficiency. Encephalopathic symptoms may be encountered. In less than 2 percent of cases, NBLs can present with paraneoplastic syndromes: opsoclonus-myoclonus-ataxia syndrome or watery diarrhea.[44] NBLs may also be discovered incidentally during scanning for other reasons, e.g. antenatal ultrasound, chest radiograph for pneumonia or screening protocols.

Urinary excretion of high levels of catecholamine metabolites occurs in 85-90 percent of patients. These metabolites are identified as vanillylmandelic acid (VMA) and homovanillic acid (HVA). The VMA/HVA ratio in patients with disseminated disease correlates with prognosis. Vanillacetic acid (VLA) in urine indicates a poor prognosis.[45]

Pathology

The tumors arise from the primitive neuroectodermal cells. Histologically, NBLs are composed of small round and rosette forming cells which may be difficult to distinguish from similar round cells seen in Ewing's sarcoma, rhabdomyosarcoma, and even leukemia. Classically three different types of neural crest tumors are described based on the degree of differentiation of these primitive cells and subsequent variable malignancy. Neuroblastoma is considered the most malignant, ganglioneuroma a benign and ganglioneuroblastoma with a mixed mature and undifferentiated histology as a "semi malignant" or intermediate manifestation of this neoplastic disease. Within a given tumor the state of maturation may change: especially in an infant, the degree of malignancy may decrease and the neoplastic process may disappear.

Staging

The age of the patient and the stage of disease at diagnosis are the two most important predictors of survival in neuroblastoma. The International Neuroblastoma Staging System (INSS)[46] is based on radiological findings, surgical resectability, lymph node involvement and bone marrow involvement (Table 16.3). Patients with stage 1 have greater than 90 percent 5-year survival. The

Table 16.3: International neuroblastoma staging system[46]
Stage 1: Localized tumor confined to the area of origin; complete gross resection with or without microscopic residual disease; identifiable ipsilateral and contralateral lymph nodes negative macroscopically.
Stage 2A: Localized tumor with incomplete gross excision, identifiable ipsilateral and contralateral lymph nodes negative microscopically.
Stage 2B: Unilateral tumor with complete or incomplete gross resection with positive ipsilateral regional lymph nodes contralateral lymph nodes negative microscopically.
Stage 3: Tumor infiltrating across the midline with or without regional lymph node involvement; unilateral tumor with contralateral regional lymph node involvement; or midline tumor with bilateral regional lymph node involvement.
Stage 4: Dissemination of tumor to distant lymph nodes, bone, bone marrow, liver, or other organs (except as defined in stage 4S).
Stage 4S: Localized primary tumor (as defined for stage 1 or 2) with dissemination limited to skin, liver, or bone marrow (<10 percent tumor cells, and MIBG scan negative in the marrow) limited to infants <1 year of age.

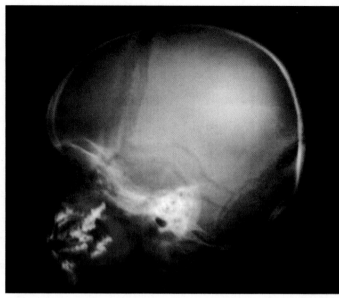

Fig. 16.12: Lateral film of the skull shows sutural widening due to underlying dural involvement

survival rate falls with increasing stage of disease, the exception being stage 4S in which the survival can be between 60-90 percent. Spontaneous regression has been demonstrated in a small group of stage 4S patients. The overall survival of patients less than 1 year of age is almost 75 percent. As the age of the patient at diagnosis increases the survival rate falls.[42]

A more recently introduced recognized variant of NBL, stage 4N (N=nodes) has been described which is not included in the INSS classification. This has been added for children with distant nodal spread, but no bony cortical involvement on account of better prognosis.[44]

Imaging

Imaging of neuroblastoma requires evaluation of the primary tumor and the metastatic extent of disease.

Plain radiographs: Abdominal radiographs may show the presence of an abdominal mass. One of the characteristic findings in neuroblastoma is calcification, which can be demonstrated in about one half of abdominal neuroblastomas (compared with only less than 10% in Wilms' tumor). The calcification is usually finely stippled but may also be linear or ring shaped and can sometimes be seen in areas of metastases such as lymph nodes or liver. Evidence of erosion of vertebral body or widened interpedicular distance suggests intraspinal extension.

If the child has presented with bone pain, it is likely that initial imaging will include skeletal radiographs. Discrete lytic areas or metaphyseal lucencies are typical of metastatic involvement and plain film appearances can simulate leukemic infiltration. However, the bones may appear normal even in the presence of metastases. Skull radiographs may also show lytic areas or sutural widening due to underlying dural involvement (Fig. 16.12).

Ultrasound: The mass is seen as a predominantly solid, poorly defined, heterogeneous, echogenic mass with few echopoor areas.

Calcification is commonly seen (Fig. 16.13A). The displaced kidney can be identified, most often inferolateral to the mass, with a well defined plane between the mass and the kidney. In rare cases a neuroblastoma may invade the kidney and then it is impossible to differentiate from Wilms' tumor. The tumor often extends across the midline and can be seen to encase and anteriorly displace the aorta, IVC and other vascular structures rather than invade them. The opposite kidney may also be displaced by large masses. US is useful in detecting differential movements of the tumor relative to the adjacent organs i.e. liver and ipsilateral kidney. If there is no differential movement, involvement is likely. Nodal and focal hepatic metastases can be identified.

Antenatal and perinatal US examination has resulted in an apparent increase in the incidence of fetal or congenital neuroblastoma. The US appearance is variable and ranges from cystic through solid to mixed with foci of calcification.[46] The differential diagnosis of this appearance is adrenal hemorrhage, extralobar pulmonary sequestration and congenital mesoblastic nephroma.

CT and MR Imaging: Further axial imaging for staging of a newly discovered NBL can be performed with either CT or MRI of the primary site. Both modalities can accurately assess the location and the size of the primary tumor, the vascular encasement and tumor resectability, but may sometimes be equivocal in the evaluation of invasive growth and lymphadenopathy. MRI is superior to CT in determining marrow infiltration and intraspinal extension of tumor.

On CT, a NBL is seen as a large, heterogeneous, lobulated soft-tissue mass that shows mild heterogeneous enhancement. Coarse, finely stippled or curvilinear calcifications are seen in more than 90% of the abdominal (Figs 16.13B and 16.14A and B) and 50% of the thoracic NBLs on CT.[44] Low attenuation areas seen within the tumor represent necrosis or hemorrhage. On MRI, the

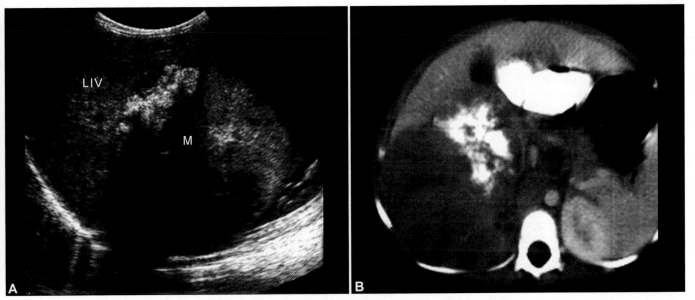

Figs 16.13A and B: Neuroblastoma. (A) US and (B) Contrast enhanced axial CT shows a solid, right adrenal mass with a large area of calcification within. Multiple retroperitoneal nodes are also seen on CT

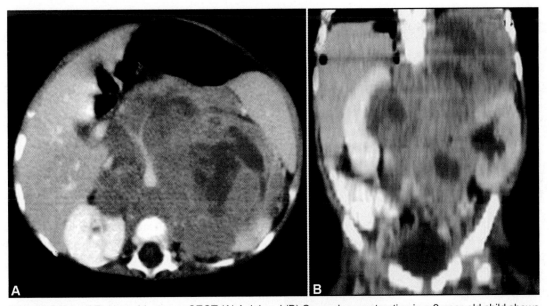

Figs 16.14A and B: Neuroblastoma. CECT (A) Axial and (B) Coronal reconstruction in a 2-year-old child shows a large lobulated left abdominal mass with few hypodense necrotic areas within. The mass elevates and encases the aorta and its branches. The IVC is displaced anteriorly and to the right. The left kidney is displaced inferolaterally and shows the negative beak sign suggesting an extra renal origin.

tumor is typically heterogeneous, with low signal on T1- and high signal intensity on T2-weighted images, and shows little or no enhancement (Figs 16.15A and B). Cystic and hemorrhagic areas within the tumor can be well identified but not calcification. On diffusion-weighted images, NBLs show increased tumor signal which is attributed to restricted diffusion of water protons within the dense tumor matrix.[47]

The tumor is usually lobulated and lacks an identifiable capsule. Involved nodes at the renal hila, porta, and in the retroperitoneum are often large. Distinguishing between the primary tumor and the adjacent nodal disease is often difficult. Adrenal tumors frequently displace the ipsilateral kidney inferiorly while paravertebral tumors may push the kidney anteriorly.

Both CT and MRI can demonstrate retrocrural and paravertebral extension and encasement and compression of the major abdominal vessels. Spinal canal extension is more common with thoracic than with abdominal tumors and the extent of extension, spinal cord displacement and compression are better seen on MRI.

Hepatic metastases have two distinct patterns—either diffuse infiltration seen in 4S infants, which maybe indiscernible on CT, but is clearly seen on MRI as characteristically bright signal on

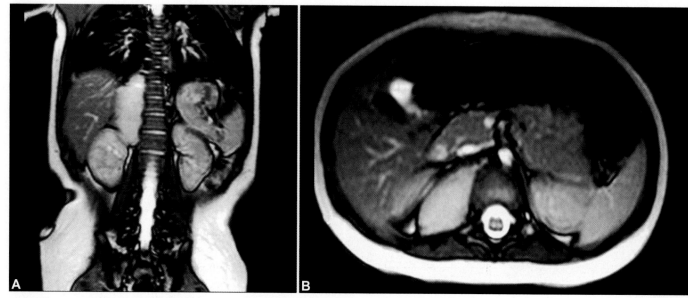

Figs 16.15A and B: Paravertebral neuroblastoma. (A) Coronal and (B) Axial T2-weighted MR images in a child presenting with opsoclonus-myoclonus syndrome show a well defined hyperintense solid mass seen in the right paravertebral region superior to the right kidney. There is no evidence of intraspinal extension of the tumor

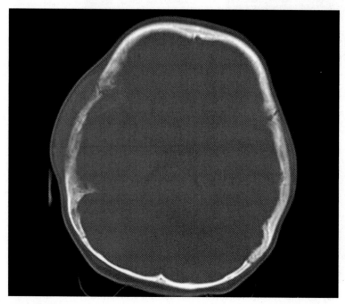

Fig. 16.16: Cranial metastasis in neuroblastoma. CT cranium shows bony erosion of the right parietal bone with overlying soft tissue thickening

T2-weighted images; or focal nodular lesions seen in older children with stage 4 disease which can be readily identified on both CT and MRI. Lung metastases are rare, occurring in approximately 3% cases.[48] MRI plays an important role is assessing disseminated disease in the bone marrow. Bone marrow disease is usually seen as diffuse infiltration but it may also present a nodular pattern with areas of low and high signal intensity on T1- and T2-weighted images, respectively. Both CT and MRI may be needed for detection and follow-up of cranial disease particularly with recurrent disease. Bony erosion is identified on CT (Fig. 16.16),

both CT and MRI can demonstrate soft tissue deposits and focal dural involvement whereas diffuse leptomeningeal disease is best seen on contrast enhanced MRI.

Some studies suggest that MRI with whole body short time inversion recovery (STIR) imaging can replace the combination of CT and bone scintigraphy for overall assessment of stage 4 disease in children with NBL, reducing the radiation exposure and the number of sedation procedures required.[49]

Nuclear scanning: Two-thirds of patients with neuroblastoma have metastatic bone disease at diagnosis. *^{99m}Technetium methylene diphosphonate (^{99m}Tc MDP) whole-body bone scintigraphy* should be performed on all patients at diagnosis. It is more sensitive than a radiographic skeletal survey. Plain radiographs should be performed on suspicious areas of abnormal increased tracer uptake. The primary tumor frequently takes up ^{99m}Tc MDP and is consequently seen on bone data acquisition.[50]

MIBG (metaiodobenzylguanidine) imaging plays an important role in diagnosis and follow-up of patients with NBL. MIBG labeled with either I^{123} or I^{131} should be done in all patients. MIBG is an analogue of catecholamine precursors and is taken up by catecholamine-producing cells and although other neuroendocrine tumors such as phaeochromocytoma, medullary carcinoma of thyroid and carcinoid tumors also take up MIBG, these are extremely rare in the pediatric population. Therefore, uptake of MIBG is considered specific for neuroblastoma.

MIBG is taken up by both—the primary tumor and metastases and shows high sensitivity (88%) and specificity (99%) in detecting primary tumor and metastatic involvement (cortical bone, bone marrow and lymph nodes) in more than 90 percent of patients.[49] MIBG scanning is less sensitive than MDP at detecting bone involvement, and using only MIBG may result in an underestimate of bone metastases. False negative MIBG scans do occur and therefore many centers combine MIBG and MDP in the diagnostic work-up of children with NBL to minimize the incidence of false-positive or false-negative results.

Positron Emission Tomography (PET), using [18]fluoro-2-deoxy-glucose, has emerged as a promising modality for revealing NBL in both soft-tissue and skeleton. FDG uptake is directly proportional to tumor burden and to tumor-cell proliferation. Primary tumor and metastatic spread concentrate FDG avidly before therapy, whereas after therapy variable patterns of accumulation have been observed. PET scanning can be useful in MIBG-negative cases and during follow-up when assessing response to treatment.[51]

Differential Diagnosis

The differential diagnosis encompasses all pediatric abdominal masses, particularly Wilms' tumor (discussed in earlier section), teratoma, lymphoma, metastatic retroperitoneal lymphadenopathy and rhabdoid tumor. A congenital neuroblastoma diagnosed in the neonatal period needs to be differentiated from neonatal adrenal hemorrhage. The diagnosis of adrenal hemorrhage is usually made by ultrasound, which identifies the mass and shows, in sequential examinations, decreasing size and cystic evolution. Color Doppler is useful to show avascularity of adrenal hemorrhage. MRI may show the classic signal intensity pattern of aging blood products, but diagnostic difficulties can occur because of bleeds of different ages. Other pediatric adrenal tumors, such as phaeochromocytoma and adrenal carcinoma, are much less common.

Management and Follow-up

Treatment depends on several factors, including stage of the disease at the time of presentation and response to initial therapy. Surgery, chemotherapy and radiation therapy all have a role to play. Primary surgical resection is done for localized tumors and initial chemotherapy for those that are unresectable, followed by delayed surgery once they decrease in size.

The imaging strategy in the follow-up period depends largely on the imaging protocols followed by various pediatric oncology set-ups. Regular follow-up is required after surgery to assess the tumor bed for local recurrence. Follow-up is also essential in non operable tumors to assess response to chemotherapy and to determine the most appropriate time for delayed surgery. Imaging includes chest radiographs, abdominal US, and CT/MRI of the primary site. [99m]Tc MDP and I[123] MIBG scanning are performed until they have returned to normal or until the end of treatment.[51]

GANGLIONEUROBLASTOMA

A ganglioneuroblastoma is intermediate in aggressiveness in the spectrum of neural crest tumors between the frankly malignant neuroblastoma and the benign ganglioneuroma. Most occur in the abdomen and thorax. Clinically, they present with effects of a mass lesion, hormonal manifestations being rare. Occasionally they can be discovered incidentally on radiographs performed for some other purpose.

Imaging and investigation are the same as described for neuroblastomas (Figs 16.17A to C). Catecholamine excretion is usually increased. Biopsy is required for diagnosis but sampling errors may occur due to variable tumor composition.[51]

GANGLIONEUROMA

This tumor is benign and is formed of nerve fibres and mature ganglion cells. Most ganglioneuromas occur in the posterior mediastinum. Only one-third occur in the abdomen, and most are paravertebral, rarely from adrenal medulla. These tumors generally occur in older children or adolescents, who are often asymptomatic. Hormonally active lesions are rare. They may be discovered incidentally on radiographs or present with mass effect.

The imaging appearances are similar to those of neuroblastoma but unlike NBLs, they are well encapsulated masses. The abdominal lesions may even encase the aorta and the inferior vena cava and their branches or invade the spinal canal. The definitive diagnosis depends on histological examination of tumor tissue. Surgical removal may be difficult particularly when the mass is encasing vital structures or with intraspinal extension. In these cases conservative management is advocated with regular clinical and imaging follow-up.[51,52]

PHEOCHROMOCYTOMA

Pheochromocytoma is an uncommon neoplasm in children.[42] Like neuroblastoma, pheochromocytoma is of neural crest origin, secretes catecholamines, and may be located in the adrenal medulla or anywhere along the sympathetic chain. In children, 70 percent of phaeochromocytomas occur in the adrenal gland and 20 percent have bilateral involvement. 30 percent have extra adrenal involvement, and most of these occur in the upper abdomen. Other less common extra adrenal sites include the sympathetic chain anywhere from base of skull to pelvis, urinary bladder, spermatic cord and vagina. Multiple lesions are present in 30-70 percent of children. Malignancy occurs in less than 10 percent.[53]

Pheochromocytoma usually presents in older children and a familial occurrence is well documented. It has been seen as a part of multiple endocrine neoplasia syndrome (MEN 2). It has also been associated with a number of diseases, including neurofibro-matosis, von Hippel-Lindau disease and Sturge-Weber syndrome.

Clinical Presentation

Clinical presentation is usually related to the secretion of catecholamines. Patients may present with hypertension, sweating, headaches, visual blurring, flushing, tachycardia, hypertensive encephalopathy, weight loss and diarrhea. Urinary catecholamines are usually markedly elevated, much more so than with neuroblastoma.[42]

Imaging

On ultrasound a phaeochromocytoma may be seen as a well defined hypoechoic mass which may be homogenous or heterogenous due to hemorrhage and necrosis (Fig. 16.18A). Calcification is uncommon. Sonography easily detects lesions in and adjacent to adrenal glands but is less sensitive than CT and MRI for lesions in

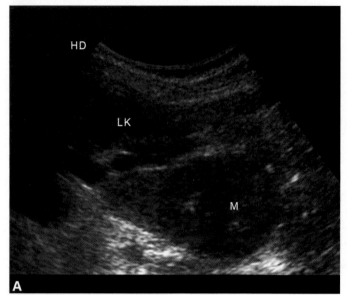

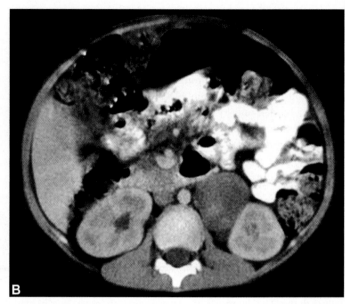

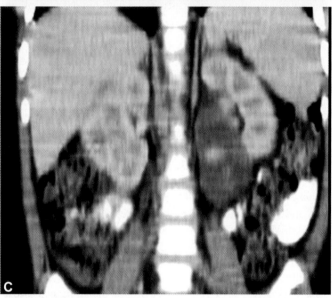

Figs 16.17A to C: Paravertebral ganglioneuroblastoma in a 10 -month infant. (A) Longitudinal US and (B and C) Contrast enhanced CT (axial and coronal reformation) shows a well defined, oval, solid mass medial and inferior to lower pole of left kidney displacing it laterally. The imaging features cannot differentiate it from a paravertebral neuroblastoma. The diagnosis was made on histopathology.

mid and lower abdomen.[52] On CT, the lesions have a soft tissue attenuation with diffuse, mottled or rim-like enhancement (Fig. 16.18B). Adrenergic blockade, to prevent a hypertensive crisis, is not required prior to nonionic contrast administration during CT scanning.[17] On MRI, phaeochromocytomas have a low signal on T1-weighted images and high signal on T2-weighted images, with intense enhancement and slow wash-out after contrast administration. Malignancy is best determined by identifying distant metastases to nonchromaffin tissues like lung, liver, bone and lymph nodes.[53] I[131] MIBG can accurately localize a phaeochromocytoma, but does not show the anatomy as well as CT or MRI. It is particularly helpful in detecting nonadrenal tumors (paragangliomas). MIBG may be positive in the abdomen even when an US is negative and MIBG should always be done prior to surgery to detect or exclude multiple sites of disease.

ADRENAL CORTICAL TUMORS

Adrenocortical tumors (ACT) are very rare in children with a worldwide annual incidence of 0.3 per million children below the age of 15 years. Seventy-five percent of children who develop adrenocortical tumors are less than 5 years old at the time of diagnosis. The incidence is higher in young girls with a female/male ratio of 2:1, whereas in adolescence the sex ratio is equal. Two syndromes have a clear association with this tumor: Li–Fraumeni syndrome is associated with mutations of the *p53* gene, and Beckwith–Wiedemann syndrome which has mutations in the 11p15 region.[54]

Clinical Features

More than 75 percent of adrenocortical tumors are functional, secreting one or more hormones (androgens, cortisol, aldosterone,

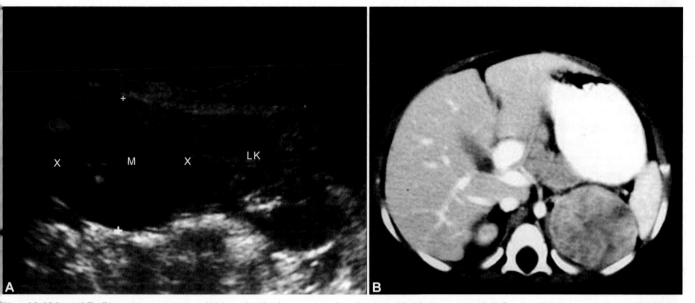

Figs 16.18A and B: Pheochromocytoma. (A) Longitudinal sonogram in a 2-year-old girl shows a well defined, solid, hypoechoic mass with few small hyperechoic foci in the left suprarenal region (M = mass, LK = left kidney). (B) Contrast-enhanced CT shows the tumor as a well defined solid mass which shows mottled enhancement.

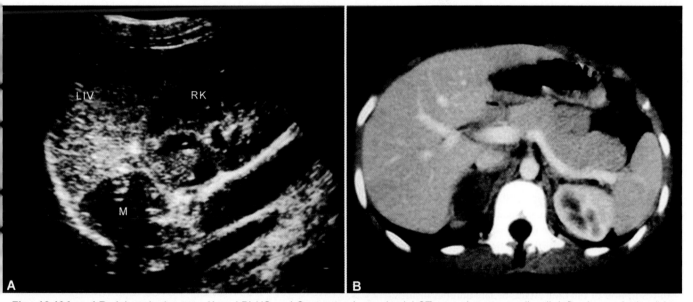

Figs 16.19A and B: Adrenal adenoma. (A and B) US and Contrast enhanced axial CT scan shows a small well defined mass in the right suprarenal region in a 12 year old boy, hypodense on CT with no evidence of calcification.

or estrogens). Virilization, with early onset of pubic hair, hypertrophy of the clitoris or penis, accelerated growth, gynaecomastia or acne, is the most common presentation. The second most common manifestation is with hypercortisolism (Cushing's syndrome), whilst presentation with a palpable abdominal mass is unusual. Hypertension may be seen in up to 43 percent at diagnosis.[55] This may be due to either mineralocorticoid or glucocorticoid excess, increased aldosterone production or simply renal artery compression by the tumor, and the hypertension usually resolves after tumor resection. Diagnosis of an ACT is supported by raised levels of androstenedione,

dehydroepiandrosterone sulphate (DHEAS), testosterone, and urinary steroids. These hormones are also useful markers for the detection of tumor recurrence during follow-up. The combination of hormone production and adrenal mass is diagnostic of an adrenocortical tumor.

Imaging Features

On all 3 modalities (US, CT and MRI), the smaller lesions tend to have a fairly homogenous appearance (Figs 16.19A and B) and areas of hemorrhage, necrosis and calcification are seen in the larger lesions. A characteristic central scar with radiating linear bands representing areas of necrosis and calcification is often seen in the large lesion.[53]

The tumor tends to be locally aggressive and frequently invades the IVC and may extend into the right atrium.[56] The tumor may also metastasize to lung, nodes, bone, and liver. MR imaging is the modality of choice and demonstrates the primary tumor, caval extension, and liver metastases.[57] Chest CT to exclude or detect pulmonary metastases should be performed at first diagnosis.

The classification of benign from malignant ACTs is not clear cut and is the subject of much debate.[17] Even established histopathological criteria and algorithms adapted from tumors in adults do not allow a clear classification in children. Differentiation between adenoma and carcinoma is in practice somewhat arbitrary, and all patients (even those with a seemingly benign adenoma completely resected) require close follow-up initially. The majority of ACTs in children are interpreted pathologically as malignant in most studies. Factors favoring malignancy include size over 5–10 cm, weight over 200 g, invasion into the periadrenal soft tissues or IVC.[17]

Surgical resection is the mainstay of treatment. Younger children, particularly those less than 5 years, with pathologically malignant ACTs, have a significantly better prognosis than older children and adolescents.[17]

ADRENAL HEMORRHAGE

Adrenal hemorrhage occurs almost exclusively in newborns in association with perinatal asphyxia, trauma or bacterial (typically meningococcal) septicemia. The precise cause is unknown but is thought to be stress related or due to birth trauma, as there is an increased frequency in larger babies or babies of diabetic mothers. The hemorrhagic process may involve the whole gland or part of one, or both adrenal glands in about 10 percent of cases.

Clinical Features

In a moderate or massive degree of adrenal hemorrhage, there is clinically a palpable flank mass due to the caudal displacement of the ipsilateral kidney from the hemorrhagic mass. The mass is usually not palpable at birth and develops over the following 24 hours. The child will often become jaundiced and present with vomiting. The mass typically regresses within days to a few weeks with resorption of the clot. Acute or late adrenal insufficiency is uncommon, even in bilateral adrenal hemorrhage.

Imaging Features

US demonstrates a suprarenal mass that is variable in echogenicity.[57] In the acute phase, the hemorrhage is usually echogenic, representing clot formation (Fig. 16.20). Over several weeks, the hemorrhage becomes echofree as the clot lyses and becomes liquefied. The hemorrhage gradually decreases in size and may result in adrenal calcification. If there is no evidence of ultrasonographic resolution after several days, other diagnoses, including neuroblastoma and its variants, but also benign conditions such as an adrenal cyst or extraadrenal abnormality from a surrounding structure including an enteric duplication cyst, need to be considered.

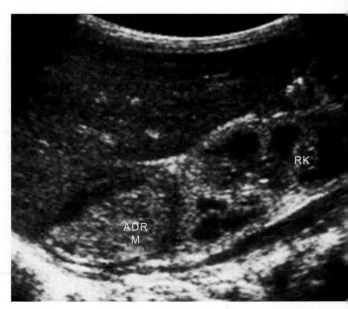

Fig. 16.20: Adrenal hemorrhage. Longitudinal US scan through the right flank in a 9 day old infant shows a well defined cystic mass in the right suprarenal regional with a fluid-fluid level.

In older children, post traumatic adrenal hemorrhage has been described to occur in some 3 percent of blunt abdominal injury and often associated with ipsilateral lesions of the liver, kidney or spleen. It seems more likely to occur on the right side, is usually asymptomatic and, also, without evidence of subsequent adrenal insufficiency.[52]

ADRENAL CYSTS

Large adrenal cysts may be found in older children. These are usually endothelial lined and found incidentally. Their importance lies in their being mistaken for adrenal neoplasms. If cross sectional imaging shows a smooth thin walled cyst without any evidence of solid components, and there is no endocrine dysfunction, hypertension, infection or metastatic disease, they can be managed conservatively because adrenal neoplasms seldom have large cystic components and never present as thin smooth walled cystic structures without solid components.

PRIMARY RETROPERITONEAL TUMORS

Primary tumors of retroperitoneum are rare tumors that originate in the retroperitoneal space but outside the major organs in that space. These neoplasms are generally derived from neurogenic cells, embryonic rests or mesenchymal cells and may be benign or malignant.

NEUROGENIC TUMORS

Neurogenic tumors may arise from tissue of the sympathetic (autonomic) nervous system and include extra-adrenal neuroblastoma (Fig. 16.15), ganglio-neuroblastoma (Fig. 16.17) and ganglioneuroma, or from neuroectoderm as in the case of a primitive peripheral neuroectodermal tumor. Extra-adrenal pheochromocytoma also arises in the retroperitoneum. The site of origin of all these tumors is in the paravertebral gutter with resultant

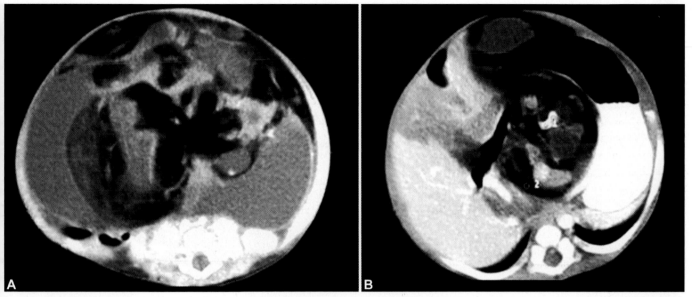

Figs 16.21A and B: Teratoma. (A) Contrast-enhanced axial CT section shows a large well defined heterogenous mass with cystic, solid and fat attenuation components in a 3-month-old child. (B) A higher section shows the presence of a tooth within the mass, clinching the diagnosis

anterior and lateral displacement of other retroperitoneal structures including kidneys, ureters and the inferior vena cava. Their imaging and investigations are similar to that of their adrenal counterparts and have been discussed above. Uncommon neuro-ectodermal tumors are paraganglioma, neurofibroma, neurofibrosarcoma, neurolemmoma, or schwannoma. Although occasionally isolated tumors, they are often seen as multiple tumors in patients with neurofibromatosis.[58]

GERM CELL TUMORS

Germ cell tumors are derived from the primordial germinal epithelial layer cells and two-thirds of these tumors are extragonadal in location. These include germinomas, embryonal carcinoma, endodermal sinus tumor, choriocarcinoma, gonadoblastoma and teratoma. *Teratomas*, the most common of germ cell tumor, account for 3.5 - 4 percent of all germ cell tumors in children. They contain all three embryonal layers – ectoderm, mesoderm and endoderm. They are the third most common tumors of the retroperitoneum in children following neuroblastoma and Wilms' tumor. The ratio of girls to boys is 2:1. Malignancy is seen in 10-15 percent cases.[60] Increase in abdominal girth is the most common presenting symptom, frequently accompanied by pain, nausea, vomiting and weight loss. The presence of a palpable abdominal mass is an almost universal finding. Occasionally, the tumor is present antenatally and diagnosed at birth, these neonatal teratomas have a higher incidence of malignancy than those in older children. Malignant teratomas can produce alpha-fetoprotein and its serum levels can be used to monitor response to therapy/recurrence.[61]

Imaging

Plain radiographs may demonstrate calcification or formed bony components such as teeth and phalanges, which are pathognomic.

The tumor may be cystic, solid, or mixed. Although US demonstrates the solid or cystic nature of the tumor, CT defines the true location and character of the mass better and is useful to delineate the extent of the disease in retroperitoneum and its relationship to major vessels (Figs 16.21A and B). Fat may be identified in about half the cases and fat fluid levels may sometimes be seen. Internal homogeneity, fat density, cyst formation, and calcification are important predictors of a benign retroperitoneal tumor on CT.[62]

MESENCHYMAL TUMORS

Lipomatous Tumors

These are often quite large at the time of diagnosis and are usually benign. They include lipoma, lipoblastoma and liposarcoma-like lipoblastomatosis. These tumors are best visualized on CT and MRI, showing homogeneous fatty attenuation at CT and homogeneous signal identical to that of fat on all MR imaging sequences. The boundaries of the mass are clearly delineated because of marked contrast in signal intensity with surrounding structures. Lipoblastoma is extensive and locally invasive, and difficult or impossible to remove completely. Its appearance on imaging studies may be similar to lipoma but some cases have shown areas of relatively increased attenuation on CT, which on pathologic examination have been shown to be regions of myxoid material. Liposarcoma is extremely rare in children, but is locally invasive and also metastatic to distant sites.

Rhabdomyosarcoma and Undifferentiated Sarcomas

Rhabdomyosarcoma (RMS) accounts for 5 to 8 percent of childhood cancer and presents in a wide variety of histologic types and patterns of spread of tumor. Retroperitoneal rhabdomyosarcomas are rare tumors. The tumors infiltrate locally, invade

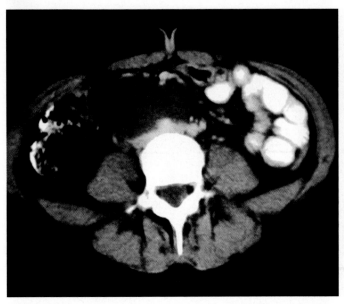

Fig. 16.22: Lymphangioma. Contrast enhanced axial CT shows a cystic mass in midline with thin imperceptible walls, just anterior to the major abdominal vessels, displacing the mesenteric vessels anteriorly

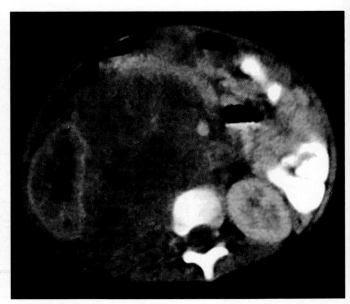

Fig. 16.23: Metastatic testicular germ cell tumor. Contrast-enhanced CT shows massive, low attenuation retroperitoneal lymphadenopathy displacing the right kidney laterally (negative beak sign seen) in a diagnosed case of testicular germ cell tumor in a 2-year-old boy

lymphatics and blood vessels, and frequently present with distant hematogenous metastases to the lungs, bone marrow, and bone. Retroperitoneal lymph nodes, bone marrow metastases, and distant hematogenous metastases to the lungs are common at presentation. Other sarcomas occasionally seen in children and adolescents include fibrosarcoma, neurofibrosarcoma, malignant fibrous histiocytoma, hemangiopericytoma and leiomyosarcoma.[59]

RETROPERITONEAL LYMPHANGIOMA

Retroperitoneal lymphangioma is a benign tumor of congenital lymphatic origin. Cystic lymphangioma or hygroma consist of multiple dilated, poorly developed lymphatic channels. The cystic spaces are lined with endothelium and contain multiple thin septa and chylous fluid. Although it may present early as a palpable abdominal mass, the soft nature of this lesion, makes it difficult to identify on physical examination. The mass may compress adjacent structures, particularly displacing and obstructing the ureters. On US, a lymphangioma is seen as a cystic mass with multiple, apparently noncommunicating, fluid containing cystic regions, separated by thin septae. CT also shows the cystic nature of the mass, although the septae are not well seen (Fig. 16.22). Rarely hemorrhage or infection may complicate a lymphangioma.

LYMPH NODE MASSES

Isolated retroperitoneal lymph node enlargement in children is unusual and associated findings help to clarify the diagnosis. Retroperitoneal lymphadenopathy can be benign, most often infective—tubercular, or it can occur with a variety of malignant processes including metastatic lymph node enlargement or lymphoma.

Metastasis to retroperitoneal nodes in children occur by spread from primary retroperitoneal malignancies such as Wilms' tumor,

neuroblastoma, or spread from testicular or ovarian malignancies (Fig. 16.23). Intra-abdominal lymphoma in children is nearly always non-Hodgkin's lymphoma, most commonly Burkitt's lymphoma. Retroperitoneal lymphadenopathy generally occurs along with bowel, hepatic or spleen involvement. Initial presentation with retroperitoneal masses is uncommon and more likely to be associated with lymphomas related to pharmacologic immunosuppression.[63]

CT is the most frequently used modality for evaluation of enlarged nodes. However, MRI, especially fat suppressed T2-weighted images are very sensitive for the detection of lymph nodes and performs better than CT particularly in children who have a paucity of fat. CT and MRI use nonspecific criterion of size and are limited in their ability to differentiate benign from malignant nodes. Contrast enhanced MR lymphography using ultrasmall supermagnetic iron oxide (USPIO) particles is a promising technique in differentiating benign from metastatic nodes and providing information on lymph node morphology and function.[64] FDG-PET may be more sensitive and specific for evaluation of lymphomas and certain retroperitoneal metastases depending on the primary.

RETROPERITONEAL ABSCESS AND HEMATOMA

Tuberculous spondylitis is the commonest cause of an iliopsoas abscess in our country. The inflammatory mass shows a variety of appearances ranging from diffuse homogeneous enlargement of the iliopsoas muscle to discrete masses containing central areas of low CT attenuation or high signal intensity on T2-weighted MR images (Figs 16.24A to C). Post contrast images show abscesses as expansile lesions with nonenhancing necrotic centers, intense peripheral enhancement and enhancement of the surrounding tissue. Calcification may occasionally be seen on CT and plain

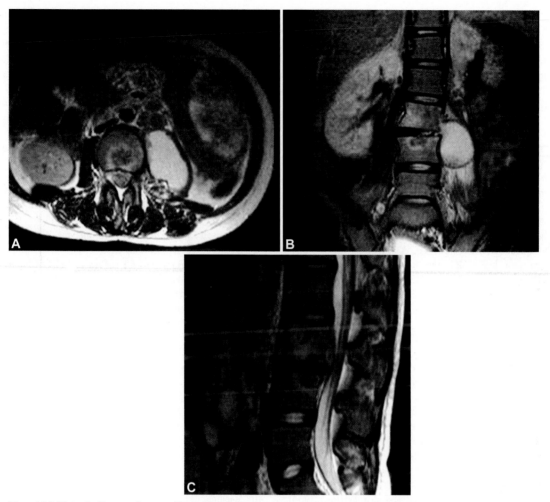

Figs 16.24A to C: Psoas abscess (A) Axial (T2W), (B) Coronal (STIR) and (C) Sagittal T2-weighted MR images show the abscess as a well defined hyperintense lesion with a smooth hypointense rim in the left psoas muscle. The whole muscle appears hyperintense. Vertebral and discal involvement is well seen. A small epidural extension of the abscess can be seen in the sagittal section

radiographs. Although vertebral involvement can be well appreciated on both CT and MRI, MRI scores over CT in detecting intraspinal extension of the inflammatory granulation tissue/abscess and cord compression). US can detect the psoas abscess as a sonolucent region within the psoas muscle with associated fluid along the margins of the psoas and can serve as a guide for diagnostic and therapeutic drainage of these abscesses.

Hematomas of the retroperitoneum are most commonly the result of severe blunt trauma or a surgical procedure. Spontaneous retroperitoneal hematomas, usually within the iliopsoas muscle, can be seen in patients with hemophilia or other bleeding diathesis. On US, CT and MRI the muscle is seen to be enlarged with characteristic changing pattern of a evolving hemorrhage within it.

CONCLUSION

Seventy to eighty percent of abdominal masses in infants and children are retroperitoneal in origin, renal being the most common. Imaging aims to diagnose the site, nature, extent and stage of the disease, so as to determine the appropriate management. The various imaging modalities available need to be used in a logical sequence as governed by the findings in an individual case and availability of facilities.

REFERENCES

1. Minami M, Ohmoto K, Chansangavej C, et al. Origin of abdominal tumors: useful findings and signs on tomographic imaging. Radiology 1996; 201:491-9.
2. Geller E, Smergel EM, Lowry PA. Renal neoplasms of childhood. RCNA 1997; 35(6):1391-1413.
3. Lowe HL, Isuani BH, Heller RM, et al. Paediatric renal masses: Wilms' tumor and beyond. Radiographics 2000; 20(6):1585-1603.
4. Breslow NE, Beckwith JB, Ciol M, et al. Age distribution of Wilms' tumor. Report from the National Wilms' tumor study. Cancer Res 1988; 48:1653-57.
5. Charles AK, Vujanic GM, Berry PJ. Renal tumors of childhood. Histopathology 1998; 32:293-309.
6. Lonergan GJ, Martinez-Leon MI, Agrons GA, Montemarano H, Suarez ES. Nephrogenic rests, nephroblastomatosis, and associated lesions of the kidney. RadioGraphics 1998; 18:947-968.

7. Bond JV: Bilateral Wilms' tumor: Age at diagnosis, associated congenital anomalies and possible patterns of inheritance. Lancet 1975; 2:482-484.

8. Yokomori K, Hori T, Takemura T, et al. Demonstration of both primary and secondary remission in renal tumors in children. J Paediatr Surg 1988; 23:403-09.

9. R White KS, Grossman H: Wilms' and associated renal tumors of childhood. Paedr Radiol 1990; 21:81-8.

10. D'Angio GJ, Evans AE, Breslow N, et al. The treatment of Wilms' tumor: Results of the second National Wilms' tumor study. Cancer 1981; 47:2302-11.

11. Fernbach SK, Feinstein KA, Donaldson JS, et al. Nephroblastomatosis: Comparison of CT with US and urography. Radiology 1988; 166:153.

12. Remain TAH, Siegel MJ, Shackeyord GD: Wilms' tumor in children: Abdominal CT and US evaluation. Radiology 1986; 160:501-05.

13. Ritchey ML, Kelalis P, Breslow NE, et al. Intracaval and atrial involvement with nephroblastoma: Review of National Wilms' Tumor Study-3. J Urol 1988; 140:1113.

14. Tongaonkar HB, Qureshi SS, Kurkure PA, Muckaden MA, Arora B, Yuvaraja TB. Wilms' tumor: An update. Indian J Urol 2007; 23:458-66.

15. Owens CM, Veys PA, Pritchard J, Levitt G, Imeson J, Dicks-Mireaux C. Role of chest computed tomography at diagnosis in the management of Wilms' tumor: A study by the United Kingdom Children's Cancer Study Group. J Clin Oncol 2002; 20:2768-73.

16. Ehrlich PF, Hamilton TE, Grundy P, Ritchey M, Haase G, Shamberger RC, et al. The value of surgery in directing therapy for patients with Wilms' tumor with pulmonary disease. A report from the National Wilms' Tumor Study Group (National Wilms' Tumor Study 5). J Pediatr Surg 2006; 41:162-7.

17. McHugh K. Renal and adrenal tumors in children. Cancer Imaging 2007; 7(1):41-51

18. Beckwith JB. Children at increased risk for Wilms' tumor: monitoring issues. J Pediatr 1998; 132:377-9.

19. White KS, Grossman H. Wilms' and associated renal tumors of childhood. Pediatr Radiol 1991; 21:81-88.

20. Carneiro RC, Fordham LA. Tumors of the Urinary Tract in Carty H, Brunelle F, Stringer DA, et al (Eds). Imaging Children (2nd Edn) Churchill Livingstone publications 2005; 1:777-804.

21. Grundy P, Perlman E, Rosen NS, et al. Current issues in Wilms' tumor management. Curr Probl Cancer 2005; 29:221–60. [PubMed]

22. Bolande RP, Brough AJ, Izant RJ Jr. Congenital mesoblastic nephroma of infancy: A report of eight cases and the relationship to Wilms' tumor. Paediatrics 1967; 40:272-278.

23. Chan HS, Cheng MY, Mancer K, et al. Congenital mesoblastic nephroma: Clinicoradiological study of 17 cases representing the pathological spectrum of the disease. J. Paediatrics 1987; 111(1): 64-70.

24. Agrons GA, Kingsman KD, Wagner BJ, Sotelo-Avila C. Rhabdoid tumor of the kidney in children: A comparative study. AJR Am J Roentgenol 1997; 168:447-451.

25. Charles AK, Vujanic GM, Berry PJ. Renal tumors of childhood. Histopathology 1998; 32:293-309.

26. Chung CJ, Lorenzo R, Rayder S, et al. Rhabdoid tumors of the kidney in children: CT findings. AJR Am J Roentgenol 1995; 164:697-700.

27. Hartman DS, Davis CJ, Jr, Madewell JE, Friedman AC. Primary malignant renal tumors in the second decade of life: Wilms' tumor versus renal cell carcinoma. J Urol 1982; 127:888-91.

28. Madewell JE, Goldman SM, Davis CJ, Hartman DS, Feigin DS, Lichtenstein JE. Multilocular cystic nephroma: A radiologic-pathologic correlation of 58 patients. Radiology 1983; 146:309-21.

29. Agrons GA, Wagner BJ, Davidson AJ, Suarez ES. Multilocular cystic renal tumor in children: Radiologic-pathologic correlation. RadioGraphics 1995; 15:653–69.

30. Wood BP, Muurahainen N, Anderson VM, et al. Multicystic nephroblastoma: Ultrasound diagnosis (with a pathologic-anatomic commentary). Pediatr Radiol 1982; 12:43–7.

31. Lemaitre L, Robert Y, Dubrulle F, et al. Renal angiomyolipoma: growth followed-up with CT and/or US. Radiology 1995; 197:598-602.

32. Kurosaki Y, Tanaka Y, Kuramoto K, et al. Improved CT fat detection in small kidney angiomyolipomas using thin sections and single voxel measurements. JCAT 1993; 17: 745-8.

33. Strouse PJ: Paediatric Renal Neoplasms. RCNA 1996; 34(6):1081-1100.

34. Vazquez JL, Barnewolt CE, Shamberger RC, Chung T, Perez-Atayde AR. Ossifying renal tumor of infancy presenting as a palpable abdominal mass. Pediatr Radiol 1998; 28:454-457.

35. Ito J, Shinohara N, Koyanagi T, Hanioka K. Ossifying renal tumor of infancy: The first Japanese case with long-term follow-up. Pathol Int 1998; 48:151-159.

36. Navarro O, Conolly B, Taylor G, Bagli DJ. Metanephric adenoma of the kidney: A case report. Pediatr Radiol 1999; 29:100-103.

37. Hartman DS, Davis CJ, Jr, Goldman SM, Friedman AC, Fritzsche P. Renal lymphoma: Radiologic-pathologic correlation of 21 cases. Radiology 1982; 144:759-66.

38. Albregts AE, Cohen MD, Gallani CA: Neuroblastoma invading the kidney. J Paediatric Surgery 1994; 29:930-933.

39. Raby WN, Kopplin P, Weitzman S. Metastatic osteosarcoma of the kidney presenting as renal haemorrhage. Journal of Paediatric Haematology/Oncology 1996; 18:321-22.

40. Kushner BH. Neuroblastoma: A disease requiring a multitude of imaging studies. J Nucl Med. 2004; 45:1172–88. [PubMed]

41. Kushner B, Cheung NK: Neuroblastoma: An overview Haem/Onc Annals 1993; 1:189-201.

42. Abramson SJ: Adrenal Neoplasms in children. RCNA 1997; 35(6):1415-51.

43. Rha SE, Byun JY, Jung SE, Chun HJ, Lee HG, Lee JM. Neurogenic tumors in the abdomen: Tumor types and imaging characteristics. Radiographics 2003; 23:29–43. [PubMed]

44. Hirons MP, Owens CM. Radiology of neuroblastoma in children. Eur Radiol 2001; 11:2071–81. [PubMed]

45. Currarino G, Wood B, Massond M: The genitourinary tract and Retroperitoneum. In Silverman FN, Kuhn JP (Eds): Caffey's Paediatric X-ray Diagnosis: An Integrated Imaging Approach. Mosby 1993; 2:1145-1375.

46. Brodeur GM, Pritchard J, Berthold F, et al. Revisions of the international criteria for neuroblastoma diagnosis, staging and response to treatment. J Clin Oncol 1993; 11:1466.

47. Ferraro EM, Fakhry J, Aruny JE, et al. Prenatal adrenal neuroblastoma. Case report with review of the literature. J ultrasound Medicine 1988; 7:275-278.

48. Uhl M, Altehoefer C, Kontny U, et al. MRI diffusion imaging of neuroblastomas: First results and correlation to histology. Eur Radiol 2002; 12:2335-38.

49. Lonergan GJ, Schwab CM, Suarez ES, et al. Neuroblastoma, ganglioneuroblastoma, and ganglioneuroma: radiologic-pathologic correlation. Radiograhics 2002; 22:911-34.

50. Laffan EE, O' Connor R, Ryan SP, et al. Whole body magnetic resonance imaging: A useful additional sequence in paediatric imaging. Paediatr Radiol 2004; 34:472-80.

51. Chaya SA. Neuroblastoma. In Grainger and Allison (Eds): Diagnostic Radiology: A Textbook of Medical Imaging (4th edn) 2001; 2:1483-86.

52. Willi UV. The adrenal glands. In Carty H, Brunelle F, Stringer DA, et al (Eds). Imaging Children (2nd Ed) Churchill Livingstone publications 2005; 1:975-96.

53. Daneman A. Adrenal Gland in Kuhn JP, Slovis TL, Haller JO (Eds) Caffey's Pediatric Diagnostic Imaging Vol 2, 10th edn. Mosby Publications 2004; 1894-1908.

54. Ein S, Wertzman S, Thorner P, et al. Paediatric malignant phaeochromocytoma. J Paediatr Surg 1994; 29:1197-1201.

55. Bonfig W, Bittman I, Bechtold S, et al. Virilizing adrenocortical tumors in children. Eur J Paedtiatr 2003; 162:623-628.

56. Michalkiewicz E, Sandrini R, Figueiredo B, et al. Clinical and outcome characteristics of children with adrenocortical tumors: A report from the International Pediatric Adrenocortical Tumor Registry. J Clin Oncol 2004; 22:838–45. [PubMed]

57. Godine L, Bordon W, Brasch R, et al. Adrenocortical carcinoma with extension into IVC and right atrium: Report of 3 cases in children. Pediatric Radiology 1990; 20:166-68.

58. Mittelstaedt CA, Volberg FM, Merten D, et al. The sonographic diagnosis of neonatal adrenal haemorrhage. Radiology 1979; 131:453-457.

59. Haller J. Retroperitoneal masses. In Kuhn JP, Slovis TL, Haller JO (Eds) Caffey's Pediatric Diagnostic Imaging Vol 2, 10th edn. Mosby Publications 2004; 1909-14.

60. Grosfield JL, Billimere DF. Teratomas in infancy and childhood. Curr Prob Cancer 1985; 9:1-53.

61. Rattan KN, Kadian YS, Nair VJ, et al. Primary retroperitoneal tumors in children: A single institution experience: African J of Paed Surg 2010; 7(1):5-8.

62. Hayasaka K, Yamada T, Saitoh Y, et al. CT evaluation of primary benign retroperitoneal tumor. Radiat. Med 1994; 12:115-20.

63. Parker BR. Leukemia and lymphoma in childhood. Radiol Clin North Am 1997; 35:1495.

64. Bellin MF, Lebleu L, Meric JB. Evaluation of retroperitoneal and Pelvic node metastases with MRI lymphangiography. Abdominal Imaging 2003; 28:155-63.

CHAPTER 17

Evaluation of Female Pelvis and Testicular Abnormalities

Kushaljit Singh Sodhi, Akshay Kumar Saxena

Female Pelvis

Ultrasonography (USG) is the most useful modality for imaging genital organs in infants and children, because it is a noninvasive and painless study which does not require sedation for the baby (in contrast to computed tomography (CT) and magnetic resonance (MR) exams). The lack of ionizing radiation makes ultrasound very attractive as a pediatric imaging modality.[1,2]

Knowledge of simple embryology and basic physiology is necessary in investigating cases of precocious puberty, amenorrhea, pelvic pain, pelvic masses, or ambiguous genitalia in children, which are key reasons for imaging of female pelvis in children.

CT remains useful for tumor staging, follow-up and in acute abdomen. Magnetic resonance imaging provides precise demonstration of anatomic features in multiple planes in cases of complex anomalies, when US findings are inconclusive.[3]

Normal US Anatomy of Genital Organs in Infants and Children

The size and shape of the ovaries and of uterus vary during childhood, are age dependent, and under hormonal influence. The maternal and placental hormones produce a relatively larger size of the neonatal uterus and ovaries. The uterus has a prominent, echogenic endometrial lining.[1,2]

During infancy, the size, shape, and echotexture of the uterus and ovaries remain relatively stable. However, the ovaries are never dormant and follicles or cysts can be seen at every age. Two to three years before the onset of puberty, the uterine volume gradually increases with accelerated growth occurring during puberty.[2]

The Uterus

Uterine anatomy changes with age of the child (Figs 17.1A to C). The neonatal uterus is prominent under the influence of maternal and placental hormones.[4,5] The cervix is larger than the fundus (fundus-to-cervix ratio= 1/2), the uterine length is approximately 3.5 cm, and the maximum thickness is approximately 1.4 cm. The endometrial lining is often echogenic. Some fluid can also be seen within the endometrial cavity. During infancy the proportion of cervix to uterine body changes to 1:1. This tubular shape is stable until 2 to 3 years before the onset of puberty.[2]

The prepubertal uterus has a tubular configuration (anteroposterior cervix equal to anteroposterior fundus) or sometimes a spade shape (anteroposterior cervix larger than anteroposterior fundus).[6-9] The endometrium is normally not apparent; however, high-frequency transducers can demonstrate the central lining in some cases. The length is 2.5–4 cm; the thickness does not exceed 10 mm.

During puberty the greatest growth occurs in the fundus and corpus, altering to a pear-shaped uterus (~25 ml). The pubertal uterus has the adult pear configuration (fundus larger than cervix) (fundus-to-cervix ratio = 2/1 to 3/1)[6-9] (Figs 17.1C) and is 5–8 cm long, 3 cm wide, and 1.5 cm thick. The endometrial lining is seen and varies with the phases of the menstrual cycle. The endometrial canal is seen as a thin echogenic interface and the endometrium demonstrates cyclical changes every cycle. The measurement of the endometrial thickness includes both endometrial lines.

Doppler ultrasound of the uterine artery can be used to confirm the onset of puberty. In prepubertal girls, the pulsed Doppler demonstrates a narrow systolic waveform without positive diastolic flow. In postpubertal girls, a broad systolic waveform is seen with positive diastolic flow.[6]

Ovaries

Ovarian size is usually described by assessment of the ovarian volume: Neonatal ovaries measure 1 to 3.6 ml.[2,6] In infants measurements are average of slightly greater than 1 cm^3 for the first year of life and 0.67 cm^3 for the second year.[10,11]

Multiple follicles in the ovaries are normal in a neonatal ovary. After birth, Follicle Stimulating Hormone (FSH) rises in the newborn period due to the abrupt lack of the placental and maternal hormones. During the second year of life the FSH level decreases, but a pulsatile secretion of FSH persists at a low level. The ovary thus contains mature follicles at all ages. Antral follicle (tertiary follicles) are fluid-filled follicles, which are round in shape and usually < 9 mm in size in the prepubertal girl.[1,2]

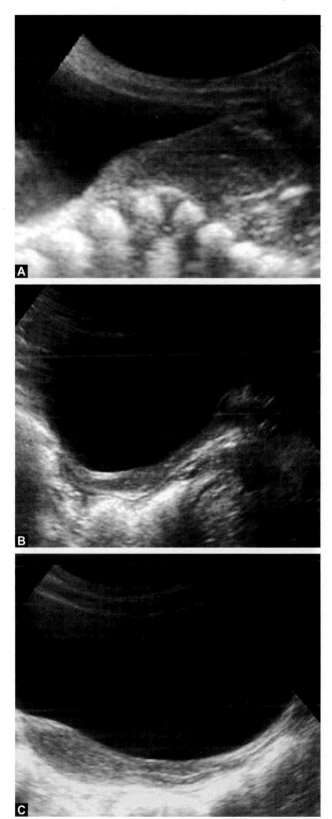

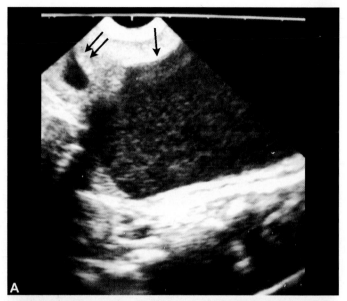

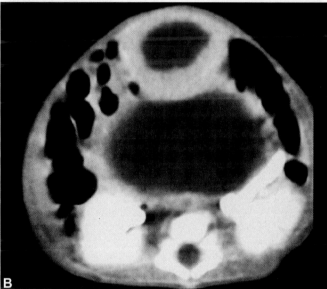

Figs 17.2A and B: Hydrometrocolpos in a 1 Year old female child with palpable midline pelvic lump. Ultrasound (A) shows a fluid filled distended vagina (arrow) and the uterine cavity with its thick myometrium (double arrow). CT scan (B) reveals two fluid filled structures separate from the displaced small urinary bladder, consistent with distended uterine cavity and vagina

Figs 17.1A to C: Neonatal Uterus (A). Longitudinal US scan shows a prominent cervix, characteristically seen in a neonate. Prepubertal uterus (B) Longitudinal US scan in a 7 year old shows a tubular uterus Post-pubertal uterus (C) Longitudinal scan in a 15-year-old shows that the fundus is larger than cervix and uterus is pear shaped

The mean ovarian volume in girls less than 6 years of age is less than or equal to 1 cm³. The increase in ovarian volume begins after 6 years of age.

In prepubertal girls (6–10 years old),ovarian volumes range from 1.2 to 2.3 cm³. In Premenarchal girls (11–12 years old), ovarian volumes range from 2 to 4 cm³. (Table 17.1) In post-menarchal girls, the ovarian volume averages 8 cm³.

Normal microcystic follicles are routinely imaged (in 84 percent of cases) from birth to 24 months of age and in 68 percent of cases between 2 and 12 years of age).[12] Practically, the following measurements can be considered as upper values for prepubertal girls: Uterine length = 4.5 cm, uterine thickness

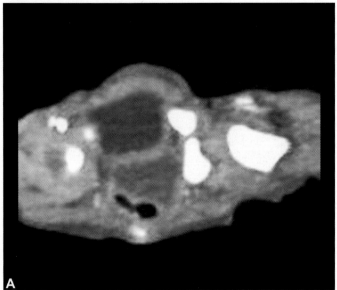

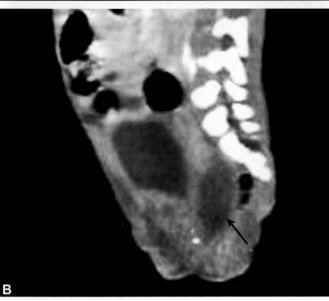

Figs 17.3A and B: CT scan: Axial (A) and Sagittal (B) images of hydrocolpos in a 4 month old IUGR child showing cystic structure (arrow) behind urinary bladder, anterior to rectum, and inferior to uterus, consistent with hydrocolpos

Age (year)	Mean volume (cm)^3	Standard deviation
1	1.05	0.7
2	0.67	0.35
3	0.7	0.2
4	0.8	0.4
5	0.9	0.02
6	1.2	0.4
7	1.3	0.6
8	1.1	0.5
9	2.0	0.8
10	2.2	0.7
11	2.5	1.3
12	3.8	1.4
13	4.2	2.3

Table 17.1: Pediatric ovarian volumes

Sources: References 10, 11

ultrasound of ovarian cysts is recommended to ensure resolution after 6 weeks or after one and a half menstrual cycles.[16-18] Maternal hormones may cause large neonatal ovarian cysts.[19] Although, retention cysts are usually asymptomatic and detected incidentally on sonograms, they may cause pain related to pressure or hemorrhage.

Follicular and corpus luteum retention cysts cannot be differentiated with imaging studies. However, corpus luteum cysts tend to be more symptomatic. Diagnosis requires correlation with the date of the last menstrual period or tissue sampling. Serial sonography is suggested, since the majority of functional cysts demonstrate cyclic changes or regress spontaneously.

On sonograms, a non-hemorrhagic functional cyst appears as a smooth, unilocular cystic mass. The sonographic features that suggest hemorrhage within a simple cyst are variable and depend on the age of the blood. Most hemorrhagic ovarian cysts are seen as complex masses with septations, low-level echoes, a fluid-debris level, or coagulated blood. Hemorrhagic cysts are a avascular on Doppler sonography. Clot lysis and resolution is an important diagnostic feature. With time, the cyst becomes more sonolucent or anechoic.[2,13]

ANOMALIES OF THE FEMALE PELVIS

Mullerian Anomalies

Mullerian anomalies are classified into: (*a*) mullerian agenesis, (*b*) disorders of lateral fusion (duplication defects) with or without obstruction, and (*c*) disorders of vertical fusion (canalization defects) with or without obstruction.[1]

Because of the frequent association between anomalies of lateral fusion and anomalies of vertical fusion, it is helpful to consider these anomalies according to the presence or absence of obstruction.

Mullerian agenesis: Mullerian agenesis (Mayer-Rokitansky-Kuster-Hauser syndrome) is the second most common cause of primary infertility/primary amenorrhea, after gonadal dysgenesis.[20,21] Mullerian agenesis is characterized by vaginal

= 1 cm (the single most useful criterion), and ovarian volume = 4–5 cm^3.[1,2]

Ovarian Cysts

Ovarian cysts can be classified as physiological, functional, or neoplastic.[13] When a normal mature follicle fails to involute and continues to enlarge, secondary to hormonal imbalance, a functional or retention cyst results. These cysts may develop from preovulatory follicles (follicular cysts) or from postovulatory follicles (corpus luteum cysts) and usually range from 4 to 10 cm in size.[13-15]

Cysts up to 2 cm are usually follicles. Larger cysts (>2 cm) may be pathologic, particularly if persistent.[2] Follow-up

atresia associated with an absent or rudimentary uterus (unicornuate or bicornuate) and normal ovaries. The karyotype is normal (46, XX). Renal anomalies (agenesis, ectopia) occur in 50 percent of cases; skeletal or spinal anomalies occur in 12 percent of cases. In 6–10 percent of patients, functioning endometrium may be present within the rudimentary uterus, resulting in unilateral hematometra.

Obstructive Mullerian Anomalies

Failure of vertical fusion or canalization of the urogenital sinus or the Müllerian duct system may result in cervical stenosis or atresia, vaginal atresia, or transverse vaginal septa. A transverse vaginal septum can occur at many levels of the vagina and creates a blockage of the vagina and uterus. In addition, hymenal tissue may be imperforate. Imperforate hymen is the most common genital outflow tract anomaly.

Most of the cases of hydrometrocolpos in the neonatal group are associated with a urogenital sinus or cloacal malformation.[22,23] Hematometrocolpos presenting in adolescent girls is secondary to vaginal obstruction by an imperforate hymen. The patient presents at puberty with primary amenorrhea and cyclic lower abdominal or pelvic pain.[24] Ultrasound typically shows a fluid-filled mass posterior to the bladder, which represents the dilated vagina (Figs 17.2A and B, 17.3A and B). The uterus may also be dilated. The dilated uterus can be differentiated from the vagina by the cervical margin and thicker wall. Not infrequently, hematometrocolpos is present with duplication anomalies.[25] In the newborn period, a bulging mass (hydrocolpos) may be noted at the introitus.

Hematometrocolpos is cured by relieving the obstruction, whereas, hematometra usually requires a hysterectomy. Approximately, 45 percent of vaginal septa occur in the upper vagina, 40 percent in the middle vagina, and 15 percent in the lower vagina. An obstructed hemivagina with a double uterus is almost always associated with ipsilateral renal agenesis. At clinical examination, cyclic abdominal pain (due to the obstruction) coexists with normal menses (through the unobstructed system).[1,2]

Nonobstructive Mullerian Anomalies

These include septate, bicornuate, didelphys, and unicornuate uterus. A longitudinal vaginal septum can be associated with uterine duplication defects (e.g., uterus didelphys, uterus bicollis with a complete vaginal septum).

Primary Amenorrhea

Primary amenorrhea is defined as (a) no menarche by 16 years of age, (b) no thelarche or adrenarche by 14 years of age, or (c) no menarche more than 3 years after adrenarche and thelarche.[1]

The presence or absence of secondary sexual development at clinical examination and mullerian structures at US is the basis for further laboratory tests. Common causes include gonadal dysgenesis (Turner syndrome) (33 percent of cases), mullerian (uterovaginal) anomalies (20%), hypothalamic-pituitary causes (15%), constitutional delay (often familial) (10%), and other causes (e.g., systemic, psychiatric) (22%).

Multiple syndromes result in primary amenorrhea including Turner syndrome, MRKH syndrome, Kallmann syndrome, Prader-Willi syndrome, Androgen Insensitivity syndrome, and Swyer syndrome.[26-28]

In Swyer syndrome (XY gonadal dysgenesis) no functional gonads are present to induce puberty, in an otherwise normal girl whose karyotype is found to be XY. The gonads are found to be nonfunctional streaks. Estrogen and progesterone therapy is commenced. The nonfunctioning gonads are removed because of their risk of developing gonadoblastoma.[2]

Turner syndrome: Patients with XO karyotype (approximately 70 percent of those with Turner syndrome) have a pre-pubertaluterus and non visualized or streaky ovaries.[29] In rare instances, especially in mosaic karyotypes, the ovaries can be normal in appearance.[29] Spontaneous puberty occurs in 5–15 percent of patients with Turner syndrome.[30]

Polycystic Ovary Syndrome (PCOS)

PCOS is an endocrine disorder resulting in chronic anovulation. PCOS is a common cause of infertility and amenorrhea. It is associated with Stein Leventhal syndrome, which includes obesity and hirsutism. On ultrasound, multiple, small follicles (over 10) may be noted with increased echogenicity of the stroma. The ovaries are often 1.5-3 times larger than normal; however, the ovarian volume may be normal in 30 percent of cases.[2] The diagnosis of PCOS is confirmed biochemically.

PELVIC MASSES IN CHILDREN

Benign Ovarian Neoplasms

Ovarian teratomas are the most common benign ovarian neoplasm in pediatric patients.[2] Mature teratomas or dermoid cysts constitute for two-thirds of pediatric ovarian tumors.[13]

Typically, they are found in adolescents. Dermoids contains two cell layers: Mesoderm and Ectoderm. Teratomas are made up of elements from all three layers, including the endoderm. Two-thirds of patients present with an abdominal mass and the rest with pain due to torsion or hemorrhage. Twenty-five percent of teratomas are bilateral. Malignancy is found in 2 to 10 percent. Teratomas may have cystic, solid, or mixed appearance on ultrasound due to its contents. They appear echogenic due to contained fat, hair, sebum, or calcium (teeth, bone). Anechoic components are due to serous fluid or sebum.[31] Approximately, 10-15 percent of benign teratomas are purely anechoic masses at sonography. Another 10-15 percent of teratomas are predominantly echogenic.

Peripheral nodules and shadowing each occur in 70 percent of teratomas in postpubertal girls. In contrast, mural nodules occur in only 40 percent of prepubertal girls and shadowing in only 15 percent.[13] Other features of teratomas include fat- or hair-fluid levels and central soft-tissue masses.[31,32]

CT and MR imaging are useful in further characterization. The most characteristic CT appearance of a benign teratoma is that of a predominantly fluid-filled lesion containing a mixture of fat,

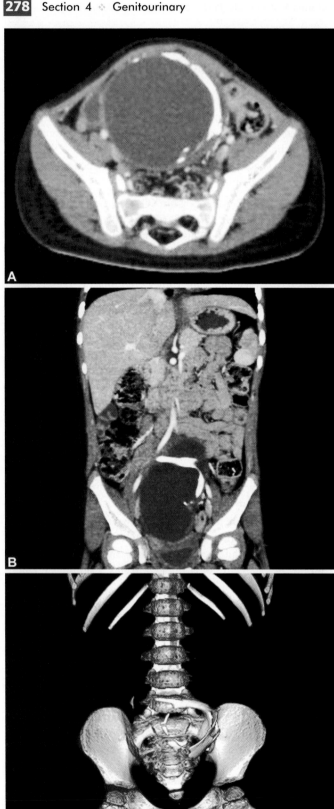

Figs 17.4A to C: CT abdomen (A to C) demonstrates a pelvic cystic tumor with bony elements in axial (A), coronal (B) and volume rendered images (C) in a case of mature teratoma in a 3-year-old girl (*For color version Fig. 17.4C see plate 6*)

hair, debris, and calcifications (Figs 17.4A to C). Calcifications (either teeth or bone) often are localized to the solid globular protuberance (i.e., mural nodule or dermoid plug) arising from the cyst wall. Rarely, a teratoma appears on CT scans as a primarily fatty mass without calcification. If fat or a combination of fat and calcium is identified within a cystic mass, a specific diagnosis of teratoma can be made. In general, two thirds of teratomas display characteristic CT features. On MR images also cystic teratomas vary in signal intensity depending on their tissue composition.[19] On T1-weighted images, fat appears as an area of high signal intensity, while serous fluid has low signal intensity. On T2-weighted images, fat and serous fluid have high signal intensity. Calcifications, bone, and hair have low signal intensity on MR images.[13]

Malignant Neoplasms

Malignant pelvic lesions in the female pelvis are rare and can arise from bone (Ewing sarcoma, coccygeal teratomas), soft tissue or muscles, uterus, or bladder (rhabdomyosarcoma) or have neurogenic origin (neuroblastoma). Some cystic and solid masses have particular diagnostic features (teratomas), but often additional imaging modalities (MR/CT) and/or histology are necessary to confirm a specific diagnosis.

Sacrococcygeal teratoma is one of the most common presacral tumors which contains derivates of three germinal layers. These tumors occur more frequently in girls and are classified into four types, according to the location. Type I is predominantly external while type IV is presacral with no external component in it. CT and MRI are useful for depiction of location, it's differentiation and extent of this tumor. (Figs 17.5A and B, 17.6A and B)

Rhabdomyosarcoma is the most common soft-tissue sarcoma in children. Peak incidence is between 2 and 6 years. The genitourinary tract is a common site of origin.

In girls, rhabdomyosarcoma can arise from the bladder, or vagina and surrounding tissues. Six percent are sarcoma botryoides, which is an embryonal rhabdomyosarcoma originating from the vagina, cervix, or bladder of young girls. The tumor characteristically resembles a bunch of grapes.

Vaginal rhabdomyosarcomas are commonly botryoid and are almost exclusively found in very young children. At US, a vaginal rhabdomyosarcoma appears as a large, solid, heterogeneous or hypoechoic mass posterior to the bladder.

Malignant Ovarian Neoplasm

Malignant pelvic neoplasms with gynecologic origin are rare in children and include sex cord stromal tumors (granulosa cell, theca cell, fibroblast, Leydig and Sertoli cells) and germ cell tumors (dysgerminoma, malignant teratoma, endodermal sinus tumor, embryonal carcinoma, choriocarcinoma) (Figs 17.7 and 17.8). Sex cord stromal tumors represent 8 percent of ovarian neoplasm and affect all age groups. The more common type is granulosa cell tumors. Due to the estrogenic effects of these tumors, females present with pseudoprecocious puberty, endometrial bleeding, and sonographic findings of enlargement of the uterus and thickening of the endometrium. The appearance

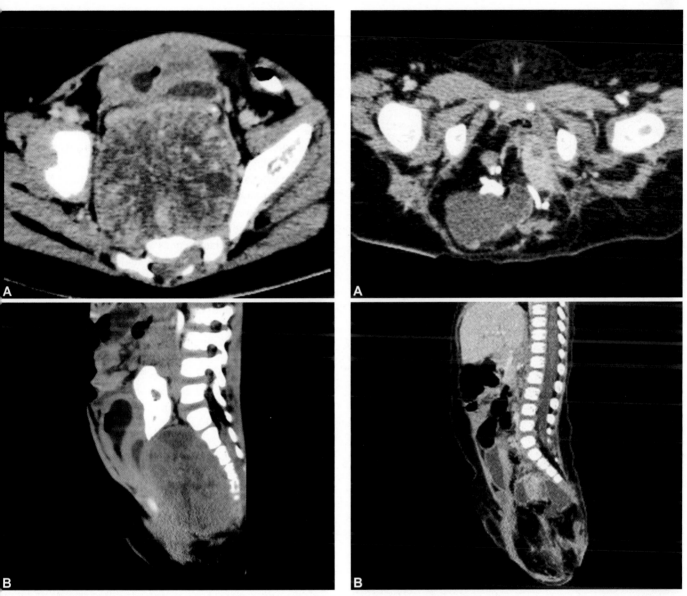

Figs 17.5A and B: CT scan: Axial (A) and Sagittal (B) images of malignant sacrococcygeal teratoma in a 2-year-old female child which also demonstrated bony involvement along with markedly raised AFP levels

Figs 17.6A and B: Axial and sagittal CT scan in another patient of sacrococcygeal teratoma which demonstrates areas of fat, calcification, and cystic components within this tumor

of sex cord tumors vary and range from large multicystic masses to small solid masses.[33]

Children with germ-cell tumors present often with asymptomatic pelvic or abdominal masses. With imaging, solid masses are found, which are echogenic on ultrasound and have soft-tissue attenuation on CT (Figs 17.7A and B). Other findings include calcifications, central necrosis, irregular walls, thick septations, papillary projections, and free abdominal and pelvic fluid. Metastasis occurs in lungs, liver, and peritoneum. Yolk sac tumor is a germ-cell tumor and is a rare, malignant tumor composed of cells that line the yolk sac of the embryo. The tumor is most often found in children before the age of 2 years. As with most other pelvic masses, ovarian yolk sac tumors grow very large before being noticed clinically.[2]

Ovarian Torsion

Ovarian torsion is the twisting of an ovary on its ligamentous supports, which can lead to a compromised blood supply.[23] Adnexal torsion is a term that includes either ovary, fallopian tube, or both. Concomitant ovarian and tubal torsion has been shown to occur in upto 67 percent of cases of adnexal torsion.[34,35]

Symptoms of ovarian torsion are often nonspecific, making it difficult to differentiate from other causes of acute abdominal pain. Ovarian torsion is frequently associated with a cyst or tumor, which is typically benign; the most common is mature cystic teratoma. Ultrasonography (US) is the primary imaging modality for evaluation of ovarian torsion.

With US, the typical findings of ovarian torsion can be visualized in patients of all ages, although they are not always

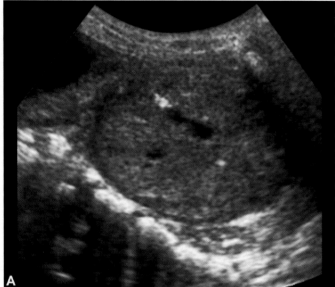

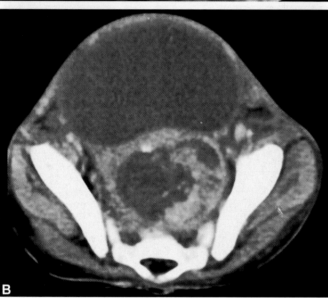

Figs 17.7A and B: Ultrasound (A) shows a well encapsulated predominantly solid adnexal mass with calcific foci and few cystic areas. Biopsy revealed Malignant Germ cell tumour. CT scan (B) reveals a large heterogeneous solid cystic pelvic mass, with a calcific focii

ovary disease and are not solely diagnostic of ovarian torsion. Multiple peripheral cysts in the setting of pain with a unilaterally enlarged ovary are helpful in diagnosing ovarian torsion.[34]

Color Doppler Imaging in Ovarian Torsion

The color Doppler flow manifestations of ovarian torsion are variable and are based, in part, on the degree of vascular compromise. The typical color Doppler sonographic finding in ovarian torsion is the absence of arterial flow. However, in one study involving patients with confirmed ovarian torsion, the absence of arterial flow was found in only 73 percent of cases.[35] In yet another study, 60 percent had normal color Doppler flow findings.[10,39] However, the most frequent finding is either decrease or absence of venous flow (93%), which may reflect the early collapse of the compliant venous walls.[35] The most promising findings incorporating both grayscale and color Doppler sonography are a twisted vascular pedicle and the whirlpool sign.[38,39] In a study by Lee et al,[39] a twisted vascular pedicle was detected in 88 percent of cases of ovarian torsion.

To summarize, US features of ovarian torsion include a unilateral enlarged ovary, uniform peripheral cystic structures, a coexistent mass within the affected ovary, free pelvic fluid, lack of arterial or venous flow, and a twisted vascular pedicle. It is important to remember that the presence of flow at color Doppler imaging does not allow exclusion of torsion but instead suggests that the ovary may be viable, especially if flow is present centrally. Absence of flow in the twisted vascular pedicle may indicate that the ovary is not viable.[34]

The role of computed tomography (CT) has expanded, and it is increasingly being used in evaluation of abdominal pain. Common CT features of ovarian torsion include an enlarged ovary, uterine deviation to the twisted side, smooth wall thickening of the twisted adnexal cystic mass, fallopian tube thickening, peripheral cystic structures, and ascites.[1,2,23] Understanding the imaging appearance of ovarian torsion will lead to conservative, ovary-sparing treatment.

Tuboovarian Abscess

Pelvic inflammatory disease more commonly affects postpubertal girls. The inflammatory process usually begins in the cervix, ascending to the endometrium; fallopian tubes; and, rarely, to the ovaries, parametrium, and peritoneal cavity. The diagnosis is made clinically, based on symptoms of pain, vaginal discharge, and fever. US, CT or MRI are useful for detecting complications such as pyosalpinx, tuboovarian abscess.[13]

Pyosalpinx appears as a hypoechoic tubular mass with internal debris, whereas tuboovarian abscess is seen as a complex mass, often with debris, septations, and irregular thick walls. After antibiotics, pelvic inflammatory disease may resolve completely or lead to sequelae such as hydrosalpinx or adhesions. CT can complement US. At CT, a tuboovarian abscess often appears as a soft-tissue mass with central areas of lower attenuation and thick walls. Occasionally, air or an air-fluid level may be seen.

present. One series studying the effectiveness of US in diagnosing ovarian torsion yielded a positive predictive value of 87.5 percent and specificity of 93.3 percent.[37] The most constant finding in ovarian torsion is a large ovary.[35] Early in the disease, even before infarction has occurred, unilateral ovarian enlargement (>4 cm) is most commonly detected. In up to 74 percent of cases, US may demonstrate multiple small (up to 25 mm), uniform cysts aligned in the periphery of the engorged ovary. This appearance is likely secondary to follicles that have been displaced to the periphery due to the marked edema and venous congestion.[34,37] Peripherally arranged follicles is also an non-specific sign and may be seen in normal ovaries of fertile women and in patients with polycystic

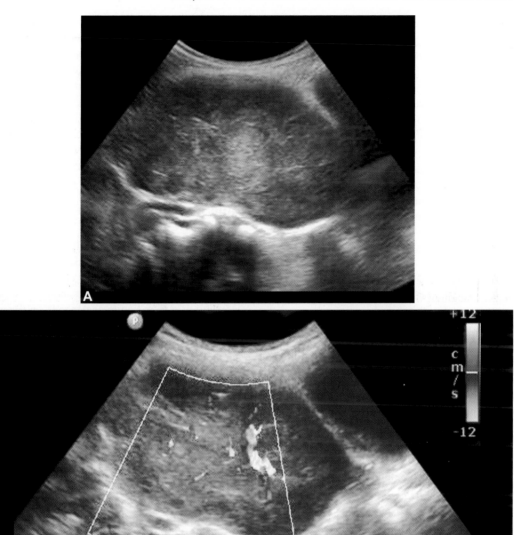

Figs 17.8A and B: Dysgerminoma right ovary. Ultrasound pelvis reveals a solid pelvic mass in the right adnexa (A), which on color Doppler (B) demonstrates mild increased central vascularity (*For color version Fig. 17.8B see plate 6*)

Ectopic Pregnancy

Ectopic pregnancy is a known but infrequent cause of pelvic mass in postpubertal girls.

The most specific US finding for diagnosing an ectopic pregnancy is the visualization of an extrauterine embryo. More often, ectopic pregnancy is manifested as a nonspecific echogenic or complex adnexal mass, often associated with cul-de-sac fluid and an enlarged uterus with a pseudogestational sac.[40,41] A pseudogestational sac has only a single echogenic ring representing parietal decidua, whereas an early intrauterine pregnancy has a double-ring appearance resulting from visualization of the inner capsulari decidua and outer parietal decidua. Because of the non-specficity of the adnexal masses, it is vital to correlate the US appearance with the level of the β subunit of human chorionicgonadotropin (hCG).

NONGYNECOLOGIC PELVIC MASSES

Pelvic masses of non-gynecologic origin include appendiceal abscesses, fluid collections, and fluid-filled bowel ,which can be confounded with primary adnexal lesions.[13]

On sonograms, periappendiceal abscess appears as a complex mass in the right lower quadrant. If an appendicolith or gas is present, bright echoes with shadowing may be noted. Positive ultrasound findings of appendicitis are diameter over 6 mm, lack of compressibility, increased vascularity of the appendical wall, appendicolith, adjacent abdominal free fluid, increased echogenicity of adjacent mesenteric fat, and enlarged lymphnodes.

Cerebrospinal fluid pseudocysts are infrequent complications of ventriculoperitoneal shunting, resulting from loculation of draining cerebrospinalfluid. On sonograms, uninfectedpseudocysts appear as hypoechoic masses. When infected, pseudocysts become more complex, containing internal echoes or septations.

Fluid-filled bowel may potentially be confused with an adnexal cyst at US. In most cases bowel can be identified due to peristalsis detected with real-time imaging. In addition, complicated fluid collections resulting from bleeding or ascites due to peritoneal metastases may be confused with ovarian masses. These collections may change with changes in patient position.

Other non-gynaecological cystic masses which can be seen in the pelvis include mesenteric cysts, duplication cysts, urachal remnants, Meckel's diverticulum, ureteroceles, dilated ureters, hydronephrosis in ectopic kidneys, vascular and lymphatic malformations, abscess, and hematoma. The larger the size of the lesion, the more difficult it is to determine its origin.

Role of MRI In Imaging of Female Pelvis

Magnetic Resonance Imaging (MRI) also plays a crucial role in diagnosis, treatment selection, treatment planning, and follow-up of both benign and malignant gynecological conditions. Advantages of MRI include superb spatial and tissue contrast resolution, lack of ionizing radiation, multiplanar capability, and fast techniques. However, optimization of MRI sequences and clinical protocols is crucial to ensure best results.[43] In pediatrics, MRI is mainly used for congenital anomalies and in evaluation of indeterminate adenexal masses.

Congenital Uterine Anomalies

Müllerian duct anomalies result from nondevelopment or varying degrees of nonfusion or nonresorption of the Müllerian ducts. The role of MRI is to provide both precise classification and demonstration of associated complications.[44] (Classification of Mullerian anomalies has been discussed at the start of this chapter).

In Mayer–Rokitansky–Kuster–Hauser syndrome, there is absence or anomalies of the uterus and upper vagina, with varying degrees of development of the lower vagina.[43]

The unicornuate uterus appears as a curved, elongated uterus with tapering of the fundal segment off midline (the"banana-like" configuration) on T2-weighted MR images.

Normal uterine zonal anatomy is maintained. The rudimentary horn, when present, usually demonstrates lower signal intensity on T2-weighted images. Communication with rudimentary horn can be easily demonstrated on MRI.

Partial fusion of the Müllerian ducts results in the bicornuate uterus. MRI shows uterine horns separated by an interveningcleft in the external fundal myometrium of longer than 1 cm. Normal zonal anatomy is seen in each horn and there is a dividing septum which is composed of myometrium.

The uterus didelphys results from nonfusion of the two Müllerian ducts. Two separate normal-sized uterine horns and cervices are demonstrated on T2-weighted MR images.

A longitudinal vaginal septum is present in 75 percent of cases, occasionally complicated by transverse septa causing obstruction. The two uterine horns are usually widely separated, with preservation of the endometrial and myometrial widths.

A septate uterus is seen when there is incomplete resorption of the final fibrous septum between the two uterine horns. The septum may be partial, or it may be complete and extend to the external cervical os. The differentiation between the septate and the bicornuate uterus is clinically important as the septate uterus is associated with a higher rate of reproductive complications. T2-weighted MR images taken parallel to the long axis of the uterus demonstrate a convex, flat, or concave (less than 1 cm) external uterine contor and the presence of the fibrous septa.[43]

Role of MRI in Characterization of Adnexal Lesions

The strength of MRI is its ability to characterize ovarian lesions, especially in the case of masses that are indeterminate on ultrasound. The signal intensity characteristics of ovarian masses can lead to a systematic approach to diagnosis. The signal intensity of a specific tumor depends on the presence, type, and extent of cystic and solid components within a lesion. Lesions that have a homogeneous low signal intensity on T1-weighted images and high signal intensity on T2-weighted images are simple fluid-filled structures and are considered benign. In general, benign epithelial ovarian neoplasms are predominantly cystic. Fat, hemorrhage, and mucin-containing lesions have high signal intensity on T1-weighted images. Fat-saturated T1-weighted images help distinguish between hemorrhage and fat within a lesion (e.g. endometriosis versus mature cystic teratoma). An adnexal mass of low or intermediate signal intensity on T1-weighted images and low signal intensity on T2-weighted images contain fibrosis and smooth muscle components. Such lesions include pedunculated leiomyoma, fibroma, fibrothecoma, cystadenofibroma, and brenner tumors. The absence of a normal ipsilateral ovary or the presence of small follicles surrounding the mass helps identify the ovarian origin of fibromas.[43-45]

It is imperative to note that as there are no MRI signal intensity characteristics, that are specific for malignant epithelial tumor, such tumors must be distinguished based on morphologic criteria. The MRI features which are most predictive of malignancy are an enhancing solid component or vegetations within a cystic lesion, presence of necrosis within a solid lesion, as well as presence of ascites and peritoneal deposits.[46,47]

Although, both ultrasound and contrast-enhanced MRI have high sensitivity (97 and 100 percent, respectively) in the identification of solid components within an adnexal mass. MRI, however, is reported to demonstrate higher accuracy (93%).[46,47]

CONCLUSION

Ultrasound has proven to be a powerful imaging tool for most clinical indications, related to the pediatric female pelvis. Knowledge of the normal physiologic and age varying appearance of the pelvic organs during childhood is essential. Most pathology within the pediatric pelvis is well delineated with ultrasound. MRI is useful in depicting congenital anomalies and in evaluation of indeterminate adenexal masses.

Imaging of Testicular Abnormalities

The clinical manifestations in testicular abnormalities include pain, swelling, redness, or a palpable mass. These include undescended testes, hydrocoele, varicocele, acute scrotum, scrotal tumors, benign testicular cysts, testicular microlithiasis, scrotal trauma, scrotal hernia and systemic diseases with testicular involvement.

Gray-scale ultrasonography (US) in combination with color or power Doppler imaging, is a well accepted technique for assessing testicular abnormalities.[48] US permits differentiation between lesions that require urgent surgery (testicular torsion, malignant tumors, and traumatic rupture) and those that can be managed conservatively (e.g. epididymoorchitis, torsion of the testicular appendages).

Undescended Testes

Various terms such as maldescended, undescended, retractile and ectopic testes have been used in the literature. Hormann M, have illustrated the entity of 'undescended testes' in their review on scrotal imaging in children.[49] The term "undescended testes" summarizes all conditions, in which the testes are absent from the scrotal sac:[50]

1. Maldescended: Testis not descended into the normal position 4 cm below the inguinal ligament.
2. Cryptorchidism: A maldescended, abdominally positioned testis.
3. Incompletely descended: Testis lying in the inguinal canal between the external and internal ring (most common site 75–80 percent).[51]
4. Obstructed testis: Testis lying in the superficial pouch.
5. Prescrotal retention: Testis lying within the scrotal sac, at a high position less than 4 cm below the inguinal ligament.
6. Retractile testis: Testis lies in normal position, retracts in cases of patent processus vaginalis and cremasteric muscle contraction.
7. Ectopic testis: Testis lying outside the normal path of descent—groin, perineum, penile root, femoral triangle, opposite scrotum (crossed ectopia).
8. Absent testis: no viable testicular tissue can be found.

Approximately, 3.5 percent of all male term infants, 20 percent of premature, and 100 percent of infants with a birth weight of less than 800 g have undescended testis. In 80 percent of these male infants, the testes are descended by the age of 1 year.[49] After 1 year of age, the descent of the undescended testis is almost not observed. Initial strategy, therefore, is to wait and reevaluate the child at age of 9–12 months and operate within this time.

Untreated undescended testes may lead to infertility when lying in the abdominal cavity. Also, undescended testes carry a significantly higher risk for development of malignancy. It is reported that 10 percent of all testicular malignancies occur in undescended testes or in testes treated for cryptorchidism.[51,52] Intra-abdominal testes carries a four times greater risk for development of malignancy than an inguinal testis.[53] The most frequent tumors in undescended testes are seminoma and embryonal cell carcinoma. The majority of undescended testes can be detected with ultrasound, as 75–80 percent are located between the internal and external inguinal ring.[51]

Higher intra-abdominal locations make detection with ultrasound more difficult. MR imaging has been recommended in such cases. MR imaging offers excellent images of the testes, although, it has the disadvantage of a relative high cost and the need for sedation or anaesthesia in small children.[49] The location of the testis influences the optimal section orientation. In the lower abdomen and inguinal canal, coronal orientation offers the best results, while intra-abdominal testes are best depicted in axial and sagittal orientations. Surgeons in many institutions prefer laparoscopy as a diagnostic and at the same time a therapeutic tool in small children in cases in which ultrasound findings are inconclusive.

Inguinal-Scrotal Hernia

Inguinal-scrotal hernia is defined as the passage of intestinal loops and/or omentum into the scrotum.[48] The prevalence of inguinal hernia is higher in preterm neonates.[26] The hernia is more frequently located on the right side, as the right processus vaginalis closes later than the left.[54] Physical examination is usually sufficient to allow diagnosis in most cases. US examination is indicated in patients with inconclusive physical findings, in patients with acute scrotum, and also to investigate contralateral involvement in patients in whom only a unilateral hernia is clinically evident.[55]

The diagnosis of hernia is achieved by visualization of air bubble movement and/or intestinal peristalsis during the real-time examination. The herniated omentum is seen as a highly echogenic structure on US. Inguinal rings larger than 4 mm are an indication for prophylactic herniorrhaphy.[55] Color or power Doppler imaging is useful in inguinal-scrotal hernia to investigate intestinal and testicular perfusion. Urgent surgery is indicated in patients with an aperistaltic akinetic dilated bowel loop (a sign of strangulation).[56]

Varicoceles

Varicoceles are seldom seen in early childhood, but occur in adolescents and adults, and are a leading cause of male infertility. A varicocele is abnormal dilatation of the veins of the spermatic cord, which is usually caused by incompetent valves of the internal spermatic vein, and results in impaired drainage into the spermatic cord veins. Varicoceles can be visible, palpable or subclinical at clinical examination. Palpable and subclinical varicoceles are diagnosed with ultrasound: On grayscale imaging they appear as multiple, serpiginous, tubular structures of varying sizes, larger than 2 mm in diameter.[49] On color and pulsed-wave Doppler images, venous flow is better demonstrated during the Valsalva maneuver (Fig. 17.9). Varicocele may affect testicular growth;[57] hence, testicular volumes should be systematically measured and any asymmetry evaluated with US.[48]

Hydrocele

Hydrocele, is collection of fluid between the visceral and parietal layers of the tunica vaginalis and/or along the spermatic cord. It is one of the most common cause of painless scrotal swelling in

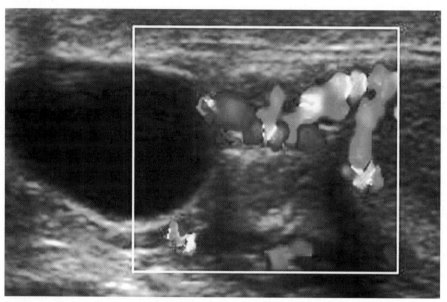

Fig. 17.9: Color Doppler ultrasound demonstrates typical dilated veins of spermatic cord, seen in child with varicocele along with encysted cord hydrocele (*For color version see plate 7*)

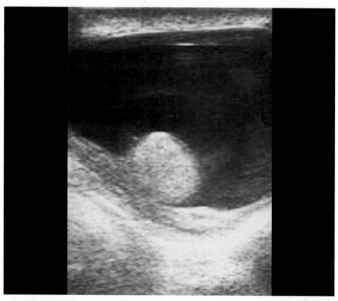

Fig. 17.10: Hydrocele. Longitudinal ultrasound of the right hemiscrotum shows a fluid collection surrounding the testes

children. In the normal scrotum, 1–2 ml of serous fluid may be observed in the potential tunica vaginalis cavity and should not be mistaken for hydrocele. Virtually all hydroceles are congenital in neonates and infants and associated with a patent processus vaginalis, which allows peritoneal fluid to enter the scrotal sac.[48,58] In older children and adolescents, hydroceles are usually acquired and are often result of an inflammatory process, testicular torsion, trauma, or a tumor.

At USG, congenital hydrocele appears as an anechoic fluid collection surrounding the anterolateral aspects of the testis, which may sometimes extend to the inguinal canal or as a fluid collection with low-level swirling echoes[58] (Fig. 17.10).

Spermatic cord cyst, a less common type of hydrocele, which more commonly appears as a fluid collection in the spermatic cord and results from closure of the processus vaginalis above the testis and below the internal inguinal ring (Figs 17.11A and B). Two types of spermatic cord hydrocole are known. The first type is encysted hydrocele of the cord, where the fluid collection does not communicate with the peritoneum or the tunica vaginalis. The second type is the funicular hydrocele , where there is a fluid collection along the cord, communicating with the peritoneum at the internal ring.

Most congenital hydroceles (80%) resolve spontaneously before the age of 2 years. However, surgical treatment is usually applied in spermatic cord and abdominoscrotal hydroceles.[48]

Cystic Dysplasia of the Testis

Cystic dysplasia of the testis is primarily incidentally found when evaluating children with renal dysplasia. It involves cystic dilatation of the rete testes. It is associated with dysplasia or agenesis of the ipsilateral kidney.[49]

Testicular Calcification (Microcalcification)

Testicular microcalcification is usually an incidental finding. Testicular microlithiasis is defined as multiple calcifications that are smaller than 2 mm and appear as hyperechoic structures throughout or in a large area of the testis.[49] They are associated with congenital syndromes (Klinefelter syndrome, pseudoherma-phroditism), with congenital anomalies (undescended testes) or they could be idiopathic; they are also seen in tumors and are of unknown cause.

The calcifications are seen as fine, bright, nonshadowing hyperechoic foci (five or more on any single view) that are uniform in size and are distributed in a diffuse pattern or in peripheral clusters.[48] As testicular microlithiasis is considered to be a

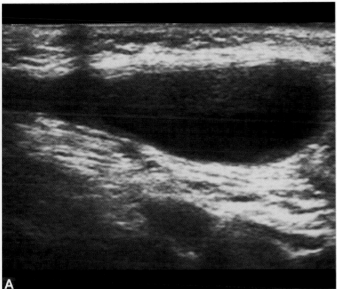

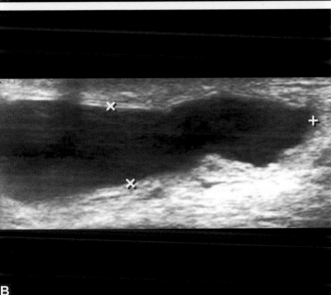

Figs 17.11A and B: Spermatic cord hydrocele (Funicular hydrocele). Longitudinal scan of the right spermatic cord of a 2-year-old child, shows a fluid collection along the cord, communicating with the peritoneum at the internal ring (A). Ultrasound in another patient (B) with spermatic cord hydrocele

premalignant condition; thus, serial scrotal US monitoring (once per year) is recommended.[59]

Acute Scrotum

Acute scrotum refers to a clinical setting of sudden-onset scrotal pain, redness, and swelling, which is most frequently caused by acute epididymo-orchitis, torsion of the testicular appendages, or testicular torsion.[48] Since scrotal involvement is usually unilateral, one should start the examination on the asymptomatic side first to have a basis for comparison. Color Doppler imaging, or power Doppler imaging should be added to gray-scale ultrasound.

Epididymo-orchitis

Epididymo-orchitis, is a common cause of acute scrotum in children.[48] It is mainly of infectious origin. The infection usually originates in the bladder or prostate gland, spreads through the vas deferens and the lymphatics of the spermatic cord to the epididymis, and finally reaches the testis, causing epididymo-orchitis. Isolated orchitis can also occur, but is rare.

There are two reported peaks of prevalence: under 2 years of age and over 6 years of age. Many conditions predispose to epididymo-orchitis, which include Imperforate anus, ureteral ectopia to the seminal vesicle, bladder exstrophy, neurogenic bladder, posterior urethral valves, and dysfunctional voiding. Chronic mild trauma can also lead to mild non-infective epididymo-orchitis.[49] Children present with pain of acute onset, which is typically not as rapid as in torsion, and with reddening of the skin and oedema. Clinical examination may be difficult because of pain, and elevating the scrotum beyond the symphysis pubis (Prehn's sign) relieves pain.[49]

The epididymal head is the most affected region, and reactive hydrocele and wall thickening are also frequently present. Increased size and, decreased, increased, or heterogeneous echogenicity of the affected organ are usually observed. On color Doppler imaging, there is increased blood flow within the epididymis, testis, or both[48] (Figs 17.12A and B and 17.13A and B).

Occasionally, the entire epididymis is affected. Malignancies such as leukemia and lymphoma, that diffusely infiltrate the testicular parenchyma, may have a US appearance similar to that of diffuse orchitis. In such cases, the clinical history is extremely important.

In cases with accompanying orchitis, the testis is also enlarged and shows a heterogeneous echotexture.[60] Color Doppler studies show hyperemia in all cases in the affected regions, and ideally should help to distinguish from torsion. However, hyperemia disappears rapidly with improvement of symptoms under therapy.[61] With spectral Doppler studies, a low-resistance waveform with decreased resistance index (RI<0.5) is observed.[62] Hyperemia of the testis also may be the result of vasculitis in Henoch–Schönlein purpura. In these cases, different presentations of vasculitis can be observed and therefore can be differentiated from inflammation of other cause.[49]

Granulomatous epididymo-orchitis is a chronic inflammation occurring in postpubertal boys.[48] The affected part of the epididymis, mainly the tail, is enlarged with heterogeneous echogenicity.[63] At color Doppler imaging, chronic epididymo-orchitis does not demonstrate the increased blood flow, typical of acute epididymitis. The sonographic features can be similar to those of epididymal adenomatoid tumor; however, patients with chronic epididymitis present with a painful mass, whereas the tumor is usually painless.

Torsion of the Testicular Appendages

The appendages are sessile structures, which thus predisposes them to torsion, and the appendix testis is most often affected.[48] Torsion of the appendix testis occurs mainly in prepubertal boys

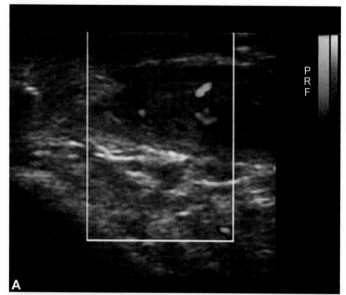

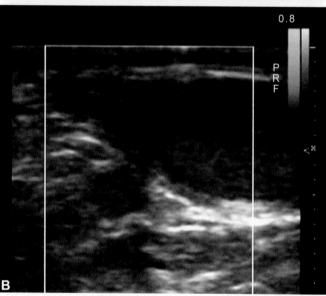

Figs 17.12A and B: Epididymitis. Epididymis is enlarged, heterogeneous and demonstrates increased flow on color Doppler (A). Normal opposite epididymis is shown for comparison (B) (*For color version see plate 7*)

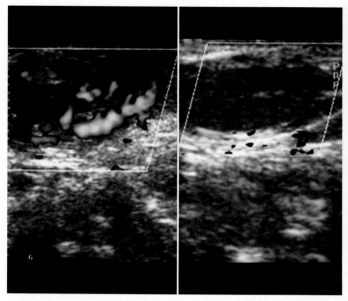

Fig. 17.13: Epididymo-orchitis in a 9-year-old boy. Ultrasound revealed enlarged epididymal head with heterogeneous echotexture of epididymus and testes, which demonstrated increased vascularity on power Doppler. Oppisite normal left testis is shown for comparison (*For color version see plate 8*)

(aged 7–14 years), is more frequent on the left side, and is a common cause of acute scrotum in this age group.[64]

Affected patients typically present with gradual or sudden intense pain, usually localized in the upper pole of the testis. At physical examination, the classic finding in these children is a small palpable nodule on the superior aspect of the testis, which is called the "blue dot" sign. This is seen in nearly one third of patients, and this is a pathognomonic feature of this entity.

At US, the twisted appendage is seen as a round extratesticular mass with high or mixed echogenicity depending on the evolution time.[65] Associated findings include an enlarged epididymal head, reactive hydrocele, and scrotal skin thickening. There is no Doppler signal in the twisted appendage, and the epididymis and

scrotal tunics are hypervascularized .Management is conservative, in contrast to torsion of the spermatic cord, and the pain resolves after 2–3 days. The appendix becomes atrophic and finally calcifies.

Testicular Torsion

Testicular torsion, entails first venous and later arterial flow obstruction. The extent of testicular ischemia in these patients depends on the degree of twisting (180°–720°) and the duration of the torsion. Testicular salvage is more likely in patients treated within 6 hours after the onset of torsion, hence the need for an urgent, immediate diagnosis.[48]

Testicular torsion are of two types: Extravaginal and intravaginal.

Extravaginal torsion or supravaginal torsion, can only occur before the tunica vaginalis and the gubernaculum become fixed to the scrotal wall, and therefore can only occur in the perinatal period.[66] At birth, the testis is infarcted and necrotic, and clinically, children present with a painless mass, swelling and discoloration of the scrotal sac. Ultrasound, typically demonstrates an enlarged heterogeneous testis, ipsilateral hydrocoele, thickening, and absent flow in the spermatic cord and testis.

Intravaginal torsion can occur at any age but is more common in adolescents. A known predisposing factor is the "bellclapper" deformity, in which the tunica vaginalis joins high on the spermatic cord, leaving the testis free to rotate.[49]

Differentiation between testicular torsion and epididymo-orchitis is important, since scrotal pain, swelling, and redness are clinical symptoms common to these two entities. Generally, pain in testicular torsion has a sudden onset, whereas in orchitis, it is more gradual. However, 5 percent of children with orchitis have sudden onset of pain, and only 50 percent of patients with testicular torsion have an acute attack.[44]

The pain is constant and does not increase with palpation or movement and is not relieved when the scrotum is elevated above the symphysis, in contrast to inflammatory conditions.

In the early phases of torsion (1–3 hours), testicular echogenicity appears normal. With progression, enlargement of the affected testis and increased or heterogeneous echogenicity are common findings. Sonographic evaluation of the spermatic cord is an essential part of the examination. The point of cord twisting can be identified at the external inguinal orifice. More than 24 hours after the onset of symptoms, there is reversion to normal echogenicity and after 10 days the testis becomes atrophic.[49] A definitive diagnosis of complete testicular torsion is made when blood flow is visualized on the normal side but is absent on the affected side.[48]

Two kinds of torsion can be differentiated: Complete torsion (>360°) and incomplete torsion (<360°).[49] In complete torsion, initially the epididymis is the first organ without flow, but after about 6 h a collateral arterial supply from the inferior epigastric artery is opened, which can mislead the examiner. Incomplete torsion refers to cord twisting of less than 360°, in which some arterial flow persists in the affected testis (seen in 20 percent cases in one series). The venous flow is obstructed. Therefore, it is important to study the testicular perforating arteries to avoid false-negative ultrasound results.[49]

Additional, information can be obtained from pulsed-wave Doppler imaging, with which decreased or reversed diastolic flow may be evident on the affected side, and from scintigraphy and MR imaging.[67,68]

Normal echogenicity with mild testicular enlargement has been reported as a good sign of viability, whereas marked enlargement, heterogeneous echotexture, and scrotal wall hypervascularity are signs of testicular infarction and necrosis.

Acute Idiopathic Scrotal Edema

Acute idiopathic scrotal edema is a self-limiting disease which is characterized by edema and erythema of the scrotum.[69] It is the fourth most common cause of acute scrotum in patients aged below 20 years, following epididymitis, testicular torsion, and torsion of appendages.[69,70] Since clinically it manifests similar to those of other surgically correctable acute scrotal disease, it is important to confirm diagnosis, using US and Doppler to avoid unnecessary surgery.

Exact etiology of this entity remains unclear, however, it is considered a variant of angioneurotic edema.[70] Patients with idiopathic scrotal edema may also show eosinophilia, which may be the result of allergic reaction. In most reported cases, all source of infection was excluded from surrounding structures. It is also known that as mostly unilateral, and perineal or inguinal erythema is coexistent in half the cases.[70-72] However, bilateral involvement was more common in one study by Lee et al, (75%) compared with previous studies.[69] The most common characteristic of is scrotal wall edema, (Fig. 17.14) which is easily visualized on US, which has also been confirmed by surgical findings.[72]

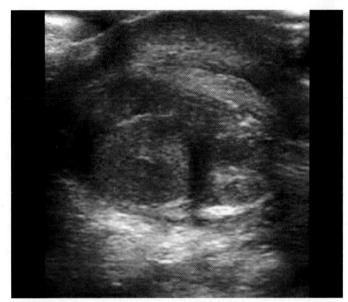

Fig. 17.14: Acute idiopathic scrotal edema. Transverse ultrasound scan of both hemiscrota shows marked thickening of scrotal walls

Several studies have described the following US and Doppler findings:

1. Marked thickening of the scrotal wall, with heterogeneous striated and edematous appearance, with increased flow.
2. Increased peritesticular blood flow.
3. Mildly reactive hydrocele.[71,72]
4. The testes and epididymis are normal in appearance and do not show increased vascularity.[73]
5. Enlargement and increased vascularity of the inguinal lymph nodes.

As, it is an self-limiting disease, surgical intervention should be avoided. US examination along with Doppler is very useful to differentiate between other acute scrotal diseases and acute idiopathic scrotal edema.

Scrotal Tumors

The incidence of scrotal tumors is estimated at 0.5–2.0 cases per 100,000 boys.[74] Scrotal tumors typically manifest as painless scrotal swelling. Owing to its excellent spatial resolution, US is highly sensitive for identifying scrotal masses.[75] This technique allows differentiation between cystic and solid tumors and classification as intra- or extratesticular. The term *paratesticular* refers to a group of extratesticular lesions that are not easily identified as originating from a particular tissue. Computed tomography (CT) is reserved for detecting spread in malignant tumors, while MR imaging is useful for characterizing the tumor content or better delineation of extratesticular solid masses.[76] Certain tumor markers (α-fetoprotein and human chorionic-gonadotropin) also help to make a more precise diagnosis.

Testicular Tumors

Testicular tumors account for 1 percent of all pediatric solid tumors.[48] They have two peaks of prevalence, first before 3 years of age and secondly, in the postpubertal period. They usually manifest as a painless scrotal mass. However, in approximately 10 percent of patients, testicular tumor is associated with pain due to hemorrhage or infarction, mimicking torsion or epididymitis. Testicular tumors are subdivided into two groups: Germ cell tumors and non–germ cell tumors.

Germ cell tumors: Germ cell tumors result from the transformation of primitive germ cells. These pluripotential cells can remain nondifferentiated (seminomas), become slightly differentiated (embryonal carcinoma), or transform into differentiated embryonal (mature or immature teratomas) or extraembryonal (choriocarcinoma) structures.[77]

For clinical purposes, germ cell tumors are also divided into two groups: seminomatous and nonseminomatous germ cell tumors.[78]

Seminomas, in comparison with nonseminomatous tumors, occur in older population,with an average patient age of 40.5 years. Seminoma is extremely radiosensitive, and radiotherapy for low-stage tumors is very effective, resulting in a 5-year survival rate of 95 percent.[78]

Nonseminomatous Germ Cell Tumors

Yolk sac tumor, also known as endodermal sinus tumor, is the most common germ cell tumor, accounts for 80 percent of childhood testicular tumors,with most cases occurring before the age of 2 years. In its pure form, yolk sac tumor is rare in adults; however, it is present in 44 percent of adult cases of mixed germ cell tumor.[79]

α-fetoprotein is normally produced by the embryonic yolk sac, and thus serum α-fetoprotein levels are elevated in greater than 90 percent of patients with yolk sac tumor.[78] These markers are also useful in follow-up to check for regression or recurrence of the tumor.

The US findings are nonspecific, usually showing a solid mass replacing the entire testis.The presence of hypoechoic areas within the tumor, which indicates areas of necrosis, is a frequent finding (Figs 17.15A to C). As with all germ cell tumors, spread is predominantly via the lymphatic system; hence, the lymphatic pathway should be included in the initial work-up.

The second most common germ cell tumor is *teratoma*, which is classified as mature, immature and those with malignant areas. Generally, teratomas occur in children less than 4 years of age.[78]

The sonographic appearance depends on the components of the three germinal layers (endodermal, mesodermal, and ectodermal). Cysts are a common feature and may be an echoic or complex, depending on the cyst contents (i.e. serous, mucoid, or keratinous fluid). Teratoma may appear as a complex mass with cystic components, or a cystic lesion with peripheral solid components or calcifications, and echogenic intratumor fat.[78] These tumors are usually benign in prepubertal children, so tissue sparing surgery may be possible; however, in adolescents they are often malignant and require orchidectomy.

Testicular epidermoid cyst is the most common benign testicular tumor with no malignant potential. Epidermoid cysts are composed of keratinizing, stratified, squamous epithelium with a well-defined fibrous wall. The cyst contains cheesy material and may resemble a solid tumor at US. Several sonographic patterns have been described: An echogenic lesion surrounded by a hypoechoic or echogenic rim, a target appearance, and an "onionring" configuration with alternating echogenic and anechoic areas within the lesion.[80] The presence of well-delineated borders and a vascularity at color Doppler imaging favors the diagnosis. In inconclusive cases, MR imaging can aid in identification. On contrast-enhanced images, they are seen as sharply demarcated, low signal-intensity, non-enhancing lesions.[81]

Although, the radiologic appearance of epidermoid cyst is quite characteristic, it is not however, pathognomonic. Teratomas and other malignant tumors may also have a similar appearance, and mass should be carefully evaluated for any irregular borders, which might suggest a malignant lesion. Because carcinoma cannot be completely excluded, orchiectomy is usually performed. However, if the lesion has been thoroughly evaluated and if there is a strong possibility that it is an epidermoid cyst, it is recommended to perform a testis sparing enucleation rather than orchiectomy.[78]

Non-germ cell tumors: Non-germ cell tumors, are less frequent than germ cell tumors,and can develop from the gonadal stroma (Leydigcell tumor), sex cord cells (Sertoli cell tumor), or sex cord cells plus stroma (gonadoblastoma).[48]

These account for nearly 4 percent of all testicular tumors.[78] The prevalence is higher in the pediatric age group, for which non-germ cell tumors constitute 10–30 percent of all testicular neoplasms.[78] Ninety percent of all non–germ cell tumors are benign. Unfortunately, no radiologic criteria allows definite differentiation of benign from malignant disease, and orchiectomy is usually performed in all cases. Even with histologic analysis, it is difficult at times, to determine the biologic behavior of these tumors.

Leydig cell tumors are the most common in this group, accounting for 1–3 percent of all testicular tumors. They can be seen in any age group, with 20 percent of cases reported to occur in patients younger than 10 years, 25 percent in patients aged 10–30 years, 30 percent in patients aged 30–50 years, and 25 percent in patients older than 50 years.[82] Nearly 30 percent of patients will have an endocrinopathy secondary to secretion of androgens or estrogens by the tumor. Leydig cell tumors are generally small solid masses, but they may show cystic areas, hemorrhage, or necrosis (Fig. 17.16).[82] Their sonographic appearance is also variable and is indistinguishable from that of germ cell tumors.

Sertoli cell tumors are less common than leydig cell tumors, and constitute less than 1 percent of testicular tumors. They are less hormonally active, but gynecomastia can occur.[82] Sertoli cell tumors are typically well-circumscribed, unilateral, round to lobulated masses. An subtype is the large-cell calcifying Sertoli cell tumor, which is most often seen in the pediatric age group. This subtype commonly manifests as multiple and bilateral masses, which, as the name implies, are distinguished by large areas of calcification that are readily seen with US.[83] This subgroup has been associated with Peutz-Jeghers syndrome and

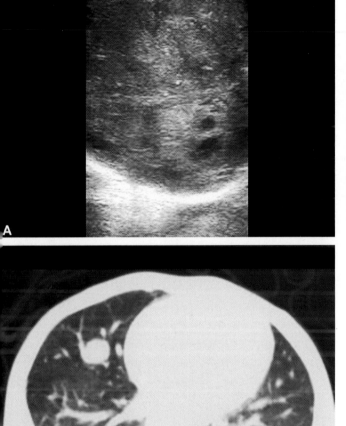

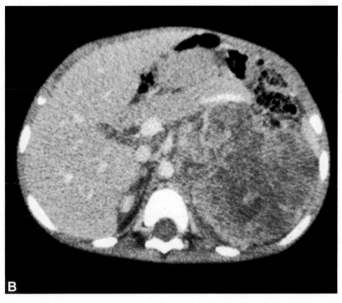

Figs 17.15A to C: Non-seminomatous germ cell tumor in a 2.5 years old male child who presented with left scrotal swelling. Ultrasound (A) revealed a large heterogeneous predominantly solid intratesticular mass. CT scan revealed left metastatic retroperitoneal mass (B) with pulmonary metastasis (C)

Carney syndrome (pituitary adenomas, mucocutaneous pigmentation, and myxomas of the heart, skin, eyelids, and breast).[78,83]

Gonadoblastoma is a dysgenetic lesion occurring in the setting of gonadal dysgenesis and intersex syndromes. Approximately, 80 percent of the patients are phenotypically female.[82,83]

Other Testicular Tumors

Primary follicular lymphoma of the testes is an infrequent tumor, with only few reported cases.[84] However, secondary involvement is common in patients with acute lymphoblastic leukemia and non-Hodgkin B-cell lymphoma.[85] At US, there are two relatively more common patterns of involvement, which are seen in both leukemia and lymphoma: the more common diffuse type, in which the testis is enlarged and hypoechoic, and the focal type, which demonstrates multiple hypoechoic nodules. Increased blood flow may be seen on color Doppler images, which may simulate an inflammatory lesion.

Primary leukemia of the testis is rare. However, the testis is a common site of leukemia recurrence in children, with 80 percent of patients being in bone marrow remission.[86,87] It is believed that the blood testis barrier allows leukemic cells to be "hidden" during chemotherapy. The clinical characteristics and sonographic appearance of leukemia of the testis can be quite varied, as the tumors may be unilateral or bilateral, diffuse or focal, hypoechoic or hyperechoic[86,87] (Figs 17.17A and B).

Metastasis of other solid tumors, such as Wilms' tumor, neuroblastoma, and retinoblastoma, that may affect the testis have also been reported.[48]

Benign testicular cysts can be located either within the tunica albuginea or the parenchyma.[78] Tunica albuginea cysts are typically peripherally located and may be single or multiple. Recognition of their classic location and appearance usually helps in making this diagnosis. Careful analysis must be done to

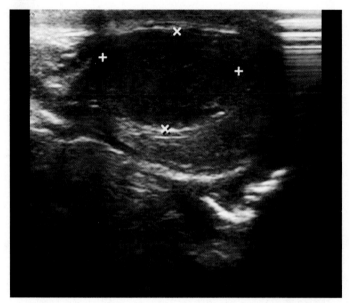

Fig. 17.16: Testicular ultrasound showing a hypoechoic intratesticular lesion in a child with leydig cell tumor of testes

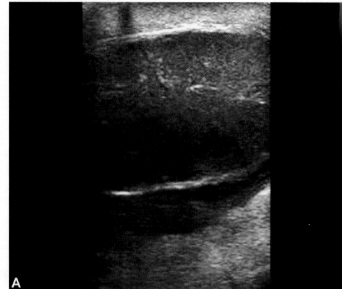

A

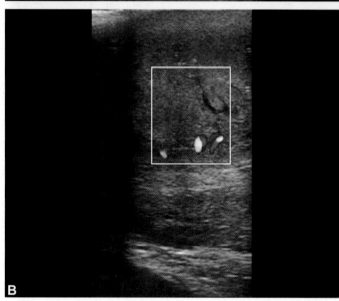

B

Figs 17.17A and B: Ultrasound (A and B) reveals diffuse leukemic infiltration of testes in a child with lymphoblastic leukemia (*For color version Fig. 17.17B see plate 8*)

differentiate these lesions from cystic neoplasms, typically teratomas. If the cystic lesion has any solid components, it should be considered malignant.

EXTRATESTICULAR TUMORS

Paratesticular Rhabdomyosarcoma

The most common extra testicular tumor is paratesticular rhabdomyosarcoma, which originates in the spermatic cord or scrotal tunics.[48] The majority of these tumors occur in the first two decades of life and belong to the embryonal histopathologic subtype. At US, paratesticular rhabdomyosarcoma is seen as a hypo- or hyperechoic solid mass that may envelop or invade the epididymis and testis, which demonstrates hypervascularity at color Doppler imaging.[88]

CT is often recommended in the initial work-up to determine tumor spread, and MR imaging can be performed, if required, to delimit the borders of the mass relative to the epididymis and testis.[89] Long-term survival is expected in patients under 10 years of age with disease confined to the scrotum.

Adenomatoid Tumor

Adenomatoid tumors are benign, solid extra testicular lesions that can originate from the epididymis, tunica vaginalis, or spermatic cord. They are the most common tumor of the epididymis and occur more often in the lower pole than in the upper pole by a ratio of 4:1.[90] Usually, an incidental finding, adenomatoid tumors manifest as a painless scrotal mass, with the majority diagnosed inpatients aged 20–50 years.[91] They are typically unilateral and occur more frequently on the left side. When they grow noninvasively into the testicular parenchyma, they can simulate intratesticular disease.

At US, they appear as a solid extratesticular mass with variable echogenicity.[91,92] Commonly, MR imaging demonstrates low signal intensity relative to the testicular parenchyma on T2-weighted images. However, the appearance is not specific and should be differentiated from granulomatous epididymitis, a chronic form of epididymitis that manifests as a painful palpable mass . At color Doppler imaging, vessels are observed within the adenomatous tumor, whereas usually no vessels are seen in granulomatous epididymitis.[48,60]

Epididymal cysts, although not true tumors, typically manifest as a palpable mass and are of lymphatic origin. Because they contain clear serous fluid, they are seen as an anechoic, well-defined mass with increased through transmission. Epididymal cysts cannot be differentiated from spermatoceles, which are secondary to obstruction and dilatation of the efferent ductal system. However, the latter occur exclusively in postpubertal boys.[91]

Primary malignant tumors of the epidydimis are rare in children; epididymal involvement is largely due to metastatic spread from B-cell acute lymphoblastic leukemia and B-cell non-Hodgkin lymphoma.[91]

Epididymal Cystadenoma

Papillary cystadenoma of the epididymis is a benign epithelial neoplasm. It is seen in up to 60 percent of men with von Hippel–Lindau disease.[91] Although, the sporadic variety is usually seen in middle-aged men, it is seen earlier in patients with von Hippel–Lindau disease. The sonographic appearance is variable. It can appear as a solid appearance with few cystic spaces or can appear as multiloculated cystic lesion with small papillary projections.[90-92] In patients with von Hippel–Lindau disease, sonographic criteria for diagnosis of epididymal cystadenoma consist of *(a)* a predominantly solid epididymal mass larger than 10 × 14 mm and *(b)* slow growth. At MR imaging, a cystic mass with septations or mural nodules can be seen.

Lipoma

Lipoma is the most common benign tumor of the spermatic cord and can occur at any age.[91] At US, it is a well-defined, homogeneous, hyperechoic paratesticular lesion.[92] At MR imaging, lipoma appears uniform and follows fat signal intensity with all sequences, including fat-suppressed sequences, which confirms the diagnosis.[93]

Fibrous Pseudotumor

Fibrous pseudotumor is considered as a benign, reactive fibrous paratesticular tissue. As it can grow up to large sizes, therefore, it can mimic a neoplasm. It commonly arises from the tunica vaginalis. The sonographic appearance is nonspecific,[90,92] and calcification is commonly seen. The lesion can dislodge and become freely mobile within the scrotal sac; such a lesion is known as a "scrotal pearl". At MR imaging, owing to the presence of fibrosis, the lesion has low signal intensity on both T1- and T2-weighted images with variable enhancement.

ADRENAL RESTS

These are a rare cause of testicular masses, which can be seen in patients with congenital adrenal hyperplasia and rarely in those with Cushing syndrome. These rests are usually less than 5 mm and can be found in the testis and surrounding tissues in 7.5–15 percent of newborns and 1.6 percent of adults.[94] If these cells are exposed to elevated levels of adrenocorticotropic hormone, they can enlarge to form masses.

These were present in 11 of 20 patients (55%) with CAH, in one series reported by Aso C et al.[48] As potential malignancy is extremely rare, testicular biopsy is not required, even when the mass increases in size.

The sonographic appearance of adrenal rests is variable, with some series describing predominantly hypoechoic masses and others reporting heterogeneously hyperechoic masses with shadowing.[94,95] On MR imaging, these have been reported to have low signal intensity on both T1- and T2-weighted images.[96] It is

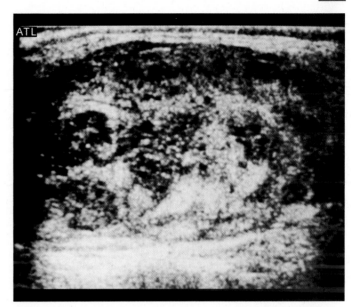

Fig. 17.18: Longitudinal ultrasonogram in a 12-year-old child (with history of scrotal injury while playing football) shows a large heterogeneous soft tissue mass in the left scrotal sac, suggestive of testicular hematoma

important to recognize these as benign lesions to avoid unnecessary orchiectomy.[78]

Sarcoidosis is a multisystem, chronic granulomatous disease that rarely affects the genital tract. Although, it more commonly affects the epididymis but can, in some cases, also involve the testis. Testicular lesions can be solitary, but they are more commonly multiple, small, bilateral masses.[97] Testicular sarcoidosis is more common in African-Americans than in other racial groups.[82]

Scrotal Involvement in Systemic Diseases

Scrotal involvement can be seen in many systemic diseases.[48] The testes are affected in 15–37 percent of patients with Henoch-Schonlein purpura.[98,99] In this disease, scrotal symptoms may even precede other manifestations. US findings include scrotal wall thickening, epididymal enlargement, and reactive hydrocele. Involvement is bilateral in the majority of cases; hence, this entity should be considered when bilateral US findings similar to those of inflammatory epididymitis are visualized.

Scrotal Trauma

Scrotal trauma, in children can result from a trivial fall, sports or motor vehicle and straddle accidents. Since physical examination is limited by swelling and pain, US is an good modality for its detection. Lesions range from extratesticular hematoma to testicular rupture. Extratesticular hematomas may be quite large and their echogenicity changes over time, being echogenic in the acute state and anechoic during follow-up. (Fig. 17.18). Conservative treatment is recommended except in cases of impaired testicular flow testicular rupture is rare, but should be suspected when the margins of the testis are poorly defined or disruption of the capsular blood flow is observed.[48,60] MR imaging increases the diagnostic confidence and is useful in pre-operative work-up of testicular rupture.[100] MRI is extremely helpful for evaluation of scrotal blunt trauma owing to its high tissue contrast, multiplanar imaging, and ability to depict hemorrhage at different stages. The low signal from the albuginea is a remarkable sign, ensuring testicular integrity.

Role of MRI in Testicular Abnormalities

MR imaging is useful as a problem-solving tool when sonographic findings are equivocal.[90] Magnetic resonance imaging (MRI) has been tested, with good results in different scrotal diseases because of its superb anatomic details, and great tissue contrast.[100-102] MRI dramatically improves the diagnostic reliability in certain given conditions, such as scrotal blunt trauma, nonpalpable lesions with an inconclusive sonographic appearance, patients with chronic scrotal pain with nonspecific sonograms, and when the US and clinical findings are discrepant.

MR imaging accurately allows characterization of scrotal masses as intratesticular or extratesticular and can demonstrate various types of lesions and tissue, including cysts or fluid, solid masses, fat, and fibrosis. MR imaging can be of additional value when the location of a scrotal mass is uncertain or when US does not allow differentiation between a solid mass and an inflammatory or vascular abnormality. Gadolinium-enhanced MR imaging can further help differentiate between a benign cystic lesion and a cystic neoplasm. Contrast enhanced MRI can also be used to demonstrate areas of absent or reduced testicular perfusion, such as in segmental testicular infarct. MR imaging can demonstrate an intra abdominal undescended testis, which can be difficult to detect with US, and is superior to US in differentiation between an undescended testis and testicular agenesis.[90]

CONCLUSION

A wide spectrum of diseases can involve the scrotum in children. Ultrasonography (US) performed by using a high-frequency transducer, with color Doppler, is the initial imaging modality of choice when evaluating testicular abnormalities. US can suggest a specific diagnosis for a wide variety of intrascrotal diseases, appropriately guiding treatment. Magnetic resonance imaging can be useful as a problem-solving tool when sonographic findings are equivocal or suboptimal. CT scan has no current role in evaluation of scrotal disorders in children, however, it is useful in staging of malignancy.

REFERENCES

1. Gare L, Dubois J, Grignon A, Filiatrault D, Vliet GV. US of the Pediatric Female Pelvis : A Clinical Perspective. Radiographics 2001; 21:1393–407.
2. Stranzinger E, Strouse PJ. Ultrasound of the Pediatric Female Pelvis Seminars In US, CT, MRI 2008; 29:98-113.
3. Lang IM, Babyn P, Oliver GD. MR imaging of pediatric uterovaginal anomalies. Pediatr Radiol 1999; 29:163–170.
4. Nussbaum AR, Sanders RC, Jones MD. Neonatal uterine morphology as seen on real-time US. Radiology 1986; 160:641-3.
5. Hata K, Nishigaki A, Makihara K, Takamiya O, Hata T, Kitao M. Ultrasonic evaluation of the normal uterus in the neonate. J Perinat Med 1989; 17:313-7.
6. Haber HP, Mayer EI. Ultrasound evaluation of uterine and ovarian size from birth to puberty. Pediatr Radiol 1994; 24:11-3.
7. Holm K, Laursen EM, Brocks V, Muller J. Pubertal maturation of the internal genitalia: An ultrasound evaluation of 166 healthy girls. Ultrasound Obstet Gynecol 1995; 6:175-81.
8. Buzi F, Pilotta A, Dordoni D, Lombardi A, Zaglio S, Adlard P. Pelvic ultrasonography in normal girls and in girls with pubertal precocity. Acta Paediatr 1998; 87:1138-45.
9. Orbak Z, Sagsoz N, Alp H, Tan H, Yildirim H, Kaya D. Pelvic ultrasound measurements in normal girls: Relation to puberty and sex hormone concentration. J Pediatr Endocrinol Metab 1998; 11:525-30.
10. Cohen HL, Shapiro MA, Mandel FS, Shapiro ML. Normal ovaries in neonates and infants: A sonographic study of 77 patients 1 day to 24 months old. AJR Am J Roentgenol 1993; 160:583-6.
11. Orsini LF, Salardi S, Pilu G, Bovicelli L, Cacciari E. Pelvic organs in premenarcheal girls: Real-time ultrasonography. Radiology 1984; 153:113-6.
12. Cohen HL, Eisenberg P, Mandel F, Haller JO. Ovarian cysts are common in premenarchal girls: A sonographic study of 101 children 2–12 years old. AJR Am J Roentgenol 1992; 159:89-91.
13. Surratt, JT, Siegel MJ. Imaging of Pediatric Ovarian Masses. Radiographics 1991; 11:533-48.
14. Fleischer AC, Daniel JF, Rodier J, Lindsay AM, James AE Jr. Sonographic monitoring of ovarian follicular development. JCU 1981; 9:275-80.
15. Ritchie WGM. Sonographic evaluation of normal and induced ovulation. Radiology 1986; 161:1-10.
16. Templeman C, Fallat ME, Blinchevsky A, et al. Non inflammatory ovarian masses in girls and young women. Obstet Gynecol 2000; 96:229-33.
17. De Silva KS, Kanumakala S, Grover SR, et al. Ovarian lesions in children and adolescents–an 11-year review. J Pediatr Endocrinol Metab 2004; 17:951-7.
18. Brandt ML, Helmrath MA. Ovarian cysts in infants and children. Semin Pediatr Surg 2005; 14:78-85.
19. Nussbaum AR, Sanders RC, Hartman DS, et al. Neonatal ovarian cysts: Sonographic-pathologic correlation. Radiology 1988; 168:817-21.
20. Rosenberg HK, Sherman NH, Tarry WF, Duckett JW, Snyder HM. Mayer-Rokitansky-Kuster-Hauser syndrome: US AID to diagnosis. Radiology 1986; 161:815-9.
21. Carranza-Lira S, Forbin K, Martinez-Chequer JC. Rokitansky syndrome and MURCS association: Clinical features and basis for diagnosis. Int J Fertil Womens Med 1999; 44:250-5.
22. Blask AR, Sanders RC, Gearhart JP. Obstructed uterovaginal anomalies: Demonstration with sonography. I. Neonates and infants. Radiology 1991; 179:79-83.
23. Banerjee AK, Clarke O, MacDonald LM. Sonographic detection of neonatal hydrometrocolpos. Br J Radiol 1992; 65:268-71.
24. Sugar NF, Graham EA. Common gynecologic problems in prepubertal girls. Pediatr Rev 2006; 27:213-23.
25. Strouse PJ. Sonographic evaluation of the child with lower abdominal or pelvic pain. Radiol Clin North Am 2006; 44:911-23.
26. Ziereisen F, Guissard G, Damry N, et al. Sonographic imaging of the pediatric female pelvis. Eur Radiol 2005; 15:1296-309.

27. Robert Y, Mestdagh P, Ziereisen F, et al. Imaging of the female pelvis in adolescence. J Radiol 2001; 82:1765-80.

28. Haber HP, Ranke MB. Pelvic ultrasonography in Turner syndrome: Standards for uterine and ovarian volume. J Ultrasound Med 1999; 18:271-6.

29. Mazzanti L, Nizzoli G, Tassinari D, et al. Spontaneous growth and pubertal development in Turner's syndrome with different karyotypes. Acta Paediatr 1994; 83:299-304.

30. Matarazzo P, Lala R, Artesani L, Franceschini PG, De Sanctis C. Sonographic appearance of ovaries and gonadotropin secretions as prognostic tools of spontaneous puberty in girls with Turner's syndrome.J Pediatr Endocrinol Metab 1995; 8:267-74.

31. Sheth S, Fishman EK, Buck JL, et al. The variable sonographic appearances of ovarian teratomas: Correlation with CT. AJR Am J Roentgenol 1988; 151:331-4.

32. Sisler CL, Siegel MJ. Ovarian teratomas: A comparison of the sonographic appearance in prepubertal and postpubertal girls. AJR 1990; 154:139-14.

33. Outwater EK, Wagner BJ, Mannion C, et al. Sex cord-stromal and steroid cell tumors of the ovary. Radiographics 1998; 18:1523-46.

34. Chang HC, Bhatt S, Dogra VS. Pearls and Pitfalls in diagnosis of Ovarian Torsion. Radiographics 2008; 28:1355-68.

35. Albayram F, Hamper UM. Ovarian and adnexal torsion: Spectrum of sonographic findings with pathologic correlation. J Ultrasound Med 2001; 20(10):1083-9.

36. Breech LL, Hillard PJ. Adnexal torsion in pediatric and adolescent girls. Curr Opin Obstet Gynecol 2005; 17(5):483-9.

37. Graif M, Itzchak Y. Sonographic evaluation of ovarian torsion in childhood and adolescence. AJR AmJ Roentgenol 1988; 150(3):647-9.

38. Vijayaraghavan SB. Sonographic whirlpool sign in ovarian torsion. J Ultrasound Med 2004; 23(12):1643-9.

39. Lee EJ, Kwon HC, Joo HJ, Suh JH, Fleischer AC. Diagnosis of ovarian torsion with color Doppler sonography: Depiction of twisted vascular pedicle. J Ultrasound Med 1998; 17(2):83-9.

40. Dashefsky SM, Lyons EA, Levi CS, Lindsay DJ. Suspected ectopic pregnancy: Endovaginal and transvesical US. Radiology 1988; 169:181-4.

41. Filly RA. Ectopic pregnancy: The role of sonography. Radiology 1987; 162:661-8.

42. Strouse PJ, DiPietro MA, Saez F. Transient small-bowel intussusceptions in children on CT. Pediatr Radiol 2003; 33:316-20.

43. Sala E. Magnetic Resonance Imaging of the Female Pelvis. Seminars in Roentogenology 2008; 290-302.

44. Carrington BM, Hricak H, Nuruddin RN, et al. Mullerian duct anomalies: MR imaging evaluation. Radiology 1990; 176:715-20.

45. Jeong YY, Outwater EK, Kang HK. Imaging evaluation of ovarian masses. Radiographics 2000; 20:1445-70.

46. Hricak H, Chen M, Coakley FV, et al. Complex adnexal masses: Detection and characterization with MR imaging–multivariate analysis. Radiology 2000; 214:39-46.

47. Tempany CM, Zou KH, Silverman SG, et al. Staging of advanced ovarian cancer: Comparison of imaging modalities—report from the Radiological Diagnostic Oncology Group. Radiology 2000; 215:761-7.

48. Aso C, Enr1´quez G, Fite M´, Tora´n N, Piro´C, Piqueras J, Lucaya J. Gray-Scale and Color Doppler Sonography of Scrotal Disorders in Children: An Update Radiographics 2005; 25:1197-214.

49. Hormann M, Balassy C, Marcel O, Philipp MO, Pumberger W. Imaging of the scrotum in children. Eur Radiol 2004; 14:974-83.

50. Whitaker RH. Undescended testes: The need for a standard classification. Br J Urol 1992; 70:1-6.

51. Oyen RH. Scrotal Ultrasound. Eur Radiol 2002; 12:19-34.

52. Nguyen HT, Coakely F, Hricak H. Cryptorchidism: Strategies in detection. Eur Radiol 1999; 9:336-43.

53. Campbell HE. The incidence of malignant growth in the undescended testicle: A reply and reevaluation. J Urol 1959; 81:663-8.

54. Siegel MJ. The acute scrotum. Radiol Clin North Am 1997; 35:959-76.

55. Chou TY, Chu CC, Diau GY, Wu CJ, Gueng MK. Inguinal hernia in children: US versus exploratory surgery and intraoperative contralateral laparoscopy. Radiology 1996; 201:385-8.

56. Ogata M, Imai S, Hosotani R, Aoyama H, Hayashi M, Ishikawa T. Abdominal ultrasonography for the diagnosis of strangulation in small bowel obstruction. Br J Surg 1994; 81:421-4.

57. Thomas JC, Elder JS. Testicular growth arrest and adolescent varicocele: Does varicocele size make a difference? J Urol 2002; 168:1689-91.

58. Gooding GA, Leonhardt WC, Marshall G, Seltzer MA, Presti JC Jr. Cholesterol crystals in hydroceles: Sonographic detection and possible significance. AJR Am J Roentgenol 1997; 169:527-9.

59. Drut R. Yolk sac tumor and testicular microlithiasis. Pediatr Pathol Mol Med 2003; 22:343-7.

60. Dogra VS, Gottlieb RH, Mayumi O, Rubens DJ. Sonography of the scrotum. Radiology 2003; 227:18-36.

61. Rifkin MD, Cochlin DLI. Scrotal masses (and scrotal enlargement). In: Rifkin MD, Cochlin DLI (Eds). Imaging of the scrotum and penis. Martin Dunitz Ltd, London 2002; pp 33-95.

62. Jee WH, Choe BY, Byun JY, Shinn KS, Hwang TK. Resistive index of the intrascrotal artery in scrotal inflammatory disease. Acta Radiol 1997; 38:1026-30.

63. Salmeron I, Ramirez-Escobar M, Puertas F, Marcos R, Garcia-Marcos F, Sanchez R. Granulomatous epididymo-orchitis: Sonographic features and clinical outcome in brucellosis, tuberculosis and idiopathic granulomatous epididymo-orchitis. J Urol 1998; 159:1954-7.

64. Monga M, Scarpero HM, Ortenberg J. Metachronous bilateral torsion of the testicular appendices.Int J Urol 1999; 6:589-91.

65. Hesser U, Rosenborg M, Gierup J, Karpe B, Nystrom A, Hedenborg L. Gray-scale sonography in torsion of the testicular appendages. Pediatr Radiol 1993; 23:529-32.

66. Brown Casillas VJ, Montalvo AM, Albores-Saavedra J. Intrauterine spermatic cord torsion in the newborn: Sonographic and pathologic correlation. Radiology 1990; 177:755-7.

67. Paltiel HJ, Connolly LP, Atala A, Paltiel AD, Zurakowski D, Treves ST. Acute scrotal symptoms in boys with an indeterminate clinical presentation: Comparison of color Doppler sonography and scintigraphy. Radiology 1998; 207:223-31.

68. Watanabe Y, Dohke M, Ohkubo K, et al. Scrotal disorders: Evaluation of testicular enhancement patterns at dynamic contrast-enhanced subtraction MR imaging. Radiology 2000; 217:219-27.

69. Lee A, Park SJ, Lee HK, Hong HS, Lee BH, Kim DH. Acute idiopathic scrotal edema: Ultrasonographic findings at an emergency unit. Eur Radiol 2009; 19:2075-80.

70. Klin B, Lotan G, Efrati Y, Zlotkevich L, Strauss S. Acute idiopathic scrotal edema in childred-revisited. J Pediatr Surg 2002; 37:1200-2.

71. Van Langen AM, Gal S, Hulsmann AR, De Nef JJ. Acute idiopathic scrotal oedema: Four cases and a shortreview. Eur J Pediatr 2001; 160:455-6.

72. Kaplan GW. Acute idiopathic scrotal edema. J Pediatr Surg 1977; 12:647-9.

73. Varga J, Zivkovic D, Grebeldinger S, Somer D. Acute scrotal pain. In children—ten years' experience. Urol Int 2007; 78:73–7.

74. Kay R. Prepubertal Testicular Tumor Registry. J Urol 1993; 150:671-4.

75. Woodward PJ, Schwab CM, Sesterhenn IA. Extratesticularscrotal masses: Radiologic-pathologic correlation. Radiographics 2003; 23:215-40.

76. Cramer BM, Schlegel EA, Thueroff JW. MR imaging in the differential diagnosis of scrotal and testicular disease. Radiographics 1991; 11:9-21.

77. Martelli H, Patte C. Gonadal tumours in children. Arch Pediatr 2003; 10:246-50.

78. Paula J. Woodward PJ, Sohaey R, O'Donoghue MJ,Green DE. Tumors and Tumorlike Lesions of the Testis: Radiologic-Pathologic Correlation. Radiographics 2002; 22:189-216.

79. Frush DP, Sheldon CA. Diagnostic imaging for pediatric scrotal disorders. Radiographics 1998; 18:969-85.

80. Schwerk WB, Schwerk WN, Rodeck G. Testicular tumors: Prospective analysis of real-time US patterns and abdominal staging. Radiology 1987; 164:369-74.

81. Cho JH, Chang JC, Park BH, Lee JG, Son CH. Sonographic and MR imaging findings of testicular epidermoid cysts. AJR Am J Roentgenol 2002; 178:743-8.

82. Ulbright TM, Amin MB, Young RH. Tumors of the testis, adnexa, spermatic cord, and scrotum. In: Atlas of tumor pathology, fasc 25, ser 3. Washington, DC: Armed Forces Institute of Pathology 1999; 1-290.

83. Chang B, Borer JG, Tan PE, Diamond DA. Large-cell calcifying Sertoli cell tumor of the testis: Case report and review of the literature. Urology 1998; 52:520-2.

84. Pileri SA, Sabattini E, Rosito P, et al. Primary follicular lymphoma of the testis in childhood: Anentity with peculiar clinical and molecular characteristics. J Clin Pathol 2002; 55:684-8.

85. Dalle JH, Mechinaud F, Michon J, et al. Testicular disease in childhood B-cell non-Hodgkin's lymphoma: The French Society of Pediatric Oncology experience. J Clin Oncol 2001; 19:2397-403.

86. Mazzu D, Jeffrey RB Jr, Ralls PW. Lymphoma and leukemia involving the testicles: Findings on gray-scale and color Doppler sonography. AJR Am J Roentgenol 1995; 164:645-7.

87. Heaney JA, Klauber GT, Conley GR. Acute leukemia: Diagnosis and management of testicular involvement. Urology 1983; 21:573-7.

88. Mak CW, Chou CK, Su CC, Huan SK, Chang JM. Ultrasound diagnosis of paratesticular rhabdomyosarcoma. Br J Radiol 2004; 77:250-2.

89. Mason BJ, Kier R. Sonographic and MR imaging appearances of paratesticular rhabdomyosarcoma. AJR Am J Roentgenol 1998; 171:523-4.

90. Kim W, Rosen MA, Langer JE, Banner MP, Siegelman ES, Ramchandani P. US–MR Imaging Correlation in Pathologic Conditions of the Scrotum. Radiographics 2007; 27:1239-53.

91. Yang DM, Kim SH, Kim HN, et al. Differential diagnosis of focal epididymal lesions with gray scale sonographic, color Doppler sonographic, and clinical features. J Ultrasound Med 2003; 22:135-42.

92. Akbar SA, Sayyed TA, Jafri SZ, Hasteh F, Neill JS. Multimodality imaging of paratesticular neoplasms and their rare mimics. Radiographics 2003; 23:1461-76.

93. Pretorius E. MRI of the male pelvis and bladder. In: Siegelman ES, Ed. Body MRI. Philadelphia, Pa: Elsevier Saunders 2005; 372–86.

94. Vanzulli A, DelMaschio A, Paesano P, et al. Testicular masses in association with adrenogenital syndrome: US findings. Radiology 1992; 183:425-9.

95. Seidenwurm D, Smathers RL, Kan P, Hoffman A. Intratesticular adrenal rests diagnosed by ultrasound. Radiology 1985; 155:479-81.

96. Berg NB, Schenkman NS, Skoog SJ, Davis CJ. Testicular masses associated with congenital adrenal hyperplasia: MRI findings. Urology 1996; 47:252-3.

97. Burke BJ, Parker SH, Parker KD, Pienkos EJ. The ultrasonographic appearance of coexistent epididymal and testicular sarcoidosis. J Clin Ultrasound 1990; 18:522-6.

98. Ben-Sira L, Laor T. Severe scrotal pain in boys with Henoch-Schonlein purpura: Incidence and sonography. Pediatr Radiol 2000; 30:125-8.

99. Laor T, Atala A, Teele RL. Scrotal ultrasonography in Henoch-Schonlein purpura. Pediatr Radiol 1992; 22:505-6.

100. Muglia V, Tucci S, Elias J, Trad CVS, Bilbey J, Cooperberg PL. Magnetic resonance imaging of scrotal diseases: When it makes the difference. UROLOGY 2002; 59:419-23.

101. Schultz-Lampel D, Bogaert G, Thuroff JW, et al. MRI for evaluation of scrotal pathology. Urol Res 1991; 19:289-92.

102. Sica GT, and Teeger S. MR imaging of scrotal, testicular and penile diseases. MRI Clin North Am 1996; 4:545-62.

CHAPTER 18

Imaging of Intersex Disorders

Sanjay Sharma, Arun Kumar Gupta

INTRODUCTION

Intersex disorders presenting with ambiguous genitalia are complex and uncommon conditions that involve intermingling of characteristics of each sex to varying degrees due to a defect in embryological development. The incidence is approximately one per 1,000 live births. Although most are not medical emergencies, they are considered psychologic emergencies. Prompt diagnosis of ambiguous genitalia is necessary to help the family and later the child to adjust psychologically. Most cases of ambiguous genitalia are discovered at birth. Knowledge of internal genital anatomy is crucial in the overall management of these patients. The role of a radiologist is to demonstrate this anatomy using different imaging techniques. An understanding of the normal sexual differentiation is essential before interpreting the pathological state.

Normal Sexual Differentiation[1]

Genital primordia of a fetus are intrinsically programed to differentiate into female sex. However, in the presence of a Y chromosome the undifferentiated gonads differentiate into testes. Anti-Müllerian hormone (AMH), which is secreted by the Sertoli cells of the testes, inhibits the development of Müllerian ducts (i.e. female structures) while testosterone secreted from Leydig cells of the testes maintain and differentiate Wolffian ducts i.e. male structures). Thus, presence of Y chromosome differentiates the genital primordia into a male. On the other hand, in the absence of Y chromosome, testicular tissue and its two hormones are absent due to which there is no inhibition of Müllerian ducts by AMH. Wolffian ducts regress because of lack of testosterone. End result is a normal female child.

Imaging of an Intersex Child[2-6]

Intersex disorders presenting with ambiguous genitalia form a challenging clinical problem. Biochemical and chromosomal assays, besides the radiological evaluation are required in order to completely address its different aspects. Genitography, Ultrasound, and MR imaging, are routinely employed. Judicious use of minimum investigations to obtain maximum information should be the goal.

Genitography[2,7]

As most of these children have a urogenital sinus, the anatomy displayed using genitography becomes essential in treatment planning as regards the corrective surgery for gender assignment. In this technique, water soluble contrast is injected retrogradely, via the external genital opening so as to outline the genital anatomy. Contrast is injected, either by placing the nozzle of a syringe (flush technique) or the tip of an end hole catheter (catheter technique), within the external genital opening (Figs 18.1A and B). It aims to address the following:

a. Degree of masculinization of the urogenital sinus and the urethra.
b. Vaginal status, i.e. its presence, size and any cervical indentation by the uterus.
c. Junctional site of vagina with the urethra, i.e. whether low, middle or high junction (Figs 18.2A to C). Low, middle or high vaginal insertion, determines the morphological female, indeterminate or the male urethral type respectively.
d. Presence of uterus/fallopian tubes, either by their direct opacification or indirectly by visualization of cervical indentation at the cranial end of the contrast filled vagina.

It must be realized that no genitographic appearance is specific for one particular type of intersex disorder. It only depicts the degree of virilization of genitalia. Genitography only provides information about the status of the derivatives of Müllerian and Wolffian ducts. Gonadal evaluation is not possible. The technique is 'invasive' and it uses ionizing radiation.

Other Imaging Modalities

Ultrasound and MRI are two non-invasive cross sectional imaging techniques available for examination of the pelvic structures. As stated earlier, role of imaging is to identify: (a) structures derived from Müllerian or Wolffian ducts and (b) status of gonads. Therefore, image analysis should include evaluation for the presence or absence of uterus, vagina, clitoris/penis, ovaries, prostate and testes. Addition of pelvic ultrasonography has been a valuable supplement to genitography and karyotyping in the work-up of an intersex child for assessing not only gonads but also the presence of uterus and cervix, but has its limitations of small field of view, poor demonstration of complex anomalies and inability to keep the child's urinary bladder adequately distended to provide a sonographic window.

Recent reports on the use of MRI in these disorders have been promising.[8,9] Strength of MRI lies in its multiplanar capability, excellent soft tissue characterization, large field of view, and non-ionizing nature. It contributes to the accurate morphological

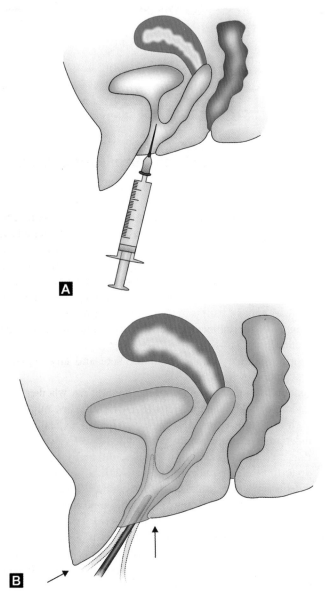

A

B

Figs 18.1A and B: Techniques of genitography, flush technique (A) and catheter technique (B). In former, tip of the syringe nozzle is within the external opening and barrel is pressed against the perineum. In latter, single hole catheter should be used and its tip should be in the common urogenital sinus. Dotted lines show the potential pitfall if the tip enters either channel selectively. Arrows in (B) indicate compression of perineal skin around the catheter to prevent reflux of contrast

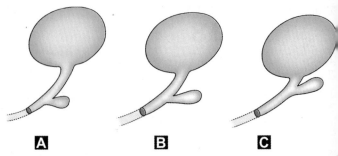

A   **B**   **C**

Figs 18.2A to C: Schematic drawing of possible junctional sites of vagina (or its remnant) with the urethra: Low (A), middle (B) and high (C). Generally higher the junctional site, more degree of masculinization will be present

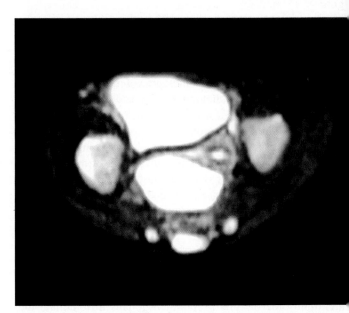

Fig. 18.3: Axial T2W MRI shows the normal zonal anatomy of uterus i.e. central hyper, outer hypo and outermost intermediate signal uterine tissues

evaluation of Müllerian and Wolffian duct structures, gonads and the development of phallus, all of which are essential for appropriate gender assignment and planning surgical reconstruction. Axial, sagittal and coronal T1 and T2W images are obtained using fast/turbo spin echo sequences. Suggested section thickness is 5 mm in patients older than 5 years and 3 mm in patients under 5 years. Secaf *et al* [8] have suggested use of an image matrix of 256 × 192 with two to four signal averages. Image analysis includes the assessment of uterus, vagina, ovaries, testes, penis and clitoris.MRI is now considered to be more valuable than ultrasound in the evaluation of internal genitalia,

especially in the newborn. In the neonatal period, the ovaries and uterus are physiologically prominent due to maternal hormonal influence. CT now has a very limited role to play due to the widespread use of MRI.

MR Appearance of Genital Structures

The normal *uterus* demonstrates clear zonal anatomy on T2W images. Three zones demonstrated on T2WI (Fig. 18.3), i.e innermost hyperintense linear area within the uterus corresponds to endometrium, the surrounding hypointense band represents the junctional zone (inner myometrium) and the outer intermediate signal intensity zone corresponds to outer myometrium.[1] However, a hypoplastic uterus is not only small but demonstrates low signal intensity of the entire myometrium on T2W images. For complete evaluation of the uterus, both axial and sagittal T2W images are most useful. The *vagina* is best visualized on axial T2W images. Sagittal images are complementary to the axial images. On T2W images, the hypointense vaginal wall can be distinguished from the bright central canal representing mucosa and surrounding adipose tissue. Demonstration of *urogenital sinus* on MRI is difficult. Normal *testes and ovaries* have medium to low signal intensity on T1W images and high signal intensity on T2W images. Gonadal tissue characterization is not always possible, unless follicles are seen in case of ovary. Ectopic gonads frequently demonstrate an outer rim of medium signal intensity on T2W images, which differentiates it from lymph nodes. Axial T1W and T2W images are useful in the evaluation of gonads. Sagittal and coronal images are also helpful. Although signal intensity of atrophic, dysgenetic, or streak gonads are not as high as that of normal gonads on T2W images, histological evaluation is necessary for differentiation between normal and abnormal gonads. Gonads are sought in the intra-scrotal, high scrotal, intracanalicular or intrapelvic location. The normal *penis* is composed of paired corpora cavernosa, corpus spongiosum, and supporting muscular structures such as bulbocavernosus, ischiocavernosus and transverse perineal muscles. Paired corpora cavernosa and corpus spongiosum have medium signal intensity on T1W images and high signal intensity on T2W images. On T2W images, these structures are easily differentiated from the supporting muscles and urethra. Presence of normal *clitoris* is established when on a T2W image, high signal intensity tissue is seen adjacent to ischium in the anatomical location of crura of corpora cavernosa (Fig. 18.4). When full length of the clitoris extends for greater than 1 cm anterior to the pubic ramus, it is considered hypertrophied.[8]

CLASSIFICATION OF INTERSEX

Over the years, a number of workers have put forth contradictory views regarding classification of intersex states. Paquin et al,[11] based on a study of 7 patients concluded that presence and appearance of urogenital sinus on imaging itself is not diagnostic of any specific type of hermaphroditism. Shopfner[12] studied 66 intersex children and classified them into six types, demonstrating progressive masculinization from type I to type VI. He believed that each genitographic type represented a specific type of intersexuality, an observation in direct contradiction to Paquin et al[11] and other subsequent workers. A French team of endocrinologists and radiologists[1,13] carried out studies in more than 120 patients and concluded, unlike Shopfner,[12] that no genitographic pattern is specific for any particular type of intersexual state. At AIIMS, our conclusion is similar to that of Paquin et al[11] and the French team.[1]

Presently, intersex patients are assigned to one of the following types:
i. Female pseudohermaphroditism (FPH)
ii. Male pseudohermaphroditism (MPH)
iii. True hermaphroditism (TH)
iv. Mixed gonadal dysgenesis (MGD)
v. Dysgenetic male pseudohermaphroditism (DMP).

Female Pseudohermaphroditism (FPH)[1,2,7,14,15]

FPH denotes a female karyotype 46XX with presence of normal ovaries, uterus and tubes. Although the external genitalia are

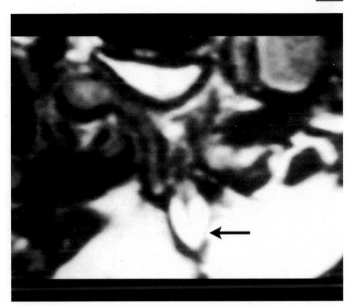

Fig. 18.4: Coronal T2W MRI shows the normal clitoral appearance. Compare this with Figure 18.11

ambiguous, the testes or internal Wolffian duct derivatives, like vas deferens and seminal vesicles are absent.

Etiology: It results from the action of an extra-gonadal testosterone on a normal female fetus resulting in virilization of genitalia to varying degrees. A number of mechanisms may be responsible but the most common one is congenital adrenal hyperplasia, resulting from an enzymatic defect (21 hydroxylase deficiency being the commonest) in adrenal steroidogenesis.

Types: Degree of virilization of the urogenital sinus and the external genitalia vary, depending upon the time of onset of the insult and the amount of androgen. Prader[15] had classified them into 5 types based on clinical and genitographic findings. Some surgeons, however, are not fully satisfied with this classification from surgical point of view. Based on the degree of virilization FPH can be classified either as complete or incomplete.

Complete virilization is equivalent to Prader type V and results from massive amounts of androgens in the early phase of embryonic development. Clinically the external genitalia, i.e. the penis and the scrotum are like that of a normal male except that the scrotum is empty. Genitography reveals a male type urethra (Fig. 18.5A), which at times may be associated with an underdeveloped vagina opening high on the vertical portion (high junction). Cervical impression is absent or difficult to appreciate. MRI or pelvic sonography would demonstrate presence of uterus and gonads (Fig. 18.5B). MRI or CT shows bilateral adrenal hyperplasia (Fig. 18.5C). Bone age is accelerated (Fig. 18.5D). It is advisable to rear these children as male.

Incomplete virilization type is equivalent to Prader types I to IV and occurs as a result of exposure to lesser amounts of androgens later during the embryonic development. Clinically, external genital appearance varies from simple clitoral hypertrophy (Prader

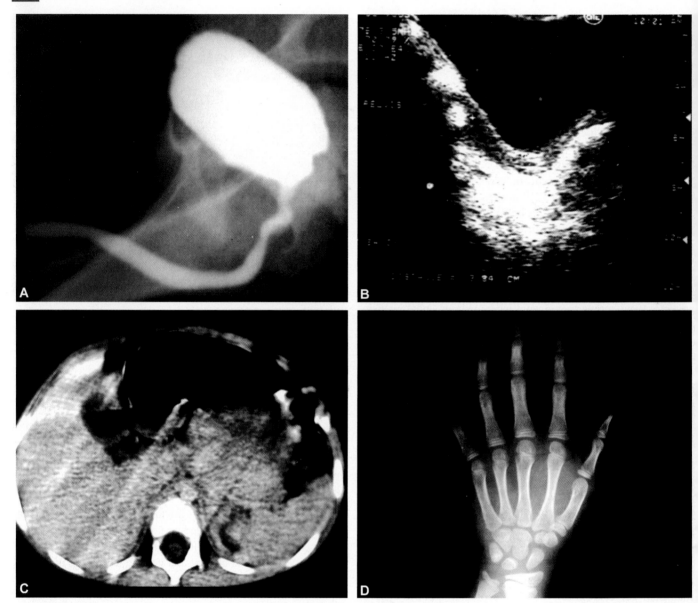

Figs 18.5A to D: A 4-year-old child with FPH, complete virilization type: Genitography (A) did not show any Müllerian duct derivative in a boy with normal external genitalia with cryptorchidism. Pelvic sonography, (B) revealed presence of a well-formed uterus. CT (C) demonstrated bilateral adrenal hyperplasia, (D) bone age is accelerated

type I) to perineal hypospadias (Prader type IV). Genitography reveals a well-developed vagina with cervical impression (Figs 18.6A and B), uterus and tubes (Figs 18.6C and D). These patients should be reared as female.

MR images demonstrate masculinized external genitalia with normal ovaries (Fig. 18.7A) and uterus (Fig. 18.7B). It may show enlarged adrenal glands due to adrenal hyperplasia. Although external genitalia of complete virilization type of FPH are similar to those of males, there are no testes at any site. In patients of incomplete virilization type of FPH, the hypertrophied clitoris mimics penis due to prominent corpora cavernosa and corpus spongiosum (Fig. 18.7C). The uterus and the vagina may be filled with clear urine due to reflux into them through the urogenital sinus.[16]

Male Pseudohermaphroditism (MPH)[1,2,7]

MPH represents a genetic male having 46 XY karyotype with normal or mildly defective testes.

Cause: Five well-recognized types based on etiology are:

i. Combined anti-Müllerian hormone (AMH) and testosterone deficiency

ii. AMH deficiency alone

iii. Androgen receptor insensitivity (testicular feminization syndrome: complete and incomplete types)

iv. Defective testosterone biosynthesis

v. 5 α-reductase deficiency resulting in decreased dihydrotestosterone production.

Final definitive diagnosis would require sophisticated laboratory facilities for estimation of these hormones.

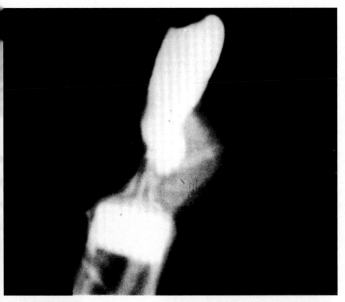

Fig. 18.6A: FPH, incomplete virilization types (different cases): (A) Flush technique genitography filled only a well-formed vagina. Note a concave upward filling defect on top of the vagina, the cervical identification, presence of which indirectly denotes a well-formed uterus

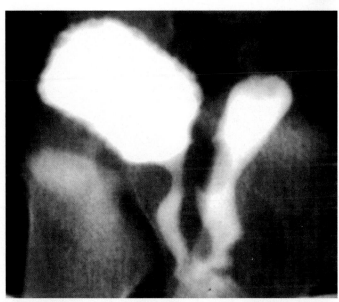

Fig. 18.6B: FPH, incomplete virilization types: (B) Both urethra and vagina, open together very low, close to the surface of perineum. Again note negative filling defect, the cervical indentation. Uterus and tubes are not opacified in both (A) and (B)

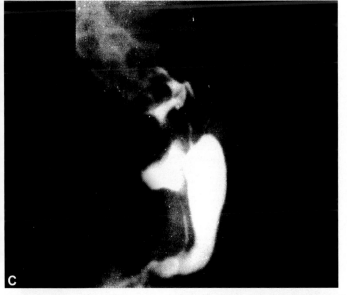

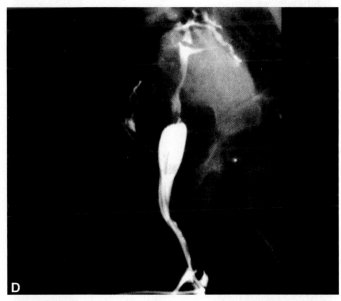

Figs 18.6C and D: FPH, incomplete virilization types: Picture is similar to (B) except that contrast has entered the uterine cavity and tubes with spill over into the peritoneal cavity

Without going into the details of each subtypes of MPH listed above, it would suffice to state that the clinical (i.e., external genitalia) and genitographic appearance (i.e. internal genitalia) of three of these MPH, i.e. incomplete testicular feminization syndrome; defective testosterone biosynthesis and steroid 5 alpha reductase deficiency, are similar, i.e. externally they all show ambiguous genitalia with perineal hypospadias while internally, on genitographic study, they show variable sized urogenital sinus and a small sized vagina without cervical impression (Figs 18.8A to C).

MRI demonstrates bilateral testes (commonly undescended) (Figs 18.9A and B) and incompletely musculinized or frankly feminized external genitalia. There is no uterus (Fig. 18.10) or ovaries. Both testes are of normal size and signal intensity and are located in the scrotum or in the inguinal canals. The corpora cavernosa and, corpus spongiosum, and the supporting muscular structures are well-demonstrated (Fig. 18.11) and the prostatic tissue appears to be present. Hypospadias is well-visualized on sagittal images. Pseudovagina may be seen on MR images.[16]

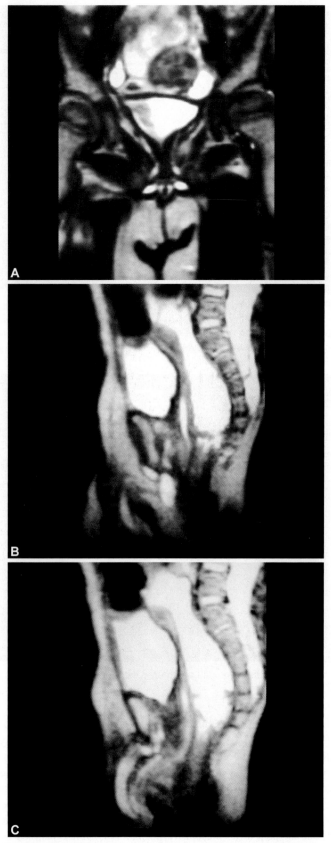

Figs 18.7A to C: MRI in FPH: (A) Coronal T2WI shows bilateral normal ovaries with high signal intensity. (B) Midline Sagittal MRI: Normal uterus well seen. (C) Externally, hypertrophied clitoris seen

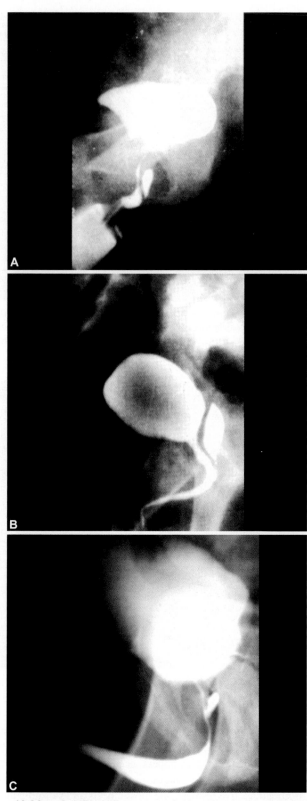

Figs 18.8A to C: MPH (different cases): Note that the junctional site is low (A), middle (B) and high (C). As the junctional site moves up, the degree of masculinization also increases which is evident by longer, male type urethra. In (C), small vaginal remnant, also called utriculus is arising from the vertical portion of the urethra. Also note absence of cervical indentation and the top of the vaginal remnants remaining round

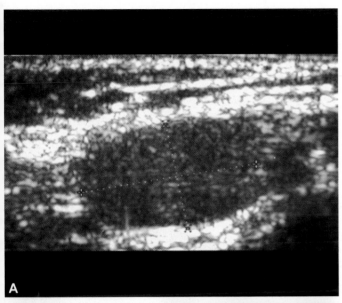

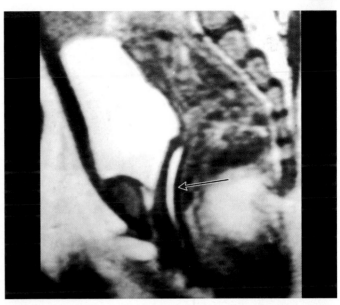

Fig. 18.10: MPH. Midline sagittal T2W MRI shows fluid filled vagina but absent uterus

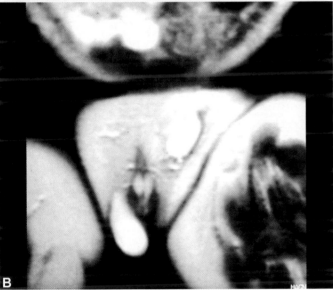

Figs 18.9A and B: MPH. Undescended testes. (A) Ultrasonography detects a gonad at inguinal canal. (B) T2W coronal MRI demonstrates bilateral undescended testes as high signal masses

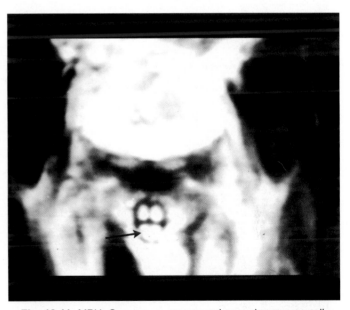

Fig. 18.11: MPH. Corpora cavernosa and spongiosum are well-demonstrated, presence of these suggest male type of anatomy

Patient with AMH deficiency is also called 'Male with uterus' because on clinical examination of the external genitalia, these patients appear as normal male with the urethra opening at the tip of a normally formed penis. They also have cryptorchidism (or inguinal hernia) and internally fully developed Müllerian duct derivatives, i.e. well-formed vagina and uterus (Figs 18.12A and B) are present.

In complete testicular feminization syndrome, on the other hand, externally there is no sexual ambiguity and the external genitalia appears as that of a normal female but genitography would demonstrate a short, blind ending vagina without any evidence of cervix and a separate urethral opening (Fig. 18.13).

If a newborn has perineal hypospadias and 46XY karyotype, it is important to assume that the child is a male with congenital urogenital malformation. In these patients, one must keep MPH in the differential diagnosis. Genitography and, if facilities are available, d-hydroxy testosterone therapeutic test, are mandatory prior to reaching at the final diagnosis and assigning a particular sex to the child.

Rarely, MPH also forms part of a syndrome called Drash's syndrome which has three components, i.e. MPH, progressive mesangial sclerosis with nephrotic syndrome and Wilms' tumor.

True Hermaphroditism (TH)[1,7]

Majority (50-80%) of true hermaphrodites are have a 46XX karyotype with both the ovary and the testicular tissue present in

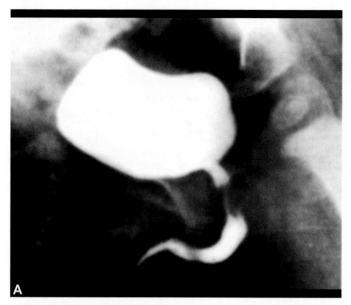
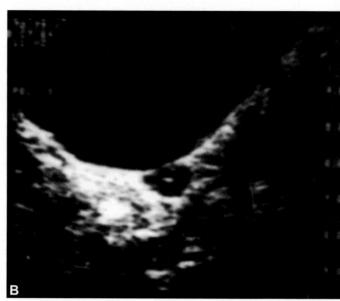

Figs 18.12A and B: MPH, AMH deficiency type. Genitography (A) documents a male type urethra only. On sonography (B), however, a good sized uterus and cervix was detected. Example of 'Male with uterus'

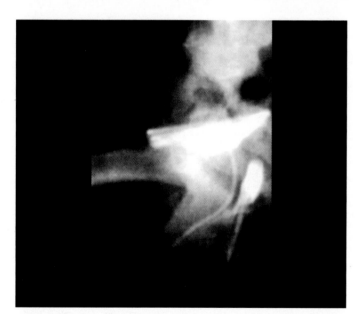

Fig. 18.13: MPH, complete testicular feminization syndrome type: Clinically, no ambiguity in the external genitalia which was female type, i.e. two separate openings, one each for urethra and vagina present. Simultaneous, separate catheterization of both the openings with retrograde contrast injection demonstrates a small, hypoplastic, blind ending vagina with rounded top and absence of cervical indentation. Sonography or MRI would show absence of uterus or cervix

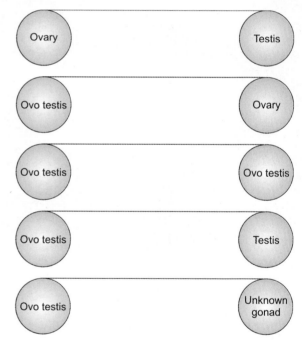

Fig. 18.14: TH: Schematic drawing to show all possible combinations of testicular and an ovarian tissue, on the two sides

the same patient or even same gonad. Various possible combinations in which these tissues may occur in TH are shown in Figure 18.14.

Clinically, before puberty, patients with TH present with an ambiguous external genitalia but later presentation may be varying such as cryptorchidism, breast development in a patient reared up as a male, hematuria (actually menstruation through the urogenital sinus opening) in those reared up as a male, amenorrhea in those reared up as female, inguinal hernia, etc.

Genitography shows a urogenital sinus of variable size with a relatively well-developed vagina which may open at varying level into the urethra. Contrast might also enter into the uterus and tubes (Fig. 18.15).

MRI demonstrates both an ovary and a testis (one or both of which may be replaced by an ovotestis) and variable internal and external genitalia.

Final diagnosis is made only after laparotomy, identification of the Müllerian and Wolffian duct derivatives and gonadal biopsy and histopathological examination of the gonads.

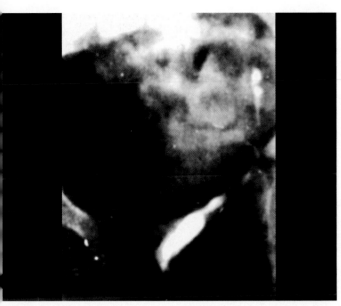

Fig. 18.15: TH, Genitography: demonstrates presence of Müllerian duct derivative only on the left side. Due to the presence of testicular tissue on the contralateral side, Müllerian duct structures do not differentiate on that side

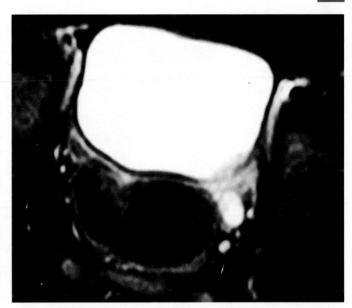

Fig. 18.17: DMP, T2W Axial MRI shows left sided gonad with high signal. Histopathologically, it was a dysgenetic gonad

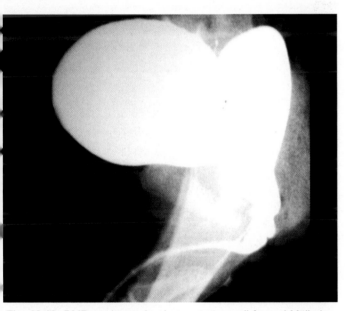

Fig. 18.16: DMP, genitography demonstrates well-formed Müllerian duct derivatives internally

Surgical management consists of excision of inappropriate gonadal tissues followed by appropriate genitoplasty of external genitalia.

Mixed Gonadal Dysgenesis (MGD) and Dysgenetic Male Pseudohermaphroditism (DMP)[1,2,7]

It is believed that MGD and DMP represent different spectra of the same condition. In both MGD and DMP, karyotypes are similar, i.e. XY; internally Müllerian ducts are always present

(Fig. 18.16) and externally hypospadias is almost always found. The only difference between the two is in the histology of the gonads (Fig. 18.17), i.e. MGD (Figs 18.18A to F) has a normal testis on one side and dysgenetic testis on the contralateral side, while DMP has dysgenetic testes on both the sides. On MRI, dysgenetic gonads have a spectrum of appearances ranging from normal size to streak gonads. Although dysgenetic gonads have intermediate signal intensity on T1W and T2W images, histological confirmation is essential for definitive diagnosis. In any case, prophylactic early gonadectomy must be performed because of a high incidence of testicular tumors developing in both these disorders. The small, hypoplastic uterus and vagina are well demonstrated on MRI.

There are only few MRI studies in the literature regarding imaging of patients with intersex disorders.[5,16] Role of MRI in patients with intersex patients seems to be two folds: (a) to delineate internal genital anatomy, including gonads, and (b) to characterize the external genital structures, especially to differentiate hypertrophied phallus from normal penis. In a study by Secaf *et al*,[8] MRI depiction of uterus was possible in 93 percent, vagina in 95 percent, penis in 10 percent, testes in 88 percent, and ovary in 74 percent patients. At AIIMS, genitography, ultrasound and MRI were performed in 33 children of intersex disorder (13 days to 17 years of age) after appropriate clinical work-up, karyotyping and hormonal analysis.[16] The ability to detect common urogenital sinus (UGS), vagina and gonads by each modality was assessed. Surgical follow-up was available in 17 cases whereas karyotype, hormonal assay and bio-chemical profile was taken as a proof of diagnosis in the remaining 16 cases. Common UGS was properly evaluated in 48 percent cases by genitography, and none by ultrasound or MRI. Vagina was detected by genitography, US and MRI in 100 percent, 39.4 percent and 78 percent respectively. Uterus was detected by

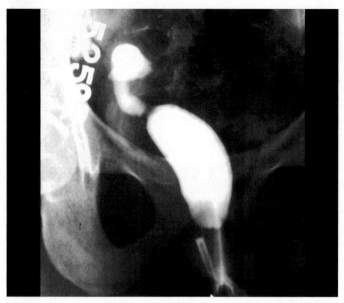

Fig. 18.18A: MGD: Genitography documents a right sided Müllerian duct structures

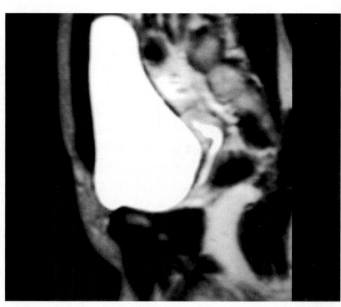

Fig. 18.18C: MGD: Sagittal T2W MRI demonstrates well-formed uterus

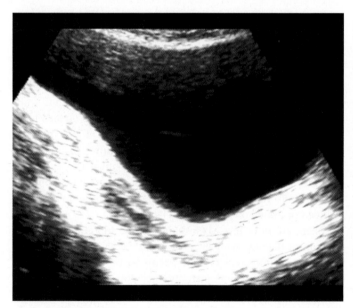

Fig. 18.18B: MGD: On US, longitudinal section uterus is seen

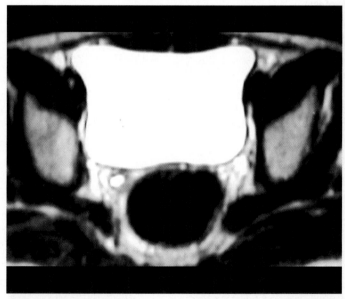

Fig. 18.18D: MGD: Axial T2W MRI localizes the uterus to right side only

genitography, US and MRI in 69 percent, 75 percent and 100 percent cases respectively. US detected 21 inguinal and 8 intra-abdominal gonads (total 44%), whereas MRI detected 40 inguinal and 11 intra-abdominal gonads (total 77.3%).[17] Relatively hypointense (even hyperintense) gonad on T2W images could be atrophic or dysgenetic gonads and requires histological analysis.

Supporting muscles of phallus, viz. bulbospongiosus (BS), ischiocavernosus (IC) and superficial transverse perinii (STP) have been stated to help to differentiate enlarged clitoris from penis on MRI.[8] In the study at AIIMS, it was found that well-developed BS and IC muscles are a better indicator of chromosomal (karyotype) than hormonal (urethral type) sex. Well-developed supporting muscles suggest a likely male karyotype. However, when these muscles are indeterminate or non-visualized, it cannot predict the chromosomal (karyotype) sex, but may suggest a female or indeterminate urethral type. STP muscle is not visualized in a large majority but when seen, it suggests a likely male karyotype. Poor or non-visualization of this muscle gives no clue about the chromosomal sex or urethral type.[18] Literature is silent on MRI findings of these muscles in different types of intersex patients.

More work in this field comparing MRI with ultrasound, genitography and correlation with surgical findings is required before a final algorithmic approach can be decided.

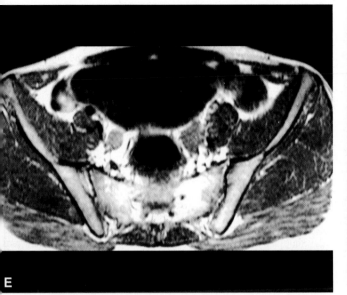
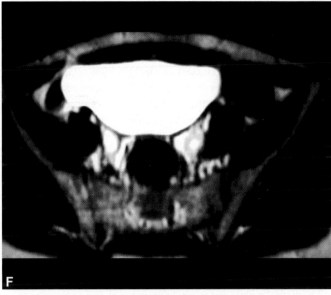

Figs 18.18E and F: MGD: Axial T1W (E) and T2W MRI (F) demonstrates bilateral gonads. Histologically both were dysgenetic

CLUES TO THE DIAGNOSIS

At most centers especially in India, laboratory facilities for a detailed investigation of a case of intersex child are lacking. Under these circumstances, by combining the information of karyotyping genitographic anatomy and MRI, one can reach at a reasonably correct "working diagnosis" within a short period of time and thus the sex of rearing can be assigned to the child at an early age. The diagnostic approach is shown in Table 18.1. MRI is now more widely used. With increasing experience in interpreting the complex anatomy of intersex disorders, it is necessary that MRI

Table 18.1: Diagnostic algorithm in an intersex child. Criteria used: Karyotyping + genitographic anatomy				
Genitographic anatomy → karyotyping ↓				
Chromatin Positive (XX)	FPH (Total virilization type)	—	—	• FPH (Partial virilization type) • TH
	MPH	MPH	MPH	• MGD • DMP
Chromatin Negative (XY)	(AMH deficiency only)	(Androgen receptor insensitivity type: complete testicular feminization syndrome)	Causes: • Deficiency of 5 alpha reductase • Defective bio-synthesis of testosterone • Incomplete testicular feminization syndrome	• MPH with combined AMH and testosterone deficiency

Key: MPH = Male pseudohermaphroditism
FPH = Female pseudohermaphroditism
TH = True hermaphroditism
MGD = Mixed gonadal dysgenesis
DMP = Dysgenetic male pseudohermaphroditism
AMH = Anti-Müllerian hormone

should form an essential component in the diagnostic work-up of these patients for reaching definitive diagnosis.

CONCLUSION

Intersex disorders are complex clinical problems. Genitography, ultrasonography and more recently MRI are important imaging tools. Except perhaps for the evaluation of urogenital sinus, most of the other information required in an intersex child can now be obtained non-invasively and reliably by MRI without use of ionizing radiation. Role of the radiologist is not to arrive at a diagnosis, but to accurately demonstrate the genital anatomy. This is often difficult as the conditions encountered are diverse in aetiology and often incompletely expressed. The final diagnosis is established by putting clinical findings with a combination of cytogenetic, biochemical and radiological studies. An early decision regarding the phenotypic sex, lessens the psychological impact on the child and is crucial in parent counselling. A close cooperation between a pediatric endocrinologist, pediatric surgeon and pediatric radiologist is vital for comprehensive management of these challenging disorders.

REFERENCES

1. Josso N, Karger, Basel (Eds). The Intersex Child of Pediatric and Adolescent Endocrinology 1981; 8.
2. Silverman F (Ed). Caffey's Pediatric X-ray Diagnosis (9th ed). Chicago: Year Book Medical Publishers Inc. 1993; 2.
3. Cohen HL, Bober SE. Imaging the pediatric pelvis: The normal and abnormal genital tract and simulators in its diseases. Urol Radiol 1992; 14:273-83.
4. Cremin BJ. Intersex states in young children: The importance of radiology in making a correct diagnosis. Clin Radiol 1974; 25:63-73.
5. Gambino J, Coldwell B, Dietrich R, et al. Congenital disorders of sexual differentiation: MR findings. Pictorial Essay AJR 1992; 158:363-7.
6. Horowity M, Glassberg KI. Ambiguous genitalia: Diagnosis, evaluation, and treatment. Urol Radiol 1992; 14:306-18.
7. Gupta AK. Imaging of intersex. In Subbarao K, Banerjee S, Aggarwal SK, et al (Eds): Diagnostic Radiology and Imaging 1997; 1:860-9.
8. Secaf E, Hricak H, Gooding CA, et al. Role of MRI in the evaluation of ambiguous genitalia. Pediatric Radiology 1994; 24:231-5.
9. Wright NB, Smith C, Rickwood AMK, et al. Review: Imaging children with ambiguous genitalia and intersex states. Clini Radio 1995; 50:823-9.
10. McCarthy S, Tauber C, Gore J. Female pelvic anatomy: MR assessment of variations during the menstrual cycle and with use of oral contraceptives. Radiology 1986; 160:119-23.
11. Paquin AJ, Baker DH, Finby N, et al. The urogenital sinus: Its demonstration and significance. J Urol 1957; 78:796-807.
12. Shopfner Ch E. In S Karger, Basel (Eds). Genitography in Intersex Problems. Progr Pediat Radiol. 1970; 3:97-115.
13. Josso N, Fortier B, Faure C. Genitography in intersexual states: A review of 86 cases with new criteria for the study of the urogenital sinus. Acuta Endocrinologica. 1969; 62:165-80,.
14. Nihoul-Fekete C. Feminising genitoplasty in the intersex child. In Josso N, Karger S, Basel (Eds): The Intersex Child. Pediatric and Adolescent Endocrinology. 1981; 8:240-60.
15. Prader A. Helv Paediat 9: 231-48 (Quoted in reference number 8) 1954.
16. Choi HK, Cho KS, Lee HW, Kim KS. MR imaging of intersexuality. Radiographics 1998; 18:83-96.
17. Haloi AK, Gupta AK, Sharma S, et al. Radiological evaluation of children with intersex disorders with ambiguous genitalia using genitography, ultrasonography and MR imaging. AJR 2001; 178:50. Abstact (Suppl).
18. Sharma S, Gupta AK, Haloi AK. MR imaging of muscles supporting the phallus : A clue to the true sex in an intersex child. Radiology 2002; 225:669, Abstract (Suppl).

CHAPTER **19**

Skeletal Dysplasias

Gaurav S Pradhan

INTRODUCTION

The skeletal dysplasias are a large heterogeneous group of genetic conditions characterized by abnormal shape, growth, number or integrity of bones. In the broadest sense, skeletal dysplasias may be divided into the osteodysplasias and the chondrodysplasias depending on the fact that the dysplasias are due to disturbance in osteoid production or in chondroid formation respectively. The dysplasias may result from the following:
1. Abnormal growth—affecting shape and size of skeleton.
2. Abnormal number of bones—either decreased or increased.
3. Abnormal texture—decreased or increased activity of remodelling process and mineral deposition.

The birth prevalence of skeletal dysplasias recognizable in the neonatal period has been estimated to be 2.4/10,000 births.[1] The lack of understanding of etiology of skeletal dysplasias resulted in classifications that were mainly descriptive and the technique most likely to identify the findings was predominantly used to categorize the anomalies.[2,3] Therefore, many definitions are based on radiological criteria with a few based on histological or clinical criteria.

TERMINOLOGY

Most skeletal dysplasias are forms of disproportionate short stature. To date about 220 well-established skeletal dysplasias are known to exist. Despite recent breakthroughs in the areas of collagen biochemistry and gene localization, the diagnosis still lies primarily in the hands of the radiologist.[4-6]

For the evaluation of skeletal dysplasias, certain basic definitions are important. Skeletal dysplasias can involve either the spine or the long bones. When the spine or any of its parts are shortened, the prefix spondylo is used. Involvement of the long bones on the other hand is subclassified into rhizomelia (proximal shortening involving the humerus and/or femur), mesomelic when, there is shortening of distal limb (radius and tibia) and micromelic when there is shortening of proximal and distal limbs. Dysostosis are skeletal abnormalities caused by embryonic developmental errors as opposed to dysplasias, which exert their effect during the entire period of skeletal growth.

These definitions are important because the terminologies of many disorders were created based on radiologic findings, although they may be confusing at times. The skeletal dysplasias are often classified according to whether the epiphysis, the metaphysis or the diaphysis is involved. Thus, it is important that the tubular bones are viewed before closure of the epiphyseal plate.

Another important consideration in dealing with skeletal dysplasia is the concept of lethality. About 25 disorders are included in the group of lethal dysplasias.

By far the most common lethal dysplasia, at or before birth, is thanatophoric dysplasia. Other relatively common lethal skeletal dysplasias include homozygous achondroplasia, osteogenesis imperfecta type II and achondrogenesis type II/hypochondrogenesis.

Usually, these conditions are lethal because the infant possesses a small chest cage as a direct result of having short ribs, leading to respiratory insufficiency and death in most cases. The chest circumference to abdominal circumference ratio in most of these cases is usually less than 0.85 and reflects the reduction of chest size. No children of asphyxiating thoracic dysplasia who have managed to live beyond 2 years have been reported to die of respiratory insufficiency. The reason for this appears to be growth of thoracic cage, resulting in adequate respiratory function. It is therefore very critical when dealing with a newborn with skeletal dysplasia to establish the diagnosis quickly and then to decide if the child should receive ventilator care.[7, 8]

The nonlethal skeletal dysplasias are a much larger group. They are considered according to the time of appearance, at birth or early infancy, or others after 2 years of age. Heterozygous achondroplasia is the most common condition that appears close to birth. The radiographic findings are specific to this disorder, which is differentiated from pseudoachondroplasia where the head is normal sized.

Most patients of nonlethal dysplasias if managed properly, could live relatively normal and productive lives.

Skeletal survey for the diagnosis of skeletal dysplasia should include the following radiographs:
- Skull – AP, lateral and Towne's
- Spine – AP and lateral
- Chest – AP view
- Pelvis – AP view
- Upper and lower extremities – AP view
- Hands and feet – AP view
- Lateral view of foot in neonatal disorders and a full body AP and lateral radiograph in postmortem examination of newborn.

Newer Imaging Modalities

Computed tomography and magnetic resonance imaging have an important role to play in the evaluation of intracranial and spinal cord anomalies in skeletal dysplasias. They are also helpful in assessing abnormalities of the cranium and the bony spinal canal. This is important in prognosticating the outcome of the dysplasia. 3-dimensional CT scan is used to evaluate craniofacial anomalies prior to reconstructive surgery while MR imaging of the spine is helpful in the presurgical planning prior to surgical treatment of spinal abnormalities.[7, 8]

Despite recent advances in imaging, fetal skeletal dysplasias are difficult to diagnose in utero. This is especially so, as there are large number of skeletal dysplasias with overlapping phenotypic features, lack of systemic approach and due to variable time of presentation of the dysplasia. The dysplasia may be suspected during routine ultrasound, if an abnormal or short bone or some other abnormal skeletal finding is detected. It is also important to evaluate chest circumference, femur length-abdominal circumference ratio to assess the possibility of lethality, besides evaluating for other craniofacial and skeletal anomalies. The bones should be evaluated for presence, curvature, degree of mineralization and fractures. The femur length-abdominal circumference ratio of less than 0.16 suggests lung hypoplasia, while femur length-foot length ratio of less than 1, suggests skeletal dysplasias. If there is disproportionate limb shortening, then the segment {rhizo, meso or acromelic} involved should be assessed.[9, 10]

The dysplasias and dysostoses group of skeletal abnormalities have been broadly classified into five major groups (Table 19.1).[11]

OSTEOCHONDRODYSPLASIAS

Defects of Growth of Tubular Bones, Spine or Both

Dysplasias Manifested at Birth

Achondrogenesis

1. Clinicopathologic features: Achondrogenesis is a phenotypically diverse group of chondrodysplasias characterised by a short trunk and micromelia. Achondrogenesis is classified into two types, type I and type II. In achondrogenesis I, the child is usually stillborn or dies soon after birth. Achondrogenesis II is not lethal and usually appears in children of consanguinous parents.
2. Imaging features: The radiologic findings in achondrogenesis I include severe lack of ossification of vertebral bodies, small deformed iliac bones, absent or poor ossification of pubic and ischial bones. There is severe micromelia involving the tubular bones, which are markedly shortened and malformed with wide cupped ends. The ribs are short and show cupped and flared ends. Rib fractures are present in some patients. The skull and other membranous bones are involved.

    Imaging features in achondrogenesis II include shortening of bones in distal extremities. The bones are curved and distal segments may be absent. The ossification of bones of hand and feet is delayed. Polydactyly of the hands and feet is

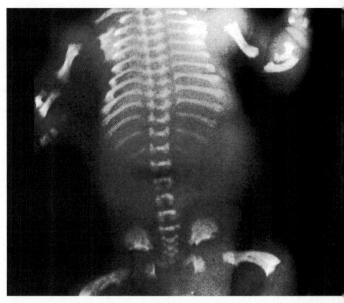

Fig. 19.1: AP projection of a Thanaophoric dwarf showing short and curved tubular bones with telephone receiver configuration of the femora. There is deficient ossification of the vertebral bodies producing an H shaped appearance. The ribs are short with undercut scapulae

common. The skull and other membranous bones are not involved, distinguishing it from type I.

Thanatophoric dysplasia

1. Clinical features: As the name implies, thanatophoric dysplasia meaning "death bearing", is the most common lethal bony dysplasia. Clinically the disease is so severe that it may be recognized *in utero*, with a family history of polyhydramnios and spontaneous abortions. The thorax is markedly narrow with resultant inability of the infant to inflate the lung. Prenatal diagnosis by sonography is possible. Polyhydraminos, poor foetal activity and presence of extra ossification pelvic centres can help in the diagnosis of the dysplasia *in utero*.[12]
2. Imaging features: The radiological features include marked rhizomelic shortening of tubular bones with presence of metaphyseal flaring, osseous widening and bowing. Bowed femora are characteristic and appear like telephone receivers (Fig. 19.1). Skull changes include frontal bossing, macrocephaly, small skull base and small foramen magnum and cloverleaf skull. Thorax is slender with short ribs with flared anterior ends. There is marked flattening of vertebral bodies with constriction of their mid portions, prominent intervertebral disc spaces against a back drop of well formed neural arches giving a typical H or inverted U appearance on AP view. Narrowing of spinal canal is most marked in lumbar region. Changes in pelvis include small rectangular iliac bones, small sacrosciatic notches with short and wide pubic and ischial bones.

    The features distinguishing this dysplasia from achondroplasia are severe universal vertebra plana in spine and short tubular bowed bones of limbs.

Table 19.1: Classification of skeletal abnormalities

1. Osteochondrodysplasias (Abnormalities of Cartilage or Bone Growth and Development)

i. Defects of growth of tubular bones, spine or both

Manifested at birth

- Achondrogenesis
- Thanatophoric dysplasia
- Achondroplasia
- Chondrodysplasia punctata
- Metatrophic dwarfism
- Diastophic dwarfism
- Chondroectodermal dysplasia
- Asphyxiating thoracic dysplasia (Jeune)
- Spondyloepiphyseal dysplasia congenita
- Cleidocranial dysplasia
- Mesomelic dwarfism

Manifested in later life

- Hypochondroplasia
- Metaphyseal chondrodysplasia
- Spondylometaphyseal dysplasia
- Multiple epiphyseal dysplasia
- Spondyloepiphyseal dysplasia tarda
- Acrodysplasia

ii. Disorganised development of cartilage and fibrous components of the skeleton

- Dysplasia epiphysealis hemimelica
- Multiple cartilaginous exostosis
- Enchondromatosis (Ollier's disease)
- Fibrous dysplasia

iii. Abnormalities in the density of cortical diaphyseal structures or metaphyseal modelling, or both

- Osteogenesis imperfecta congenita
- Osteogenesis imperfecta tarda
- Osteopetrosis
- Pycnodysostosis
- Osteopoikilosis
- Osteopathia striata
- Melorheostosis
- Diaphyseal dysplasia
- Metaphyseal dysplasia
- Craniodiaphyseal dysplasia
- Craniometaphyseal dysplasia
- Frontometaphyseal dysplasia

2. Dysostoses (Malformation of Individual Bone, Singly or in Combination)

i. Dysostoses with cranial and facial involvement

- Craniosynostosis
- Craniofacial synostosis

ii. Dysostosis with predominantly axial involvement

- Vertebral segmentation defects
- Sprengel's deformity
- Osteo-onychodysostosis

iii. Dysostosis with predominant involvement of extremities

- Amelia
- Hemimelia
- Phocomelia
- Radioulnar synostosis
- Polysyndactyly
- Clinodactyly

3. Idiopathic Osteolysis

- Acro-osteolysis (phalangeal type, tarsocarpal type)
- Multicentric osteolysis

4. Primary Disturbances of Growth

- Cornelia de Lange syndrome
- Progeria

5. Constitutional Diseases of Bone with Known Pathogenesis

i. Chromosomal aberrations

ii. Primary metabolic abnormalities

- Calcium phosphorous metabolism (Hypophosphatasia)
- Mucopolysaccharidosis
- Mucolipidosis and lipidosis

iii. Bone abnormalities secondary to disturbances of extra-skeleton systems

- Endocrine
- Hematologic
- Neurologic
- Renal
- Gastrointestinal
- Cardiopulmonary

Achondroplasia

1. Clinicopathological features: Achondroplasia is the most common type of nonlethal dysplasia presenting with dwarfism. It is a hereditary condition with an autosomal dominant mode of transmission, though now most cases may be due to mutation of gene in older fathers, in 85% of cases. It presents at birth and is characterized clinically by a large head with brachycephaly, prominent frontal bones with nasal bridge recession, rhizomelic dwarfism, constricted thorax and trident hands due to separation of second and third digits. There is generalized defect in enchondral bone formation. The apophyseal growth is deficient towards the metaphysis, resulting in a V-shaped defect in which the epiphysis is incorporated. A fibrous band growing from periosteum can interpose between epiphysis and the ossifying cartilage, with resultant stunting of longitudinal growth.

2. Imaging features: The radiographic findings include a large cranium with respect to size of face with defective growth of base of skull giving a pinched appearance. The foramen magnum is small and funnel shaped. CT and MRI of cranio-

cervical region show associated abnormalities of the cervicomedullary junction. Anteroposterior diameter of chest is decreased due to short ribs. Spinal abnormalities include reduction in inter-pedicular distances in lumbar region with short pedicles, narrow spinal canal and posterior vertebral scalloping (Fig. 19.2A). Vertebral bodies are flattened and can appear bullet shaped in infancy and early childhood. Changes in pelvis include square iliac bones with posteriorly set horizontal acetabular roof and small sacrosciatic notches giving classical "tombstone appearance" (Fig. 19.2B). Rhizomelic shortening of proximal bones, with deepseated epiphysis in flared metaphysis gives a V shaped appearance (Fig. 19.2C). Shortening and widening of tubular bones of hand and feet, with typical involvement of proximal and middle phalanges can also be seen.

With advancing age, severe spinal cord compromise and disc protrusions become especially important and are best evaluated by MRI. (Figs 19.2D and E)

In hypochondroplasia, the radiologic findings are similar but less severe than those of achondroplasia and the skull is never affected.

Achondroplasia needs to be differentiated from thanatophoric dysplasia, spondyloepiphyseal dysplasia, diastrophic dwarfism, metatrophic dwarfism, asphyxiating thoracic dysplasia, Ellis-van-Creveld syndrome, cartilage hair hypoplasia and metaphyseal dysostosis.

Chondrodysplasia Punctata (CDP) Group

1. Clinical pathological features: It is transmitted as an autosomal recessive trait, with a female preponderance. Most of the cases are manifest clinically before two years of age. There is craniofacial dysmorphism, ocular abnormalities, severe mental retardation, spastic tetraplegia and joint contractures with shortening of one or more limbs. There is a benign non-rhizomelic group with good prognosis with little residual deformity, and a potentially lethal rhizomelic group. Death occurs in the rhizomelic group due to tracheal stenosis or spinal cord compression usually within the first decade. Mucoid degeneration in epiphyseal centre has been seen histologically which leads to fragmentation of the epiphysis. This becomes a nidus for calcareous deposits or punctate ossification.

2. Imaging features: Radiologic findings include stippled calcification of the cartilage at the end of bones. There is symmetric rhizomelic or mesomelic limb shortening with metaphyseal splaying.[13] There can be delayed ossification of carpal bones. There is hypoplasia of bones of mid-face with nasal flattening. Changes in spine include defective vertebral ossification, flattening of vertebral column, transient lucent vertebral defect, and abnormalities of segmentation, kyphosis and scoliosis. Neurologic abnormalities such as Dandy-Walker frequently co-exist. Iliac blades lack normal flaring. Calcifications in and around epiphysis are frequently seen in region of acetabulum, femur, spine and carpal and tarsal bones in Conradi-Hünermann type.

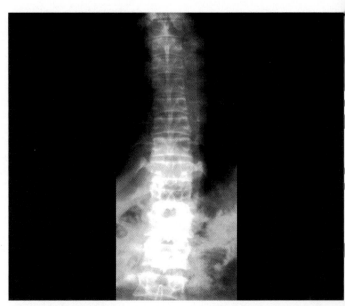

Fig. 19.2A: Reduction of interpedicular distances in lumbar spine on AP view, in a case of achondroplasia.

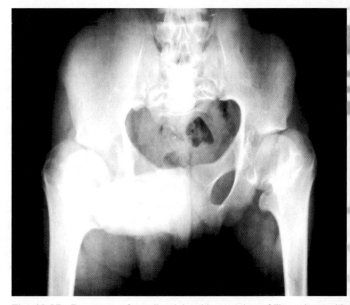

Fig. 19.2B: Presence of small pelvis with squaring of iliac wings with horizontal acetabular roof giving tombstone appearance, in a case of achondroplasia

The radiologic appearance is characteristic and should not be confused with other conditions (Fig. 19.3). In cretins, there can be epiphyseal fragmentation which is however larger and conforms to the expected shadow of the epiphysis.

Metatrophic Dysplasia

1. Clinical features: Metatrophic dysplasia is characterized by short extremities and a normal trunk at birth, and short trunk with kyphoscoliosis later in life.

2. Imaging features: The radiologic findings include marked metaphyseal widening with short bones of extremity giving a dumbbell appearance. The trochanters are large, typically the

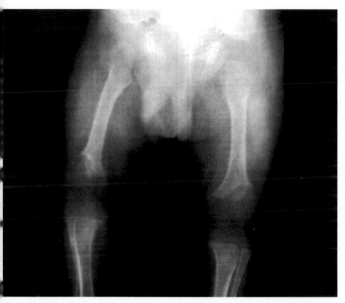

Fig. 19.2C: X-ray of lower extremities showing rhizomelic shortening of femora with V shaped defect of the distal femoral metaphysis, in a case of achondroplasia

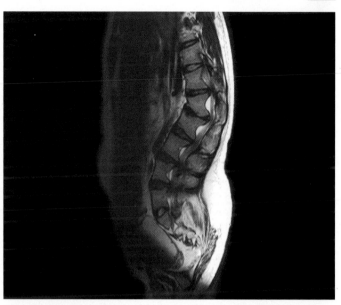

Fig. 19.2E: Sagittal MR image of the same patient showing marked wedging of vertebrae with posterior scalloping of vertebral bodies with prominent subarachnoid spaces anterior to the cauda equina, well seen on T2 weighted image

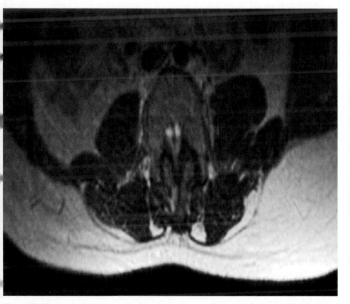

Fig. 19.2D: Axial MR image showing triangular configration of the spinal canal in a case of heterozygous achondroplasia, presenting with progressive spinal deformity

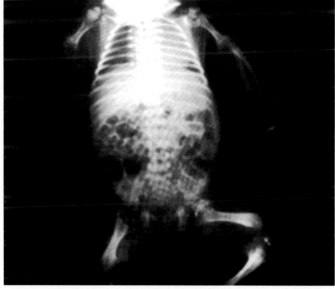

Fig. 19.3: Rhizomelic dwarfism with stippled epiphyseal calcification in a newborn, in a case of chondrodysplasia punctata

lesser trochanter with the appearance simulating a battle-axe. The epiphyses show delayed appearance and are small and deformed. The vertebral bodies are markedly reduced in height and appear rectangular or diamond shaped and can show anterior wedging. The intervertebral disc spaces consequently appear large. The neural arches are well developed. There may be hypoplasia of the dens with resultant atlantoaxial instability. The thorax is elongated with decreased AP diameter due to short ribs in infancy. There is severe anterior bowing of sternum

with development of kyphoscoliosis in childhood. Changes in pelvis include short ilia with curved lateral margins, flat acetabular roof, wide Y shaped triradiate cartilage and small sacrosciatic notches.

Diastrophic dysplasia group

1. Clinical features: The term diastrophic meaning twisted or crooked has been used to highlight the phenotype resulting from this autosomal recessive disorder. This dysplasia group has a mutation in the sulfate transporter gene. It is

characterized by short stature, progressive scoliosis, kyphosis, clubfeet, Hitchiker's thumb, multiple contractures, dislocations, deformed ears and cleft palate.

2. Imaging features: There is micromelic dwarfism with marked shortening of tubular bones with metaphyseal widening and rounding. The first metacarpal is oval and usually hypoplastic. There is delayed appearance of the epiphysis with flattening and deformity, seen characteristically in proximal and distal femora. Epiphysis in hand and foot bones may be irregular, distorted and deformed. A disproportionate shortening of ulna and fibula can be present. Narrowing of joint spaces especially of hip and elbows can be seen. Femora may have broad inter trochanteric regions with short femoral necks. Scoliosis is progressive leading to spinal abnormalities, instability, cord compression, and death.

Diastrophic dysplasia needs to be differentiated from achondroplasia and Morquio's syndrome. The oval metacarpal of diastrophic dwarfism is the most distinguishing feature. The presence of a basal segment of innominate bone and the lack of narrowing of the interpedicular distances in the lumbar region distinguish it from achondroplasia. The characteristic spinal changes in form of anterior beaking of lumbar vertebrae and "simian shaped" pelvis in Morquio's syndrome help in differentiating it from diastrophic dysplasia.

Chondroectodermal dysplasia
1. Clinical features: This is a short-limbed dwarfism characterised by ectodermal dysplasia, polydactyly and congenital heart disease. There is distal shortening of limbs, absent or hypoplastic nails, abnormal hair, dysplastic teeth and upper lip abnormalities. It is inherited as an autosomal recessive trait and is evident at birth. Death is common in childhood due to cardiac and pulmonary complications.

2. Imaging features: In addition to changes in asphyxiating thoracic dysplasia, there is presence of carpal fusion, postaxial poly and syndactyly, enlargement of proximal end of ulna and distal end of radius giving drumstick appearance with anterior dislocation of radial heads. Medial tibial exostoses, wide but hypoplastic lateral aspect of proximal tibia, genu valgum and fibular shortening are other typical features. Atrial septal defect is a commonly associated cardiac abnormality. The spine and skull are normal.

Asphyxiating thoracic dysplasia (Jeune Syndrome)
1. Clinical features: This is an autosomal recessive condition, which is evident at birth. The infants have characteristically constricted chests with shortening of the extremities. There is in addition, marked pulmonary hypoplasia. Most infants die due to respiratory distress while renal failure is frequent in those that survive.

2. Imaging features: The significant radiological features include high handle bar appearance of clavicles along with narrow thorax, short horizontal ribs and wide irregular costochondral junctions. Changes in pelvis include short ilia with flat acetabular roof and downward spike like projections giving trident appearance to the acetabulum. Premature ossification of capital femoral epiphysis is fairly common with presence of metaphyseal irregularity. Epiphysis in hand bones can be cone shaped and fuse prematurely, producing shortening of middle and distal phalanges. Skull and spine are normal. It is not associated with congenital heart disease.[14]

It can be differentiated from chondroectodermal dysplasia by the presence of short ribs, hepatic fibrosis and higher incidence of progressive renal disease. In addition, there is less frequent polydactyly and less frequent nail changes.

Spondyloepiphyseal dysplasia congenita
1. Clinical features: Spondyloepiphyseal dysplasia congenita is a hereditary dysplasia transmitted as an autosomal dominant trait that affects the spine and proximal epiphysis of long bones at birth. This short limb dwarfism is characterised by mild shortening of the limbs, cleft palate, flat face, short neck and increased anteroposterior chest diameter. Progressive kyphoscoliosis occurs as the child grows. Knock-knees and bowleg deformities are common. The hands and feet are normal.

2. Imaging features: The height of vertebral bodies is decreased with pear shaped vertebrae seen in infancy due to lack of development of the posterior portion of vertebral bodies. Anterior wedging, irregularity and generalised flattening can be present in childhood with development of kyphoscoliosis and lumbar lordosis. The interpedicular distances are narrowed in lumbar region. Atlanto-axial dislocation due to hypoplasia of dens can also be present. The chest is broad and bell shaped and of decreased height. There is in addition, short squared scapulae with flared anterior ends of ribs, delay in sternal ossification and pectus-carinatum. There is marked delay in ossification of the pubic bones and proximal portion of femora. The femoral heads often ossify from multiple centres and progressive coxa vara develops with premature osteoarthritis. Prominent shortening of neck of femora with small femoral heads well below the level of greater trochanter can be seen. The epiphyses are irregular and the metaphyses show flaring and irregularity in long tubular bones. The ossification may be delayed (Fig. 19.4).

Spondyloepiphyseal dysplasia congenita needs to be differentiated from Morquio's disease, diastrophic dwarfism, metatrophic dwarfism and multiple epiphyseal dysplasias.

Cleidocranial dysplasia
1. Clinical features: It is an uncommon autosomal dominant condition characterised by delayed or incomplete calvarial ossification and clavicular hypoplasia or aplasia. Midline structures are primarily affected in this dysplasia and the disease manifests in infancy. Mild shortening of the stature may also be present in cleidocranial dysplasia.

2. Imaging features: Radiologic findings include poor ossification of skull bones with presence of multiple wormian bones and wide sutures. The parietal bone ossification may be absent at birth. The foramen magnum is large and deformed, basilar invagination may occur. The clavicle is deficient in its outer or middle parts, though rarely it may be totally absent (Fig. 19.5A). The thorax is narrow and bell

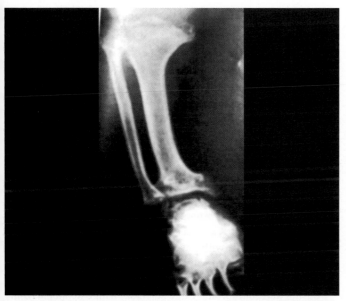

Fig. 19.4: Epiphyseal and metaphyseal irregularities with metaphyseal widening involving both tibia and fibula with angular deformity at the ankle joint, in a case of spondyloepiphyseal dysplasia congenita

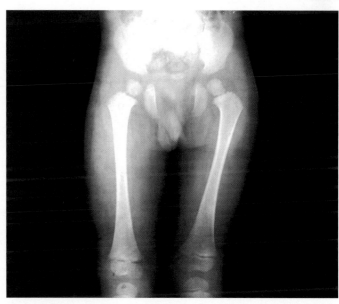

Fig. 19.5B: X-ray pelvis showing delayed ossification of pubic bones with wide pubic symphysis, giving a see-through appearance, in a case of cleidocranial dysplasia

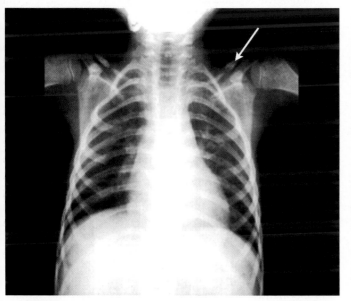

Fig. 19.5A: X-ray chest of an infant showing absence of both the clavicles in their middle parts, in a case of cleidocranial dysplasia

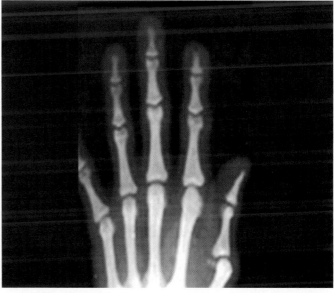

Fig. 19.5C: X-ray of hands and forearm in a case of cleidocranial dysplasia showing acro-osteolysis involving multiple terminal phalanges of both hands

shaped with a small hypoplastic scapula.[14,15] Pelvic abnormalities are common and include delayed ossification of pubic bones, narrow iliac wings and wide pubic symphysis giving a 'see-through' appearance (Fig. 19.5B). Coxa valga deformity is frequently present. The changes in spine include failure of fusion of neural arches, wedging of vertebral bodies with scoliosis, multiple ossification centres of thoracic vertebral bodies, defect in pars interarticularis in lumbar spine and spina bifida occulta in cervical and thoracic vertebrae.[16] There can be mild widening of the metaphysis and narrowing

of the diaphysis of tubular bones. Hand changes include long 2nd and 5th metacarpals with supernummery ossification centers and short 2nd and 5th phalanges, small middle and small tapered distal phalanges, pseudoepiphysis in metacarpal bones, and cone shaped epiphysis and retarded ossification of the carpal bones (Fig. 19.5C). Tibiotalar slant and short fibulae may also be present.

Yunis-Varon syndrome comprises cleidocranial dysostosis, micrognathia, absence of thumbs and first metatarsals and distal aphalangia.

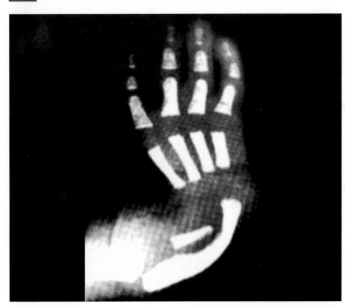

Fig. 19.6: Newborn infant with hypoplastic radius, curved ulna with absent thumb in a case of mesomelic dysplasia

Mesomelic dysplasias

Dyschondrosteosis is the most common mesomelic dysplasia.

It is transmitted as an autosomal dominant trait with a female predominance. Dorsal dislocation of distal ulna is present with limited elbow and wrist movement.

1. Radiological features: It is characterised by mesomelic limb shortening with Madelung deformity of the forearm. It is also called as Léri-Weill syndrome. There is shortening of radius with bowing deformity and subluxated distal end of ulna. The lack of development of distal radial epiphysis results in tilting of the distal end of radius in a volar and ulnar direction. The radial head can also dislocate. Similar changes in lower leg can result in deformity of ankle mortice.

   Nievergelt type is the most severe type of mesomelic dysplasia, which is also accompanied by bony prominences in the lower legs. Hypoplasia of bones of forearm and leg is common (Fig. 19.6). Dysplasia of tibia may result in triangular or rhomboid configuration of tibia and slanting of the growth plate of tibia. Proximal radioulnar synostosis with elbow dislocation and fusion of carpal bones may also be seen.

Dysplasias Manifested in Later Life

Hypochondroplasia

1. Clinical features: This dysplasia is transmitted in an autosomal dominant mode. The clinical features include short stature with relatively long trunk and disproportionate short limbs. The head is normal, which distinguishes it from achondroplasia.
2. Imaging features: The radiologic features include rhizomelia with metaphyseal flaring, spinal stenosis due to reduced interpedicular distances, small pelvis and lordotic sacrum. There is broadening of femoral neck and the distal fibula is overgrown as compared to proximal fibula. The differential diagnosis includes achondroplasia, diastrophic dwarfism,

spondyloepiphyseal dysplasia and chondroectodermal dysplasia.

Metaphyseal chondrodysplasia

Metaphyseal chondrodysplasias are a large heterogeneous groups of disorders.

1. Jansen Type:
   Clinical features: This is a rare severe dysplasia due to excessive proliferating hypertrophic cartilage in the metaphysis. There is marked dwarfism, swelling of joints and bowed legs and forearms detectable at birth.
   Imaging features: In infancy there is marked irregularity of the metaphysis, widened growth plate and bowing of tubular bones with diffuse osteopenia. Subperiosteal resorption of bones and fractures also occur in childhood. There is cupping of the metaphysis with a wide zone of irregular calcification. There is resultant dwarfism with metaphyseal flaring and bowed bones. Spine shows minimal platyspondyly. There is basilar and supraorbital ridge sclerosis with osteopenia of the skull vault.

   In the early cases, differential diagnosis includes renal osteodystrophy and hypophosphatasia, however the radiological features are diagnostic.

2. Schmid Type:
   Clinical features: Presents in early childhood, and this is often misdiagnosed as rickets because of metaphyseal changes.

   It is transmitted as an autosomal dominant trait and manifests as mild dwarfism. The skeletal abnormalities are not evident at birth but appear in third and fourth year of life. Radiological findings include growth plate widening, metaphyseal irregularity, and flaring especially in knee and hip joints. Coxa-vara is common due to involvement of metaphyses of proximal femora. The spine and hands are not involved.

   Patients with cartilage hair hypoplasia also show irregular metaphyses with bowing and dwarfism, but the brittle, short hair accompanying the syndrome help in differentiating the two conditions.

Spondylometaphyseal dysplasias (SMD)

1. Clinical features: This dysplasia is characterised by abnormalities in the vertebrae and metaphyses of tubular bones. In Kozlowski type there is short stature, kyphosis and scoliosis, diminutive hands, and feet with bowing of bones.
2. Imaging features: Radiological findings include markedly retarded skeletal maturation with degenerative changes in joints. There is flattening of vertebral bodies with pedicles located medially and altered spinal curvatures (Fig. 19.7A). Metaphyseal irregularity is most evident at the ends of long bones (Fig. 19.7B). Proximal femora are commonly involved with resultant coxa-vara. The iliac bones are shortened with small sacrosciatic notches and horizontal acetabular roof. In Sutcliffe type there are small triangular bony fragments at the periphery of metaphysis adjacent to growth plate (corner fracture appearance) and severe coxa vara. In spine, the findings include exaggerated end plate convexity, anterior wedging of vertebral bodies and square or ovoid vertebral bodies.[17]

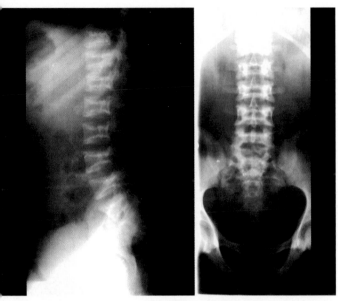

Fig. 19.7A: X-ray lumbar spine AP and lateral views showing platyspondyly with endplate irregularity and sclerosis

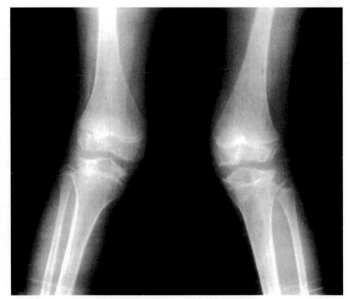

Fig. 19.8: X-ray of both knees AP view showing epiphyseal flattening with irregularity of both distal femora and proximal tibia with mild fibular flattening and resultant genu-valgum, in a case of multiple epiphyseal dysplasia

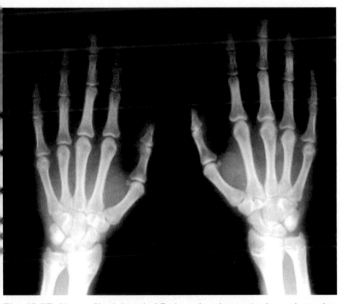

Fig. 19.7B: X-ray of both hands AP view showing metaphyseal cupping and irregularity involving distal metaphysis of radius and ulna, in a case of spondylometaphyseal dysplasia

Multiple epiphyseal dysplasia (MED)

1. Clinical features: It is transmitted in an autosomal dominant manner in most of the cases. Mild dwarfism with flexion deformities and degenerative arthritis are frequently present.
2. Imaging features: Radiographic findings are especially prominent in hip, knee, wrist and ankles. The ossification centres appear late, show delayed mineralisation and are fragmented. They ossify from multiple centres and can have a "mulberry appearance". The secondary centres are small and flattened. Fusion of ossification centres is also delayed, and a fragmented piece of the centre may result in the formation of loose body. In older patients slipped epiphysis may result

with resultant deformities of joint, such as tibio-talar slant, genu valgum and premature osteoarthritis (Fig. 19.8). The metaphyseal changes are especially noticeable in metacarpal and metatarsal bones. There are short broad phalanges with irregularity of epiphyseal ends of bones. The spine is affected in two-thirds of patients and changes include mild platyspondyly, anterior wedging with irregularity of anterior aspect of end plates associated with scoliosis, typically in mid thoracic spine.

The involvement of multiple epiphyses with lack of metaphyseal change helps in differentiating this condition from Perthes' disease.

In cretins, the bone age is severely retarded, which is a helpful differentiating feature.

X-linked spondyloepiphyseal dysplasia tarda

1. Clinical features: This condition is seen exclusively in males as it is transmitted as a sex-linked trait. It becomes evident after five years of age due to impaired growth of spine. The dwarfism is of the short limb type. Premature hip osteoarthritis with pain and limited motion is noticed around puberty.
2. Imaging features: Radiologically, platyspondyly is prominently present in the spine (Figs 19.9A and B). Other features include hump shaped area of dense bone on the central and posterior portion of the end plates. The disc spaces consequently appear wide anteriorly and narrow posteriorly. The odontoid process may be deformed. There may be disc protrusions in the thoracic region. There is relative increase in the antero-posterior diameter of chest. Degenerative changes in spine develop in early adult life. Pelvic bones and femoral necks may be small with presence of coxa vara. Osteoarthritis involving hip can be disabling (Fig. 19.9C).

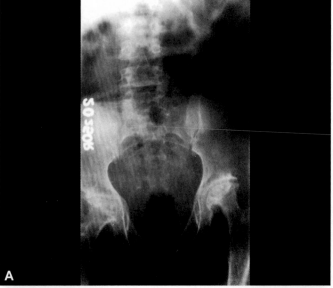

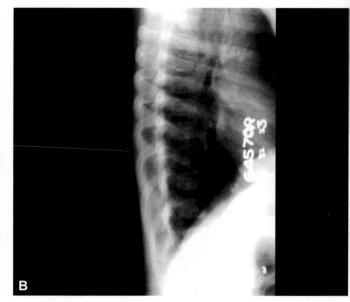

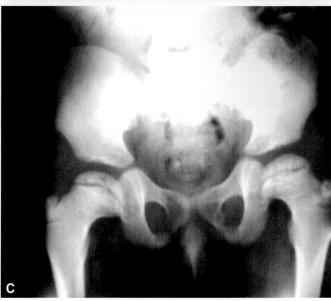

Figs 19.9A to C: (A) X-ray spine AP and (B) Lateral views showing generalized platyspondyly. (C) X-ray pelvis AP view-rounded flared ilia with distal tapering and bilateral symmetrical capital femoral epiphyseal flattening, sclerosis and fissuring, in a case of spondyloepiphyseal dysplasia tarda

Morquio's disease can be excluded by the absence of severe platyspondyly and severe dysplasia of the peripheral epiphyses.

Acrodysplasia—trichorhinophalangeal dysplasia

1. Clinical features: It is transmitted as an autosomal dominant trait. Clinical features include sparse scalp hair, pear shaped nose, short stature, joint laxity and deformity of proximal interphalangeal joints. Three types of dysplasias have been described.
2. Imaging features: The characteristic radiologic findings in type I dysplasia include cone shaped epiphysis in hands producing a U-shaped pattern with osseous shortening, especially in middle phalanges of second and third digit with ivory epiphysis being common in the distal phalanges. The proximal femoral epiphyses are small and often demonstrate changes resembling Perthes' disease. Pectus carinatum, scoliosis and kyphosis can also be seen. In type II dysplasia, there are cone

shaped epiphyses in thumb and other digits with presence of multiple exostoses, which distort and expand the bone. There is asymmetric limb growth, tibiofibular synostosis, short fibula, wide femoral neck and changes similar to Perthes' disease. Segmentation errors in spine and macrocephaly may occasionally be present. In type III dysplasia, there is severe generalised shortening of all the phalanges and metacarpals without the presence of exostosis.[18]

Disorganized Development of Cartilage and Fibrous Components of the Skeleton

Dysplasia Epiphysealis Hemimelica

1. Clinical features: The clinical features consist of pain, deformity, and restricted motion of affected joints.
2. Imaging features: The radiological features of this dysplasia include early appearance and excessive growth of epiphysis with irregularly calcified mass projecting from the epiphysis.

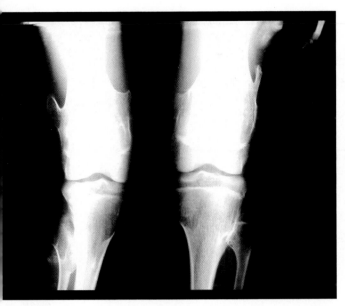

Fig. 19.10: Multiple bony exostosis seen involving both lower femora and upper ends of tibia and fibulae with metaphyseal modeling deformity

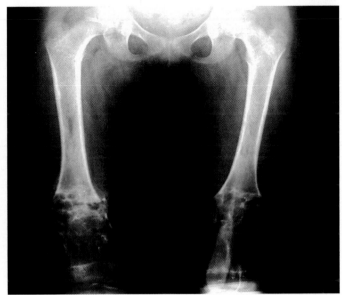

Fig. 19.11: X-ray of both knees AP view showing marked bony expansion with loss of cortical integrity of the distal femoral metaphysis with intramedullary calcification and lucencies, in a case of Ollier disease

The irregular mass may initially appear distinct from the surrounding bone, though eventually, it fuses with the adjacent epiphysis. Distal femur and distal tibia are among the common sites of involvement. Epiphyseal involvement on one side of body may be associated with hemihypertrophy. Spinal abnormalities including scoliosis can occur.

Multiple Cartilaginous Exostoses

1. Clinical features: This condition also called diaphyseal aclasis is characterised by cartilage capped exostosis. It occurs more commonly in boys, who develop painless lumps near ends of long bones. They have mild shortness of stature.
2. Imaging features: The radiological appearance and size of exostosis is variable. They arise on metaphyseal side of growth plate and point away from the epiphyses with associated metaphyseal expansion and deformity (Fig. 19.10). In hands, however the origin can be in the epiphysis. The forearms are frequently deformed as a consequence of bowing of radius, dislocation of radial head, ulnar angulation of distal end of radius and shortening of ulna. The long tubular bones are frequently involved, however ribs, scapula and pelvis can also be affected. Vertebral involvement though uncommon, can lead to compression of spinal cord or nerve roots. Complications related to osteochondroma include interference with growth, compression of adjacent structures and malignant transformation. Malignant transformation may be indicated by continued growth of osteochondroma even after cessation of normal growth, changing appearance of calcification in cartilage cap and irregular outline or bony destruction of exostosis.

Enchondromatosis (Ollier's disease)

1. Clinical features: Clinically there is asymmetrical limb shortening with expansion of affected bone and occasionally pathological fracture.
2. Imaging features: The radiological features include radiolucent masses, which may be round or triangular in the tubular bones of hand, which may show considerable expansion and pathological fracture. Focal area of calcification can be present in the mass (Fig. 19.11). Cartilaginous areas extending from physis lead to interference with growth and resultant shortening and deformity. The femur and tibia are most commonly involved. In pelvis V shaped radiolucent areas are seen in iliac bones. The enchondromas typically stabilise or even regress in adulthood. Malignant transformation to chondrosarcoma in one-fourth of patients can occur.

Enchondromatosis with Hemangiomas (Maffucci's Syndrome)

The radiological features are similar to Ollier's disease with the additional presence of phleboliths and soft tissue masses due to haemangiomas, more commonly in hands and feet (Fig. 19.12). The haemangiomas can disappear, and they need not overlie the bone lesions. A higher incidence of malignant transformation is seen compared to Ollier's disease.

Fibrous Dysplasia

1. Clinical features: This dysplasia is seen in the first three decades with a female preponderance. There is deformity and pain related to involved bones, with pathological fracture at times. The lesions tend to be unilateral. Histologically, medullary bone

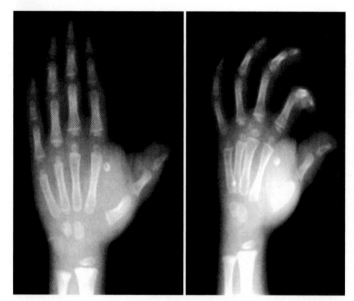

Fig. 19.12: X-ray of right hand AP view showing soft tissue swelling with presence of calcified phelboliths suggestive of hemangioma between the metacarpal bones, in a case of Maffucci'syndrome. Enchondromatosis may not be present in the region of hemangioma, as in this case

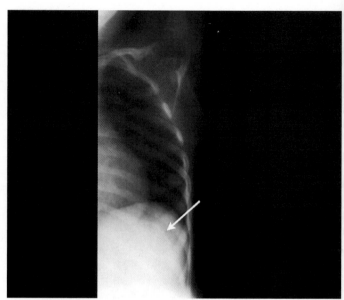

Fig. 19.13A: Bony expansion with lysis and groundglass haze in a case of fibrous dysplasia involving the 10th rib posteriorly

is seen to be replaced by fibrous tissue and cysts. This dysplasia can be monostotic or polyostotic. The association of polyostotic fibrous dysplasia, sexual precocity, café-au-lait pigmentation in females, constitutes the McCune Albright syndrome. Sarcomatous degeneration can occur in about 1 percent of cases.

2. Imaging features: The radiological features include "ground glass" appearance or radiolucent areas of altered trabeculae in the ribs and long bones with associated patchy sclerosis and expansion (Fig. 19.13A). There is endosteal scalloping and cortical thinning. Localised or asymmetrical overgrowth of bones may be seen. Pathological fractures and deformities due to bone softening such as 'shepherd's crook deformity' can occur. The skull shows asymmetrical thickening of the vault with sclerosis of the base with obliteration of the paranasal sinuses (Fig. 19.13B) and marked facial deformity giving a "leontiasis ossea" appearance.[19]

Abnormalities of the Density of Cortical Diaphyseal Structure or Metaphyseal Modelling, or Both

Dysplasias with Decreased Bone Density

Osteogenesis imperfecta

1. Clinical features: Clinically there is thin skin with ligamentous laxity and easy bruising, blue sclerae, dentinogenesis imperfecta, premature otosclerosis, with presence of hydrocephalus. The dysplasia is seen to result from abnormality of type I collagen. Osteogenesis imperfecta congenita occurs early in life while osteogenesis imperfecta tarda is less severe and occurs later in life. Clinical features in osteogenesis imperfecta congenita include paper thin soft

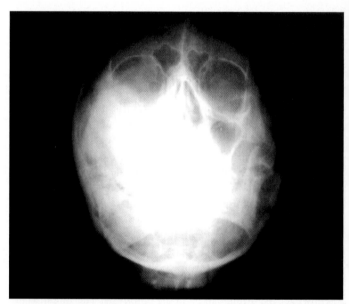

Fig. 19.13B: Bony expansion with groundglass haze and uniformly increased density seen involving the right maxillay sinus, right zygoma and right hemimandible on Water's view

skull with short broad extremities with deformities due to multiple fractures.

2. Imaging features: There is diffuse decrease in bone density in both axial and appendicular skeleton. Based on radiographic appearance of the extremities, Fairbank classified osteogenesis imperfecta into three groups. The first group includes patients with thin gracile bones (Fig. 19.14A). This is the most common expression of the disease. The bone cortices and shafts are thin with poorly defined trabeculae. The second group includes those patients with short thick limbs. The term thick bone type is a misnomer, as the cortices are thin with reduced bony density. In this group, there is severe

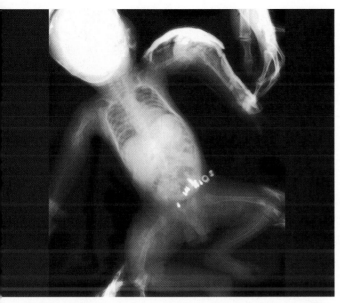

Fig. 19.14A: Infantogram showing a case of osteogenesis imperfecta congenita [thin bone type] with bone with thin cortices and decreased bone density with presence of fractures in diaphysis of both humeri and right femora with exhuberant callous formation.

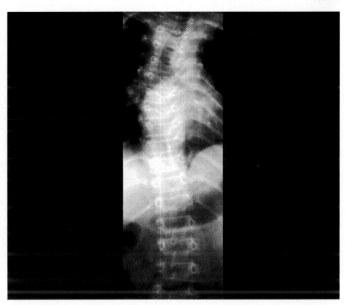

Fig. 19.14C: Radiograph of the lumbar spine [AP view] showing generalized decrease in bone density with platyspondyly, in a case of osteogenesis imperfecta tarda.

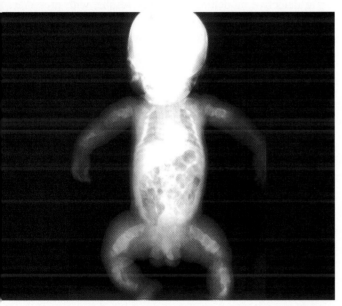

Fig. 19.14B: Infantogram showing a classical case of osteogenesis imperfecta congenita[thick bone type] with short and broad bones and decreased bony density, platyspondyly, multiple diaphyseal fractures in all the long bones of the extremities and ribs with callous formation.

micromelia with an increase in the width of the bones (Fig. 19.14B). This group has a poor prognosis. Third and least common, is a group of cases with cystic changes in the extremities with altered modelling of the bone. These occur in severely affected patients and other features include flared hyperlucent metaphyses traversed by coarse trabeculae giving a honeycomb appearance. Patients who survive infancy often undergo change from the thick limb type to the cystic or gracile type.[17]

Fractures in osteogenesis imperfecta occur most commonly in the lower limbs. Microfractures can occur at the junction of metaphysis and epiphysis. These fractures are asymmetrical and are seen as dense lines due to repeated trauma. Avulsion injury due to normal muscle pull can occur. Multiple telescoping fractures, which begin to occur *in utero*, lead to micromelia and bowing deformities. Fracture healing is usually normal, but tumoral callus and pseudoarthoses can occur. Hyperplastic callus usually occurs after trauma or surgical intervention. Multiple radiolucent scalloped areas with sclerotic margins referred to as popcorn calcifications can occur in metaphysis or epiphysis in severely affected patients. This is thought to result from traumatic fragmentation of cartilage growth plate. Laxity, tendon ruptures, fractures deformities and premature degenerative processes all contribute to wide scale deformities.

In the skull, changes include enlargement of mastoid and frontal sinuses. Wormian bones are commonly seen, arranged in mosaic pattern, along the lambdoid suture. Platybasia with or without basilar impression is a frequent deformity. Basilar impression with platybasia is referred to as *"Tam-o-Shanter"* skull. Premature otosclerosis can also result, due to thickening of stapes footplate, stapedial crural fractures, obliteration of oval window and flattening of cochlea, which can be well depicted by computed tomography. Dental abnormalities include teeth with absent pulp chambers and root canals, deformed and twisted roots and absence of enamel. Jaw fractures with excessive callus can follow dental extraction.

Spinal changes include flattened vertebral bodies, which can be biconcave or wedged anteriorly, with severe kyphoscoliosis, which is progressive (Fig. 19.14C). Pelvis is frequently triradiate with presence of compression fractures

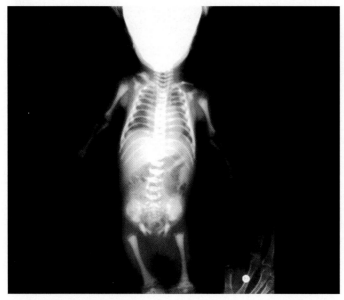

Fig. 19.15A: Generalized increase of bone density involving vertebrae, pelvic bones and extremities with transverse metaphyseal lucencies in a case of osteopetrosis, infantile type.

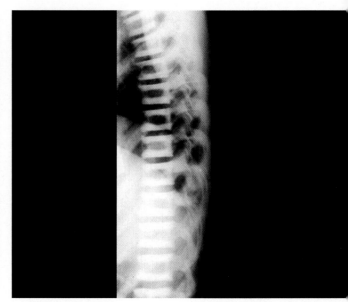

Fig. 19.15B: Generalized increase of bone density involving axial skeleton evident as endplate sclerosis in multiple dorsal and lumbar vertebrae.

and protrusio acetabulae. Shepherd's crook deformity can also be present. Sonographic detection of disease is possible *in utero* by using three diagnostic criteria described by Münoz and associates, that is:

i.   Detection of crumpled or wrinkled appearance due to fractures of long bones,

ii. Detection of severe demineralisation of calvaria, which is associated with excellent visualisation of intracranial contents, and

iii. Shortening of femur to more than three standard deviations below mean value. Other features can also be detected which include platyspondyly, beaded ribs, small thoracic circumference and wormian bones. Serial scans are important, as they can help in determining prognosis and in planning type of delivery.[20]

Increased Bone Density without Modification of Bone Shape

Osteopetrosis

1. Clinicopathological features: The primary defect is the failure of osteoclastic activity. There is enlargement of liver and spleen, anaemia and cranial nerve palsies. There can be variable modes of inheritance, both autosomal recessive and dominant types have been described.

   Four different types can be commonly recognised, which include the precocious type, the delayed type, the intermediate type and the tubular acidosis type.

2. Imaging features: The radiological findings in precocious type include generalised osteosclerosis, failure of corticomedullary differentiation and defective modelling of bones. This defective modelling of distal femora leads to the deformity called as "Erlenmeyer Flask deformity".[21] A club like appearance due

to defective modelling frequently results, with presence of transverse striations (Fig. 19.15A). Alternating areas of mature bone and sclerotic osseous tissue can give a "bone within bone" appearance.

The entire skull is involved with the cartilaginous portion of the base being most severely involved. Calvaria is thick with dense inner and outer tables, broad diploic spaces with hair-on-end appearance and small cranial foramina. The skull base shows appreciable marrow activity, well shown by MR imaging. Osteomyelitis of the mandible is fairly common. The changes in spine include radiodense vertebral bodies with end plate sclerosis.

In the delayed type, the findings are less severe compared to the precocious type. Osteosclerosis, defective undertubulation with thick cortex and a bone within bone appearance, characterise this type of osteopetrosis (Figs 19.15B and C).

In intermediate type, there is bone sclerosis, primarily of the skull base with involvement of facial bones. Interference with normal bone modelling, bone within bone appearance and ischaemic necrosis of femoral head can also be present.

In the tubular acidosis type, there is osteopetrosis with renal tubular acidosis and intracerebral calcifications, primarily in basal ganglia and periventricular region. Other radiologic findings include obliteration of medullary cavity and pathologic fractures. A significant aspect of this type is progressive improvement of the abnormalities.

Pycnodysostosis

1. Clinical features: It is transmitted as an autosomal recessive trait. Clinically there are short limbs with tendency to fracture, irregular dentition and respiratory problems. Patients are usually short and less than 150 cm in height.

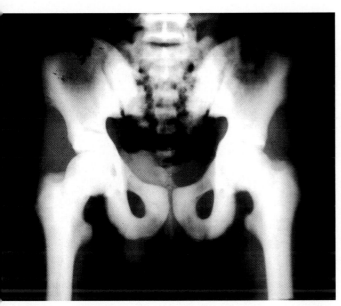

Fig. 19.15C: X-ray pelvis of the same patient showing generalized increase of bone density in a case of osteopetrosis, adolescent type.

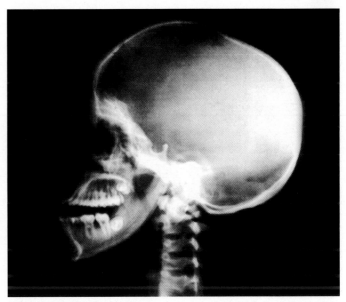

Fig. 19.16A: Skull lateral view showing widely open sutures, open anterior and posterior fontanelles with absent angle of mandible in a case of pyknodysostosis.

2. Imaging features: The radiologic findings include generalised osteosclerosis with thick sclerotic skull base. There is marked delay in closure of sutures with presence of wormian bones. The mandible is frequently hypoplastic with loss of normal angulation (Fig. 19.16A). Changes in spine include sclerosis of vertebral bodies, segmentation anomalies and spondylolisthesis (Fig. 19.16B). The bones of hand are short with hypoplasia or osteolysis of the distal phalanges (Fig. 19.16C). The medullary cavity of tubular bones may be mildly narrow.

Osteopoikilosis
1. Clinical features: This condition is asymptomatic and does not produce physical deformity. Male preponderance is seen. The condition has been found to be associated with linear scleroderma. The disease is of little clinical consequence.
2. Imaging features: Punctate, rounded, and sometimes linear sclerotic densities of one to ten millimeters are seen in medullary cavities of compact bone. These densities predominate towards ends of long bones. The pelvis is affected frequently (Fig. 19.17). The skull, ribs and spine are usually spared in this condition.

Osteopathia striata
1. Clinical features: The condition is usually asymptomatic, although sometimes it may be associated with vague joint pains.
2. Imaging features: There are multiple linear densities of varying width having an axial distribution, prominently seen in the ends of long bones. They usually extend into the epiphysis, where punctate and confluent opacities can occur (Fig. 19.18). Except for skull and clavicles, the remaining skeleton can all be involved. It is a disease of little clinical consequence.

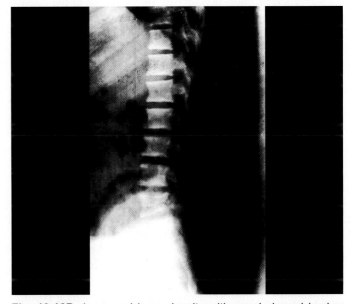

Fig. 19.16B: Increased bone density with spool shaped lumbar vertebral bodies alongwith fractures involving pars interarticularis at multiple levels.

Melorheostosis
1. Clinical features: It is also called Leri's disease. It is usually observed after three years of age. Severe pain is often the presenting symptom. Thickness and fibrosis of overlying skin is present. Tumours or malformations of blood vessels and lymphatics can be other cutaneous associations.
2. Imaging features: Multiple areas of dense hyperostosis are observed with a linear and segmental distribution corresponding to one or more dermatomes in this condition.

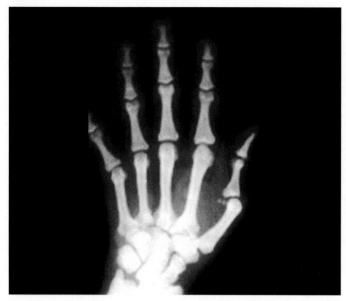

Fig. 19.16C: Increased bone density with acro-osteolysis, in a case of pyknodysostosis

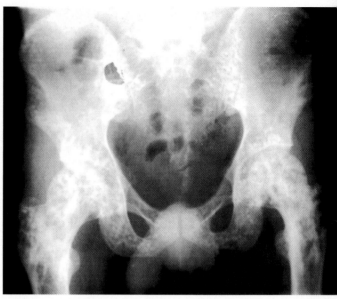

Fig. 19.17: Numerous small dense rounded opacities symmetrically involving the pubic bones and both femora, in a case of osteopoikilosis

Superficial cortical deposits are the rule, though the disease may also encroach the medullary cavity (Fig. 19.19). The resulting contour has been likened to candle wax flowing down the margin of the bone. The disease is usually monomelic and involves bones in one limb. Bony overgrowth can occur. Soft tissue ossification commonly occurs in the periarticular region between two affected bones of a limb.

Increased Bone Density with Diaphyseal Involvement

Diaphyseal dysplasia

1. Clinical features: It is an autosomal dominant disorder with variability of expression with symptoms usually occurring in or after second decade, such as bone enlargement, abnormal gait, leg pain and muscle weakness. It is a generalised, bilaterally symmetric dysplasia of bone primarily involving the diaphysis and sparing the epiphysis. It is also called Camurati Engelmann disease.
2. Imaging features: The radiologic features include cortical thickening and diaphyseal sclerosis. The endosteal involvement is more than the periosteal involvement (Fig. 19.20). Tibia, femur and humerus are commonly involved in decreasing order of frequency, while any bone can be involved. Sclerosis of skull base is common with encroachment of cranial nerves with associated complications. Changes in the spine include vertebral sclerosis especially in the posterior parts of vertebral bodies and neural arches.

Craniodiaphyseal dysplasia

1. Clinical features: It is autosomal recessive disorder characterised by deformity of face, nasal and lacrimal obstruction and cranial nerve palsies.
2. Imaging features: The radiologic features include massive and progressive hyperostosis of the skull and facial bones with obliteration of the paranasal sinuses. Involvement of the long

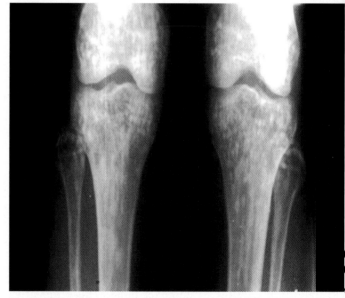

Fig. 19.18: Multiple linear opacities running vertically through the metadiaphysis and epiphysis with punctate opacities, in a case of osteopathia striata

bones varies in severity, although cortical thickening and lack of normal modelling are typical. The ribs, clavicles and ilia are wide and sclerotic, whereas the changes in spine are mild and preferentially located in the vertebral arches.

Increased Bone Density with Metaphyseal Involvement

Pyle's dysplasia

It is a rare disorder with variable modes of transmission, and mild clinical symptoms such as, joint pain, muscular weakness, bone fragility and dental malocclusion.

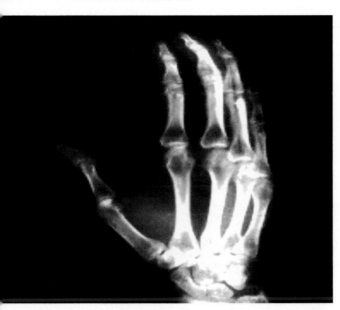

Fig. 19.19: Hyperostosis encroaching on the medulla of the proximal phalanges of the ring and middle fingers, in a case of melorrheostosis

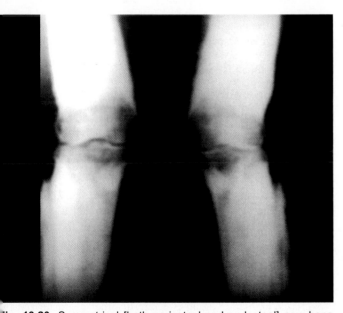

Fig. 19.20: Symmetrical [both periosteal and endosteal] new bone formation, obliterating the medullary cavity, sparing only the ends of the bones, in a case of diastrophic dysplasia

The radiologic features of *Pyle's dysplasia* include marked expansion of the metaphyseal segments of the tubular bones leading to an Erlenmeyer flask appearance, especially in the distal portions of femur and proximal portions of the tibia and fibula. The changes in upper limb are milder. There is an abrupt transition between the cylindrical and flared portions of the bone. Minor involvement of skull can occur and includes mild sclerosis of vault and prominence of supraorbital region. The spine may show platyspondyly or biconcave vertebrae. The bones of pelvis, medial portions of the clavicles, and sternal ends of ribs are frequently expanded.

Craniometaphyseal dysplasia
1. Clinical features: It is clinically characterised by facial deformity, hypertelorism, broad mass at base of nose, nasal obstruction, deafness and dental malocclusion.
2. Imaging features: There is progressive sclerosis around the sutures with sclerosis of the skull base. In addition, there is obliteration of paranasal sinuses and loss of lamina dura of teeth. Osteosclerosis in diaphysis of tubular bones is noted in infancy, which later disappears and is replaced by modelling defects. There is an addition metaphyseal expansion and club shaped epiphysis. Ribs and medial part of clavicles can be widened. Spine is rarely affected.

Frontometaphyseal dysplasia
1. Clinical features: Clinical manifestations include childhood onset, short trunk with long extremities, prominent supraorbital ridges, micrognathia and joint contractures.
2. Imaging features: The radiologic features of this dysplasia include calvarial hyperostosis, prominent supraorbital ridge, absent frontal sinuses, hypoplasia of angle and condylar processes of mandible, antegonial notching of body of mandible, flaring of the iliac wings with widening of ischial bones. Changes in tubular bones include fibular waviness and bowing, tibia recurvatum, elongation of metacarpal bones and phalanges with erosion and fusion of carpal and tarsal bones.

DYSOSTOSES

Dysostoses with Cranial and Facial Involvement

Craniosynostosis
1. Clinical features: There is local cessation of growth and distortion of calvarial configuration due to premature fusion of one or more cranial sutures.
2. Imaging features: Isolated closure of sagittal suture is encountered most frequently. Unilateral closure of lambdoid suture leads to flattening of back of head or plagiocephaly. Cloverleaf skull is associated with premature synostosis of multiple sutures.

Craniofacial Synostosis
1. Clinical features: Crouzon's syndrome is characterised by craniosynostosis, exophthalmos and midface recession. The disorder is caused by mutation in the gene for fibroblast growth factor. The skull is brachycephalic, with fusion of coronal, sagittal and lambdoid sutures, usually seen by three years of age. Hypertelorism, hypoplastic maxilla, hydrocephalus and spinal anomalies can also occur.

Dysostoses with Predominant Axial Involvement

Vertebral segmentation defects, Sprengel's deformity: Various vertebral segmentation defects can occur. Multiple block vertebrae are seen in cervico oculo-acoustic syndrome or Wildervanck syndrome. Sprengel's deformity can occur as an isolated abnormality of the scapula, which is small, triangular, elevated and rotated, so that its medial border faces spine, or as a part of Klippel-Feil syndrome.

Osteo-onychodysostosis

Nail-patella dysplasia (Hereditary osteo-onychodysostosis) The radiological features include dysplastic abnormalities of knee, iliac bone, and elbow. Hypoplasia or absence of one or both patellae and asymmetry of condyles of the femur, tibia and humerus are characteristic. Flaring of the iliac crests associated with iliac horns is pathognomonic of this syndrome. The medial femoral condyle is enlarged while the lateral condyle is hypoplastic resulting in patellar instability and genu valgum. The elbow characteristically shows hypoplasia of the radial head, which is frequently subluxated with narrow neck of radius. The abnormalities in knee and elbow are more common than the abnormality of iliac bone. However, the iliac horns arising from posterior aspect of iliac bones near sacroiliac joint are generally bilateral and pathognomonic of this condition. The iliac bones by themselves are hypoplastic. Hypoplasia of scapula, carpal bones, presence of eleven pair of ribs and Madelung's deformity are less common findings.

Dysostosis with Predominant Involvement of Extremities

Dysostosis with predominant involvement of extremities can occur alone, or as a part of a widespread dysplasia. There can be various deformities affecting the limbs, for example, there can be partial or complete absence of limbs or fingers, radioulnar synostosis, polysyndactyly, clinodactyly.

Certain neonatal anomalies in hand, foot and arm can be a pointer to the presence of skeletal dysplasia. For instance, clinodactyly (finger curvature in medial or lateral plane) can be seen in Cornelia de Lange syndrome, Down's syndrome, Nail-patella syndrome, radial hypoplasia or aplasia can be seen in Cornelia de Lange syndrome, Trisomy 18 (Fig. 19.21), metacarpal hypoplasia can be seen in chondrodystrophia calcificans congenita, polydactyly in chondrodystrophia calcificans congenita, Ellis-van Creveld syndrome, syndactyly in acrocephalosyndactyly (Apert's syndrome), chondrodystrophia calcificans congenita, Cornelia de Lange syndrome, broad thumb in acrocephalosyndactyly camptodactyly (permanent finger flexion at the proximal interphalangeal joint due to contractures or fascial abnormality) in Morquio's syndrome and nail-patella syndrome.

IDIOPATHIC MULTICENTRIC OSTEOLYSIS

1. Clinical features: The carpotarsal osteolysis syndromes include multicentric osteolysis with nephropathy, hereditary multicentric osteolysis and miscellaneous conditions characterised by localised osteolysis involving carpal and tarsal bones. Histologically, there is proliferation and hyperplasia of smooth muscle cells of synovial arterioles suggesting underlying vascular abnormity. The articular cartilage is replaced by fibrous tissue.
2. Imaging features: Radiologically, it is seen as progressive dissolution and disappearance of carpal and tarsal bones.

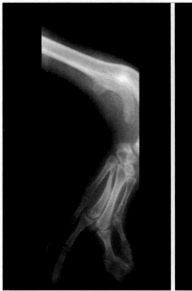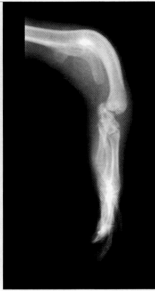

Fig. 19.21: Radial aplasia with curved ulna and absent thumb in a case of Trisomy 18

Multicentric osteolysis with nephropathy is characteristically associated with tapering of adjacent tubular bones.

PRIMARY DISTURBANCE OF GROWTH

Cornelia de Lange Syndrome

1. Clinical features: Clinical features include bushy eyebrows meeting in midline, high forehead, depressed nasal bridge excessive distance between nose and lips and antimongoloid slant.
2. Imaging features: Radiologic findings include small brachycephalic skull, small cervical spine, short proximally placed thumbs, clinodactyly involving fifth finger, small distal phalanges, hypoplasia of long bones, absent forearm bones with resultant elbow dislocation and retarded skeletal maturation.

Progeria

Progeria or premature aging is a rare disorder characterized by absence of hair, atrophic skin and failure to grow at normal rate. In first two years of life, the child develops degeneration of hair follicles, loss of subcutaneous fat, joint stiffness and poor growth. Skeletal hypoplasia is most evident in facial bones, mandible and hands. Fontanelle ossification is delayed. The tubular bones, ribs and calvaria are thin. The distal phalanges and clavicles are hypoplastic.

CONSTITUTIONAL DISEASES OF BONE WITH KNOWN PATHOGENESIS

Chromosomal Aberrations

Chromosomal aberrations due to morphologic change in the individual chromosomes with addition or deletion have been associated with diseases having effect on bony skeleton but have been kept out of definition of bony dysplasias, which in contrast continue to exert their effect throughout life. Failure of proper disjunction of sex chromosomes is seen in Turner and Klinefelter syndrome. Autosomal trisomy defects are usually result of non-disjunction or due to translocation involving autosomal chromosomes, as is seen in mongolism.

In Turner's syndrome clinically there is agenesis of the gonads, webbing of the neck and cubitus valgus. Radiological features include decreased density of bones, maldeveloped clavicles and slender ribs, depressed medial tibial condyle and shortening of the fourth metacarpal.

Down's syndrome occurs due to chromosomal aberration involving 21 chromosome. The radiological features include brachycephalic skull with decreased interorbital distance, hypoplasia of nasal bones, eleven pairs of ribs, clinodactyly involving middle phalanx of fifth digit besides widespread defects including cardiac and gastrointestinal defects.

Primary Metabolic Abnormalities

Calcium Phosphorous Metabolism (Hypophosphatasia)

Four clinical groups are recognized, although distinction between them is not always possible due to the variability in presentation due to variable deficiency of alkaline phosphatase. These include the neonatal, infantile, childhood and adult form. The neonatal form presents soon after birth, the infants dying within six months of age, while most infants usually survive in infantile form of hypophosphatasia. The childhood form presents between six months and two years of age and is clinically less severe. Bone fragility and dental abnormalities are frequent in adult form of hypophosphatasia.

1. Imaging features: The radiological features in neonatal form include diffuse profound defective ossification with broad, irregular metaphyses, seen prominently at the wrists, knee and costochondral junctions. The cranial sutures also appear wide due to defective ossification. Fractures are common.

    Infantile form is characterised by widening of cartilaginous growth plate and frayed and cupped metaphysis with the epiphysis showing spotty demineralisation. Mild irregularity of the diaphysis can also be evident due to defective mineralisation. The skull shows premature fusion with subsequent craniosynostosis, often with a brachycephalic configuration.[18]

    The characteristic features in childhood form include bowed legs or knock knees, mild rachitic changes, premature loss of deciduous teeth and dental caries. Craniosynostosis is usually not present.

    The adult form is characterised by presence of osteopaenia, Looser's zones and actual fractures.

    The differential diagnosis of the neonatal form includes other fatal short limb dwarfism, osteogenesis imperfecta and severe rickets.

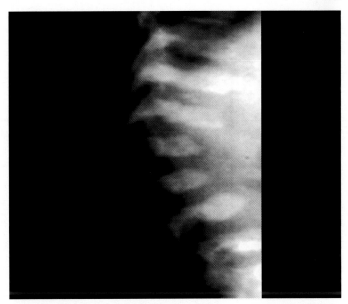

Fig. 19.22: Case of MPS-1 [Hurler syndrome] spine lateral view showing characteristic anteroinferior beaking in lumbar vertebrae

Mucopolysaccharidoses and Mucolipidoses

They are complex carbohydrate metabolism abnormalities. They can be diagnosed by means of specific metabolic test such as fibroblast culture and assay. The role of radiologist in this group of disorders is limited but important.

Mucopolysaccharidosis-I (Hurler's syndrome)

1. Clinical features: It is a rare disorder of mucopolysaccharide metabolism and is transmitted as an autosomal dominant trait. Clinical features manifest in early infancy and include large head with eyes wide apart, shrunken bridge of the nose, everted lips, protruding tongue, poorly formed teeth, hepatosplenomegaly and dorsolumbar kyphosis. Progressive mental retardation and corneal opacities are invariably present with death occurring at a younger age compared to other mucopolysaccharidoses.

2. Imaging features: The radiological features of this disorder include macrocephaly, craniostenosis, J shaped sella, atlantoaxial subluxation, ovoid vertebral bodies, hypoplasia of vertebra around thoracolumbar region (Fig. 19.22). The changes in pelvis include hypoplasia of base of ilia, pseudo-enlargement of acetabula and coxa valga. In the hands changes include pointing of proximal ends of metacarpal bones and shortening and widening of short tubular bones. Progressive hydrocephalus and deficient myelination can often be present. Hurler's syndrome may be confused with Morquio's syndrome, but changes in the spine, skull and long bones help in differentiating between the two conditions.

Mucopolysaccharidosis-IV (Morquio's syndrome)

1. Clinical features: Clinical features include dwarfism with low dorsal kyphosis, flexion deformities of both hips and knees, knock knees and flat feet. The head is thrust forward and

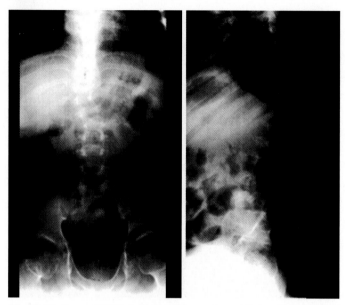

Fig. 19.23: Case of MPS-1V [Morquio's syndrome] Spine AP and lateral views showing generalized platyspondyly and characteristic central anterior tongue like beak in multiple lumbar vertebrae with ape shaped pelvis

appears shrunken between high shoulders. Deformities become noticeable after one year of age.

2. Imaging features: The radiological features of this disorder are characteristic and include slightly rounded vertebral bodies in infancy with small anterior beak. In childhood, a central tongue or projection appears from the anterior aspect of vertebral bodies (Fig. 19.23). In adults, the vertebrae are flat and rectangular with irregular margins. Hypoplasia of the dens is often present. There is anterior bowing of sternum with increased diameter of chest. Changes in pelvis include flaring of iliac wings with increased obliquity of acetabular roofs. The femoral capital epiphysis is dysplastic with resultant coxa valga. There is widening of metacarpals with pointed anterior ends and small and irregular carpals with slanting of distal articular surfaces of radius and ulna at the wrist. The long tubular bones show diminished growth, epiphyseal deformity and metaphyseal flaring.

Differential diagnosis of Morquio's syndrome includes Hurler's syndrome, Spondyloepiphyseal dysplasia and diastrophic dwarfism.

Mucolipidosis

These are inherited as autosomal recessive trait and this group exhibits clinical features depending on the deficiency of the enzyme involved. The radiologic features resemble those of mucopolysaccharidosis except that urinary excretion of mucopolysaccharides is not increased.

Bone Abnormalities Secondary to Disturbances of Extraskeleton Systems

Bone abnormalities can result secondary to endocrine, haematologic, neurologic, renal, gastrointestinal and cardio-pulmonary diseases. These diseases of bone classified under "constitutional diseases of bone" are secondary abnormalities and not classified under skeletal dysplasias.

CONCLUSION

Methodical evaluation in some and pathogonomonic features in others can lead to a specific diagnosis of skeletal dysplasia.

The establishment of a precise diagnosis is important for numerous reasons such as, genetic counselling, accurate recurrence risk, prenatal diagnosis in future pregnancies, prediction of adult height and most importantly, clinical management including prevention of complications and disabilities.

REFERENCES

1. Camera G, Mastroiacovo P: Birth prevalence of skeletal dysplasias in the Italian multi-centric monitoring system for birth defects. In Papadatos CJ, Bartsocas CS (Eds): Skeletal Dysplasias New York: Alan R. Liss 1982; 441-49.
2. Spranger J: International classification of osteochondrodysplasias. Eur Pediatr 1992; 151:407-15.
3. Lachman Ralph S: International nomenclature and classification of the osteochondrodysplasias. Pediatr Radiol 1998; 28:737-44.
4. Frézal Jean, Le Merrer M, Chauvet ML: Osteochondrodysplasias, dysostosis, disorders of calcium metabolism, congenital malformations syndromes and other disorders. Pediatr Radiol 1997; 27:366-87.
5. Horton W: Advances in the genetics of human chondrodysplasias. Pediatr Radiol 1997; 27:422-27.
6. Superti-Furga Andrea, Bonafé Luisa, Rimoin David L: Molecular pathogenetic classification of genetic disorders of the skeleton. Am J Med Gene (Semin Med Genet) 2001; 106:282-93.
7. Behrman Richard E, Kliegman Robert M, Jenson Hal B: Nelson Textbook of Pediatrics (16th ed) India reprint. Noida Harcourt Asia Pte Ltd, Thompson press(I) Ltd 2000; 2113-36.
8. Kirks Donald R, Thorne Griscom N: Practical Pediatric Imaging-Diagnostic Radiology of Infants and Children (3rd ed). Philadelphia, New York: Lippincott-Raven Publishers, 1999.
9. Deborah Krakow, Yasemin Alanay, Lauren P. Rimoin, et al: Evaluation of prenatal onset osteochondrodysplasias by ultrasonography; A retrospective and prospective analysis. Am J Med Genet A. August 2008; 1;146A[15]:1917-1924.
10. Deborah Krakow, Ralph S Lachman and David L. Rimoin: Guidelines for prenatal diagnosis of fetal skeletal dysplasias. Genet Med. February 2009; 11[2]:127-133.
11. Edeiken's Roentgen Diagnosis of Diseases of Bone, (4th ed) Williams and Wilkins 1990; 2.
12. Kitoch Hiroshi, Lachman Ralph S, Brodie Steven G, et al: Extrapelvic ossification centers in thanatophoric dysplasia and platyspondylic lethal skeletal dysplasia. Pediatr Radiol 1998; 28:759-63.
13. Pozanski AK: Punctate epiphysis: A radiological sign not a disease. Pediatr Radiol 1994; 24:418-24.
14. Taybi H, Lachman RS: Radiology of syndromes, metabolic disorders and skeletal dysplasias. St Louis: Mosby Year Book Publications, 1996.
15. Sutton David: Textbook of Radiology and Imaging (7th ed). Churchill Livingstone 2003; 2.

16. Lachman Ralph S: The cervical spine in the skeletal dysplasias and associated disorders. Pediatr Radiol 1997; 27:402-08.

17. Resnick Donald: Diagnosis of Bone and Joint Disorders (4th ed). W.B. Saunders Company. An imprint of Elsevier Science 2002; 5.

18. Gledion Andres: Phalangeal cone shaped epiphyses of the hand: Their history, diagnostic sensitivity and specificity in cartilage hair dysplasia and the trichorhinophalangeal syndrome I and II. Pediatr Radiol 1998; 28:751-58.

19. Arabella I Leet and Mchael T Collins: Current approach to Fibrous Dysplasia and McCune Albright syndrome J Child Orthop; 1[1]: 3-17, March 2007. Grainger Ronald G, Allison David: Grainger and Allison's Diagnostic Radiology: A Textbook of Medical Imaging (3rd ed), Churchill Livingstone, 1997.

20. Murray Ronald O, Jacobson Harold G, Stoker Dennis J: The Radiology of Skeletal Disorders, Exercises in Diagnosis (3rd ed). Churchill Livingstone 1990; 2.

21. Maha A Faden, Deborah Krakow, et al: Erlenmeyer Flask bone deformity in the skeletal dysplasias. Am J Med Genet A, 149 A [6]: 1334-1345, June 2009.

CHAPTER 20

Skeletal Maturity Assessment

Arun Kumar Gupta

From the moment one is born until the time one has grown up, the bones go through a set of characteristic changes – the skeletal maturity or sometimes also referred to as bone age. Therefore, skeletal maturity is the only indicator of development that is available from birth to full maturity.[1] Skeletal maturity in pathological terms denotes consolidation of new tissues by calcification of the fibrous and cartilaginous elements. It is distinct from growth. In clinical terms one may describe each individual passing from a stage of "wholly immature" to a stage of "wholly mature" through a normal growth process. At any particular stage, one individual might be more or less mature than another individual.

MEASUREMENT OF MATURITY

Maturity can be measured by observing certain events which occur in all individuals along the "Road to full maturity". These are called Developmental milestones[2] which could be dental, skeletal or pubertal development (secondary sexual characters, i.e. pubic hair, breast development, penis development).

In an ideal situation, the developmental milestones should occur in *all* the individuals, invariably in the *same order* and should cover the entire developmental span *evenly and completely*. Only skeletal maturity provides developmental milestones closest to such an ideal situation. It is, therefore, the most commonly used parameter of maturity in clinical practice.

In addition, the method employed to assess 'skeletal maturity' is non-invasive, inexpensive and independent of body size, weight and chronological age. All these advantages make assessment of maturity by 'skeletal maturity' method an ideal clinical tool.

Skeletal Maturity Assessment: Why is it Necessary?

Skeletal maturity assessment is required in clinical practice for two major reasons:

A. In pediatric endocrinological problems and growth disorders
B. For medicolegal reasons.

A. In the field of *pediatric endocrinology*, skeletal maturity assessment is not only essential but highly crucial for a number of reasons:[2]

- For diagnosing underlying cause in short stature children with growth delay (Fig. 20.1)
- For reassuring young people with non-pathological but unusual growth delay

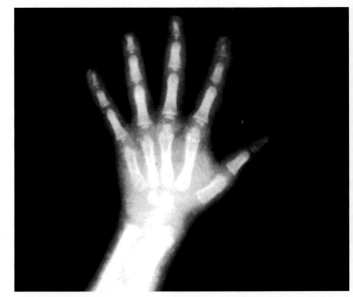

Fig. 20.1: Radiograph of left hand and wrist of a male child. Chronological age: 9 years and 9 months. Bone age, TW2 method: RUS-2.9 years, CS-2.3 years, 20 Bone Bone age-2.7 years
(RUS = Radius, ulna and short bones; CS = Carpal score)

- Monitoring growth hormone and anabolic steroid therapy
- Monitoring treatment in various endocrinopathies, e.g. hypothyroidism, congenital adrenal hyperplasia
- In the differential diagnosis of sexual precocity
- For prediction of adult height
- For selection of children in sports
- Public health reasons—Comparison of environmental, dietary and other factors between different populations.

B. For *medicolegal reasons*, estimation of age of an individual is important both for the medical jurist and lawyers. The gravity of offence is dependent upon particular age and also certain rights are given to the persons only at certain age.[3] Estimation of age, is therefore, of considerable importance from the point of view of administration of justice. This is important in a number of situations: identification, employment, criminal responsibility, judicial punishment, consent for marriage, rape, criminal abortion, prostitution, etc.[3]

Most difficult problem arises in estimation of age of adolescent girls. Period of adolescence extends from puberty to full maturity.

Factors to be taken into consideration for estimation of age are:[3]

a. dentition, i.e. number of teeth in each jaw
b. appearance of hair in the armpits and on pubis
c. development of breasts
d. appearance of first menstrual period
e. height, weight, general configuration and development of body
f. radiological examination of joints.

Methods to Assess Skeletal Maturity

Skeletal maturity in an individual child is assessed by comparing his or her state of bone development with the standards that have already been evolved from examination of radiographs of normal children.[2-4] Different methods use different standards for determining skeletal maturity. The three important methods are:

a. Appearance and fusion of ossification centers
b. Greulich and Pyle atlas method (G-P method)
c. Tanner and Whitehouse II method (TW2 method).

Appearance and Fusion of Ossification Centers

The earliest method for assessing skeletal maturity was by observing the time of appearance and fusion of various ossification centers.

Although this method has the *advantage* of being simple, quick and easy to calculate, it has significant *drawbacks*[5-7] and the two major ones are: ossification centers especially those of carpal bones may have extremely variable appearance and fusion time (Fig. 20.2) even on the two sides of the same individual, and secondly the bone age calculated by this method usually has a wide range, thereby, diminishing its clinical usefulness in pediatric endocrine diseases.

For these reasons, it became apparent that this method was neither valid nor reliable and hence inadequate and unsatisfactory

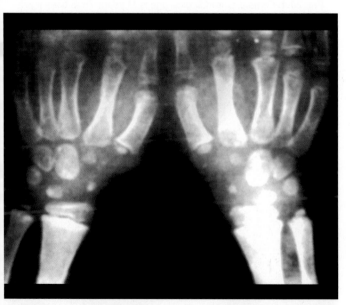

Fig. 20.2: Posteroanterior radiograph of both wrists of a 14 years male. Note asymmetrical appearance of carpal centers on the two sides, a major drawback of the technique using 'appearance-fusion' of centers as the basis

for estimating skeletal maturity in children with pediatric endocrine diseases where crucial decisions for treatment are based to a large extent on this information.[7]

However, this method still has its utility in medicolegal cases.[3,8] This is more so in adolescent girls involved in rape, kidnapping and prostitution where courts directive will change depending on age. Also, whether to try a boy or girl involved in some offence under juvenile act or not will depend on his/her age.

Radiology plays a crucial role in all these cases.[3] However, it is important to remember that radiological bone age must be interpreted along with other clinical parameters of growth before final decision.

For Indian children, standards have been established by a number of workers.[3,7-11] Using prepared charts the degree of skeletal development or 'bone age' can be calculated readily. Different sets of radiographs are required for bone age estimation depending upon the chronological age, e.g.

• PA radiograph of wrist and hand
• Elbow, knee, shoulder—either one or both ends depending upon expected age
• Pelvis AP for iliac crest appearance and fusion.

At AIIMS two published data for children from Delhi are followed[8,9] for calculating bone age by this method.

Greulich and Pyle (G-P) Method

In 1940 Greulich and Pyle published an atlas of standards of skeletal maturity based on longitudinal studies in 1930s of a relatively small number of Euro-American children living in Cleveland who were above average in economic and educational status.[12] This atlas was the turning point in establishing scientific standards of skeletal maturity. It is still the most widely used method in the Western countries due to its relative simplicity to use.

The atlas consists of a set of standard (*typical*) radiographs of the wrist and hand representing a particular bone age at some thirty points along the maturity scale. Standards for boys and girls are separate since girls mature earlier than boys. In order to determine the skeletal maturity of a child, the user should match the radiograph under question "as close as possible" to one of the plates in the atlas and the closest match represents that child's bone age. Thus a bone age of "12" means the child is as mature as the 'average 12 years old'.

Although the atlas for G-P method is most commonly used as described above but the same atlas also describes 'maturity indicators' for individual bones which forms the basis for the Tanner and Whitehouse method.

Popularity of G-P method is due to its simple methodology providing accurate information and similar reproducibility.[13] However, two important drawbacks are:[2] subjectivity of matching process and the scale used for expressing maturity, i.e. maturity is expressed by 'most likely' chronological age after the matching process and this 'most likely' age is then designated as 'bone age'. Some studies found G-P method to be inaccurate.[14]

Tanner and Whitehouse Method

Tanner *et al* in 1962 revolutionized skeletal maturity assessment by introducing the bone specific scoring system.[2] The study was carried out in an average socioeconomic level British (Scottish) children in 1950s. It was later modified to TW2 method in 1975. The conclusion drawn from the greatest drawback of G-P method was that the maturity scale should be defined in a manner which does not refer directly to age. In TW2 method this disadvantage was eliminated.[2] Till date this is the most accurate and reliable method for skeletal maturity assessment.

TW2 method is based on the principle that each bone develops to a reasonable, constant final shape and a sequence of recognizable state can be defined right from the appearance to the final shape all along the developmental journey. Each bone is thus classified into eight or nine stages (A to H or I) to which weighted scores are assigned. Boys and girls have different scores for the same stage of a bone. Each stage differs from the next by 'maturity indicators', i.e. slight change in shape which is presented both in visual form as well as written descriptions by the side of each stage in the atlas. While calculating skeletal maturity, both the visual *and* the descriptive information are used for assigning the stage but in case of any doubt, latter, i.e. descriptive information is used for making the final decision.

Technique

For TW2 method a posteroanterior radiograph of the left hand and wrist is used. During positioning it is important to keep the long axis of the middle finger, forearm and arm in direct line and also upper arm and forearm in the same horizontal plane. Centering is done on the third metacarpal head at a film focus distance of 30 inches (75 cm).

X-ray plate is put up for viewing with fingers pointing upwards and thumb on the right side of the viewer (Fig. 20.3).

In this method twenty bones are assessed and score is assigned to them. The scores are summed up. Three separate maturity scoring systems are derived, i.e. carpal score (CS) for the 7 carpals (out of the eight carpals pisiform is not considered for calculations), the Radius-Ulna-Short bone (RUS) score for 13 bones comprising

the radius, ulna and short bones of hand (I, III and V fingers only) and finally the TW2-20 bone score which combines both the carpal and the RUS components. For each of these three scoring systems, different 'weighted scores' are assigned. At the end of the atlas a series of tables as well as centile standard curves are given for each of these three bone age scores from which 'bone age' can be directly read for a given total score (Figs 20.4 to 20.6).

Finally three bone ages are thus obtained:

   i. RUS bone age
  ii. Carpal bone age
 iii. 20 bone–bone age

TW2 method is useful till the age of 18 years (RUS and 20 bone-bone age) in boys and till 16 years in girls (RUS and 20 bone-

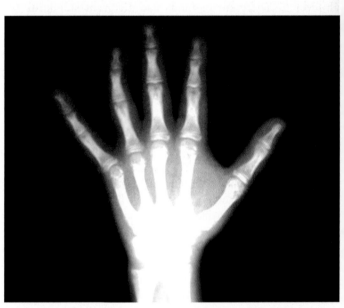

Fig. 20.4: Female: Chronological age is 11 years. RUS bone age is 11.9 years. Both matching

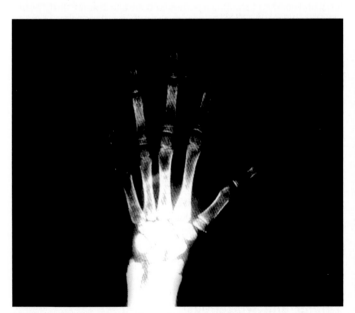

Fig. 20.3: While reviewing the radiograph of left hand and wrist by TW2 method, X-ray plate is put up with fingers pointing upwards and thumb directed to viewer's right side

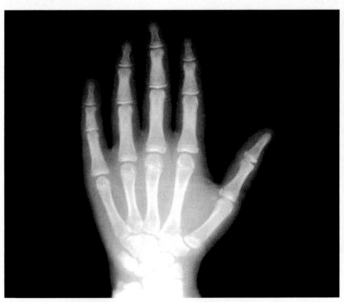

Fig. 20.5: 8 years female. RUS bone age is 13.2 years. Accelerated bone age

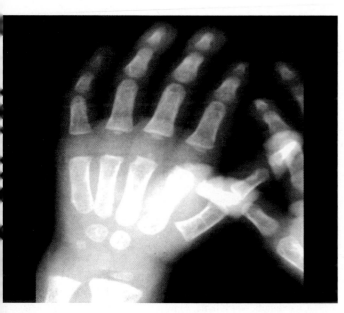

Fig. 20.6: Advantage of TW2 over conventional. By conventional method age is 3.7 +/-1.5 years. RUS age is 1.8 years. Chronological age 1.6 matches with RUS

bone age). However, upper limit for carpal bone age is 15 years in boys and 13 years in girls.

Comparison of G-P and TW2 Methods

A number of studies have compared the two standard methods. G-P method is easy and faster to do while TW2 is a more laborious, time consuming technique and requires more training. Bone age was found to be closer to chronological age by TW2 method.[15] However, TW2 was less reproducible between observers in this study.[15] The conclusion of most studies[13-17] is to use one method, preferably TW2 method, when performing serial measurements on an individual patient.

Computer-assisted Skeletal Age Scores

To eliminate the various sources of inter- and intraobserver errors associated with TW2 method (as well as for G-P method and even for carpal bone maturation) a number of studies[18-22] have reported use of computer systems. Almost all of them found computer aided systems to be reliable with results close to that with experts interpretation. With time, TW2 method may become easy and a routine procedure with the help of these computer programmes.

Ultrasound Based Bone Age Calculation

In November 2003, a German company called Sunlight introduced an ultrasound based device to test skeletal age in children and adolescents.[23] In this method of bone age estimation the child need not be referred to some specialized center but can be performed at the pediatrician's clinic with results in years and months available on the spot. Results are reported to be closely related to those produced by traditional method of Greulich and Pyle atlas.

But this needs larger studies at various centers by independent workers before finally it can be accepted as a routine technique.

Indian Scene

Skeletal maturation is dependent not only on intrinsic factors such as genetic, racial, familial and hormonal but also on extrinsic factors like socioeconomic status, nutrition, chronic illness and climate. When there is interplay of so many factors then the standards for one population may not be applicable to another population. Ideally each country, even within each country different regions, should establish their own standards through longitudinal (or at least cross sectional) studies of normal children. However, due to an ethical issue of exposing normal children to radiation hazard such studies have not been carried out in large numbers. The next best thing is to apply well established methods to our own population and compare the results. From India few studies[7, 24] have been carried out using both G-P and TW2 methods to assess skeletal maturity. Maniar[7] assessed Indian children with G-P method but found progressively increasing delay after second year of life. This method was therefore not found applicable to Indian children by the author.[7]

On the other hand Maniar[7] applied the same set of radiographs as above to TW2 method. At any age between one to seven years, the difference was found to be less than 0.8 years. Hence, TW2 method was found to be by far the best method applicable to Indian children. Our experience at AIIMS[25] in 100 normal healthy children is similar (unpublished data) and we concluded that TW2 method can be directly applied to Indian children. TW2 has been a standard method used in all pediatric endocrinology OPD patients at AIIMS for the last two decades.

To conclude, despite the difficulties of assessing bone age, and the assumptions on which various methods are based, skeletal maturity assessment is clinically relevant in that it provides the only means of assessing rates of maturational change throughout the growing period.[1] Of the various methods available, TW2 is the most accurate method and it can be applied directly to Indian population. However, this method requires correct positioning, precise radiographic technique and skilled interpretation. Awareness amongst the pediatricians and radiologists of India about TW2 method and its advantages is essential before it can become part of routine workup in every department all over the country. For medicolegal purposes however method of appearance and fusion of ossification centers continues to be in use because age groups covered under MLC problems cannot be evaluated by other two methods.

REFERENCES

1. Cox LA. The biology of bone maturation and ageing. Acta Paediatr Suppl 1997; 423:107-08.
2. Tanner JM, Whitehouse RH, Cameron N, et al. Assessment of Skeletal Maturity and Prediction of Adult Height (TW2 method) (2nd ed). London: Academic Press, 1983.
3. Kangne RN, Sami SA, Deshpande VL. Age estimation of adolescent girls by radiography. JFMT 1999; 16(1):20-26.
4. How is skeletal age measured? http://vms.cc.wmich. edu/~Anemone/anth354/tsld091.htm.
5. Kovi R, Korner A, Varkony J, et al. Bone age discrepancy on hand radiographs. Pediatr Radiol 2000; 30(7):500.
6. Marshall WA. Individual variations in rate of skeletal maturation. Nature 1969; 221(195):91.
7. Maniar B. Skeletal maturity in Indian children. The Indian J of Pediatr 1987; 54:295-302.

8. Modi's Medical Jurisprudence and Toxicology, 1999.

9. Jain S. Estimation of age from 13 to 21 years. JFMT 1999; 16(1):27-30.

10. Bajaj ID, Bhardwaj OP, Bhardwaj S. Appearance and fusion of important ossification centers. A study in Delhi population. Indian J Med Res 1967; 55:1064-7.

11. Sharat S, Khanduja PC, Agarwal KN, et al. Skeletal growth in school children. Indian Pediatric 1970; 7:98-108.

12. Greulich WW, Pyle SI. Radiographic atlas of skeletal development of hand and wrist. Stanford: Stanford University Press, 1950.

13. King DG, Steventon DM, O'Sullivan MP, et al. Reproducibility of bone ages when performed by radiology registrars: An audit of Tanner and Whitehouse II versus Greulich and Pyle methods. BJR 1994; 801(67):848-51.

14. Gilli G. The assessment of skeletal maturation. Horm Res 1996; 45(2):49-52.

15. Cole AJ, Webb L, Cole TJ. Bone age estimation: A comparison of methods. BJR 1988; 728(61):683-6.

16. Benso L, Vannelli S, et al. Main problems associated with bone age and maturity evaluation. Horm Res 1996; 45(2):42-8.

17. Bull RK, Edwards PD, Kemp PM, et al. Bone age assessment: A large scale comparison of the Greulich and Pyle, and Tanner and Whitehouse (TW2) methods. Arch Dis Child 1999; 81:172-3.

18. Canovas F, Banegas C, Cyteval M, et al. Carpal bone maturation assessment by image analysis from computed tomography scans. Horm Res 2000; 54:6-13.

19. Drayer NM, Cox LA. Assessment of bone age by Tanner and Whitehouse method using a computer–aided system. Acta Paediatr Suppl 1994; 406:77-80.

20. Frisch H, Riedl S, Wadhor T. Computer-aided estimation of skeletal age and comparison with bone age evaluation by the method of Greulich-Pyle and Tanner-Whitehouse. Pediatr Radiol 1996; 26(3):226-31.

21. Sato A, Ashizawa K, et al. Setting up an automated system for evaluation of bone age. Endocr J 1999; 46:597-600.

22. Tanner JM, Gibbons RD. A computerized image analysis system for estimating Tanner–Whitehouse 2 bone age. Horm Res 1994; 42(6):282-7.

23. Sunlight introduces Ultrasound–based bone age testing. http://www9.medica.de/cgi-bin/md.../content.cgi?lang=2 and ticket=g_u_e_s_t and oid= 11275 and print= 1/1/99.

24. Prakash S, Cameron N. Skeletal maturity of well-off children in Chandigarh, North India. Ann Hum Biol 1981; 8:175-80.

25. Gupta AK, Menon PSN, Seth V. Skeletal maturity by TW2 method in normal, healthy children at AIIMS (unpublished data).

CHAPTER 21

Spinal Dysraphism

Raju Sharma, Ankur Gadodia

INTRODUCTION

Spinal dysraphism is one of the most common congenital disorders associated with significant morbidity and mortality with estimated incidence of approximately 0.05 to 0.25 per 1000 births.[1] It can be defined as an incomplete fusion of midline mesenchymal, bony and neural structures.[2]

Spinal dysraphism is broadly classified into open and closed type. Most of the open spinal dysraphic states can be detected prenatally using ultrasound or fetal MRI. Post-natal imaging is usually performed to look for associated CNS anomalies (hydrocephalus, chiari malformation), and in postoperative patients presenting with progressive neurological deficit to look for any treatable cause. Most of the closed spinal dysraphic states remain asymptomatic at birth and are suspected in the presence of high risk cutaneous markers, or when these children present with neurological deficit later in life.[3]

MRI is the modality of choice for evaluating spinal dysraphism.[4-6] It is helpful in the classification, diagnosis and treatment planning of these disorders.

CLASSIFICATION

Most of the dysraphic spinal states can be explained on the basis of specific abnormality in early embryonic development which spans over the period of 3rd to 8th week of intrauterine life, and classification based on embryology has been proposed (Table 21.1). Since, our understanding of human embryology is likely to evolve, this classification is also likely to change over a period of time. Recently Paolo Tortori-Donati et al[5,6] proposed a classification system based on clinico-radiological features (Fig. 21.1), which is now widely accepted and followed. Spinal dysraphism is classified into two categories: Open spinal dysraphism (OSD) and closed spinal dysraphism (CSD). Neural tissue is exposed to the environment in OSDs, whereas CSDs are covered by skin, with cutaneous markers present in up to 50% of cases.

First step in the evaluation of patient with dysraphism is thorough clinical assessment (Fig. 21.2). The child's back should be evaluated to look for presence/absence of skin covering, back mass and cutaneous stigmata of dysraphism (Table 21.2).[3,5,6]

EMBRYOLOGY

It is vital to know the development of the spinal cord to understand the different types of spinal dysraphism. The development of the bony spine and intraspinal contents begins in the first month of gestation.[7,8] The spinal cord develops from ectoderm and the development occurs during three stages: neurulation, canalization and retrogressive differentiation. During the first week of gestation, there is a proliferation of ectodermal cells along the surface of the embryo to form the primitive streak. This is the neural plate which forms a groove in the midline and during the third week of gestation it begins to fold laterally. The folds begin to approach each other dorsally near the midline at the neural groove and the neural plate thus closes to form the neural tube. This is referred to as the stage of neurulation.

Simultaneous with the stage of neurulation, the overlying ectoderm of the skin separates from the neural tube and fuses in

Table 21.1: Embryological classification of spinal dysraphism
Anomalies of gastrulation
Disorders of notochordal integration
Dorsal enteric fistula
Neurenteric cysts
Split cord malformations (diastematomyelia)
Dermal sinus
Disorders of notochord formation
Caudal regression syndrome
Segmental spinal dysgenesis
Anomalies of primary neurulation
Myelomeningocele
Myeloschisis
Lipomas with dural defect
Lipomyelomeningocele
Lipomyeloschisis
Intradural lipoma
Anomalies of secondary neurulation and retrogressive differentiation
Filar lipoma
Tight filum terminale
Abnormally elongated spinal cord
Persistent terminal ventricle
Terminal myelocystocele
Anomalies of unknown origin
Cervical myelocystocele
Meningocele

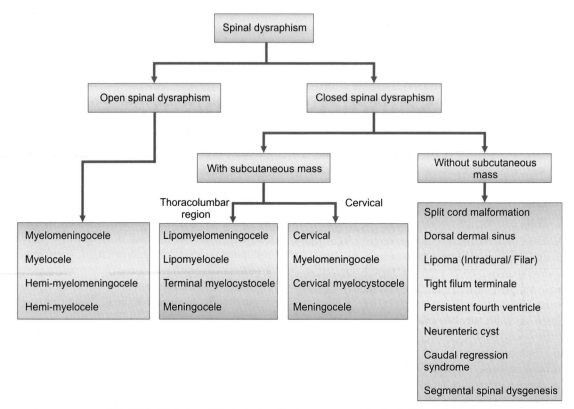

Fig. 21.1: Clinico-radiological classification proposed by Tortori-Donati et al

Table 21.2: Cutaneous lesions associated with spinal dysraphism
High Index of Suspicion
Hypertrichosis
Atypical dimples
Acrochordons/pseudo-tails/true tails
Lipomas
Hemangiomas
Aplasia cutis or scar
Dermoid cyst or sinus
Low Index of Suspicion
Telangiectasia
Capillary malformation (port-wine stain)
Hyperpigmentation
Melanocytic nevi
Teratomas

give rise to intradural lipoma, sacral teratoma and tethered low lying spinal cord.

Finally, during the stage of retrogressive differentiation (between 5-6 weeks), there is a decrease in the size of the central lumen and in the caudal cell mass and formation of the spinal cord, conus medullaris and filum terminale. The underlying cause for different types of spinal dysraphism is thought to be an insult — either genetic or acquired, that interferes with the normal process of neurulation, canalization or retrogressive differentiation.

IMAGING MODALITIES

MRI is the imaging modality of choice in the diagnosis and characterization of spinal dysraphism. Other modalities play a supplemental role.

Plain radiographs (anteroposterior and lateral views) are mandatory for evaluation of the vertebral column.[5,9] The findings seen on plain radiographs include focal spina bifida, widened spinal canal, scoliosis, segmentation anomalies like block vertebrae, butterfly vertebrae and other congenital abnormalities. Bony spur may be seen in cases of diastematomyelia. Radiographs are used as preliminary screening examination that can help to guide the further imaging work up.

Ultrasonography is primarily useful in the antenatal diagnosis of spinal dysraphism (Figs 21.3 to 21.5) and is also of some use in the neonate and infant.[4] It becomes progressively less useful as ossification of posterior elements proceeds during the first year of life. Prenatal sonography can detect the open widened neural arch

the midline. The perineural mesenchyme grows around the neural tube to form the meninges, bone and muscle. Majority of the dysraphic states including myelomeningocele, myelocele and lipomyelomeningocele are thought to occur at this stage of development of the spine and spinal cord.

During the next stage called canalization, the caudal end of the neural tube elongates into a caudal cell mass and ependyma lines a central tubular structure. It is believed that persistence of portions or abnormal development of the caudal cell mass may

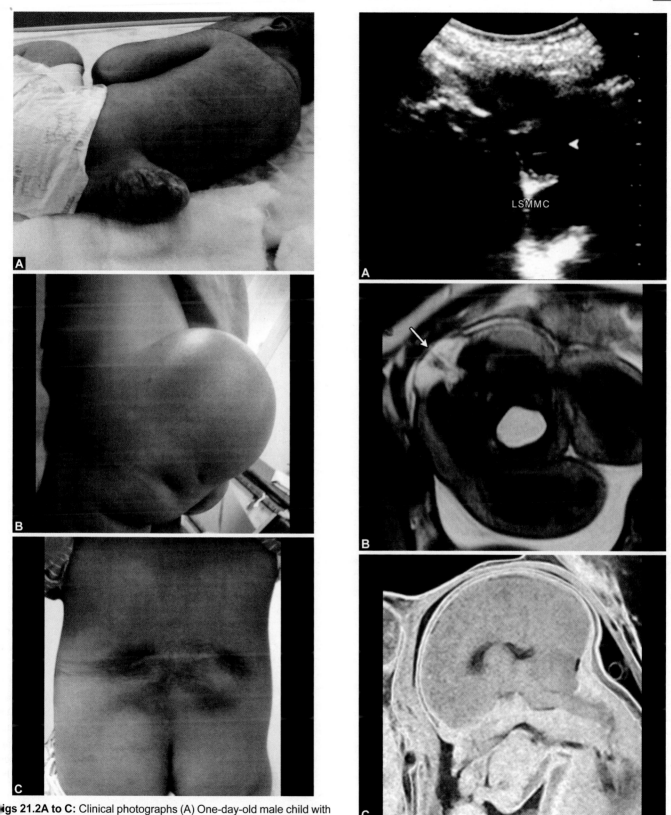

Figs 21.2A to C: Clinical photographs (A) One-day-old male child with meningomyelocele (Open spinal dysraphism). (B) Six-month old child with skin covered mass in lumbo sacral region showing associated abnormal skin dimples. Findings are suggestive of lipomyelo-meningocele (CSD with subcutaneous mass). (C) Five-year-old child with split cord malformation showing tuft of hair at high lumbar region CSD without subcutaneous mass) *(For color version see plate 8)*

Figs 21.3A to C: Myelomeningocele with chiari 2 in a 32-week-old fetus. Antenatal axial ultrasound, (A) axial T2W MR (B) images demonstrate herniation of meninges and nerve roots (arrowhead) suggestive of open spinal dysraphism Sagittal T2W MR (C) image shows chiari 2 malformation

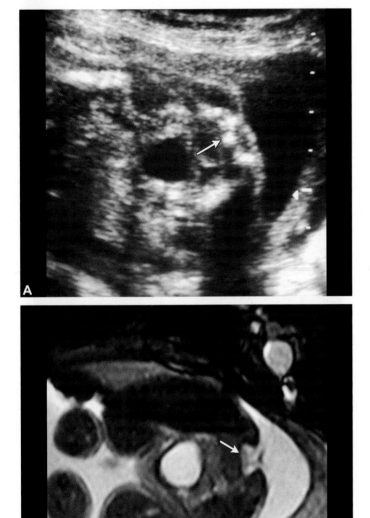

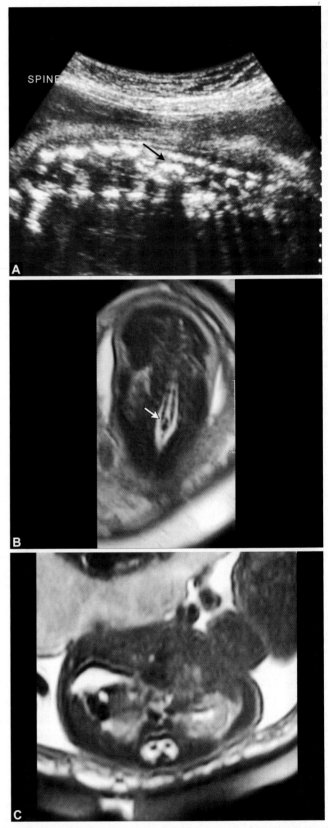

Figs 21.4A and B: Myelocele with Chiari 2 in a 26-week-old fetus. Antenatal axial ultrasound (A) axial T2W (B) images demonstrate widening of the spinal canal with absence of posterior elements. Neural placode is flushed with the skin surface (arrow)

with flared laminae, can show the meningomyelocele sac and detect hydrocephalus and other associated cranial anomalies. Direct sonography of the sac in children using high frequency transducers can provide information regarding the contents of the sac. However, for complete and more detailed information, an MR scan is usually required.

CT is useful in demonstration of the bony spur in cases of split cord malformation. Myelography and Postmyelogram CT were used prior to the advent of MRI.

MRI provides an accurate and non-invasive method for evaluating spinal dysraphism, making it the modality of choice. The excellent contrast resolution, wide field of view and multiplanar images allow evaluation of the entire spinal cord, contents of the back mass; detect cord tethering, associated syringomyelia, Chiari

Figs 21.5A to C: Split cord malformation in a 28-week-old fetus. Antenata axial ultrasound (A) image shows widening of the spinal canal with linear echogenic focus (s/o bony spur) within the spinal canal. Corona (B) and axial (C) T2W MR images demonstrate the split of the cord int two with an intervening bony spur (arrow)

malformation and other associated abnormalities. T1W images (sagittal, axial and coronal plane) demonstrate the malformation in the majority of the cases. T2W images are helpful in the demonstration of syrinx and associated pathologies like dermoid and epidermoid cyst.[6,9] Patients with spinal dysraphism may have multiple spinal anomalies. For instance, a patient with myelomeningocele may have associated syringohydromyelia and Chiari malformation. Therefore, it cannot be overemphasised that the entire spine needs to be imaged if a cutaneous or vertebral anomaly suggests the presence of a malformation. Fetal MRI is used as complimentary modality to USG (Figs 21.3 to 21.5), for the antenatal diagnosis of spinal anomalies and associated hydrocephalus.[10,11]

OPEN SPINAL DYSRAPHISM (OSD)

OSD implies exposure of neural tissue or its covering meninges to external environment without any cutaneous covering. Exposed non-neurulated neural tissue is called placode.[5] This category includes myelomeningocele, myelocele, hemimeningocele and hemimyelomeningocele. Myelomeningocele accounts for approximately 99% cases of OSD while myelocele, hemimeningocele and hemimyelomeningocele are distinctively rare.

Myelocele and Myelomeningocele

Myelomeningocele and myelocele are the most common form of OSD, occurring in upto 2 per 1000 live births and females are affected slightly more than males.[5] The incidence has decreased in the last two decades because of the use of folate supplementation in pregnant mothers in the period before conception to six weeks after conception.[4,12] The mechanism of preventive action of folate is not fully understood.

Superficial ectoderm does not disjoin from the neuroectoderm, thereby producing a midline defect. The neural tube remains open and the neural folds remain in continuity with the cutaneous ectoderm at the skin surface.[5,6] The affected newborn is identified by the presence of a placode of reddish neural tissue in the middle of the back that is exposed to air because of the absence of overlying skin. Most common location of OSDs is lumbo-sacral region (44%) followed by thoracolumbar region (32%). In contrast to lumbar meningomyelocele, cervical meningomyelocele is a classified as a closed spinal dysraphism. Imaging is usually not done as the diagnosis is clinically obvious and is a neurosurgical emergency.

Some authors suggest that MRI should be performed whenever possible as it can characterize the various components of the malformation, evaluate associated abnormalities (hydromyelia, Chiari II malformation, and hydrocephalus) and identify hemimyelomeningocele and hemimyeloceles.[13] Imaging of untreated OSDs demonstrates dehiscense of skin, subcutaneous fat, muscle and bone at the level of spina bifida (Figs 21.6 and 21.7). In a meningomyelocele the ventral subarachnoid space is distended displacing the neural placode posteriorly (Fig. 21.6), while myelocele lies flush with the skin surface without CSF space expansion (Figs 21.7A to C).

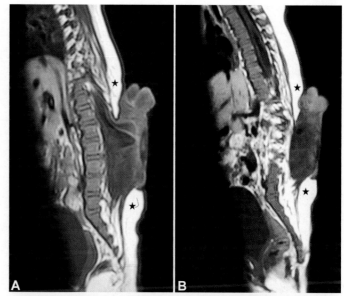

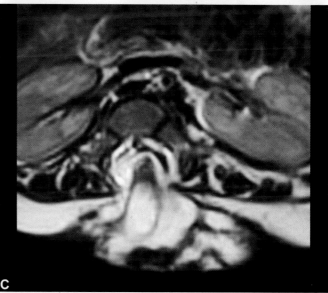

Figs 21.6A to C: Lumbosacral meningomyelocele in a 2-day-old female. Sagittal T1W (A, B) images show a large mass in lower lumbar region without skin covering. Axial T2W image (C) shows exposed neural placode with traversing dorsal and ventral nerve roots. Notice dehiscent subcutaneous fat (asterisk). Ventral subarachnoid space is distended in contrast to myelocele which lies flush with the skin surface without CSF space expansion. Also note small syrinx in the cord at thoracic level

After surgery the infants have a neurological defect that is stable. Imaging is indicated if the patient deteriorates neurologically despite adequate treatment of associated hydrocephalus or if the neurological examination findings are unusual.[14,15] MRI done in the postoperative setting may show the cord to be low lying and covered by skin graft; the stretched spinal cord may be tethered at this level (Figs 21.8 and 21.9). The spinal cord may be thinned out and may show cavitation at any level (Fig. 21.8). Intraspinal mass (epidermoid or dermoid cyst) may be associated.[15] Dermoid differs

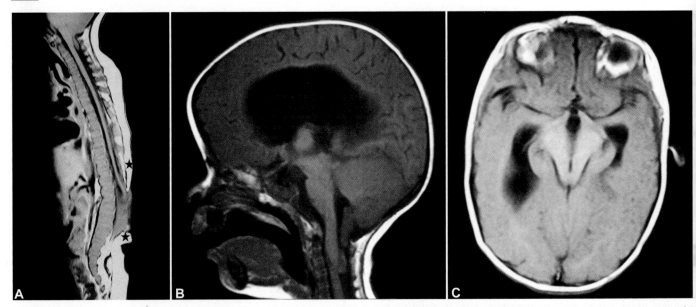

Figs 21.7A to C: Myelocele with chiari 2 malformation in a 1-day-old newborn. Sagittal T1W (A) image shows dehiscence of the subcutaneous fat (asterisks). Neural placode is exposed and flush with the skin surface without expansion of the subarachnoid space. Sagittal T1W image (B) of brain shows small posterior fossa with herniation of cerebellar tonsil behind cervical cord (black arrow). Axial T1W image (C) at mid brain level shows abnormal posterior tectal beaking (white arrow) with dilated temporal horns

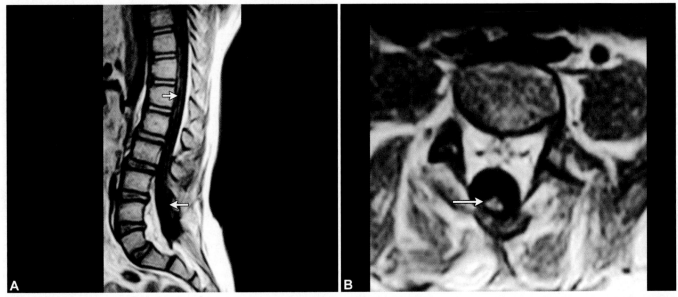

Figs 21.8A and B: Tethered cord with hydromyelia in a 2-year-old male after surgery for lumbosacral meningocele. Sagittal T1W (A) and axial T1W (B) images show low lying tethered cord reaching up to L4-L5 disc level with thinning (arrow) and hydromelia (short arrow) with abnormal eccentric location of cord indicating adhesion

from epidermoid by the presence of appendages of skin. On imaging both conditions appear similar. These lesions usually appear hypointense on T1W images, and hyperintense on T2W images similar to CSF (Fig. 21.10). They may have complex signal intensity when there is hemorrhage or when the cyst becomes infected.

Causes of postoperative neurological deterioration include retethering (Figs 21.8 and 21.9), cord ischemia, spinal cord cysts and cavitation (Figs 21.8A and B), diastematomyelia and

hydrocephalus. All these are easily amenable to detection by MR.[14] Surgical release of the adherent cord is effective and leads to improved motor function in almost 80 percent patients. Upto 85 percent of OSD patients have a concurrent hydrocephalus, and nearly all patients have an associated Chiari II malformation.[5,16]

Chiari II Malformation

Various theories have been put forward to explain this entity, but the recent theory by McLone and Knepper[17] best explains this

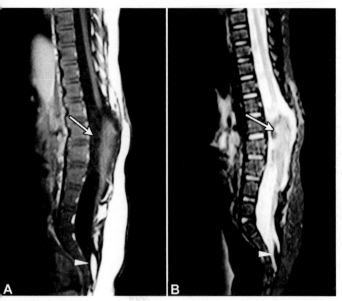

Figs 21.9A and B: Postoperative fibrosis following meningomyelocele closure in a 5-year-old female. Sagittal T1W (A) and T2W (B) images demonstrate low-lying cord tethered by fibrotic tissue, hypointense on T1W and T2W images (arrow). Also note presence of filar lipoma (arrowhead) showing hyperintensity on T1W and hypointensity on T2W fat suppressed images

association which is shown in Figure 21.11, and it has also been shown that most of these CNS anomalies can be reversed or even prevented by early intrauterine repair of the defect which highlights the importance of early diagnosis of this condition.[18,19] As against less pronounced tonsilar herniation seen with chiari I, in chiari II there is marked tonsilar herniation (Figs 21.4 and 21.7). Tectal beaking, low lying torcular herophile, and hydrocephalus are usual associations with this malformation. Tonsilar herniation should be assessed on mid-sagittal non-fat suppressed T1W image. Anatomical landmark followed is a line connecting basion with opisthion.[20] While drawing the line signal intensity of bone, not marrow should be used. Since there is gradual ascent of cerebellar tonsil with age, criteria for tonsilar ectopia changes with age (≥ 6 mm–0-10 years; ≥ 5 mm–10-30 years; ≥ 4 mm–30-80 years; ≥ 3 mm–more than 80 years).

Hemimyelocele/Hemi-myelomeningocele

This is the rarest form of OSD and results when split cord malformation is associated with defective primary neurulation of one of the hemicord which forms part of myelomeningocele. Hemimyelocele/myelomeningocele (Figs 21.12 and 21.13), also has associated chiari malformation in upto 40 percent of cases.[21,22] Clinical clues to the diagnosis include asymmetrical neurological deficit and presence of hirsutism along one side of the exposed neural defect.[23]

CLOSED SPINAL DYSRAPHISM (CSD)

CSD is a heterogenous group of disorders. In patients with CSD, early diagnosis may be useful, as SD may lead to distortion of the nerve roots with growth, resulting in neurological sequelae in the lower extremities. Early diagnosis is necessary to prevent neurological sequelae by performing early surgical procedures.

CSD with Subcutaneous Mass

CSDs with subcutaneous mass at lumbosacral region include lipomyelocele, lipomeningomyelocele, meningocele, myelocystocele. Among these lipomyelocele and lipomyelomeningocele are common entities and lipomyelocele is twice as common as lipomyelomeningocele. At cervical level differential diagnosis of CSD with subcutaneous mass includes cervical meningomyelocele, meningocele and myelocystocele.[5,6]

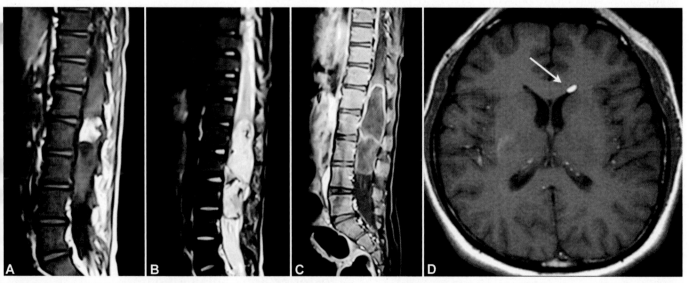

Figs 21.10A to D: Infected dermoid cyst in a 12-year-old child with history of meningomyelocele repair. Sagittal T1W (A), T2W (B) and post gadolinium (C) images show focal expansion of spinal cord at level of conus by a hyperintense (on T2W) mass with foci of T1 hyperintensity suggesting fat. Note: peripheral rim enhancement following gadolinium indicating infected cyst. Axial T1W image of brain (D) demonstrates a hyperintense focus in left frontal horn (arrow). Findings are suggestive of infected dermoid cyst with rupture

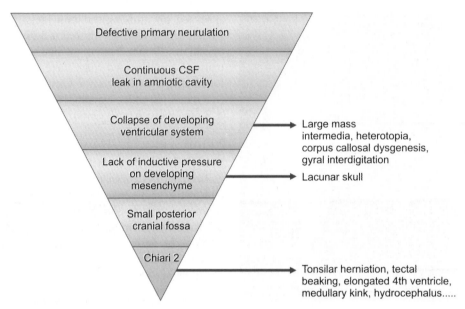

Fig. 21.11: McLone and Knepper theory explaining the pathogenesis of Chiari 2 malformation

Lipoma with Dural Defect (Lipomyelocele and Lipomyelomeningocele)

Lipomyelomeningocele consists of a large subcutaneous skin covered mass in lumbosacral region that contains fat, neural tissue, CSF and meninges.[24] This results from premature separation of surface ectoderm from neural ectoderm prior to formation of proper neural tube which allows ingress of intervening mesoderm into neural tube which in turn prevents further neurulation.[8] These mesodermal components specifically differentiate towards adipose tissue and form fatty component of these disorders. Clinically there is a mid-line soft non-tender mass above level of the intergluteal crease which extends asymmetrically into one buttock. Associated cutaneous malformation is seen in 50% cases. Differentiation of lipomyelocele from lipomyelomeningocele is by position of lipoma-placode interface. In lipomyelomeningocele the lipoma-placode interface is outside the confines of spinal canal (Figs 21.14A to C), whereas in lipomyelocele interface is either inside or at the edge of spinal canal (Figs 21.15A to C). In lipomyelocele, size of the subarachnoid space ventral to the cord is normal; however, the size of the canal may be increased depending on size of the lipoma. On the other hand in the lipomyelomeningocele there is ballooning of subarachnoid space ventral to the cord. This condition is associated with tethered cord, hydromyelia and Chiari I malformation.[9]

Meningocele

Meningocele is characterized by herniation of meninges through bony defect covered externally by the skin. The embryological basis remains unexplained.[8] As per definition the mass should not contain any of spinal cord segments or nerve root as content (Figs 21.16A and B). Rarely filum terminale may remain tethered within the sac. On imaging, CSF filled dural outpouching is seen to herniate via the spina bifida, intervertebral foramen or sacral foramen. More than 80 percent meningoceles are located in the lumbosacral spine. The bony defect may involve the posterior elements, anterior aspect of sacrum, lateral aspect of spine or distal sacrum (intrasacral meningocele).

Anterior Sacral Meningocele

Anterior sacral meningocele is characterized by herniation of meninges through anterior sacral defect, forming cyst like structure filled with CSF continuous with subarachnoid space of spinal cord. When this condition is associated with anorectal anomaly it is called Currarino's triad. Majority of cases remains asymptomatic and are detected incidentally either on pelvic examination or imaging.[25] Differential diagnosis includes cystic sacrococcygeal teratoma, large ovarian cyst and neurenteric cyst. Demonstration of continuity of cyst with thecal sac ensures diagnosis of anterior sacral meningocele (Figs 21.17A to C).

Myelocystocele

This rare entity constitutes about 5% cases of CSD and its embryological basis is not fully understood.[5,8] It could represent severe disruptive form of terminal ventricle, a defect in secondary neurulation. It has three components: skin covered posterior meningocele, hydromelic terminal cord into meningocele and posterior spina bifida. Myelocystocele may be terminal or segmental (cervical). Differential diagnosis includes simple dorsal meningocele and myelomeningocele. Continuity of the dilated central canal with the caudal cyst is diagnostic of myelocystocele and helps to differentiate it from other entities.[26]

CSD WITHOUT SUBCUTANEOUS MASS

This group includes wide variety of abnormalities in which imaging plays a crucial role in making the diagnosis.

Posterior Bony Spina Bifida

This is the simplest form of CSD and is characterized by defective fusion of posterior bony element. Isolated posterior spina bifida is seen in upto 5 percent of the general population. Usually,

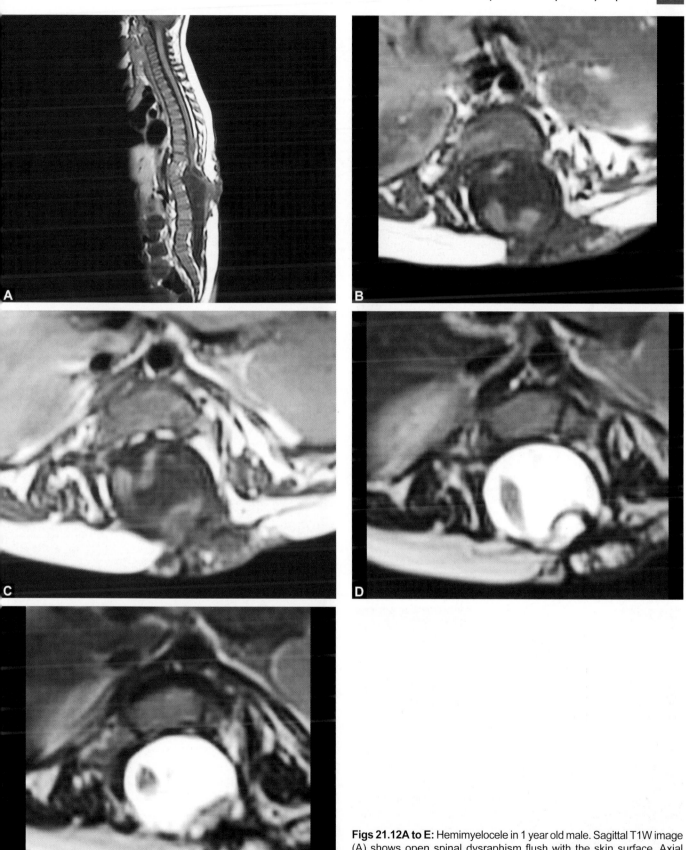

Figs 21.12A to E: Hemimyelocele in 1 year old male. Sagittal T1W image (A) shows open spinal dysraphism flush with the skin surface. Axial T1W (B, C) and T2W (D, E) images show two hemicords with left hemicord forming the neural placode which is flush with skin. Also note syrinx in the left cord

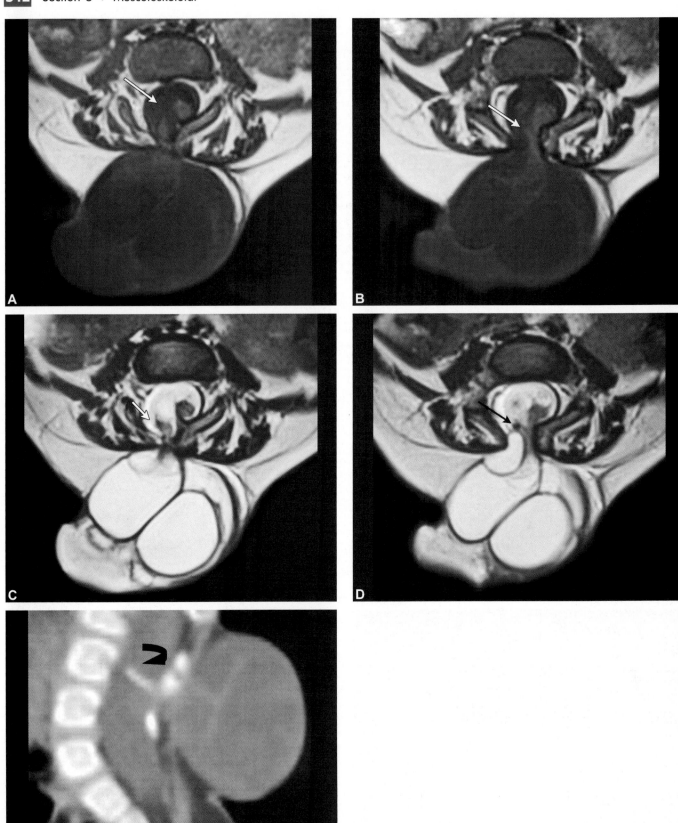

Figs 21.13A to E: Hemimeningomyelocele in a 2-year-old female. Axial T1W (A, B) and T2W images (C, D) show two hemicords with herniation of right hemicord and meninges through posterior bony defect forming large mass (arrow). Sagittal MPR CT image (E) depicts the bony spur better (curved arrow)

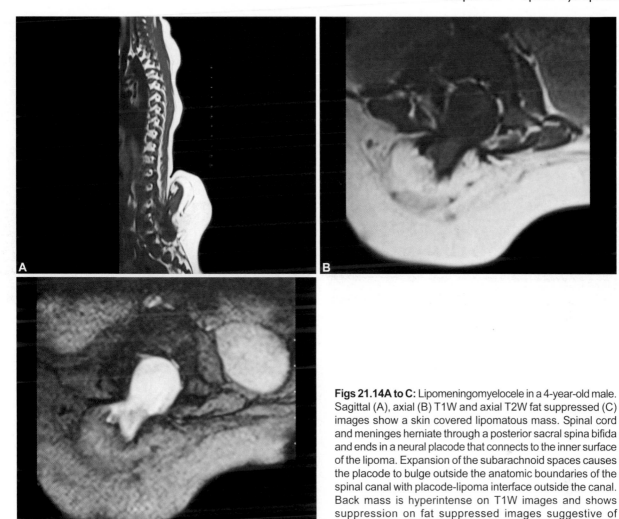

Figs 21.14A to C: Lipomeningomyelocele in a 4-year-old male. Sagittal (A), axial (B) T1W and axial T2W fat suppressed (C) images show a skin covered lipomatous mass. Spinal cord and meninges herniate through a posterior sacral spina bifida and ends in a neural placode that connects to the inner surface of the lipoma. Expansion of the subarachnoid spaces causes the placode to bulge outside the anatomic boundaries of the spinal canal with placode-lipoma interface outside the canal. Back mass is hyperintense on T1W images and shows suppression on fat suppressed images suggestive of lipomatous component

Figs 21.15A to C: Lipomyelocele in a 2-year-old male. Sagittal T1W (A) and T2W (B) images show T1 hyperintense intraspinal mass adherent to cord continuous with subcutaneous fat through wide spina bifida. Axial (C) T1W image better depicts intraspinal fatty component. Note lipoma–placode interface within confines of the spinal canal (arrow)

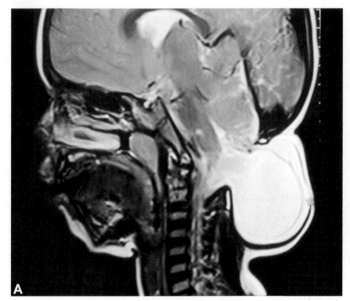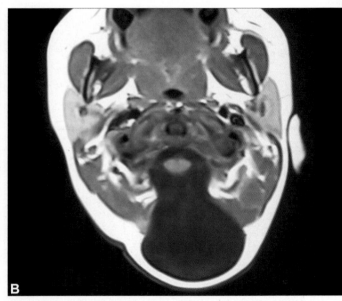

Figs 21.16A and B: Posterior cervical meningocele in a 6-month-old-male. Sagittal T2W (A) and Axial T1W (B) images show herniation of the meninges in the upper cervical region. Note associated skin covering and lack of herniation of neural elements

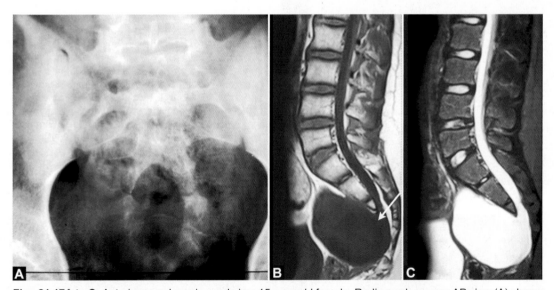

Figs 21.17A to C: Anterior sacral meningocele in a 15-year-old female. Radiograph sacrum AP view (A) shows scimitar sacrum (arrow). Sagittal T1W (B) and T2W (C) images show a large presacral cyst contiguous with the spinal canal (arrow). Also note sacral hypogenesis

insignificant, further imaging is not indicated unless there is neurological deficit or high risk cutaneous markers are present (Table 21.2). Defect is commonly seen at L5-S1 level (Fig. 21.18). Care should be taken not to diagnose this entity in children less than 6 years since it is physiological to see unfused posterior elements in lumbosacral region upto 6 years of age.[9]

Lipoma (Intradural and Intramedullary)

Lipoma results from early disjunction between neuroectoderm and ectoderm.[8] Lipoma is most commonly seen at lumbosacral level and is usually subpial in location. They occur more commonly in females, peak in the first five years of life and usually present with tethered cord syndrome. Lipomas are contained within intact dural sac and are located in midline dorsally. On MR, lipoma appears as a mass which follows signal intensity of subcutaneous fat on all pulse sequences (high signal intensity on T1W and FSE T2W images, hypointense on fat saturated images).

Filum Terminale Lipoma

Filum terminale lipoma probably results from defective secondary neurulation which leads to persistence of mesodermal elements within filum terminale which later differentiate towards adipose tissue.[5,8] Incidental detection of fatty signal (hyperintense on T1W) in the filum is a normal finding seen in upto 5% of general

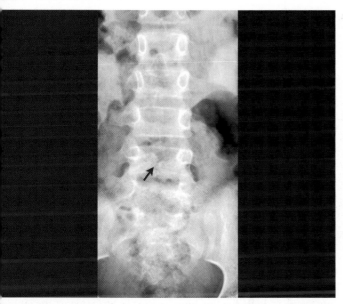

Fig. 21.18: Isolated Spina bifida in an 8-year-old male. Radiograph lumbosacral spine AP view shows absence of fusion of posterior elements of L4 & L5 (arrow)

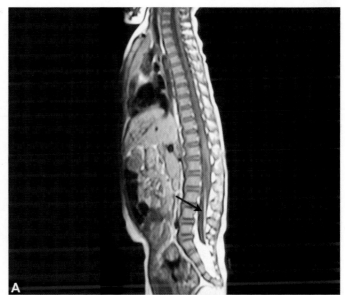

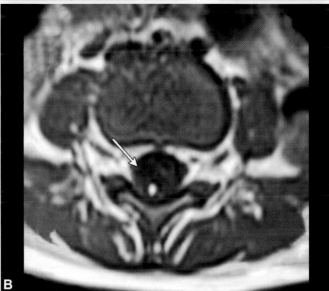

Figs 21.19A and B: Filum terminale lipoma in a 10-month-old female. Sagittal T1W (A) and axial T2W (B) images show thickened filum terminale with T1 hyperintensity indicating fat in filum terminale (arrow)

population and is referred as fatty filum.[27] Diagnosis of filum terminale lipoma should be made when the fatty filum measures more than 2 mm (Figs 21.9 and 21.19A and B). This condition may or may not be associated with cord tethering.

Tight Filum Terminale Syndrome

Tight filum terminale syndrome occurs due to defective retrogressive differentiation of neural tube formed by the process of secondary neurulation resulting in short and thick filum terminale (> 2 mm) which causes abnormal stretching of spinal cord with secondary neurological deficit.[5,6,9] Associated anomalies include posterior spina bifida, scoliosis and kyphoscoliosis. According to some authors tight filum terminale is a clinical syndrome and not an imaging diagnosis. It can be seen with anomalous filum terminale, split cord malformation and in postoperative period after surgery for open spinal dysraphism (Figs 21.20A and B). The treatment is surgical section of the filum terminale.

Persistent Terminal Ventricle

Persistent terminal ventricle results from defect in the process of secondary neurulation, resulting in the formation of small ependymal lined cavity with in conus medullaris. Usually, asymptomatic but may present with low backache and bladder dysfunction. There is dilatation of ependymal canal immediately above the filum terminale with slight expansion of conus. This condition needs to be differentiated from intramedullary tumour which can be done by its central location, CSF isointense signal intensity, and by noting lack of contrast enhancement following gadolinium and on follow up imaging.[6,9]

Neurenteric Cyst

Neurenteric cyst results from incomplete regression of neuro-enteric canal. Complete failure of regression manifest as dorsal

enteric fistula which is very rare.[8] They are enteric lined cysts that present within the spinal canal and exhibit a definite connection with the spinal cord and/or vertebra. They may communicate with an extra-spinal component of cyst in the mediastinum or mesentery through a dysraphic vertebra or they may attach by a fibrous stalk to the vertebra or gut.[5,28] The peak incidence is during the first two decades of life, and the most common location is thoracic spine followed by cervical spine. Vertebral anomalies are common though not invariable. Most cysts lie in the cervicothoracic junction or close to the conus medullaris.

Typically neurenteric cysts are located ventral to the cervicothoracic cord. Diagnosis should be thought, whenever a posterior mediastinal mass is seen along with congenital vertebral anomalies (Figs 21.21A to C). Neurenteric cysts are isointense to CSF on T1W images and hyperintense on T2W images.[28] No

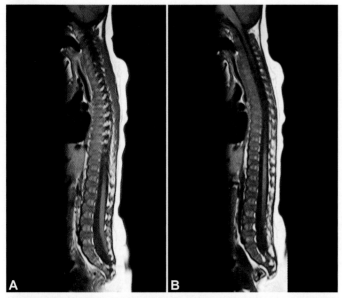

Figs 21.20A and B: Tight filum terminale (Tethered cord syndrome) in an 8-month-old female. Sagittal T1W images (A, B) show thickened filum terminale with tethered, low conus medullaris (arrow)

enhancement occurs after contrast administration. Usually, the child is asymptomatic, but can present with symptoms related to compression of airways, oesophagus, or atrium. Neurological deficit occurs secondary to intraspinal component of cyst and demonstration of this component and associated vertebral segmentation anomaly is critical in establishing the diagnosis.

SPLIT CORD MALFORMATION (SCM)

In SCM, the spinal cord is partially or completely spilt into two hemicords by either an osteocartilaginous septum or by a fibrous septum. Usually, these hemicord unite distally after splitting into two. Each segment has a central canal, and dorsal and ventral nerve roots. Over 90 percent of the cases occur in female patients. SCM

most commonly occurs in the thoraco-lumbar region (between D9 and S1 vertebral levels) and approximately 50–75% of patients have cutaneous stigmata at the site of cord split.[4-6]

SCM is classified as type 1 and type 2 based on state of the dural tube and nature of the medial septum.[21] In Pang type 1 (Figs 21.22A to F), each hemicord has a separate dural and arachnoid covering separated by a bony spur or septum (osteocartilaginous). In type 2 (Figs 21.23A to F), the hemicord are contained in a single dural sac and arachnoid covering without a rigid median septum (60% cases). Medial septum may be complete or incomplete and may course obliquely dividing the cord asymmetrically. Cleft is located at caudal end of splitting in majority of cases. SCM may be difficult to appreciate on sagittal MR images. Axial and coronal images show cord splitting as well as septum. However, fibrous septum may be very thin and is best demonstrated using thin axial/coronal T2W images.[9] SCM is suspected clinically in the presence of asymmetric neurological deficit and in presence of hairy tuft high along the back. It is important to look for this abnormality in all cases of dysraphic spine because of its frequent association. If not recognized prior to repair, it may be responsible for neurological deficit secondary to cord tethering. Commonly associated anomalies include: cord tethering seen in around 75% of patients and syringohydromyelia (50% patients). It may affect the normal cord above or below the cleft and extend into one or both hemicords. Intramedullary tumours (Figs 21.24A to C), have also been reported in the hemicord.[29] Vertebral anomalies are a rule and include spina-bifida, widened interpedicular distance, hemivertebrae and fused vertebrae.

DORSAL DERMAL SINUS (DDS)

Dorsal dermal sinus is an epithelium lined tract beginning at the skin surface which can communicate with the CNS and its meningeal coating. This results from defective disjunction of surface ectoderm from developing neural tube which leads to persistence of ectodermal connection between spinal cord and

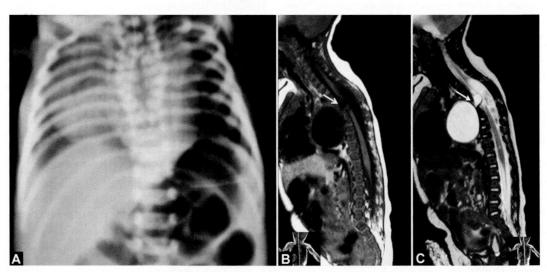

Figs 21.21A to C: Neurenteric cyst in a 1-month-old male. Chest radiograph AP view (A) shows vertebral segmentation anomalies with large posterior mediastinal mass. Sagittal T1W (B) and T2W (C) images demonstrate a dumbbell shaped mass extending from mediastinum into the spinal canal. Posterior subarachnoid space is dilated

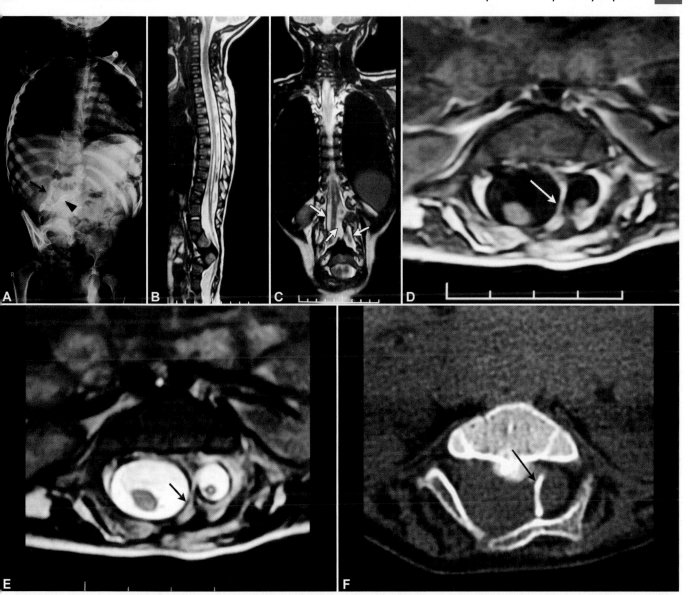

Figs 21.22A to F: Type 1 split cord malformation in an 8-year-old boy. Radiograph whole spine (A) demonstrates vertebral segmentation anomalies with intersegmental bar (arrow). Presence of vertical intersegmental bar strongly suggests split cord malformation. Also, note presence of bony spur (arrowhead). Sagittal T2W (B) image demonstrates thinning of cord with hydromyelia. Cord is also low-lying and tethered. Coronal T2W image (C), axial T1W (D) and T2W (E) images show asymmetric split of cord (arrow) into two hemicords with bony spur (arrowhead) in between. Axial CT (F) shows bony spur better

external skin.[8] Sinus tract usually ends at a level above the external opening because of the ascent of the spinal cord. The points of attachment of skin and spinal cord remain segmental or metameric, so the dermatome of involvement predicts the site of neural abnormality. Males and females are affected equally. The sinus ostium is typically midline and small hemangiomas may surround the ostium. The sinus tract extends deeply through the subcutaneous layer and between the bifid laminae toward the dura. It may end superficial to the dura, at the dura or deep to the dura.

Clinically dimples below top of the intergluteal crease end blindly whereas dimples above the level of intergluteal crease are

highly suspicious. Patients become symptomatic either by infection or due to associated dermoid and epidermoid tumours.[30] Dorsal dermal sinus will be seen as hypointense tract in both T1 and T2 weighted images extending from skin surface to spinal canal (Figs 21.25A and B). Sagittal and axial MR sequences are good to demonstrate the extraspinal portion of the dermal sinus tract, though the intraspinal portion is hard to identify. In such cases 3D MR Myelography can better delineate the tract and its intraspinal component. The differential diagnosis of DDS includes low sacrococcygeal midline dimple and pilonidal sinus, both of which do not enter spinal canal.

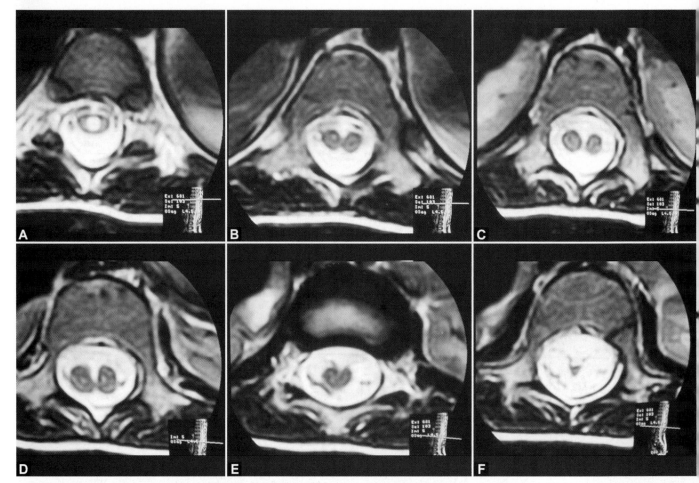

Figs 21.23A to F: Type 2 split cord malformation in a 10-year-old male. Axial T2W images (A-F) show two hemicords spur contained within a single dural sac. Syrinx is seen in the cord proximal to split and there is no bony/fibrous spur

CAUDAL AGENESIS (CAUDAL REGRESSION SYNDROME, CRS)

This is an uncommon malformation seen in 0.1-0.25:10,000 of normal pregnancies. However, it occurs in about one in 350 infants of diabetic mothers, representing an increase of about 200 times.[31] This syndrome is characterized by partial agenesis of lumbosacral spine, imperforate anus, malformed external genitalia, renal aplasia, extrophy bladder, etc. Plain films are adequate for demonstrating bony hypogenesis but do not show associated cord abnormalities. Sagittal T1W MR images are excellent for evaluating caudal vertebral agenesis, level and shape of conus and cord tethering.[6,31]

The anatomy and position of the conus defines two distinct types of abnormalities.[32] In Type I (Fig. 21.26), the conus ends above the level of L1, is typically deformed and terminates abruptly at D11 or D12, as if the normal distal tip were absent (nearly always club or wedge shaped). In this type with high conus the sacral deficit is typically large and the sacrum typically ends at or above S1. More severe the malformation, greater the number of absent vertebra and more cephalic is cord termination. In Type II (Fig. 21.27), the conus ends lower (below L1) and is elongated, stretched caudally and tethered by a thick filum or transitional lipoma. In these patients the sacrum tends to be relatively well-preserved, with identifiable portions of S2 or lower vertebral segments. Type 1 is associated with significant neurological deficit when compared to type 2 caudal agenesis.

Lumbosacral agenesis has also been classified into five different types depending on the nature and severity of agenesis. Type I is total sacral agenesis with some lumbar vertebra also missing. Type II is total sacral agenesis but the lumbar vertebra are not involved, while type III is subtotal sacral agenesis and atleast S1 is present. Type IV is a hemisacrum whereas type V is coccygeal agenesis.[4]

SEGMENTAL SPINAL DYSGENESIS (SSD)

SSD is a rare form of dysraphic spinal state resulting from defective development of segment of notochord during preneurulation stage. This is characterized by segmental agenesis of spine with dysgenesis of spinal cord at the level of bony abnormality. Severity of this anomaly varies from minimal segmental thinning of cord to complete loss of segment of spinal cord.[33]

CONCLUSION

Spinal dysraphism is a heterogeneous group of developmental abnormalities in which there is a defective closure of the neural

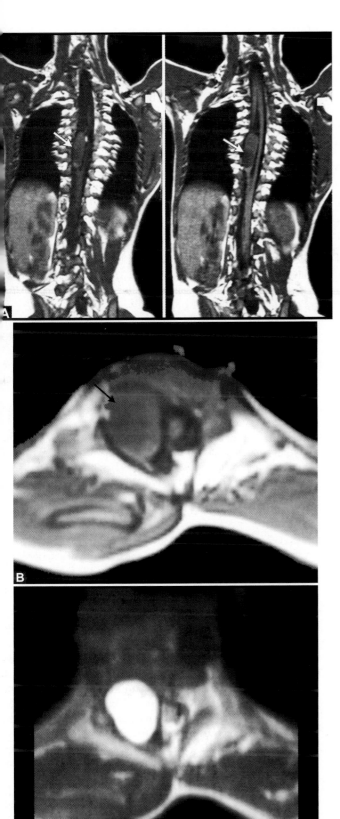

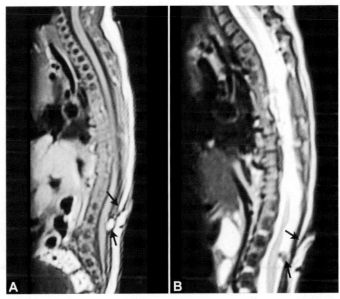

Figs 21.25A and B: Dorsal dermal sinus in a 9-day-old child with skin dimple at back. Sagittal T1W (A) and T2W (B) images show a hypointense linear tract (arrowhead) extending from skin till dura and terminates in a well defined T1 hyperintense oval lesion (arrow) suggestive of dermoid cyst

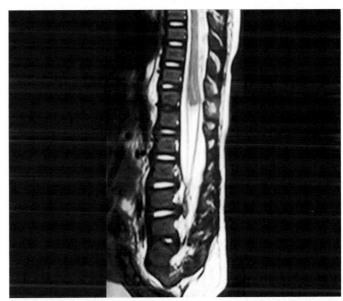

Fig. 21.26: Caudal agenesis Type-1 in a 8-month-old male. Sagittal T2W image shows absence of the sacral segments below S1 with abrupt bulbous termination of cord at D12-L1 disc level with abnormal distal nerve roots

Figs 21.24A to C: Split cord malformation with a dermoid in the right hemicord. T1W coronal (A) and axial (B) images show a split cord with an intramedullary tumour involving the right hemicord which is hypointense on T1W scans and hyperintense on the T2W axial (C) scan

tube. MRI is a single stop-shop imaging modality in majority of cases and also helps to classify them based on the commonly followed clinico-radiological classification proposed by Torotti et al. It is important for the radiologist and clinicians to be familiar with normal embryologic development of spine and MR findings of spinal dysraphism. Various other congenital anomalies are frequently associated and should be meticulously looked for when dysraphism is detected.

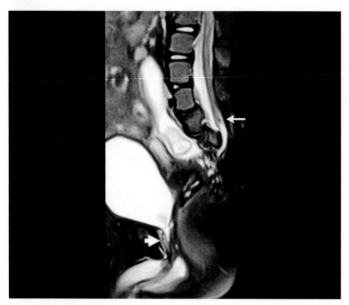

Fig. 21.27: Caudal agenesis Type-2 in a 2-year-old male. Sagittal T2W image demonstrates abnormal low lying cord reaching upto S1 (arrow) with agenesis of distal sacral segments. Bladder neck is patulous (arrowhead) suggestive of neurogenic bladder

REFERENCES

1. Warder DE. Tethered cord syndrome and occult spinal dysraphism. Neurosurg Focus 2001; 15:10:e1.

2. Byrd SR, Darling CP, Mclone DG: Developmental disorders of the pediatric spine. Radiol Cl North Am 1991; 29:9-21.

3. B. Drolet, Birthmarks to worry about. Cutaneous markers of dysraphism. Dermatol. Clin. 1998; 16:447–53.

4. Silverman FN, et al. Spinal dysraphism. In Silverman FN, Kuhn JP (Eds): Caffey's Pediatric X-ray Diagnosis (9th edn). Lippincott Williams and Wilkins 1993; 1:312-24.

5. P. Tortori-Donati, A. Rossi and A. Cama, Spinal dysraphism: A review of neuroradiological features with embryological correlations and proposal for a new classification. Neuroradiology 2000; 42: 471-91.

6. P. Tortori-Donati, A. Rossi, R. Biancheri and A. Cama, Magnetic resonance imaging of spinal dysraphism. Top. Magn. Reson. Imaging 2001; 12:375–409.

7. R.A.J. Nievelstein, N.G. Hartwig, C. Vermeji-Keers and J. Valk, Embryonic development of the mammalian caudal neural tube. Teratology 1993; 48:21–31.

8. B.N. French, The embryology of spinal dysraphism. Clin. Neurosurg. 1983; 30:295–340.

9. Rossi A, Biancheri R, Cama A, Piatelli G, Ravegnani M, Tortori-Donati P. Imaging in spine and spinal cord malformations. Eur J Radiol 2004; 50(2):177-200.

10. Bulas D. Fetal evaluation of spine dysraphism. Pediatr Radiol 2010; 40(6):1029-37.

11. Von Koch CS, Glenn OA, Goldstein RB, Barkovich AJ. Fetal magnetic resonance imaging enhances detection of spinal cord anomalies in patients with sonographically detected bony anomalies of the spine. J Ultrasound Med 2005; 24(6):781-9.

12. Hahn YS. Open myelomeningocele. Neurosurg Cl North Am 1995; 6:231-41.

13. Tortori-Donati P, Cama A, Fondelli MP, Rossi A. Le malformazioni di Chiari. In: Tortori-Donati P, Taccone A, Longo M. (Eds.), Malformazioni cranio-encefaliche. Neuroradiologia. Turin: Minerva Medica 1996; p. 209–36.

14. DG McLone and MS Dias, Complications of myelomeningocele closure. Pediatr. Neurosurg 1991; 17:267–73.

15. R.M. Scott, S.M. Wolpert, L.F. Bartoshesky, S. Zimbler and G.T Klauber, Dermoid tumors occurring at the site of previous myelomeningocele repair. J Neurosurg 1986; 65:779–83.

16. A. Cama, P. Tortori-Donati, G.L. Piatelli, M.P. Fondelli and L Andreussi, Chiari complex in children. Neuroradiological diagnosis, neurosurgical treatment and proposal of a new classification (312 cases). Eur. J Pediatr. Surg 1995; 5 Suppl 1:35–8.

17. McLone DG, Knepper PA. The cause of Chiari II malformation: A unified theory. Pediatr Neurosci 1989; 15(1):1-12.

18. Fichter MA, Dornseifer U, Henke J, Schneider KT, Kovacs L, Biemer E, Bruner J, Adzick NS, Harrison MR, Papadopulos NA. Fetal spina bifida repair—current trends and prospects of intrauterine neurosurgery. Fetal Diagn Ther 2008; 23(4):271-86.

19. Hirose S, Farmer DL. Fetal surgery for myelomeningocele. Clin Perinatol 2009; 36(2):431-8,

20. T.P. Naidich, D.G. McLone and F. Fulling, The Chiari II malformation. Part IV. The hindbrain deformity. Neuroradiology 1983; 25:179–97.

21. D. Pang, M.S. Dias and M. Ahab-Barmada, Split cord malformation Part I: A unified theory of embryogenesis for double spinal cord malformations. Neurosurgery 1992; 31:451–80.

22. D. Pang, Split cord malformation. Part II: Clinical syndrome Neurosurgery 1992; 31:481–500.

23. G.N. Breningstall, S.M. Marker and D.E. Tubman, Hydrosyringomyelia and diastematomyelia detected by MRI in myelomeningocele. Pediatr. Neurol 1992; 8:267–71.

24. T.P. Naidich, D.G. McLone and S. Mutleur, A new understanding of dorsal dysraphism with lipoma (lipomyeloschisis): Radiological evaluation and surgical correction. AJNR Am. J Neuroradiol 1983; 4:103–16.

25. K.S. Lee, D.J. Gower, J.M. McWhorter and D.A. Albertson, The role of MR imaging in the diagnosis and treatment of anterior sacral meningocele. Report of 2 cases. J Neurosurg 1988; 69:628–31.

26. Byrd SE, Darling CF, McLone DG, Tomita T. MR imaging of the pediatric spine. Magn Reson Imaging Clin N Am 1996; 4:797-833

27. E. Brown, J.C. Matthes, C. Bazan, III and J.R. Jinkins, Prevalence of incidental intraspinal lipoma of the lumbosacral spine as determined by MRI. Spine 1994; 19:833–6.

28. Gadodia A, Sharma R, Jeyaseelan N, Aggarwala S, Gupta P. Prenatal diagnosis of mediastinal neurentric cyst with an intraspinal component. J Pediatr Surg 2010; 45(6):1377-9.

29. Sharma A, Sharma R, Goyal M, Vashisht S, Berry M. Diastematomyelia associated with intramedullary tumour in a hemicord: A report of two cases. Australas Radiol 1997; 41(2):185-7

30. A.J. Barkovich, M.S.B. Edwards and P.H. Cogen, MR evaluation of spinal dermal sinus tracts in children. AJNR Am J Neuroradiol 1991; 12:123–9.

31. R.A.J. Nievelstein, J. Valk, L.M.E. Smit and C. Vermeji-Keers, MR of the caudal regression syndrome: Embryologic implications. AJNR Am J Neuroradiol 1994; 15:1021–9.

32. Pang D: Sacral agenesis and caudal spinal cord malfor-mations. Neurosurg 1993; 32:755-79.

33. P. Tortori-Donati, M.P. Fondelli, A. Rossi, C.A. Raybaud, A. Cama and V. Capra, Segmental spinal dysgenesis. Neuroradiologic findings with clinical and embryologic correlation. AJNR Am J Neuroradiol 1999; 20:445–56.

CHAPTER 22

Imaging of Pediatric Hip

Anjali Prakash

INTRODUCTION

The hip joint is a large and complex ball and socket joint consisting of a cup like acetabulum and a spherical femoral head.

Normal hip growth occurs as a result of genetically determined balanced growth of the acetabular and triradiate cartilages and the presence of a properly located femoral head. Absence of normal femoral head within the acetabulum during acetabular growth results in a flat shape of both the femoral head and acetabulum. The concave shape of the normal acetabulum is attributed to the presence of a spherical femoral head in close apposition to the acetabulum. Most acetabular development occurs by 8 years of age. The head, neck and greater trochanter of the infant hip is cartilaginous with early ossification of the femoral head seen between 3 to 6 months in girls and 6 to 9 months in boys.

Normal Anatomy

The acetabulum is formed of two fifths ischium, two fifths ilium and one fifth pubis joined by the triradiate cartilage (Fig. 22.1). Acetabulum at birth has a rim of hyaline cartilage. A fibrocartilaginous rim, the labrum that forms lateral extension of the acetabular roof, extends the acetabulum peripherally. The strong transverse ligament completes the inferior gap in the labrum. The ligamentum teres connects the acetabulum to the femoral head. A dense capsule encloses the joint and attaches superiorly to labrum on the ilium and distally along the intertrochanteric line of the femur. The joint surfaces are lined by a synovial membrane containing synovial fluid. The entire joint is surrounded and stabilized by large (extensor, flexor and adductor) muscle groups arising from the pelvis.

METHODS OF INVESTIGATION

Conventional Radiography

Hip radiography should include an anteroposterior view of the pelvis which allows quick comparison with the normal hip for subtle changes. The frog lateral view is X-ray lateral view of both hips taken together in abduction and external rotation (Fig. 22.2). Additional views may include oblique or a weight bearing view for dynamic evaluation of the joint space.

Various measurements are made on conventional radiography to assess alignment across the hip joint. Hilgenreiner line[1,2] is a YY line drawn through the center of the triradiate cartilage on both sides. Perkin's line is drawn through the superior lateral aspect of the acetabulum perpendicular to the YY line. The

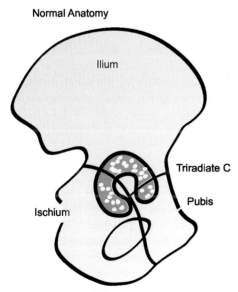

Fig. 22.1: Schematic diagram of anatomy of the acetabulum

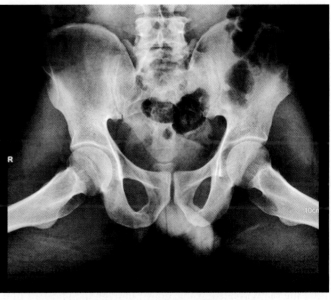

Fig. 22.2: X-ray both hips—frog-leg view

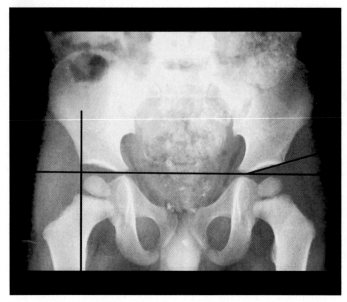

Fig. 22.3: X-ray pelvis—depicting Hilgenreiner's line and Perkin's line, femoral epiphysis lies in the medial inferior quadrant

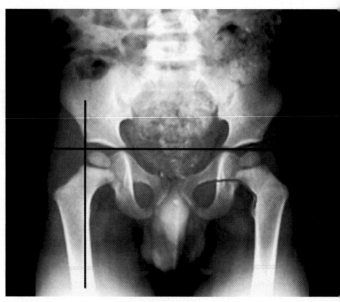

Fig. 22.5: X-ray pelvis showing acetabular angle and smooth unbroken Shenton's line

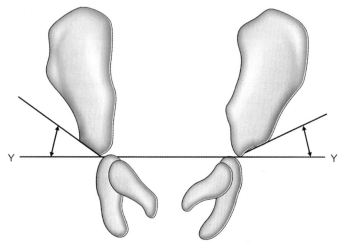

Fig. 22.4: Schematic diagram showing method for measurement of acetabular angle

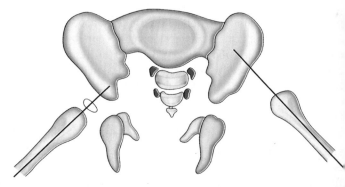

Fig. 22.6: Andren and von Rosen's method for detection of congenital dislocation of the hip before appearance of the capital femoral epiphysis

extended, cross the spine at the level of lumbosacral junction (Fig. 22.6). Andren and von Rosen view may have false negative results because of the inability to image the cartilaginous portions of the infant hip joint. False positive results may occur due to improper positioning and rotation of the pelvis.

These classical landmarks, lines and measurements were established as criteria for plain radiographic depiction of dislocation of the hip.

Ultrasonography (US)

Real time sonography has gained wide acceptance as the method of choice for imaging the infant hip. Sonography is particularly appropriate as it can image the cartilaginous femoral head and acetabulum without the use of radiation. Cartilage forms the major part of the femoral head and acetabulum in the first 6 months of life and this is not visible on plain radiograph. Not only can the detailed anatomy be demonstrated but the hip can be observed by the dynamic technique of hip sonography which incorporates motion and stress maneuvers that are based on accepted clinical examination technique. Ultrasonography is also valuable to assess

position of the femoral head can be surmised by evaluating the intersection of the Hilgenreiner line with the Perkin's line. In a normally positioned hip the femoral capital epiphysis primarily occupies the medial inferior quadrant (Fig. 22.3). The acetabular angle is the angle subtended between the Hilgenreiner line and a line parallel to the acetabular roof with the normal acetabular angle,[1] being less than 30° (Fig. 22.4).

The Shenton's line is a smooth unbroken curved line bridging the medial femoral metaphysis and the inferior margin of the superior pubic ramus. Disruption of this normally curved line suggests hip dislocation (Fig. 22.5).

Andren and von Rosen,[3] described an anteroposterior projection in which the child is supine with knees extended, hip extended and abducted to 45° from the midline and the femora fully internally rotated. A line drawn through the midshaft of an undislocated femur will pass within the acetabulum and will, if

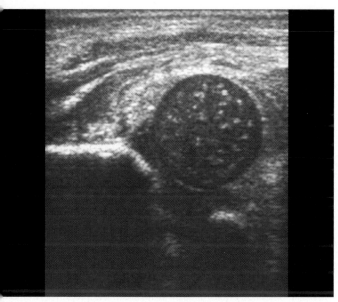

Fig. 22.7: USG-Coronal view—Femoral epiphysis shows low echogenicity with fine stippled echoes

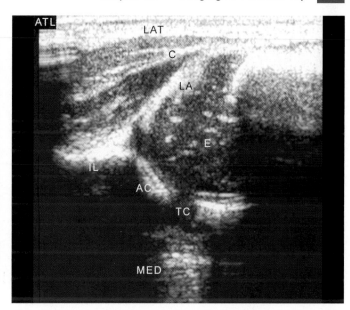

Fig. 22.9: USG (Coronal) depicting normal structures IL (Ilium). AC (Acetabulum), LA (Labrum), C (Capsule), TC (Triradiate cartilage)

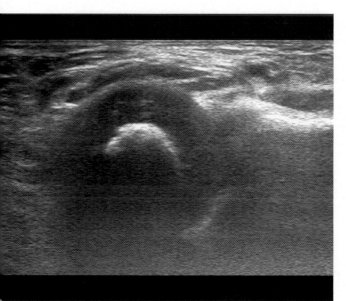

Fig. 22.8: USG—Beginning of ossification of femoral epiphysis from center

he hip in older children presenting with hip pain or limp. The procedure is noninvasive, involves no radiation, is easily available, nexpensive and in most patients sedation is not required.

Normal Sonoanatomy of the Hip

A linear array transducer with good near field resolution should be used. For infants, less than 7 months of age a 7.5 MHz transducer is appropriate and a 5 MHz transducer is used for infants between 7 to 12 months of age.

Sonographically, the normal cartilaginous femoral head is spherical measuring 1.2 to 2.1 cm in diameter in the neonatal age group. It is echopoor with finely stippled echoes, due to vascular channels (Fig. 22.7). The greater trochanter is of the same echogenicity and sonographically continuous with the femoral head. The femoral ossific nucleus is highly echogenic and becomes visible by 2-8 months of age[4] (Fig. 22.8).

The femoral head should be seated within the bony acetabulum formed by the ossification centers of ilium, ischium and pubis which are separated by the triradiate cartilage. The triangular cartilaginous roof of the acetabulum extends laterally beyond the bony acetabulum. This is echopoor except for a small fibrocartilaginous tip that is echogenic – labrum. The labrum appears as an echogenic triangle, caudal and lateral to the hypoechoic hyaline cartilage. The synovial membrane, fibrous capsule and supportive ligaments cover the limbus externally (Fig. 22.9).

In transverse images acetabulum appears as a V shaped structure with shadowing from bony anterior (pubic) and posterior (ischial) parts and echoes penetrating the vertical part of the triradiate cartilage (Fig. 22.10). The ischial component is larger than pubic part and femoral head is bisected by line continuous with the echoes penetrating the mid acetabulum.

The ligamentum teres is seen as a broad echogenic structure attached to the medial aspect of the femoral head in infants. In older children, it is obscured by the ossified femoral head. In neonates, the two layers of the synovial membrane are not distinct while in older children; some synovial fluid is normally present.

The joint capsule and ligaments are visualized as echogenic fibrous structures, which are closely approximated and cannot be separated on sonography. The hip is studied in two planes from the lateral approach, coronal and transverse with respect to the bony pelvis. The anterior approach in the parasagittal plane parallel to the femoral neck is used for evaluation of joint effusion. On anterior approach, the capsule ligament complex has a concave shape paralleling the underlying femoral neck (Figs 22.11 and 22.12).

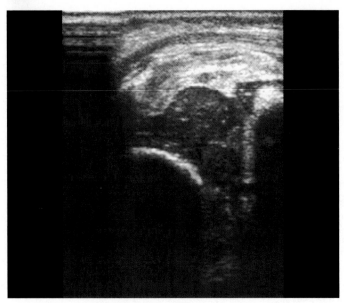

Fig. 22.10: USG Transverse image—Triradiate cartilage is seen between pubis anteriorly and ischium posteriorly

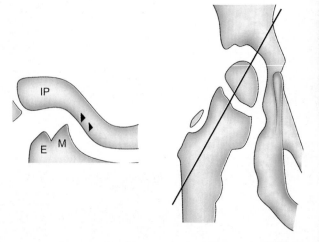

Fig. 22.11: Diagram showing plane of section obtained when the transducer is positioned parallel to the femoral neck and anatomy of the hip for detection of joint effusion in the anterior approach (E: Femoral epiphysis, M: Metaphysis; IP: Iliopsoas, Arrow head: joint capsule/Iliofemoral ligament)

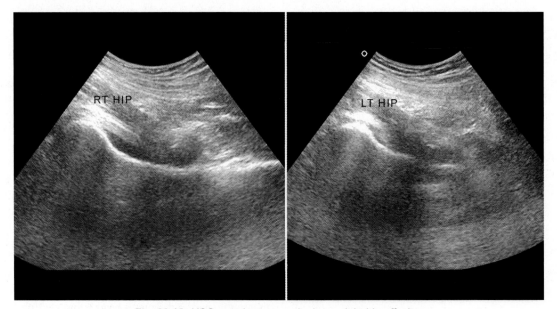

Fig. 22.12: USG anterior approach shows right hip effusion

Arthrography

Arthrography, although ideal for visualization of joint anatomy has limited use in infants due to high morbidity and risks of general anesthesia and infection. Intraoperative arthrography in conjunction with arthroscopic procedures provides precise direct visualization of anatomy and biopsy specimens but is impractical for children who require serial or frequent investigation.

Scintigraphy

Radionuclide bone scintigraphy is a sensitive, but relatively nonspecific modality for detection and characterization of articular diseases. ^{99m}Technetium–labeled polyphosphate is the most commonly used radionuclide which shows increased uptake in areas of bone turnover regardless of etiology, i.e. the growth plate in children and at abnormal sites, such as in tumor, infection, fracture, arthritis and periostitis. In osteonecrosis of the hip, it can demonstrate infarctive, reparative and inactive stages.

Computed Tomography (CT)

The use of helical CT has made three-dimensional reconstruction possible which optimizes visualization of hip articulations. CT allows accurate evaluation regarding reduction of hip in complicated cases, in the postoperative period and in presence of a spica cast.[5] Pediatric protocols that involve reduced dose can be used and study can be tailored for individual cases. A CT examination is, however, unnecessary for the treatment of the neonate or young infant with easily reducible dislocation of the hip.

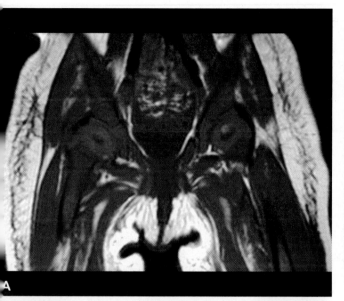

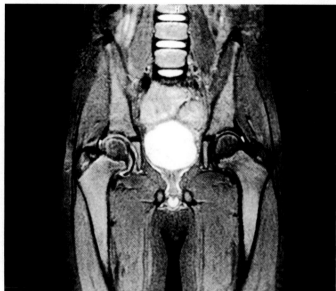

Fig. 22.13C: STIR coronal with suppression of signal from the fat

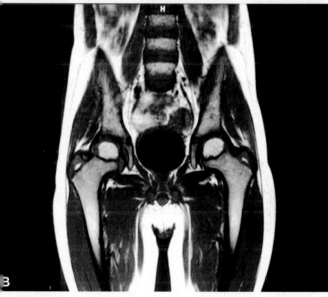

Figs 22.13A and B: MRI of a small child (4 months) T1W coronal (A), cartilaginous femoral epiphysis is seen with a small ossific nucleus. MRI-T1 weighted coronal (B) in an older child shows normal hyperintense signal of fatty marrow in epiphysis and intermediate signal of the cartilage

Magnetic Resonance Imaging (MRI)

Magnetic resonance imaging has become increasingly important in the evaluation of pediatric musculoskeletal diseases. The advantages being no known deleterious biological effect, no radiation, contrast resolution of soft tissue and muscle is superior to any other modality and fatty as well as cellular marrow components can be imaged.

Cortical bone produces a thin sharply defined black line surrounding the medullary cavity. The nonossified epiphyseal cartilage of the child is homogeneous and moderately high in signal intensity. Maturation replaces the cartilage with fatty marrow resulting in high signal of the femoral head on T1W

images. The immature metaphysis contains hematopoietic marrow and has an intermediate signal on all sequences (Figs 22.13 A to C).

Axial, coronal and sagittal MRI, using body or surface coils are useful in evaluation of hip joint. Coronal images allow assessment of shape of the acetabulum and femoral head coverage. MR images improve visualization of surrounding soft tissue structures – labrum, iliopsoas tendon, capsular tissue, ligamentum teres, transverse acetabular ligament and associated fibrofatty pulvinar. Ligaments and labrum have a low signal on all pulse sequences.

Fat saturation techniques and sequences like STIR (short tau inversion recovery) may be used to decrease the high signal intensity of the fat and enhance visualization of abnormal tissue and oedema within the marrow.

Dynamic multipositional (neutral and 2° flexion and abduction) MR in an open magnet configuration is being used to assess femoral head containment and joint congruency. This can also be used to position the femoral head, under direct visualization.[6]

MR arthrography, with direct intra-articular injection of dilute Gd-DTPA is a combination of joint distension and multiplanar imaging which provides detailed assessment of intra-articular structures especially acetabular labrum. This creates an arthrographic effect by delineating the synovial space.[7]

MR is particularly useful in cases of failed reduction of a dislocated hip to ascertain exact cause.

PEDIATRIC HIP DISORDERS

The most frequently encountered pediatric hip disorders are:
1. Dislocation
   a. Developmental dysplasia of the hip
   b. Traumatic hip dislocation

2. Hip disorders causing effusion-painful hip
   a. Septic arthritis
   b. Tubercular arthritis
   c. Transient synovitis
3. Miscellaneous
   a. Legg-Calve-Perthes disease
   b. Slipped capital femoral epiphysis
   c. Proximal focal femoral deficiency
   d. Rotational deformities

DEVELOPMENTAL DYSPLASIA OF THE HIP

The terminology congenital dislocation of the hip is now referred to as developmental dysplasia of the hip (DDH).[8] This broader term includes all the variants of the disorder during embryologic, foetal and infantile growth. DDH implies a dynamic disorder, that maybe unstable, subluxated or dislocated. DDH is composed of two elements—(1) Instability and (2) Abnormal morphology. Some authors observed that instability resulting in displacement of the femoral head prevents the acetabulum from developing properly, while other authors found that a primary deficiency in development of acetabulum allows the hip to become displaced, creating instability.

The hip is at risk for dislocation at several critical periods in utero, including shortly after its formation is complete at 12 weeks and at 18 weeks, when the hip muscles develop. The early in utero dislocations are often associated with other anomalies and are termed teratologic dislocations. These are fixed and secondary to paralysis from myelodysplasia, arthrogryposis or other neuromuscular disorders. The vast majority of cases of DDH result from forces acting on vulnerable, unstable, but otherwise normal hip in the immediate prenatal or postnatal period. These forces alter the relative proportion of ossified to cartilaginous portions of the acetabular roof in favor of structurally weaker cartilage, predisposing to dislocation.

NATURAL HISTORY AND PATHOLOGY

The hip joint is entirely cartilaginous at birth, the proximal femur has growth areas including the physeal plate, growth plate of the greater trochanter and along the isthmus of the femoral neck .The normal concave cup shaped acetabulum develops in response to the presence of a spheric femoral head. In DDH, there is a shallow saucer shaped acetabulum that is not congruent with the femoral head and there is persistent femoral anteversion.Secondary changes can be observed in the surrounding soft tissue, with contractures, thickening of the ligamentum teres, increased pulvinar fat, interposition of iliopsoas tendon and hip joint capsule. Soft tissue adaptations can develop at the acetabulum labrum with the formation of a neolimbus with superior migration of the femoral head; there is gradual eversion of the labrum with capsular tissue interposed between it and the outer wall of the acetabulum. In the older infants with DDH, the labrum may be deformed, elongated, inverted and may impede reduction. With abnormal pressure on the labrum there is formation of fibrous tissue that merges with the hyaline cartilage of the acetabulum to form the neolimbus.[9]

The reported incidence of fixed dislocation is 1 in 1000 whereas it is 0.4 to 0.6 in 1000 for late dislocation, subluxation and dysplasia. DDH is more common in girls (M: F = 1:6). The condition is usually unilateral (left > right 11:1), but both hips may be involved. Causes of DDH are multifactorial, with a combination of hormonal, familial and mechanical factors. The hormonal factor may explain the 6:1 female–male incidence and 20 percent familial incidence. The mechanical factor involves *in utero* spatial constraint and compression of the foetus as can be seen in oligohydramnios and breech position. Other risk factors include, talipes, arthrogryposis, and spinal dysraphism and generalized ligamentous laxity.

Early detection of DDH results in an excellent outcome failing which the condition can cause significant long-term morbidity.

Clinical Examination

DDH may be suspected clinically in the newborn, when a physical examination reveals asymmetrical skin folds, shortened thigh and irritability of the hip.

A "click" during the Ortolani reduction test performed by flexing the hip 90° with gentle abduction or an abnormal Barlow dislocation test performed by grasping the thigh in abduction with downward pressure on the hip indicates instability.

Radiological Diagnosis and Screening of DDH

The maximum potential for acetabular maturation is within the first 3 months of life; hence DDH should be diagnosed and treated before this time. It is important to be aware that a certain amount of instability in the hips of newborns, representing capsular laxity is normal in both boys and girls. This resolves spontaneously by 4 weeks. Delaying hip ultrasound till 6 weeks of age allow resolution of the same, and hence ultrasound of clinically normal hips should be done at 4-6 weeks of age, while a clinically unstable hip should be scanned at approximately 2 weeks.[10]

The absolute indications for hip imaging include:

(a) Family history of DDH, (b) Neonatal hip instability, (c) Limb shortening, (d) Limitation of hip abduction in flexion.

The relative indications, if more than two are present, imaging should be done are: (a) Breech presentation, (b) First born child (c) Cesarean section, (d) Other congenital anomalies, (e) Excessive fetal moulding.

IMAGING IN DDH

Conventional Radiography

As the neonatal hip is composed entirely of cartilage radiographs of the hip are frequently normal, especially if instability alone is present. An AP projection is obtained; the infant must be placed so that the pelvis is in neutral position and not rotated with hip slightly flexed. By 4-6 months, once the femoral head ossifies radiographs become more reliable.

The site of non-ossified epiphysis may be inferred as lying superior to the femoral epiphyseal plate. The superoinferior and lateral displacement of the femur can be determined by Perkin's

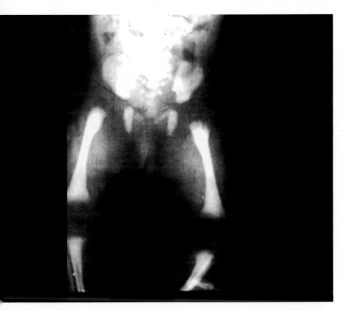

Fig. 22.14A: X-ray pelvis—Congenital dislocation of the right hip in a newborn before reduction

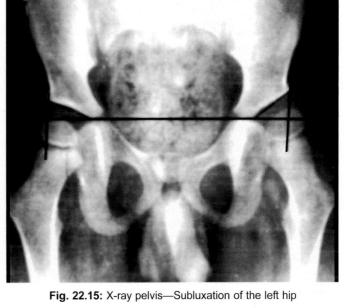

Fig. 22.15: X-ray pelvis—Subluxation of the left hip

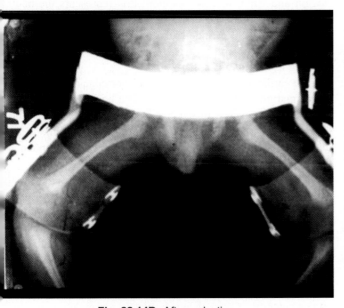

Fig. 22.14B: After reduction

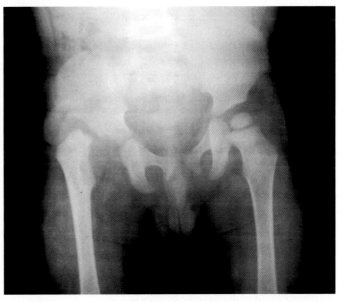

Fig. 22.16: X-ray pelvis with both hips – AP view shows a neglected DDH on the right side, with pseudoacetabulum formation

ine. The Shenton's line is disrupted in cases of dislocation. In dislocated hip, a line through the femoral shaft will point outside the acetabulum and will cross the spine at a higher level than normal as described in the Andrew and von Rosen method Figs 22.14A and B).

From the age of six months onwards, radiological diagnosis s usually easy. The femoral head is displaced upwards and outwards with delayed ossification of its epiphysis. The acetabulum is shallow with its roof sloping upwards and outwards with an increased acetabular angle (Fig. 22.15). A false acetabulum can develop in a frankly dislocated hip and is a pathognomonic sign of dislocated hip (Fig. 22.16).

In older children, other radiographic measurements may be useful. In children older than 5 years center edge angle is used. This is obtained by drawing a vertical line through the center of femoral head and perpendicular to the Hilgenrerner line. A second line is drawn obliquely from the outer edge of the acetabulum through the center of the femoral head (Fig. 22.17). The resulting angle reflects the degree of acetabulum coverage in dysplasia and the degree of femoral head displacement in an unstable hip. The center edge angle less than 20° is abnormal.

Conventional radiography suffers from the following drawbacks – the cartilage is not directly visualized and its position has to be inferred from the bony landmarks, the standard

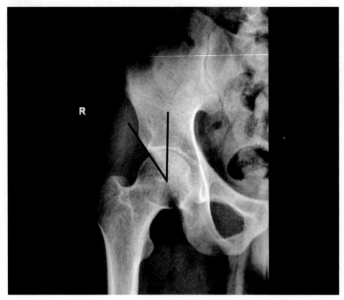

Fig. 22.17: X-ray of right hip–measurement of center–edge angle

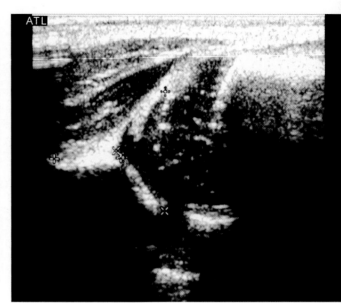

Fig. 22.18: USG–coronal view 'ball on spoon' appearance

radiographs are taken in a position in which subluxation is least likely to occur and the examination is static.

Ultrasonography in DDH

Sonography is now the primary imaging technique in the diagnosis and follow-up of DDH and has been shown to be more accurate than either clinical or radiographic assessment with a sensitivity of 100 percent and a specificity of 98 percent.[11] Ultrasound examination has the following advantages—it visualizes the nonossified cartilage of the femoral epiphyses and the cartilaginous labrum and permits dynamic assessment of stability. It cannot be used over the age of 12 months due to acoustic shadowing from the developing ossification center of the epiphysis.

The sonographic features to be noted in an infant hip include the following:

a. Position of femoral head, its coverage, and change in position with stress.
b. Assessment of acetabular dysplasia.
c. Acetabular roof–horizontal or inclined.
d. Acetabular edge—sharp, rounded or flattened.
e. Labrum everted or inverted.
f. Acetabular fossa for presence of interposed soft tissues such as excessive fat or hypertrophied ligamentum teres.

The use of ultrasound in evaluation of DDH was first described by Graf[12] in 1978 and Harcke[13] et al soon after. Modifications of these methods- by Rosendahl, Morin have been suggested and are used at some centers.

Graf assessed acetabular morphology and devised a classification system based on angles of inclination of the bony and cartilaginous roof.

A static coronal image of the hip is obtained for interpretation. The baby is supported in a lateral decubitus position, knees slightly flexed. The hip is positioned in approximately 20° of flexion and slight internal rotation; this represents the neutral position for an infant. The transducer is positioned over the greater trochanter and held perpendicular to the skin and parallel to the table in order to obtain a coronal image of the acetabulum showing its maximum depth.

The cardinal landmarks are the inferior edge of the ilium, the lateral margin of the ilium projected as a horizontal line and the acetabular labrum. The appearance of this standard plane has been likened to a "ball on spoon" appearance, with the femoral head representing the ball, the acetabulum, the bowl of the spoon and the ilium the handle of the spoon (Fig. 22.18).

The proper coronal view contains three elements (a) the echoes from the bony ilium should be in a straight line parallel to the transducer (b) the transition between the os ilium and the triradiate cartilage should be seen definitively (c) the echogenic tip of the labrum should be in the same plane as the other two. Minor anterior or posterior adjustment may be required until the standard plane is obtained. False positive diagnosis of dysplasia may be made when the transducer is not in mid plane and is rotated anteriorly. Conversely a dysplastic acetabulum may appear normal if the transducer is rotated posteriorly.

Graf demonstrated that in normal hips the round, hypoechoic speckled femoral head lies centered in the acetabulum. His protocol had 3 lines drawn on the coronal view about the acetabulum from which the α and β angles could be measured. The first baseline A is drawn along the straight lateral margin of the ilium, where the perichondrium meets the ilium. A second inclination line B connects osseous convexity to labrum and the third roof line C connects lower edge of acetabular roof medially to osseous convexity. One between acetabular roofline and baseline measures the α angle, which denotes inclination of the acetabular. A small alpha indicates a shallow bony acetabulum (Figs 22.19A and B).

The β angle is measured between the baseline and the line of inclination, giving an indication of coverage of femoral head by

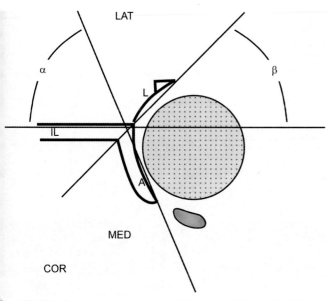

Fig. 22.19A: Schematic diagram depicting straight bony iliac interface (IL), bony acetabulum (A) and echogenic labrum (L), the α (Alpha) and β (Beta) angles are shown

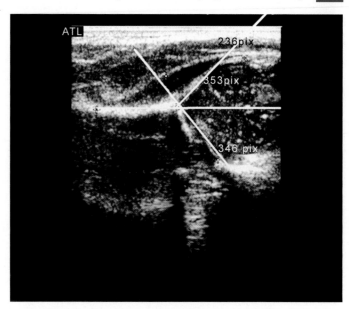

Fig. 22.19B: Sonogram depicting base line, inclination line and acetabular roof lines – normal hip Type I

Type	Description	α	β	Comments	Treatment
	Table 22.1: Graf hip types				
I	Normal hip	>60°	< 55°	Stable	None
II	Concentric position				
	a. Physiological immaturity (age < 3 mon)	50°-60°	<77°	—	Observed till change to type 1
	b. Delayed ossification (age > 3 mon)	50°-60°	55°-77°	—	Evaluation by orthopedic surgeon
	c. Concentric position	43°-49°	—	—	Evaluation by orthopedic surgeon
	d. Subluxation	43°-49°	> 77°	Labrum everted	Required
III	Low dislocation	<43°	>70°	Bony roof deficient labrum everted	Required
IV	High dislocation	Not measurable		Flat bony acetabulum, interposed labrum	Required

cartilaginous acetabular rim. A large β angle indicates lateral migration of femoral head. Classification of hip types on ultrasound studies is given in Table 22.1.

Calculation of α and β angles is not possible if the femoral head is dislocated in anterior or posterior direction. Graf described type I and II a/b as inherently stable and types II d, III and IV as inherently unstable and found that it is only necessary to test for stability with type IIc (Figs 22.20 and 22.21).

Coronal images are also used to evaluate the position of the femoral head within the acetabulum. If the acetabular cup accommodates less than one-third of the femoral head, than acetabular dysplasia is definitely present and must be suspected, if only half to one-third is accommodated (Fig. 22.22).

Harcke and Grisson[14] advocate the use of dynamic sonography of the infant hip, based on the premise that the position and stability of the femoral head are key factors in the diagnosis and management of DDH. If the femoral head is

properly positioned and stability is achieved, then acetabular development will proceed.

The US examination is modeled after clinical examination and based on provocative tests for dislocating the unstable hip and the reduction of the dislocated hip. The standard US examination should consist of two particular views: Transverse neutral and coronal-flexion (Fig. 22.23). The value of the coronal flexion view is that it reflects the position in which the physician places the hips during the dynamic physical examination. The ossific nucleus is graded for size (0= no center present, 1= center size <= 0.5 cm; 2= center size of > 0.5 cm but acetabulum visible; 3= center size large enough to prevent visualization) (Fig. 22.23).

In the transverse plane, with the infant's hip flexed, the hypoechoic cartilaginous femoral head is viewed between two echogenic limbs of a 'V' (in adduction) or U (in abduction). Stability can also be assessed in the coronal plane while pistoning the hip anteroposteriorly (knees flexed), (Fig. 22.24).

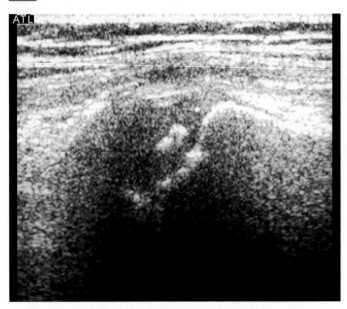

Fig. 22.20: USG—Gross superolateral hip dislocation with complete disruption in alignment with the acetabulum (Type IV CDH)

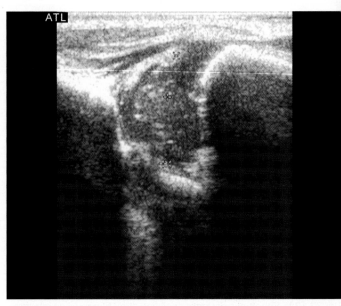

Fig. 22.22: USG—62 percent coverage of the femoral head within the acetabular cup

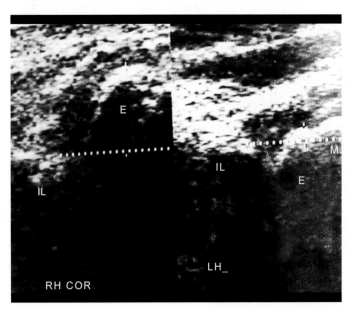

Fig. 22.21: USG old neglected CDH on the right with normal left hip

Rosendahl and co workers in 1992 described a modified Graf's method classifying hip morphology and hip stability separately. Hip morphology (alpha angle) was assessed using the standard coronal view with the femoral head centered. In cases of decentered or dislocated hips-Graf type 2c, D, 3, 4a, the femoral head was relocated by mild traction on the thigh before morphology could be studied. A Barlow maneuver was applied to assess a coexisting instability. A technique for assessing the degree of lateralization of the femoral head on the basis of Harcke's coronal flexion view was proposed by Morin et al. in 1985. Based on two lines paralleling Graf's baseline, one tangent to the lateral part of the femoral head and one tangent to the medial junction of the head and acetabular fossa were drawn, they measured distance between medial and iliac lines (d) and between the medial and lateral lines (D). The ratio of d to D multiplied by 100 indicated the percentage of the femoral head covered by the bony acetabulum.[15]

Pediatric radiologists are relying increasingly on the use of dynamic sonography as this allows real time observation of

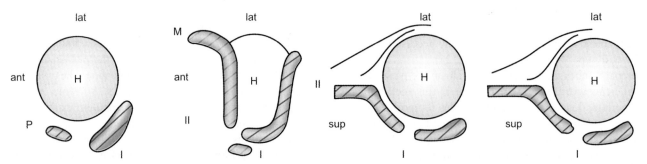

Fig. 22.23: Schematic diagram of Harcke's dynamic four step method. (A) Transverse neutral view (B) Transverse flexion view (C) Coronal flexion view (D) Coronal neutral view. Ant – Anterior, Lat – Lateral, P – Pubis, I - Ischium A = Femoral head, T – Triradiate carlitage, M – Femoral metaphysis, IL. Ilium.

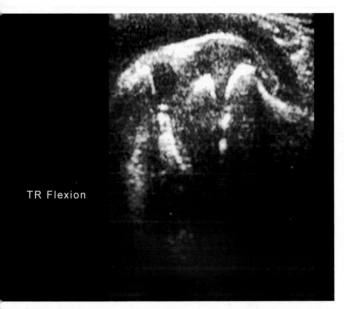

Fig. 22.24: USG—hip flexed transverse plane—femoral head viewed between two echogenic limbs of pubis and ischium in adduction ('V')

maneuvers allowing a more accurate depiction of the femoral head in relation to the acetabulum as the hip position is changed. Hence, it allows not only depiction of DDH but is also able to assess whether a particular closed reduction is appropriate.

Sonography can also be used to monitor treatment of patients with DDH in a spica cast, brace or Pavlik harness. The long axis anterior approach may be useful in a patient with a spica cast in which a window cannot be cut for lateral scanning. The window should be repositioned and the cast repaired to avoid posterior hip dislocation. The sonographic follow-up of patients being treated in a Pavlik harness is however easy as it permits movement within a safe zone while the degree of restriction prevents subluxation or dislocation. Improvement should be seen within 3 weeks of treatment. Duplex Doppler US has been used to assess vascularity of the femoral head in an infant undergoing abduction treatment. The normal spectral waveform of arterioles in the femoral head of an infant is a slow flow, low resistance arterial pattern with resistive indices ranging from 0.2 to 0.68 (mean 0.48 ± 0.11).[16] Power Doppler can be used to visualize blood flow in the cartilaginous femoral head to ensure that flow is not compromised during treatment.

CT

CT is useful for the evaluation of concentricity of closed reduction, detection of iliopsoas muscle deformity or intra-articular soft tissue obstacles such as hypertrophied fibrofatty pulvinar which can make it difficult to achieve concentric reduction by the closed method, for detection when the surgical procedures are to be performed and for the determination of femoral torsion and acetabular configuration. It can be performed even when the patient is casted (Figs 22.25A & B and 22.26). CT is most useful in postoperative assessment of reduction. Injection of contrast medium into joint is often performed during intraoperative reduction. CT done soon after allows the

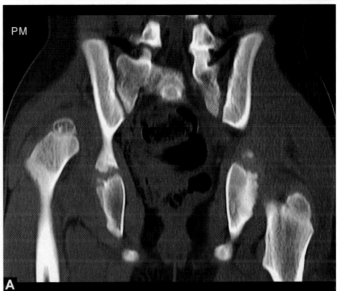

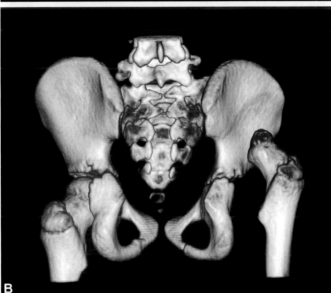

Figs 22.25A and B: CT-MPR (A) and VRT (B) shows right femoral epiphysis dislocated superiorly and posteriorly *(For color version Fig. 22.25B see plate 8)*

contrast medium surrounding the nonossified femoral head to be identified. This helps in assessment of the alignment of the femoral head and its relationship to the acetabulum.

The use of three-dimensional imaging allows direct assessment of the amount of anterior and posterior acetabular coverage. Standard CT protocols allow images to be obtained in the standard frog leg position. Even though the femoral head may not be ossified the position of the femoral metaphysis relative to the midportion of acetabulum can be evaluated.

CT scanning allows differentiation of lateral from posterior hip dislocations. Lateral displacement shows the labrum and capsule unfolded secondary to a tight iliopsoas tendon. In posterior dislocation approximation of the femoral metaphysis and acetabulum, projection of a mass behind the ischium and posterior displacement of pregluteal fat plane is seen. Acetabular

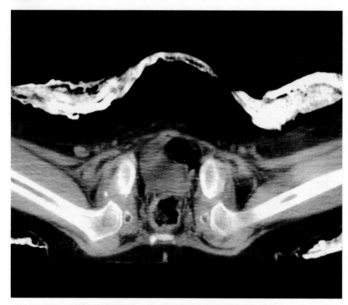

Fig. 22.26: CT case of DDH with hip spica

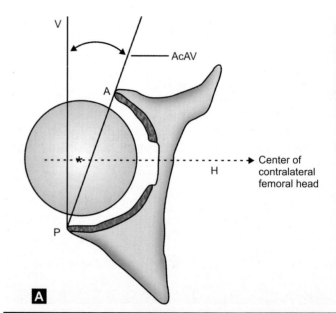

A

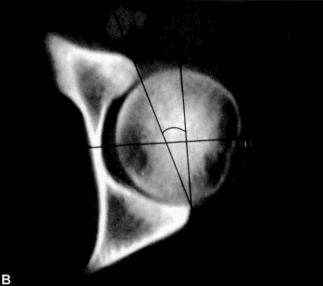

B

anteversion is measured by determining the angle of the anterior and posterior rim relative to the vertical axis of the pelvis (Figs 22.27A and B). Increased acetabular anteversion has been noted in dysplastic hips and also in some healthy volunteers. Acetabular sector angles are more specific to the presence of hip dysplasia (Figs 22.28A and B). Anterior and posterior sector angles reflect the degree of anterior and posterior acetabular support.[17] The sector angles are determined by measurement of the angle drawn between the center of the femoral head and the anterior and posterior acetabular rim relative to the horizontal axis of the pelvis. A normal anterior angle is greater than 50° and a normal posterior angle is greater than 90°. These angles are reduced in developmental dysplasia, which reflects acetabular support. Measurements of acetabular angles, have however not been found predictive of the outcome of DDH.[18]

MR

MR is used in the evaluation of dysplasia of the hip when there is (i) a complex dysplasia, (ii) there has been inadequate response to treatment, (iii) in late presentation and (iv) teratological dislocation. Axial and coronal MR images are most useful and small surface coils with high spatial resolution are necessary to evaluate DDH.

The value of MR imaging in preoperative planning is due to its ability to portray the cartilaginous part of the pelvis and also analyze the relationship of the femoral head to the acetabulum and labrum. The femoral head is variably laterally displaced in DDH, with posterior and superior reduction. MR shows femoral head coverage in both coronal and axial planes without need for complex radiographic projections or magnification correction. The degree of coverage by the cartilaginous acetabulum and labrum can be evaluated by MR. MR imaging can show changes in the shape of the acetabulum, not demonstrated on CT sonography or radiography. In DDH, the acetabulum becomes elongated

Figs 22.27A and B: Schematic diagram (A) and CT (B). Measurement of femoral anteversion from an axial CT slice. H = Horizontal line through femoral head center, P = Posterior margin of acetabulum, A = Anterior margin of acetabulum, V = Line perpendicular to line H through point PAC, AV = angle of anteversion

posteriorly or superiorly. The rim of the acetabulum becomes oval and the acetabular cartilage becomes thickened and may become displaced.[19]

Any obstruction to the reduction can be visualized, especially in cases where there is a history of failed closed reduction these include a flipped labrum, prominent pulvinar and a redundant ligamentum teres;capsule or illiopsoas tendon or transverse acetabular ligament, which may be interposed into the joint (Figs 22.29A and B). Prominent pulvinar is visualized as fibro fatty material in the joint, which does not allow normal seating of the femoral head within the joint. There can be a small amount of pulvinar normally present with the head being slightly laterally

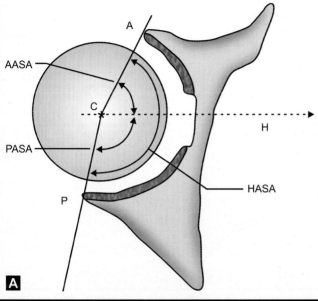

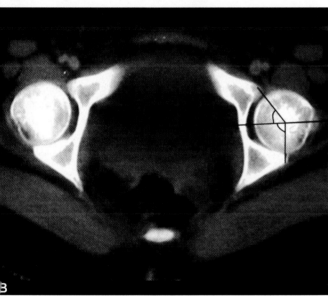

Figs 22.28A and B: Schematic diagram (A) and CT (B). Measurement of acetabular sector angles. H = Horizontal line through femoral head center, P = Posterior margin of acetabulum, A = Anterior margin of acetabulum, C = Center of femoral head, HASA = Horizontal sector angle, AASA = Anterior sector angle, PASA = Posterior sector angle

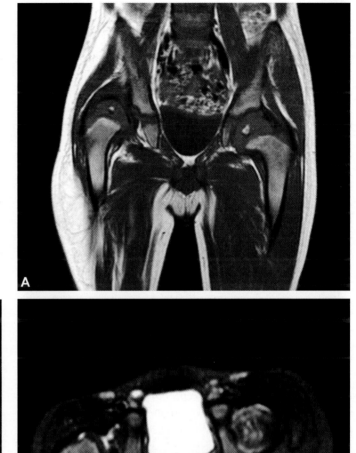

Figs 22.29A and B: MRI T1 coronal (A) and T2 axial (B) shows dislocated femoral epiphysis with hypertrophied ligamentum teres preventing relocation

displaced. If the head is encompassed by the confines of the acetabulum and pointing at the triradiate cartilage, the pulvinar usually atrophies. Gadolinium enhanced magnetic resonance arthrography visualizes the labrum, ligamentum teres, transverse acetabular ligament and the pulvinar.[20]

In the immediate postoperative period, MR imaging is useful in evaluation of proper reduction of the dislocated femoral head and its vascular health.

Recently dynamic interventional MRI in an open configuration scanner has been used in the management of developmental dysplasia. The hip can be visualized during reduction and spica can be applied within the scanner itself.[21]

Differential Diagnosis of DDH

Radiographic features such as shallow acetabulam with high angled roof lateral and cephalad displacement of the upper end of the femur and small ossification center for the head can be seen in congenital hypothyroidism. Following appropriate therapy, spontaneous resolution may occur.

Traumatic epiphyseal separation of the femoral neck in very young infants may simulate congenital dislocation. The possibility of trauma may be considered if there is history of an abnormal presentation/difficult labor. Acquired non traumatic dislocation may develop in pyoarthrosis of hip. In such a case there will be clinical sign of infection will be present.

The Painful Hip

Hip pain in a child is always potentially serious and presents a diagnostic challenge since clinical differentiation between septic arthritis; transient synovitis and Perthes' disease may be difficult. The principle concern is to distinguish sepsis of the hip joint from an irritable hip, as untreated sepsis can destroy the hip within days. The presentation may be mild and atypical and therefore imaging plays an important role in the management of such cases.

Septic Arthritis

Acute purulent infection of the joints is more common in infancy and early childhood because of greater blood flow to the joints during active growth. Hematogenous seeding is the most common cause related to an upper respiratory tract infection or pyoderma. Infection may also spread from adjacent osteomyelitis in metaphysis (specially in hip, where metaphysis is intra-articular) or from cellulitis, abscess, etc. During infancy, septic arthritis frequently complicates osteomyelitis because capillaries from the metaphysis traverses the physis into the epiphysis. Infants with immune dysfunction, indewelling cathetars, vascular lines are at increased risk. Over 90 percent of cases of septic arthritis are monoarticular with hip being one of the most commonly affected joints.

Staphylococcus aureus is the most common cause of bacterial arthritis, with group B *Streptococcus* seen in neonates. *H. influenzae* in the 1-4 years age group. Children with chickenpox are at increased risk of developing septic arthritis and other musculoskeletal infections secondary to group A Streptococcus. Pneumococcal joint infection may be seen in children with splenic dysfunction. Over 90 percent of cases of septic arthritis are monoarticular with the hip being most commonly involved.

Clinically there is fever, joint pain and swelling. Boys are affected twice as frequently as girls. It is a medical emergency as it may lead to joint destruction and impairment, if not immediately and adequately treated.

Pathology

The joint cartilage is a vascular and the synovial fluid cushions, lubricates, and nourishes the joint cartilage. Bacteria may seed into the synovial space through the highly vascular synovial membrane. Initially, there is edema and hypertrophy of the synovial membrane with joint effusion, which distends the joint. Hyperemia and immobilization leads to demineralization and osteoporosis. The ensuing inflammatory reaction results in destruction of the cartilage matrix leading to reduction of the joint space. Inflammatory pannus destroys the articular cortex, which is eroded. Severe cases are characterized by massive destruction, separation of bone ends, subluxation and dislocation. During recovery bones recalcify and bony and fibrous ankylosis may occur.

Imaging

Imaging evaluation is initially by **conventional radiography**. Plain films may be normal or demonstrate joint space widening with adjacent soft tissue swelling and disruption of normal tissue

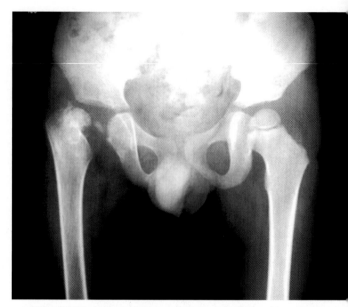

Fig. 22.30: X-ray pelvis erosions in right femoral head with dislocation and widening of joint space septic arthritis

planes. It may show joint space loss and erosions with relative preservation of mineralization (Fig. 22.30).

Radionuclide imaging is more sensitive than radiographs. A bone scan localizes the site of infection and is positive as early as 2 days after the onset of symptoms. In septic arthritis there is increased articular activity in the blood flow and blood pool phases. Reduced uptake within the epiphysis may be as a result of ischemia.

Ultrasonography can clearly delineate presence and nature of joint fluid by direct visualization,[22] and can be used to guide needle aspiration. The anterior approach along the plane of the neck is used as this is the most easily distensible part of the joint and fluid first accumulates in this area. In normal hip, the joint capsule is seen as a continuous concave reflective line paralleling the anterior aspect of the femoral neck and capital femoral epiphysis. Synovial thickening or an effusion causes the joint capsule to become convex and bulge anteriorly. A difference of 2 mm in the Anterior Capsule Distance (ACD) is indicative of effusion. Asymmetry is an unreliable parameter as effusion may be bilateral. The normal ACD increases with age and the upper limit of normal are 5 mm (<4 years) 6 mm (4-7 years) and 7 mm (8 years or over).[4]

Ultrasound can detect as little as 1 mm of fluid and all cases of septic arthritis have effusion (Figs 22.31 and 22.32A & B). Neither the size nor the relative echogenicity of fluid can be used to distinguish an infected from a simple effusion. **Power Doppler** ultrasound has been used to differentiate septic arthritis from sterile synovitis. Strouse et al found that though increased flow in the hip suggested infection, findings of normal flow do not exclude infection and should not preclude hip joint aspiration.[23]

MR imaging is extremely sensitive for detection of even a very minimal effusion with sensitivity and specificity of Gd-DTPA enhanced MR imaging of 100 percent and 77 percent in detection of septic arthritis.[24,25] Patients with both septic arthritis and

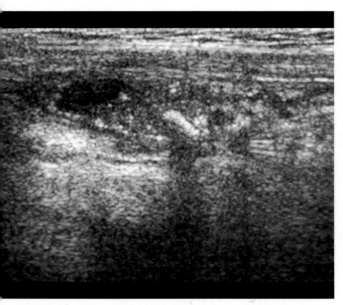

Fig. 22.31: USG—Collection with echogenic debris following infection

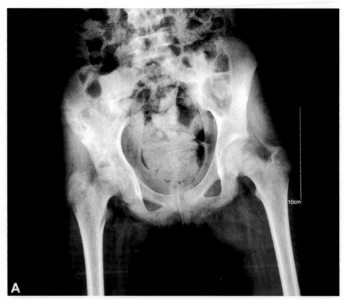

A

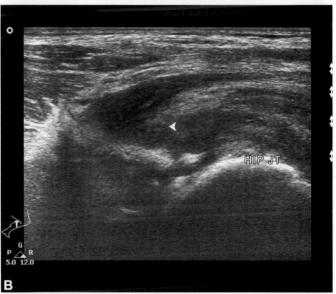

B

Figs 22.32A and B: X-ray (A) – Reduced Rt hip joint space with irregularity of articular outline. Ultrasound hip (B) of the same patient—shows disorganized joint with effusion that shows debris – a case of septic arthritis

transient synovitis may show joint effusion, intense enhancement, and hypertrophy of the synovial membrane. Patients with septic arthritis, however, also show signal abnormalities in adjacent bone marrow on fat suppressed CE MRI, a finding not seen in patients with transient synovitis. The joint space becomes an abscess cavity. Pyogenic abscess in a joint space can be differentiated from reactive fluid based on diffusion MR. A pyogenic abscess shows an increased signal intensity on diffusion weighted imaging whereas a reactive effusion shows a low signal.[26]

The earliest MR finding of acute osteomyelitis is marrow edema with decreased signal on T1 and increased signal on T2 and STIR images.[27] As infection progresses periosteal soft tissue inflammation and cortical abnormalities may be seen (Fig. 22.33). Differentiation of pyogenic from tubercular joint infection is important as treatment is different in both. Serology and joint fluid analysis form the basis of diagnosis. MR imaging may offer some clues to the diagnosis.[28] The presence of bone erosions, absence of subchondral marrow signal intensity abnormality favors a diagnosis of tubercular arthritis. A thin and smooth abscess rim favors tubercular arthritis, where as a thick and irregularly enhancing rim is indicative of pyogenic arthritis.

Septic arthritis is a surgical emergency and a delay in diagnosis and therapy may lead to femoral head destruction, arthritis and deformity (Fig. 22.34). Once an effusion has been detected, prompt arthrocentesis should be carried out. A needle with a central stylet such as spinal needle is recommended to avoid the theoretical risk of creating an implantation dermoid.

Tuberculosis of the Hip Joint

Tuberculosis of the skeletal system is widespread in our country and accounts for 15 percent of all (adults and children) patients of osteoarticular TB,[29] hip involvement, being second to spine. The patient may present with a limp, pain, or fullness around the hip with referred pain to the knee. The initial focus of tuberculous lesion may start in the acetabular roof, epiphysis, metaphysis, greater trochanter or synovial membrane. The destruction of articular cartilage is characteristically slow; consequently the cartilage space is preserved for long joint involvement is late and the patient may then present with extensive bony destruction.

Pathology and Imaging

The different stages of tuberculosis are:[30,31]

Stage I—Tubercular Synovitis

Synovial edema and outpouring of a large fibrinous exudate results in joint effusion and soft tissue swelling (Fig. 22.35).

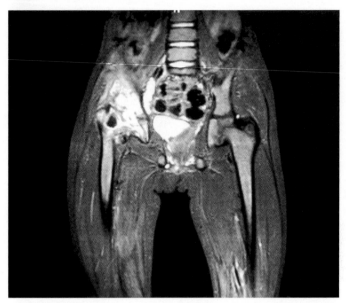

Fig. 22.33: MRI-STIR coronal—Hyperintensity within femoral head and acetabulum with joint effusion—septic arthritis

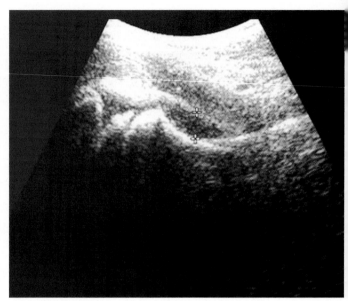

Fig. 22.35: Hip joint effusion—a case of early tubercular arthritis

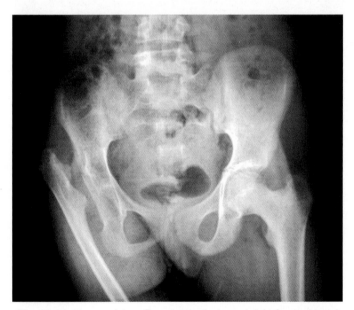

Fig. 22.34: X-ray pelvis – Completely destroyed right femoral head with dislocation – sequelae of septic arthritis

Osteopenia may be noted 12-18 months after onset of symptoms. Flexion deformity of the hip may be seen.

Stage II—Tubercular Arthritis with Damage to Articular Cartilage

There is destruction of the articular cartilage and erosion of the acetabular margins and femoral head. Periarticular osteopenia may be seen with reduction of the joint space multiple lesions, involving the epiphysis of the neck and acetabulum may be noted due to common blood supply (Figs 22.36 to 22.38).

Stage III—Advanced Arthritis

There is gross destruction of the articular cartilage, bone of femoral head and the acetabulum. Subluxation and dislocation of the joint may be seen. This leads to a broken Shenton's line with bird beak appearance of the femoral head and a mortar and pestle appearance of the joint. There may be 'wandering acetabulum'. In this there is a lesion in the acetabular roof which may result in subluxation with the femur being displaced upwards and dorsally with clinical features of limb shortening.

Ultrasound can be used to guide aspiration and evaluate femoral head destruction and joint congruency. Erosive changes are better delineated on CT. MRI can detect early tubercular involvement as it is highly sensitive to marrow pathology (Figs 22.39 to 22.41).

TRANSIENT SYNOVITIS OF HIP

Transient synovitis is a self limited inflammatory condition specific to the hip. It affects boys more commonly than girls in all age ranges, but is more common between 3-6 years. The etiology is unknown; some children have a preceding history of upper respiratory infection or trauma. Patients present with acute onset of pain, limp, refusal to bear weight None of the symptoms or laboratory investigation is pathgnomic. ESR may be raised and symptoms usually regress within ten days with simple bed rest, prolonged immobilization and traction are very rarely needed.

Only 1% have bilateral disease. Transient synovitis is a diagnosis of exclusion with the most common differentials being traumatic synovitis, JRA and perthes disease. Treatment consists of rest and NSAIDs. Long term sequlae are rare.

Radiographs are usually normal but may show joint effusion with mild widening of joint space. Sonography is sensitive to the presence of effusion.[19] Joint effusion is not a specific finding and

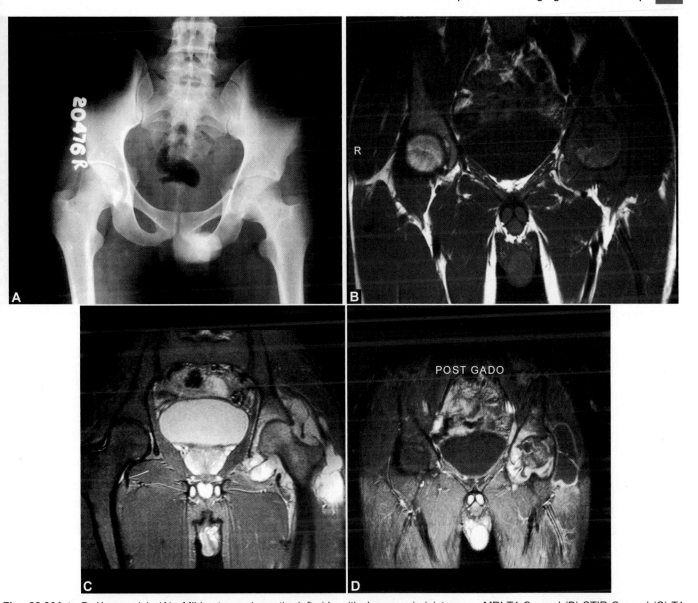

Figs 22.36A to D: X-ray pelvis (A) –Mild osteopenia on the left side with decrease in joint space. MRI T1 Coronal (B) STIR Coronal (C) T1 Coronal post gado (D). Marrow signal alteration with lytic lesion in Lt femoral head and acetabular margin, hypointense on T1, hyperintense on T2, with cortical irregularity. Heterogeneous enhancement is noted. There is a large multilocular, peripherally enhancing collection in the adjacent muscles – TB hip

aspiration is required to rule out infection. On MRI, there is evidence of joint effusion, but there is no concomitant bony abnormality[27] (Figs 22.42A and B). Scintigraphy may demonstrate a transient decrease in isotope uptake for the first week followed by rebound hyperemia within a month. Biopsies performed on these joints reveals nonspecific synovial inflammation and hypertrophy with joint effusion and normal articular cartilage and joint capsule.

LEGG-CALVE-PERTHES' DISEASE

Legg-Calve-Perthes' disease is a self-limiting osteonecrosis of the femoral head epiphysis which typically occurs between the ages

of 3 to 12 years, more common in boys (M:F = 5:1). Both hips are involved in 15 percent of patients, with involvement being asymmetric. If there is a symmetric involvement, hypothyroidism or multiple epiphyseal dysplasias should be excluded. The first symptom is a limp sometimes painless, but usually associated with pain in groin, lateral hip or knee.

The origin of LCP remains unknown. It is believed to represent multiple vascular occlusive episodes that involve the femoral head, causing changes of AVN with a long ongoing process of vascular changes and repair. This differs from AVN seen in adults, because in most cases, there is remodeling and healing with little residual deformity of the femoral head. If the

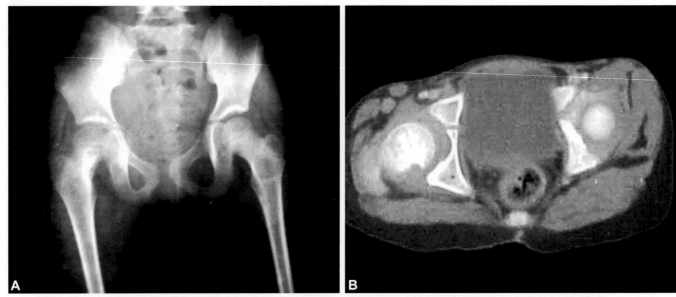

Figs 22.37A and B: X-ray pelvis (A)—Erosion of head and medial aspect of femoral neck. (B) CT pelvis—Cortical erosion of Femoral head-TB

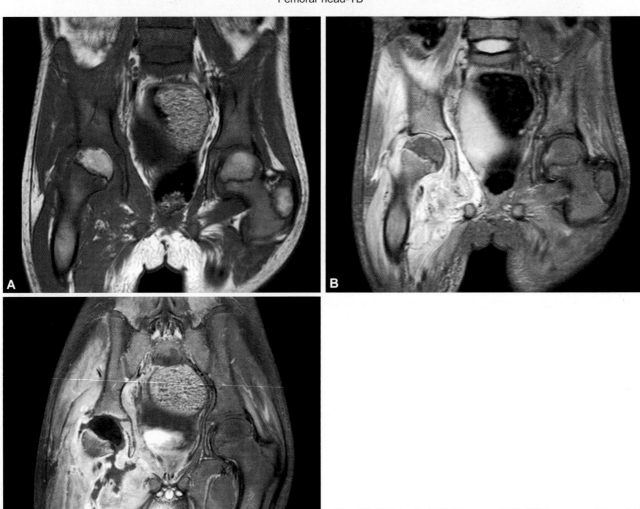

Figs 22.38A to C: MRI T1 coronal (A) STIR coronal (B) and T1 post gado (C) shows subtle erosion of the femoral head, altered signal of the acetabulum. There is enhancing collection in the muscle, hypoperfusion of the right femoral head is also noted – TB hip

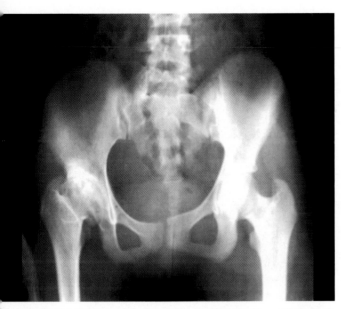

Fig. 22.39: X-ray pelvis—Advanced TB arthritis—Erosion and sclerosis of femoral head with partial collapse and decreased joint space

age of the patient at the onset of disease is more than 9 years and the shape of femoral head at skeletal maturity is non-spherical a worse outcome can be expected.

Following ischemia, the ossific nucleus of the epiphysis undergoes necrosis, causing growth arrest. The overlying cartilage, supplied by synovial fluid, survives and thickens medially and laterally in the non-weight bearing regions. Creeping substitution eventually occurs in the ossific nucleus, which becomes dense.[32]

Imaging

The goal of imaging in Perthes's is early diagnosis, assessment of the extent and location of epiphyseal involvement and of the femoral head coverage. Imaging is also required to follow healing of the disease and measure sphericity of the femoral head at completion of healing.

Radiographs remain the mainstay of diagnosis, classification and follow-up of the disease. Most children of LCP present with an abnormal radiograph. The earliest radiographic abnormality includes asymmetry of the intergluteal fat planes, growth retardation and reduced size of the capital femoral epiphysis. Subchondral fractures are noted and best seen in the frog lateral view. Increased radiographic density of the femoral ossific nucleus occurs due to trabecular compression, dystrophic calcification in the debris and creeping substitution. The classical triad comprises of condensation, collapse and fragmentation. The amount of subchondral fissuring of the femoral head on the radiograph during the initial stages, is thought to be predictive of later involvement of the femoral head. A poor prognosis is associated with subchondral fissuring more than 50 percent of the head (Figs 22.43 to 22.45).

There is a radiographic staging described by Waldenstrom which is as follows:

Initial stage – Increased head socket distance, subchondal plate thinning, dense epiphysis

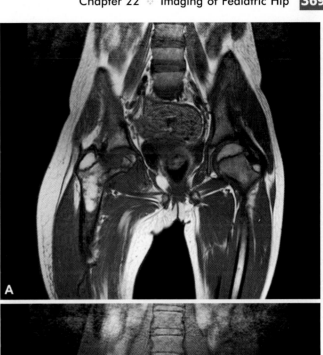

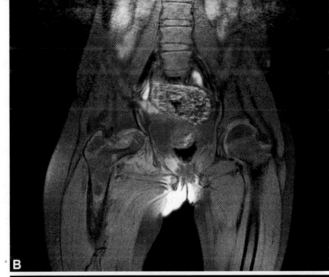

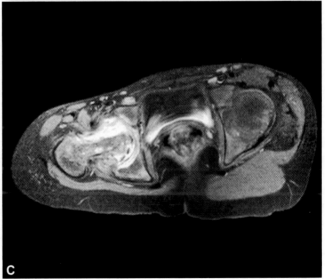

Figs 22.40A to C: MRI of the pelvis (A), STIR (B), T1 post gado (C) lytic destruction of the femoral head, neck and with enhancing synovium – Mortar and Pestle appearance –Tubercular arthritis

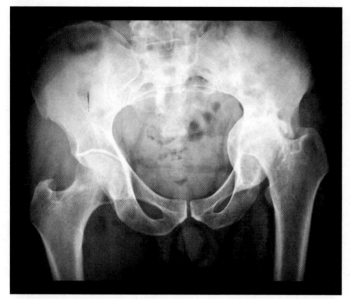

Fig. 22.41: X-ray pelvis – protusio acetabuli seen on the left in a case of tubercular hip arthritis

Fragmentation stage – Subchondral fracture in homogeneous dense epiphysis, metaphyseal cysts/pseudocysts

Reparative stage – Removal of sclerotic bone and replacement with normal bone, epiphysis more homogeneous.

Growth stage – Approach the final stage

Definative stage – Final shape – Congruent or incongruent hip joint.

To classify the extent of ischemic process for purpose of prognostication, based on plain X-rays. Catterall[33] has described four groups, estimating the extent of involvement of the head by ischemia, deformity of the head by lateral displacement, collapse and resorption of bone in the head.

Group I–Only the anterior part of the epiphysis is involved. Collapse does not occur and healing begins from the periphery of the defect.

Group II—More of the anterior epiphysis is involved which collapses and a dense sequestrum form. The unaffected segment retains its height and reaches epiphyseal plate normally. Metaphyseal changes are minor and the involved segment heals by ossification from the periphery.

Group III—Only a small uninvolved part remains posteriorly. Subchondral fissuring is prominent. Speckled ossification occurs in cartilage around the nucleus. Metaphyseal changes are more, collapse and deformity is present.

Group IV—The whole epiphysis is involved and flattened to a thin dense line. All quadrants are flattened and a mushroom deformity remains.

Herring system[34] is based on lateral pillar involvement (Lateral pillar is defined as the lateral 5-30% of epiphysis).

A – LP uninvolved

B < 50% LP loss of height

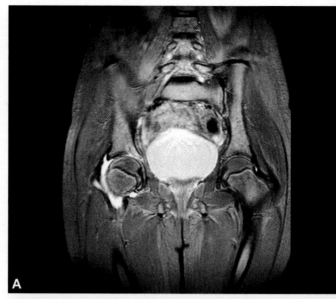

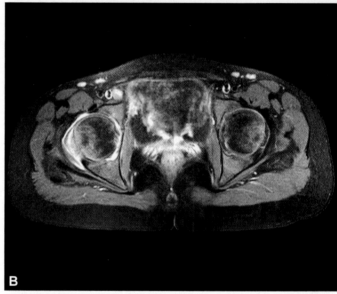

Figs 22.42A and B: MRI – T2 coronal (A) and T1 post gado (B) Shows minimal joint effusion and enhancing synouim - ? Transient synovitis

B/C Border group – Narrow LP 75% original height, poorly ossified LP with at least 50% original height or exactly 50% that is depressed relative to the central pillar.

C – 75% LP loss of height

Sonography can be used as an adjuvant to other imaging modalities. The following parameters are assessed ultrasono-graphically: (i) medial joint space, (ii) epiphyseal changes and flattening, condensation and fragmentation, (iii) metaphyseal changes such as fissures, widening and sclerosis. The earliest ultrasound appearance is of hip joint effusion. Although this is a nonspecific finding, persistence of a hip joint effusion for more than 2 weeks should raise the possibility of Perthes' disease.[5] Synovial thickening is often more marked than is seen in transient

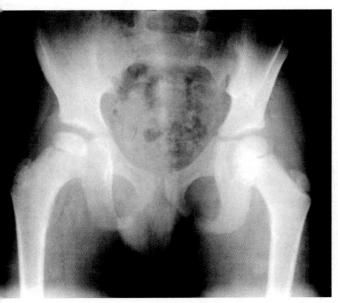

Fig. 22.43: X-ray pelvis – subtle flattening of the right femoral epiphysis. No subchondral fracture appreciated

ynovitis and thickening of the articular cartilage may be seen at n earlier stage. Ultrasound may demonstrate irregularity, flattening and fragmentation of the capital femoral epiphysis, steoid new bone, and recalcification in the healing phase. The rticular cartilage thickens. Contrast-enhanced Power Doppler has een used to demonstrate changes of the revascularization process n LCP, particularly within the physis.[35]

In very early stages of disease, the plain films may be normal nd **scintigraphy** is helpful in making the diagnosis. A focal area f decreased uptake of the isotope is seen within the femoral head, he size of the scintigraphic defect is believed to correlate with he eventual amount of involvement of the femoral head.

CT and MRI in Perthes' Disease

CT depicts changes of Perthes' disease. The area of femoral head ecrosis is usually located in the superior anterior aspect with haracteristic marginal sclerosis.[36]

MR imaging is a sensitive and specific imaging technique for he evaluation of LCP. This condition can be diagnosed evening he setting of normal or equivocal radiographs. In a suspected case f LCP, MR should include imaging in all the three planes. The oronal plane allows comparative analysis of both hips; sagittal lane is the most accurate in estimating the volume of necrotic one as well as the angular span of involvement.[37] Axial plane is mited in the evaluation of LCP because the superior portion of he head is often inadequately visualized because of partial olume averaging. MR imaging can be used during manual ositioning of the hip or multipositional MR imaging, in an open agnet configuration to study femoral head containment, articular ongruency and femoral head deformity.[38] It is comparable to rthrography for demonstration of femoral head containment and ongruency of articular surface of the hip.

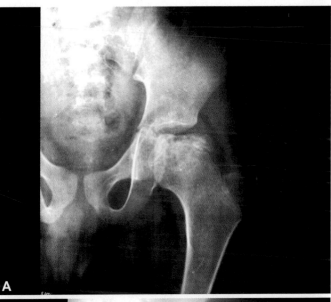

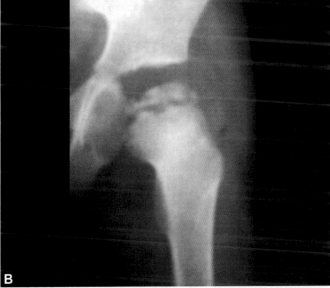

Figs 22.44A and B: X-ray pelvis—Flattening and sclerosis with fissuring of femoral head and metaphyseal changes—Perthes' disease

The typical MR appearance in the **avascular phase** is loss of the normally bright signal intensity of the femoral epiphysis on T1 weighted images (Figs 22.46A and B). Loss of signal may be subtle and needs to be compared to the contralateral hip (Figs 22.47A and B). T2 weighted/STIR imaging shows variable signal intensity, including hyperintensity representing bone marrow edema. Curvilinear subchondral T2 hyperintensity and T1 hypointensity may be observed in the anterosuperior aspect of the femoral head. This finding, referred to as the **crescent or Caffey sign,** suggests presence of a subchondral fracture. The normal hip shows rapid enhancement after IV gadolinium. In Perthes disease, there may be partial or complete nonenhancement of the proximal femoral epiphysis in the avascular phase. This is best depicted approximately 2 minutes after injection using subtraction

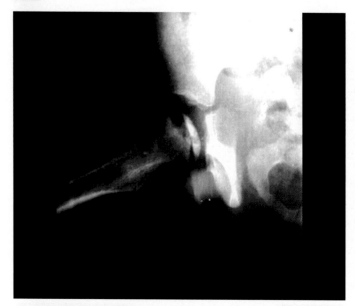

Fig. 22.45: X-ray left hip—Severe flattening of femoral head involving the entire epiphysis and sclerosis—Perthes' disease

techniques. Asymmeteric involvement is noted with the anterior portion frequently and most prominently involved. There may also be flattening of the head. This is due to combination of necrotic trabecular bone collapse and resorption. Articular cartilage and labrum hypertrophy as they continue to derive nutrition from synovium. Periarticular T2/STIR hyperintensity and contrast enhancement may be seen due to associated synovitis.

In the **revascularization and reparative phase** of the disease, MRI reveals heterogeneous proximal femoral epiphyseal signal. revascularized areas show T2/STIR hyperintensity and contrast enhancement.[39,40] Areas of revascularized epiphysis may hyperenhance after the I/V administration of contrast when compared with areas that were never avascular. Revascularized areas may also show persistent enhancement on delayed imaging.

Dynamic gadolinium-enhanced subtraction MR allows early detection of epiphyseal ischemia and accurate analysis of revascularization patterns which can aid therapeutic decision-making.[41] Nonionic gadoteriol is the preferred contrast agent.[42] Acquisition is usually obtained in coronal plane. The acquisition should be early as the enhancement of the early vascular phase decreases after 2-5 minutes post injection. The disparity between normal and abnormal side becomes less clear. The lack of perfusion, in an acute setting, does not necessarily mean that necrosis has occurred, or will occur as therapeutic intervention may interrupt the ischemic pathway.[43] Dynamic postcontrast imaging accurately quantifies the viable bone which enhances brightly. Early enhancement of the lateral pillar (the lateral one-third of the femoral head) is associated with better prognosis.

Morphological changes related to epiphyseal necrosis may include articular surface flattening (coxa plana) and fragmentation. There may be lateral subluxation of the femoral head or loss of containment. This finding is due to cartilage thickening, joint effusion and synovial thickening.

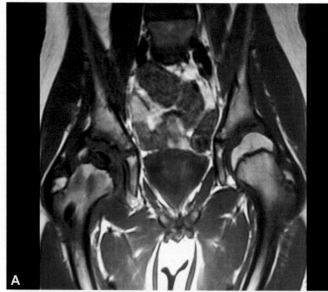

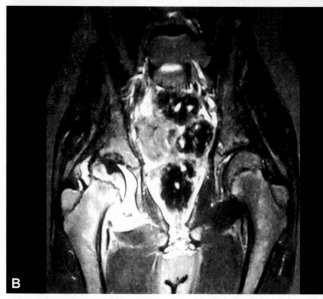

Figs 22.46A and B: MRI-T1 coronal (A) and STIR coronal (B) Flattening of femoral head with loss of normal hyperintense signal of femora epiphysis—Perthes

Abnormality of the proximal femoral physis is also seen. This may be due to the primary ischemic insult or secondary to abnormal mechanical loads. Physeal abnormalities include increased undulation of the growth plate (W or M shaped deepening of the growth plate, epiphyseal-metaphyseal osseus fusion or physeal cystic changes. this may lead to premature growth arrest of the femur). Metaphyseal lesions can be a cystic fluid collection in the metaphysis adjacent to the physis Metaphyseal signal abnormality representing cartilaginous metaphyseal ingrowth indicates higher possibility of growth abnormalities.

Subsequently, in the fragmentation stage, the involved area takes on speckled appearance, an indication of non-homogeneous revascularization of necrotic zone. As revascularization and

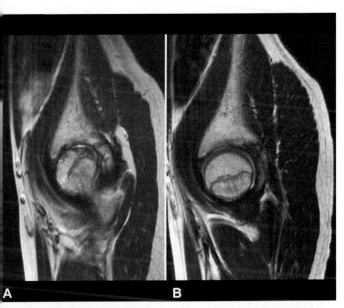

Figs 22.47A and B: T1 sag of the affected (A), and normal (B) Hip in a case of Perthes seen as decrease in size of the femoral epiphysis on the affected side

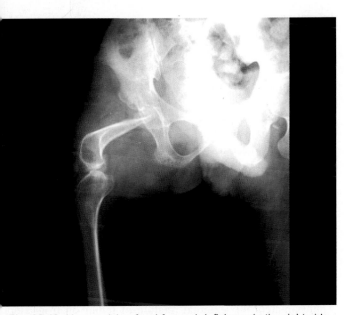

Fig. 22.48: X-ray pelvis—focal femoral deficiency in the right side

reossification progresses, the epiphysis regains a more uniform signal.

With healing, proximal femoral epiphyseal height is slowly restored, ossific fragments coalesce and mature trabecular bone again constitutes the entire ossific nucleus. After approximately six years, the epiphysis shows normal MR signal.

The extent and distribution of epiphyseal necrosis has prognostic implications. As the extent of femoral head necrosis increases, overall prognosis worsens. Prognosis is also adversely affected by the involvement of the lateral pillar, the lateral most one-third of the femoral head. Distubance of the physis is the single most important predictor of growth disturbance. Extensive

epiphyseal necrosis can sometimes be predicted by MRI in very early Perthes disease. The two features predicting the same are (a) decreased signal intensity on both T1 and T2W images covering over two thirds of the epiphysis and (b) diffuse bone marrow edema of the femoral neck and metaphysis.[44] Factors that predict early degeneration of the hip joint include later age of disease onset and abnormal shape of the femoral head at the time of skeletal maturity.

Prognostic evaluation of Legg-Calve-Perthes's disease by MRI has been proposed and takes into account the predictive value of four MRI indices – extension of necrosis, lateral extrusion, physeal involvement and metaphyseal changes. The extent of necrosis (up to or >50%) separates the two main groups A and B.[45]

DWI may be a noninvasive means of distinguishing between Perthes disease with favorable and unfavorable prognosis. Femoral epiphysis showed increased diffusivity in the affected hip. Increased metaphyseal diffusivity was found in all cases with absent lateral pillar enhancement at dynamic post contrast MR,[46] signifying poor prognosis.

The main differential diagnosis of LCP are toxic synovitis, septic hip, juvenile chronic arthritis and juvenile osteonecrosis (AVN due to a known cause-sickle cell anemia, thalassemia).

Proximal Femoral Focal Deficiency (PFFD)

PFFD is a malformation in which complete growth and development of upper femur fails to occur. It encompasses spectrum ranging from mild shortening of an otherwise normal femur to severe handicap of absent femur, except for condyles accompanied by acetabular aplasia and thigh muscular dysplasia.

Imaging

The radiographic findings consist of failure of development and delayed ossification of a lesser or greater part of the proximal femur. Hence, a short femur that is laterally situated and proximally displaced is demonstrated at birth. The distal femur is by definition always present (Figs 22.48 and 22.49), there is a misshapen femoral head and neck, upper end of disconnected distal femur- either bulbous or pointed. The femoral head is situated low in the acetabulum with a woolly outline. Secondary deformity of the acetabulum may result. In later cases, the greater trochanter will be found to curve like a beak and it may articulate with the ilium. Pelvis may show enlarged obturator foramen with a supra acetabular bump or horizontal/dysplastic roof of the acetabulum. If radiographs show a normal acetabulam at birth, presence of normal cartilaginous femoral head is likely.

Hip sonography plays a role in the classification of PFFD and in confirming the location of the femoral head with respect to the acetabulum, especially when no proximal femur is seen on radiography. US may reveal a cartilaginous head and neck.[47] Ultrasonography may be useful in prenatal diagnosis and in infants to identify the femoral head. Mobility of the femoral head within the acetabulum may also be assessed.[48]

MR imaging can identify correctly the size and position of the femoral head present. Thin section coronal and axial imaging is of use in locating a small femur head. Continuity to the rest of

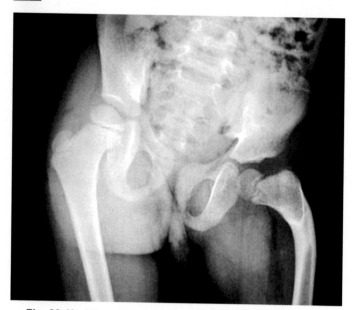

Fig. 22.49: Aitken class A PFFD: Femoral head is present and connected to the shaft of femur

the femur may also be assessed. Presurgical evaluation is important to guide the orthopedic surgeon in reconstruction. There may be a wide variation in the gap between femoral head and subtrochanteric femur. The gap may be small with pseudoarthrosis or be filled with fibro-osseous tissue. It can also be devoid of any connective tissue. This and the resultant coxa vara deformity cannot be adequately seen on a radiograph as the gap is radiolucent. On CT, the nonossified areas have soft tissue attenuation. On MRI, the femoral head, if present exhibits the intensity of yellow marrow, whereas fibrous tissue is low in signal intensity on all pulse sequence.

The prognosis and treatment options depend on grading of the abnormalities. The most commonly used system is the Aitken classification which assigns types A to D to the abnormality depending in the presence or absence of the femoral head and the acetabulum and osseous integrity of the remainder of the femoral shaft. In patients with type A PFFD, the femoral is short. The femoral head and acetabulum are present. In type D the femur is very short and head and acetabulum are absent. Acetabular deformity is correlated with the presence or absence of the femur which can be inferred from the relative development of the acetabulum.

The **differential diagnosis** can be a congenital short femur (no specific abnormalities of head, neck and shaft),

Congenital coxa vara- Head, neck normal

Developmental dysplasia of hip-Graf type 4

Traumatic femoral capital epiphysiolysis in newborn – Pain plus edema of inguinal crease and upper thigh is noted.

Slipped Capital Femoral Epiphysis

Slipped capital femoral epiphysis (SCFE) is an uncommon skeletal disorder of adolescence often overlooked because of its non-specific presentation. It is a unique disorder because no other bone shows similar changes. It is usually seen during adolescent growth spurt in overweight children, with the incidence of bilaterality being 25 percent. There is a morphological change in the relationship of the femoral head to the femoral neck centered at the physeal level probably caused by obesity. The femoral head becomes relatively retroverted at the physeal level placing the head and physis at a mechanical disadvantage when subjected to stress.

It is Salter 1 fracture through the proximal femoral physis with displacement of the capital femoral epiphysis. In most cases, the displacement of the head is usually medial and posterior relative to the metaphysis. In a few cases, there may be a valgus slip with the head rotating superiorly and posteriorly relative to the neck. This term does not include traumatic Salter-harris 1 as the etiology and management are different.

The most common sign/symptom is limp, painful limitation of hip motion while walking/running .It coincides with adolescent growth and is related to endocrine disorders like hypothyroidism, pituitary dysfunction.

The slip is classified as stable or unstable with the criterion being the ability to bear weight with or without crutches. The incidence of complications is higher with unstable variety.

Imaging

Radiographs remain the prime method of diagnosing SCFE, though it may be difficult to diagnose on anterior projection alone. Medial displacement of the capital epiphysis is seen on the antero posterior projection. A line drawn along the lateral border of the femoral neck (Klein line) in a normal individual intercepts the epiphyseal ossification center so that a small portion of the head remains lateral to this line (Fig. 22.50A and B). With SCFE, no part of femoral head ossification center is seen lateral to the line. On the anterior projection, there may be mild widening, lucency and irregularity of the physis. The femoral head may appear foreshortened and there may be apparent sclerosis in the regional femoral neck as the femoral head rotates posteriorly. In the frogleg or true lateral position, the anterior and posterior corners of the epiphysis and metaphysis line up closely in a normal patient, whereas they are displaced in SCFE (Figs 22.51 and 22.52A & B). Posterior displacement is seen on frog lateral radiograph as medial displacement of epiphysis relative to metaphysis. Approximately 90° external rotation of femur on frog-lateral means what is actually a posterior displacement of epiphysis looks like medial displacement on radiograph. On the cross table lateral radiograph with 25 flexion, it is seen as true posterior displacement of epiphysis. Metaphysis shows scalloping, irregularity, sclerosis and posterior beaking. One needs to be careful when using opposite asymptomatic hip as control for radiographic evaluation of painful one as the opposite side may have unrecognized SCFE.

Staging of radiographic findings is mild- moderate- severe based on the displacement of ossification center by < 1/3 – 1/3 – 2/3 – > 2/3 metaphyseal diameter.

Ultrasound may suggest malalignment of the capital femoral epiphysis relative to the metaphysis.[4] The alignment of the epiphysis relative to the metaphysis should be assessed as part

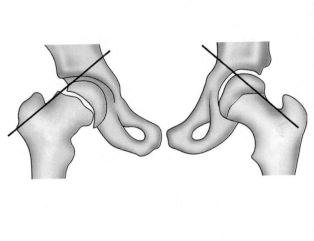

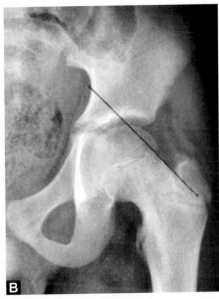

Figs 22.50A and B: Schematic representation: (A) of hip shows Klein's line that normally intersects lateral 1/3rd of the femoral epiphysis on the left, whereas in slipped epiphysis, no part of the epiphysis in lateral to it as seen on the right. X-ray pelvis. (B) Depicting the normal position of the femoral head in relation to the Klein's line

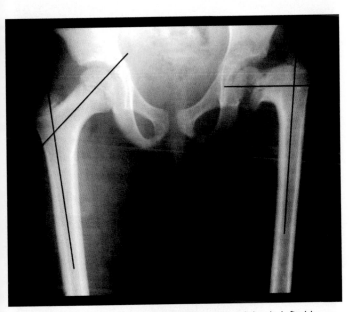

Fig. 22.51: X-ray pelvis—Slipped capital epiphysis left side

of hip ultrasound study. Joint effusion, which may accompany SCFE, is recognized by US. US can be used as follow-up of SCFE due to risk of slippage in the contralateral hip.[49]

CT demonstrates the slip and the reduced femoral anteversion, which may be quantified CT head/neck angles range from 4-57 degrees in symptomatic and 0-14° in asymptomatic patient.[50] It may also demonstrate metaphyseal scalloping and beaking (Figs 22.53A to C).

MR imaging relies on identification of the morphological change at head/neck function and the abnormal signal intensity centered on the physis, indicating stress and edema. Physeal widening is a constant feature and can be seen on MR before being apparent on radiographs. 3D volume acquisition can be used to reconstruct sagittal oblique images along the axis of the femoral neck to identify any retroversion. MR image can be oriented to a plane orthogonal to the plane of the physis to assess the width of the same. Physeal widening is seen on T1 weighted MRI, whereas synovitis and marrow oedema are appreciated on T2 weighted images (Figs 22.54A and B). MRI can also demonstrate physeal widening in the center or posteromedial origin of the physis in a contralateral asymptomatic hip, providing for prophylactic treatment of the same.[51] Hyperintensity on fluid sensitive images at the physis is indicative of a chronic slip condition. Subtle abnormalities include edema on the metaphyseal side, usually at the extreme medial end of the physis.

The complications of SCFE are avascular necrosis, occurring in 20-45 percent of cases and chondrolysis. Treatment consists of preventing further displacement and to cause closure of the physis. Chondrolysis is less common than AVN and is recognized by progressive thinning of the medial joint space on the radiographs. Premature closure of the physis of the greater trochanter is considered as predictive sign for chondrolysis. Premature osteo arthritis may develop in ¼-1/3 of patient with SCFE. Prognosis is poorer with unstable variety.

The differential diagnosis includes

- Legg-Calve-Perthes's disease—the patient is younger with irritable hip progressing to sclerosis and collapse of epiphysis, there is a hairline fracture with marrow edema:
- Hip joint inflammation
- Osteoid osteoma
- Traumatic SCFE

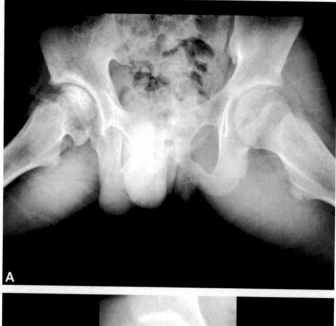

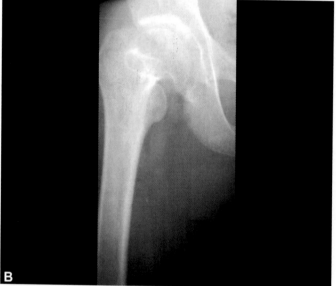

Figs 22.52A and B: X-ray frog's leg view (A) and AP view(B) —shows medial and inferior displacement of the right capital epiphysis with widening of the physis

Developmental Coxa Vara

The normal femoral neck shaft angle changes from about 150 degrees in the infant decreasing to 120° in the adult. The femoral neck is valgus in infants because of relatively increased growth in the medial portion of the physis in the perinatal period. During childhood there is a greater amount of growth in the lateral portion of the femoral physis that is influenced by weight bearing. Coxa vara is defined as femoral neck shaft angle of less than 120°.[52]

True coxa vara may be secondary to congenital anomalies, osteomalacia, or syndromes. Functional coxa vara occurs as a result of overgrowth of the greater trochanter secondary to AVN, infection or trauma. Developmental coxa vara, bilateral in 40 percent of cases, presents at 2 years of age with an abnormal

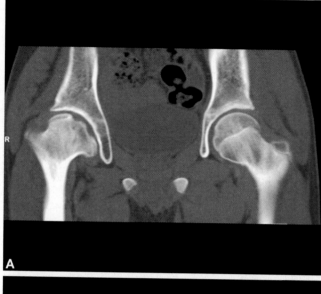

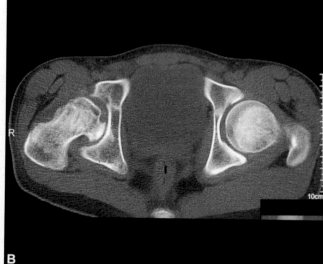

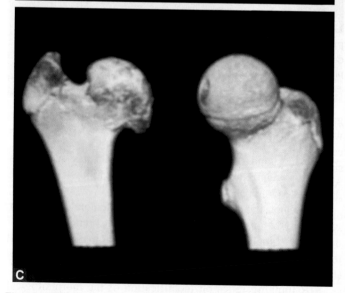

Figs 22.53A to C: CT – Coronal MPR (A), Axial (B) and VRT (C) Medial and posterior slip of the femoral epiphysis of the right hip with complication of avascular necrosis as seen by flattened head of femur

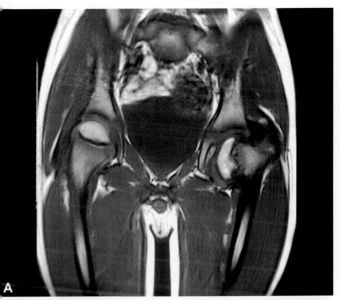

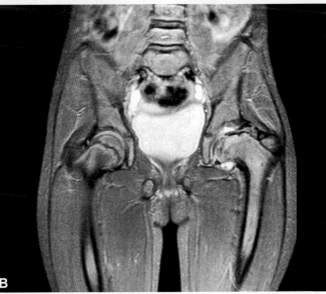

Figs 22.54A and B: (A) MRI-T1 weighted coronal and (B) STIR coronal depicting widening and irregularity of the physis on the left side with physeal slip—Slipped capital femoral epiphysis

gait. It is caused by an abnormality of bone growth at the physis with a greater rate of growth of the lateral aspect of the physis causing the physis to be more vertical than usual. Radiographs show a widened and an abnormally oriented physis (Fig. 22.55). As stress occurs along the physis multiple small steps occurs and small triangular corner fractures develop along the medial aspect of the physis. MR imaging demonstrates widening of the physis with expansion of the cartilage.

Pediatric Hip Trauma

Traumatic hip dislocations rarely occur in childhood. Posterior hip dislocations comprise majority of such dislocations.[53] A soft pliable acetabulum and ligamentous laxity may predispose the

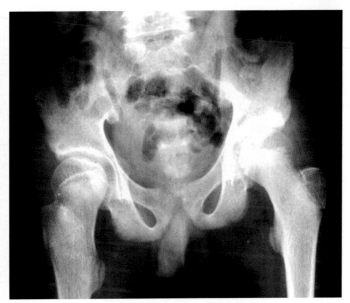

Fig. 22.55: Right coxa vara

immature hip joint to a dislocation secondary to minimal trauma. Potential associated injuries include fracture and neurovascular injury while avascular necrosis and degenerative joint disease are potential sequelae. Osteochondral fractures may be difficult to recognize on plain radiography. CT is useful in the definition of the extent and displacement of complex and impacted fractures around the hip joint.

Growth plate injuries are important to recognize as they have potential implications for growth arrest. Growth disturbance of the proximal femur can be post-traumatic or may be secondary to ischaemia following hyperabduction for DDH, Legg-Calve-Perthes' disease and rapidly developing effusions. The proximal femur physis is particularly vulnerable because the epiphyseal artery is intraarticular physeal widening or narrowing may be seen on radiographs. MR imaging is the modality of choice. T1 weighted images demonstrate low signal intensity growth recovery line and variable signal intensity bony bridge on GRE sequences, a bridge appears as a low signal intensity interruption in high signal physeal cartilage. Physeal widening on GRE and T2 weighted images implies physeal dysfunction. Medial physeal impairment leads to a short wide femoral neck and coxa vara deformity whereas vertex arrest causes Coxa valga[54] (Figs 22.56A & B and 22.57).

Neuromuscular Hip Dysplasia

Children who suffer from cerebral palsy or other neuromuscular disorders, who are unable to walk have a 58 percent incidence of hip dislocations. With muscle imbalance and lack of weight bearing, there is a coxa valga deformity with persistence of a straight neck shaft angle, which leads to hip dislocation.

Simulated standing radiographs show pelvic tilt, valgus deformity of the femoral neck, abnormal shape and placement of the femoral head. CT is helpful in evaluate the shape of the acetabulum and the degree of femoral articulation.

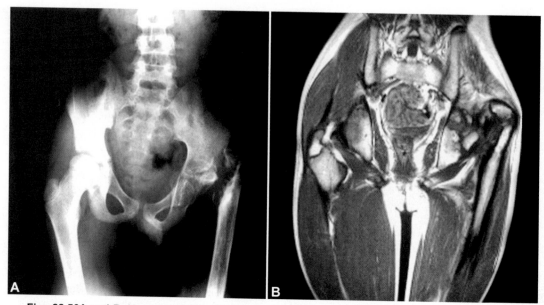

Figs 22.56A and B: X-ray pelvis (A)—Traumatic posterosuperior dislocation of the left femur, MRI-T1 coronal (B) depicting the superior and posterior dislocation

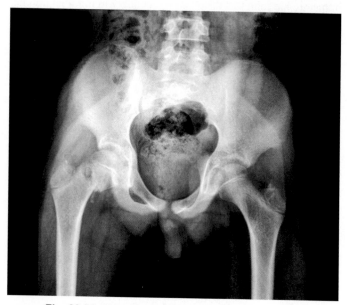

Fig. 22.57: X-ray pelvis—Fracture right femoral neck

Childhood Idiopathic Chondrolysis of the Hip

This is a rare disorder, which causes progressive destruction of the articular cartilage of the hip joint with associated bone remodeling. Cartilage loss, bone remodeling, and small joint effusions along with muscle wasting are seen.[55]

Calcification of Cartilage and Joints

Idiopathic calcification of the cartilages of the hips, i.e. acetabular rims and femoral hands has been reported in children and the patients may be asymptomatic or have a limp with restricted hip movements. This is believed to be an acquired pathology due to local chemical trauma from partial extravasation of an intravenous injection via the femoral route. On serial studies, calcification may remain unchanged, increase, or show gradual resorption with early fusion of the femoral head and neck.

The hip joint may also be involved as part of a large number of skeletal dysplasias or systemic disorders as in nutritional disorders, neoplasia like leukaemia, metastatic neuroblastoma.

Developmental and acquired abnormalities of the hip are relatively common in childhood. Radiographs, ultrasonography, MR imaging, computed tomography and nuclear medicine play an important role in the diagnosis and management of these disorders.

Femoroacetabular Impingement

The geometry of femoral neck and acetabulum plays a role in the etiology of degenerative disease.[56,57]

Normally, the femoral neck has a definite narrowing or waist which allows the femur to abduct fully without impingement on the lateral aspect of the acetabulum. In patients with FAI, the femoral neck is not tabulated normally. Instead of having an identifiable constriction, a pistol grip deformity is seen in which tabulation is lacking. A small bump or protuberance may be identified on the anterior femoral neck. Slipped capital femoral epiphysis may be a contributing factor (Fig. 22.58).

Axial oblique images prescribed along the axis of the femoral neck or reconstruction of 3D volume acquisition into axial oblique plane allows for measurement of α angle. First the center of the femoral head is identified using the contour of the head to fit a circle to outline and define the position of the center of the head. Two lines are extended from the center point of the head, one down the axis of the femoral neck and the second to the intersection point between the head and the neck, when the convexity of the femoral head becomes the concavity of the femoral neck. Angles less than 55° are abnormal or if the

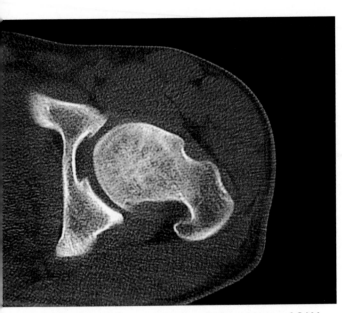

Fig. 22.58: CT—Oblique axial image shows evidence of CAM impingement with a bump at the femoral neck

head-neck line measures greater than the radius of the circle defining the femoral head, then a femoral waist deficiency is present.

FAI may also be caused by over coverage of the femoral head and neck. This may be caused by acetabular retroversion. Normally the acetabulum has its lateral opening directed slightly anteriorly. In abnormal cases, the anterolateral edge of the acetabulum extends further laterally than the posterolateral edge so that the acetabular opening is directed posteriorly. On radiographs,this is visualized as the cross over sign. This is present when the anterior lip of the acetabulum crosses over the posterior lip on a standard frontal film. This limits the ability to flex at the hip as the femoral neck impinges on the anterior acetabulum.

Abnormal morphology in the pediatric age group may not reflect the pathological abnormalities seen in adulthood, however subtle osseous abnormalities can help guide prognosis.

REFERENCES

1. Jacobs P, Renton P. Congenital anomalies: Skeletal dysplasias; chromosomal disorders. In Sutton D(Ed): Textbook of Radiology and Imaging (4th edn). Churchill Livingstone 1987; 1:2-50.
2. Hilgenreiner H. Zur Fruhdiagnose and Fruhbehandlung derangegorenen Huftgelenkrerrenkueg Med Klink 1925; 21:1385-88,1425-29.
3. Andren L, von Rosen S. The diagnosis of dislocation of hip in newborns and the preliminary results of immediate treatment. Acta Radiol 1958; 49:89-95.
4. Gibbon Wayne W, Long G. In Meire H, Cosgrove D, Dewbury K, et al (Eds): Musculoskeletal System: Abdominal and General Ultrasound (2nd edn). London: Churchill Livingstone 2000; 2.
5. Fayed LM, Johnson P, Fishman EK. Multidetector CT of musculoskeletal disease in pediatric patient;principles,techniques and clinical applications. Radiographics 2005; 25:603-61.
6. Jaramillo D, Galen TA, Winalski CS, et al. Legg-Calve-Perthes disease: MR imaging evaluation during manual positioning of the hip-comparison with conventional arthrography. Radiology 1999; 212(2):519-25.
7. Aubry S, Belanger D, Giguere C. Magnetic resonance arthrography of the hip: Insights Imaging 2010;1:72-82.
8. Klisie PJ. Congenital dislocation of the hip: A misleading term. J Bone Joint Surg Br 1981;63:38-42.
9. Kuhn JP, et al. Caffey's Pediatric Diagnostic Imaging. 10th edn 2277-9,2004: Mosby. The joints BabynPS, RansOm MD 2435-93.
10. Havije HT, Waller RS. Ultrasound screening for dysplasia of the hip (Letter). Pediatrics 1995; 95:799-800.
11. Zieger M. Ultrasound of the infant hip Part 2 validity of the method. Pediatric Radiol 1986; 16:488-92.
12. Graf R. Classification of hip joint dysplasia by means of sonography. Arch Orthop Trauma Surg 1984; 102:248.
13. Harcke HT, Lee MS, Born P, et al. Examination of the infant hip with real time ultrasonography. J Ultrasound Med 1984; 3:131.
14. Harcke HT, Grissom LE. Performing dynamic sonography of the infant hip. AJR Am J Roentgenol 1990; 155:837.
15. Rosendahl k, Toma P. Ultrasound in the diagnosis of developmental dysplasia of the new borns. The European approach. A review of methods, accuracy and clinical validity: Eur Radiol 2007; 17:1960-7.
16. Schwartz DS, Kellar MS, Fields JM, et al. Arterial waveforms of the femoral heads of healthy neonates. AJR Am J Roentgenol 1998; 170:465-66.
17. Browing WH, Rosenkrantz H, Tarquinio T. Computed Tomography in congenital hip dislocation. J Bone Joint Surgery (AM) 1982; 64:27-31.
18. Hubbard AM. Imaging of pediatric hip disorders. Rad Clin North Am 2001; 39(4).
19. Dwek JR. The Hip: MR Imaging of Uniquely Pediatric Disorders: Radiol Clin North Am 2009; 47:997-1008.
20 Kawaguchi AT, Otsuka NY, Deigado ED, et al. Magnetic resonance arthrography in children with developmental hip dysplasia. Clin Orthop 2000; 374:235-46.
21. Tennant S, Kinmant C, Lamb G, et al. The use of dynamic interventional MRI in developmental dysplasia of the hip. J Bone Joint Surg B 1999; 81(3):392-97.
22. Jawin J, Hoffer F, Rand F, et al. Joint effusion in children with an irritable hip: Ultrasound diagnosis and aspiration. Radiology 1993; 1987:459.
23. Strouse PJ, Di Pietro MA, Adler RS. Hip Effusions: Evaluation with Power Doppler Sonography. Radiology 1998; 206:731-35.
24. Hopkins K, Li K, Bergmon G. Gadolinium DTPA enhanced magnetic resonance imaging of musculoskeletal infections processes. Skeletal Radiol 1995; 24:325.
25. Lee SK, Suh KJ, Kim YW, et al. Septic arthritis, versus transient synovitis at MR imaging preliminary assessment with signal intensity alterations in bone marrow. Radiology 1999; 211:459.
26. Park JK, Kim BS, Choi G, et al. Distinction of reactive joint fluid from pyogenic abscess by diffusion–weighted imaging. J. Magn Reson Imaging 2007; 25(4):859-61.
27. Daldrup-Link HE, Steinbach L. MR imaging of Pediatric arthritis Radiol Clin N Am 2009; 47:939-55.
28. Hong SH, Kim SM, Ahn JM, et al. Tuberculous versus pyogenic arthritis: MR imaging evaluation. Radiology 2001; 218:843-53.
29. Sawhney S, Jain R. Tuberculosis of the bones and joints. In Berry, Chowdhury, Suri (Eds): Diagnostic Radiology-Musculoskeletal and Breast imaging (1st edn). Jaypee Brothers 1998.
30. Chapman H, Murray RD, Stoken OJ. Tuberculosis of the bone and joints. Semin Roentgenol 1979; 19:26-282.

31. Murray RO, Jacobson HG. Infections: Radiology of Skeletal Disorders (2nd edn). Churchill Livingstone 1997; 1.

32. Jacobs P, Renton P. Avascular necrosis of bone: Osteochondritis: Miscellaneous bone lesions. In Sutton D (Ed): Textbook of Radiology and Imaging (4th edn). Churchill Livingstone 1987; 1:77-94.

33. Caterall A. Legg-Calve-Perthes disease. New York, Churchill Livingston 1982.

34. O'hara SM. Benton C-abnormalities of hip in Diagnostic Imaging-Donelly. Amirsys 2005.

35. Doria AS, Guarniero R, Gunha FG, et al. Contrast enhanced power Doppler Sonography: Assessment of revascularization flow in Legg-Calve-Perthes' disease. Ultrasound Med Biol 2002; 28(2):171-82.

36. Strouse PJ. Musculoskeletal system. In Haaga JR, Lanzieri, Gilkeson (Eds): CT and MR Imaging of the Whole Body (4th edn) 2002; 2:2095-122.

37. Ha As, Wells J, Jaramillo D. Importance of sagittal MR imaging in nontraumatic femoral head osteonecrosis in children. Pediatr Radiol 2008; 38(ii):1195-200.

38. Jaramillo D, Galen TA, Winalski CS, et al. Legg-Calve-Perthes' disease: MR imaging evaluation during manual positioning of the hip. Comparison with conventional arthrography. Radiology 1999; 212(2):519-25.

39. Dillman JR, Hernandez RJ. MRI of Legg-Calve-Perthes disease. AJR 2009; 193:1394-1407.

40. Mahnken AH, Staatz G, Ihme IV, et al. MR signal intensity characteristics in Legg-Calve-Perthes' disease value of fat suppressed (STIR) images and contrast enhanced T1 weighted images. Acta Radiol 2002; 43(3):329-35.

41. Lamer S, Dogeret S, Khairouni A, et al. Femoral head vascularization in Legg-Calve-Perthes' disease Comparison of dynamic gadolinium enhanced substraction MRI with bone scintigraphy. Pediatric Radiol 2002; 32(8):580-85.

42. Menezes NM, Olear EA, Li X, et al. Gadolinium enhanced MR images of the growing piglet skeleton: Ionic versus. Nonionic contrast agent. Radiology 2006; 239(2):406-14.

43. Menezes NM, Connolly SA, Shapiro P, et al. Early ischemia in growing piglet skeleton. MR diffusion and perfusion imaging. Radiology 2007; 242(1):129-36.

44. Lahdes-Vasama T, Lamminen A, Merikanto J, et al. The Value of MRI in early Perthes' disease: An MRI study with a 2 year follow up. Pediatric Radiol 1997; 27(6):517-22.

45. De Sanctis N, Rega AN, Rondinella F. Prognostic evaluation of Legg-Calve-Perthes' disease by MRI-Pathomorphogenesis and new classification. J Pediatr Orthop 2000; 20(4):403-70.

46. Merlinic L, Combescure C, De Rosa V, et al. Diffusion – weighted imaging findings in perthes disease with dynamic gadolinuim – enhanced subtracted (DGS) with MR correlation – a preliminary study Pediatr Radiol 2010; 40(3):31.

47. Grissom LE, Harcke HT. Sonography in congenital deficiency of the femur. J Paediatr Orthop 1994; 14:29-33.

48. Kayser R, et al. Proximalfocal femoral deficiency – rare entity in the sonographic differential diagnosis of developmental dysplasia of the hip. J Pedia tr 2005; 146(1):141.

49. Castriota-Scandfrberg A, Orsi E. Slipped capital femoral epiphysis ultrasonographic findings skeletal. Radiol 1993; 22(3):191-93.

50. Umans H, Liebling MS, Moy L, et al. Slipped capital femoral epiphysis: A physeal lesion diagnosed by MRI with radiographic and CT correlation. Skeletal Radiol 1998; 27(3):139-44.

51. Futami T, Suzuki S, Seto Y, et al. Sequential magnetic resonance imaging in slipped capital femoral epiphysis, assessment of prestep in the contralateral hip. J Paediatr Orthop B 2001; 10(4):298-303.

52. Ozonof MB. Pediatric Orthopaedic. Radiology Philadelphia: WB Saunders 1992.

53. Petrie SG, Harris MB, Willis RB. Traumatic hip dislocation during childhood. A case report and review of the literature. Am J Ortho 1996; 25(a):645-49.

54. Ecklund K, Jaramillo D. Imaging of growth disturbance in children. Radiol Clin North Am 2001; 39(4):823-42.

55. Johnson K, Haigh SF, Ehtisham S, et al. Childhood Idiopathic Chondrolysis of the hip: MRI features. Paediatr Radiol 2003; 33(3):194-99.

56. Pfirrmann CW, Mengiardi B, Dara C, et al. Ca M and pincer femora acetabular impingement: Characteristic MR authrographic findings in 50 patients. Radiology 2006; 240(3):778-85.

57. Gam R, Parvizi J, Beck M, et al. Femoracetabular impingement: A cause of osteo arthritis of the hip. Clin Orthop Relat Res 2003; 417:112-20.

CHAPTER 23

Benign Bone and Soft Tissue Tumors and Conditions

Mahesh Prakash, Kushaljit Singh Sodhi

Benign bone tumor and tumor like lesions are very common in children. More than half of all childhood bone neoplasms are benign.[1] It is important that radiologists recognize the typical imaging features of benign tumors so that patient can avoid unnecessary diagnostic and surgical procedures.

The differential diagnosis of bone tumors can be narrowed, based on knowledge of age of the patient, gender, constitutional complaints, location of the lesion in body and bone and general radiographic characteristics.[2] Plain film radiographs remain the primary tool for evaluating bone tumors. However, other imaging methods, particularly magnetic resonance imaging (MRI) and in some cases computed tomography (CT) and nuclear studies, provide support for initial diagnosis by demonstrating specific features.[1,2] Common benign bone lesions in children are osteochondroma, nonossifying fibroma, Langerhans' cell histiocytosis, unicameral bone cyst and aneurysmal bone cyst. Benign bone tumors and tumor like lesions in children may be classified as follows:[1]

1. Cartilaginous tumors
   a. Osteochondroma
   b. Enchondroma
   c. Chondroblastoma
   d. Chondromyxoid fibroma
2. Osseous tumors
   a. Osteoid osteoma
   b. Osteoblastoma
3. Fibrous tumors
   a. Nonossifying fibroma
   b. Fibrous dysplasia
   c. Osteofibrous dysplasia
4. Langerhans cell histiocytosis
5. Giant cell tumor
6. Tumor like lesions
   a. Simple bone cyst
   b. Aneurysmal bone cyst
   c. Pseudotumor of hemophilia

CARTILAGINOUS TUMORS

Osteochondroma

Osteochondromas are common lesions of the growing skeleton, occurring in approximately 1 percent of the general population. It is the most common benign neoplasm and constitutes 20-50 percent of all benign tumors.[3] They arise from bony metaphysis with cartilage cap covering (Fig. 23.1). These tumors are either pedunculated or sessile. The long axis of the osteochondroma pedicle or stalk is almost always directed away from the adjacent joint. The direct communication between the osteochondroma and the cortex and marrow cavity of the bone from which it arises is a distinctive feature, that is particularly well demonstrated on computed tomography and magnetic resonance imaging. T2

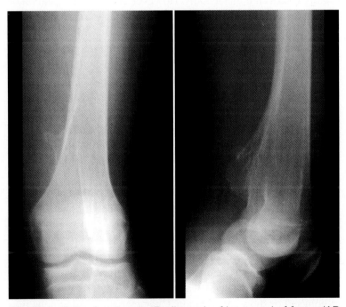

Fig. 23.1: Osteochondroma—Radiograph of lower end of femur (AP and Lat view) shows large well defined bony outgrowth, with broad based attachment to femur

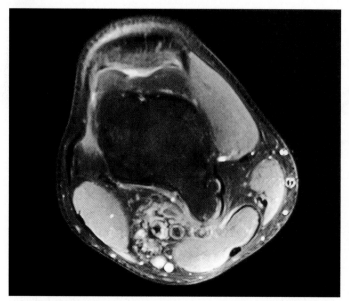

Fig. 23.2: MRI (T1W fat sat), Axial section of the same patient shows clear demonstration of continuity of marrow and cortex of host bone into osteochondroma with covering cartilage cap

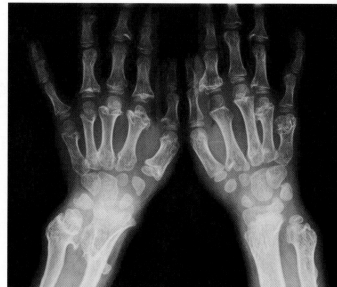

Fig. 23.3: Diaphyseal aclasia—PA radiograph of bilateral hands show multiple pedunculated osteochondromas, involving multiple bones o hands and forearm

weighted MR images is useful to demonstrate an cartilaginous cap (Fig. 23.2). The cap can be quite thick in early childhood and like the normal physis, becomes thinner with age. After epiphyseal closure, growth of the osteochondroma ceases. Multiple osteochondroma occur as a manifestation of diaphyseal aclasia, an inherited disorder with autosomal dominance (Fig. 23.3). Because most osteochondromas are asymptomatic, they are usually discovered incidentally. However, mechanical irritation of adjacent soft tissues or nerves, vascular injuries, fracture of the stalk, or malignant transformation can produce symptoms.

Malignant transformation into low grade chondrosarcoma occurs in 1 percent of osteochondromas, however, the risk is 10 to 30 percent in cases of multiple osteochondromatosis.[3,4] Malignant transformation should be considered when the osteochondroma grows after epiphyseal closure. Malignancy occurs in the cartilaginous cap, which becomes thickened. The cap of an osteochondroma usually measures less than 1 cm in thickness, whereas that of a chondrosarcoma often exceeds 2 cm.

Enchondroma

Enchondromas accounts for 12 percent of benign bone tumors.[3] These are most frequently located in the large and small tubular bones of the limbs, particularly those of the hand (Fig. 23.4). Like other cartilaginous tumors, enchondromas exhibit a lobulated growth pattern, that results in asymmetric expansion of the medullary cavity and endosteal scalloping. Tumor matrix may be radiolucent or show calcification. Characteristic cartilaginous ring and arc pattern of calcifications is seen on radiographs and CT images. On MR imaging, the tumor is isointense to muscle on T1 weighted and exhibits a heterogeneous, predominantly high T2 weighted signal.[5] Contrast enhanced MRI may demonstrate a pattern of thin arcs and rings.

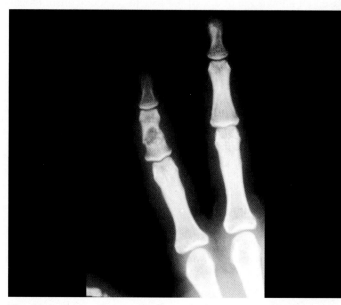

Fig. 23.4: Enchondroma—Radiograph shows a sharply demarcated expansile lytic lesion with pathological fracture in the middle phalanx of index finger

Ollier's disease is a nonheritable disorder of cartilage proliferation in which enchondromas involve multiple bones, especially those of the hands and may result in severe skeletal deformity. Enchondromatosis accompanied by multiple hemangiomas is known as Maffucci's syndrome. Calcified phleboliths may be demonstrated radiographically in the hemangiomatous soft tissue masses. Lesions associated with both Ollier's disease and Maffucci's syndrome carry a significant risk of malignant degeneration (30-70%).[6]

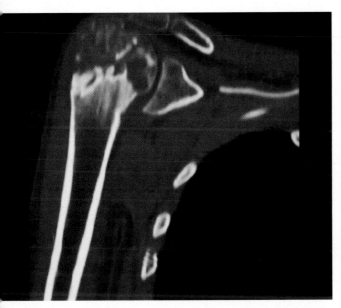

Fig. 23.5: Chondroblastoma—CT (coronal reformation) shows lytic lesion in epiphysis of upper humerus with matrix calcification

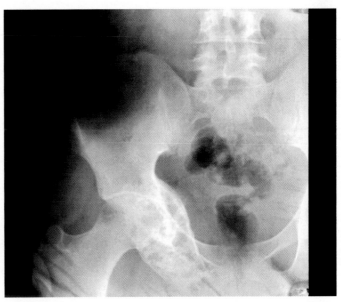

Fig. 23.6: Chondromyxoid fibroma—Radiograph of right hip shows large expansile lesion with sclerotic border involving right acetabulum

Chondroblastoma

It is less common than enchondroma. Chondroblastoma is composed of primitive cartilage cells, usually occurs in the age group of 10-20 years. It is typically located in epiphysis and apophysis of bone, most often the proximal humerus, distal femur, or proximal tibia. On plain X-ray, chondroblastoma is an eccentric, lucent, well defined lesion with sclerotic borders. Periosteal reaction, far from the lesion is another common feature suggesting an accompanying inflammatory process. Approximately one third of chondrobastoma have a calcified matrix which can be better seen on CT scan (Fig. 23.5).

The tumor shows signal intensity similar to that of muscle on MR imaging; however, the rim of the tumor has lower signal intensity. On T2 weighted images, the signal intensity of the tumor is low to intermediate. This tumor also shows extensive surrounding inflammation which may be confused with more aggressive lesion. Malignant transformation of chondroblastoma is extremely uncommon.[7]

Chondromyxoid Fibroma

Chondromyxoid fibroma is less common than chondroblastoma, affecting predominantly males in the age group of 15 to 35 years.[8] Histologically it is composed of chondroid, myxoid and fibrous tissue in varying amounts. The common locations of tumor are ilium and the bones of the knee and foot. These tumors are located characteristically in metadiaphyseal location unlike chondroblastoma and do not cross an open growth plate. On plain radiograph, it appears as a well marginated central or eccentric lucent lesion, with sclerotic margins and cortical expansion (Fig. 23.6). Half of the lesions may show parallel orientation to the long axis of the involved bone. Matrix calcification and periosteal new bone formation usually do not occur.

OSSEOUS TUMORS

Osteoid Osteoma

Osteoid osteoma is a fairly common tumor, accounting for approximately 10-12 percent of all benign tumors.[9] These tumors usually affect boys in the second decade of life. Clinically most patients presents with pain that is especially severe at night and relieved by aspirin or other nonsteroidal antiinflammatory agents.

More than half of tumors are located in proximal femur and tibia. They occur less frequently in the upper extremities than in the lower extremities. Osteoid osteomas also frequently affect the tubular bones of the hands and feet. They are however less common in the spine, where they affect the posterior arches of the vertebra. Histologically, the lesion consists of a nidus which is usually surrounded by dense sclerotic bone. The nidus contains interlacing trabeculae at various stages of ossification within a stroma of loose, vascular connective tissue. Osteoid osteoma can be cortical (the most common type), cancellous or medullary, and subperiosteal. The latter two types produce less sclerotic bone than those in the cortex do, making radiologic diagnosis difficult.

Radiographically, the lesion appears as well defined lytic lesion, surrounded by reactive sclerosis (Figs 23.7A and B). Solid or lamellated periosteal reaction is seen in 60 percent of patients. Nidus may be purely radiolucent or contain a dense center. Intra-articular osteoid osteomas may be either cancellous or periosteal and have little reactive bone or periosteal new bone formation.

CT is very useful in showing the nidus, which can vary in its degree of ossification. CT appears to display the nidus better than MRI. The tumor nidus typically shows hypo to intermediate signal on T1W images and low to high signal on T2W images. The nidus shows enhancement with gadolinium.[10] Intra-articular osteoid osteomas produce joint effusions and synovial proliferation. Radionuclide bone scans have been used for many years to help

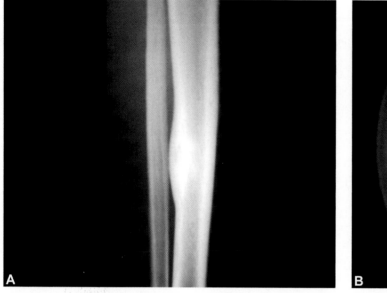 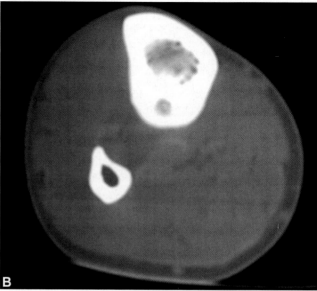

Figs 23.7A and B: Osteoid osteoma—Radiograph of leg (A) shows dense sclerosis and solid periosteal reaction in the diaphysis of tibia. CT scan axial sections reveals well defined lytic lesion with calcified nidus with gross adjacent sclerosis (B)

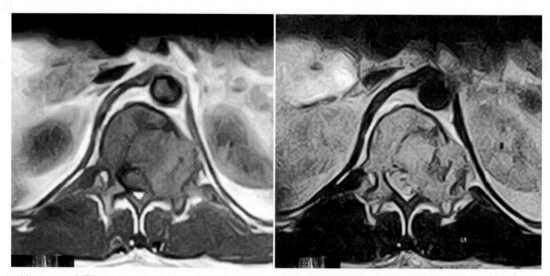

Fig. 23.8: Osteoblastoma—MRI axial section, T1 and T2WI images reveals heterogeneous signal lesion, predominantly involving posterior elements of vertebra with extension into spinal canal and left paravertebral location

diagnosis of osteoid osteomas. Bone scintigraphy, which is a highly sensitive method of detecting osteoid osteoma typically shows increased flow to the lesion on immediate images and a focus of increased activity on skeletal equilibrium images with double density sign. Many times, osteomyelitis can mimick osteoid osteoma clinically as well radiographically, however, presence of soft tissue extension favors the diagnosis of osteomyelitis. The traditional treatment of choice has been surgical excision, however, it can also be successfully treated by radiofrequency ablation under image guidance.[11]

Osteoblastoma

Osteoblastoma constitutes 2 to 6 percent of all bone tumors and most commonly occurs in patients in the second and third decade

of life.[12] This tumor is more common in males than in females. Histologically, the osteoblastoma is closely related to osteoid osteomas except that bony trabeculae are broader and longer with absence of surrounding sclerotic halo. Size is an important consideration in distinguishing between these two types of tumors. If the size of lesion is less than 1.5 cm in diameter than it is likely to be osteoid osteomas, whereas tumors larger than 1.5 cm are usually osteoblastoma.

The most common location of osteoblastoma is spine where it classically affects posterior elements (33%)[12] (Fig. 23.8). The other common locations are proximal femur and talus. On plain X-ray, spinal osteoblastoma is osteolytic lesion with destruction of overlying cortex and may extend to in the spinal canal. In the long bones, osteoblastoma appear radiologically as round or oval

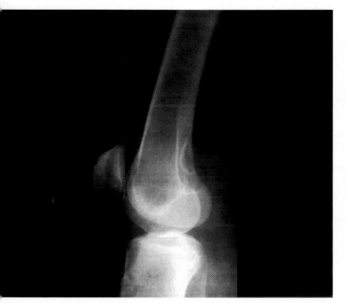

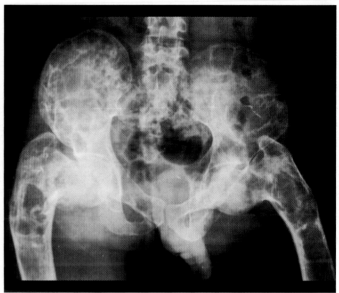

Fig. 23.9: Nonossifying fibroma—Radiograph of knee joint (Lat view) shows well defined lytic lesion with sclerotic margin in characteristic location of lower end of femur

Fig. 23.10: Fibrous dysplasia—Radiograph of pelvis shows multiple lytic lesions involving all the visualized bones with characteristic Shepherd's crook deformity

lucent tumors in the medulla. Periosteal reaction is common. Edema in the soft tissues or marrow appears hyperintense on T2 weighted images but the signal characteristics are not specific. Treatment is by surgical excision or curettage, but there is a moderate recurrence rate after these procedures.

FIBROUS TUMORS

Nonossifying Fibroma

Nonossifying fibroma is a benign fibroblastic mass that occurs in long bones of children and represents continuation of growth of fibrous cortical defect. It occurs eccentrically in the medullary cavity. The common location of lesion is in the bones around the knee joints. These lesions are usually asymptomatic and do not require specific treatment. On plain radiography, the lesion appears as well marginated eccentric lytic lesion with scalloped margin (Fig. 23.9). Its inner border is often sclerotic and may appear multilocular due to corrugations. Differential diagnosis includes unicameral bone cyst, aneurysmal bone cyst, fibrous dysplasia, and chondromyxoid fibroma. The signal intensity of nonossifying fibroma is equal to or less than muscle on T1 weighted MR images and hypointense to fat on T2 weighted images. Postcontrast images usually show heterogeneous enhancement.

Fibrous Dysplasia

Fibrous dysplasia is disorders where bone is replaced by abnormal fibrous tissue. Fibrous dysplasia can be monostotic, polyostotic, monomelic, or polymelic. It is more common in young females. It is occasionally seen in the first decade of life. In a small percentage of cases (2-3%), fibrous dysplasia is associated with endocrine disorders, especially precocious puberty in girls (McCune-Albright syndrome).[13] Although it is not a true

neoplasm, fibrous dysplasia involving a long bone may mimic a bone tumor or cyst. This type of fibrous dysplasia causes expansion of the medullary cavity of tubular bones, endosteal scalloping and trabeculation. The margin is sclerotic. The lesion may appear as ground glass or radiolucent, and this depends upon amount of fibrous tissue within the lesion. Bowing of the affected long bone may occur; when the affected bone is femur, the resulting deformity is called a "Shepherd's crook" (Fig. 23.10). Thinning and destruction of the bony cortex may be seen on CT or MR images. Soft tissue extension of the lesion is unusual. On T1-weighted MR images, the signal intensity of fibrous dysplasia is similar to that of skeletal muscle. Although, the signal of pure fibrous tissue is hypointense on T2-weighted images, the signal of fibrous dysplasia is variable.

Osteofibrous Dysplasia

It is a rare lesion that is usually confined to the tibia but can also involve the fibula. Most cases occur during the first decade of life. On plain X-ray, the lesion appears as an eccentric, lucent, solitary or multiloculated, lesion involving the anterior aspect of tibia. CT is very helpful in determining its intracortical location, an important feature in distinguishing osteofibrous dysplasia from fibrous dysplasia.[14]

HISTIOCYTOSIS X (LANGERHANS CELL HISTIOCYTOSIS)

Histiocytosis X is a syndrome that consists of group of clinical pathological entities: eosinophilic granuloma, Hand-Schüler-Christian disease and Letterer-Siwe disease. Eosinophilic granuloma is localized skeletal disease and is one of the commonly occurring bone tumors of boys in the first decade of life.[15] The skull is the most frequent location, followed by the femur, mandible, pelvis, ribs and spine. The lesions are usually

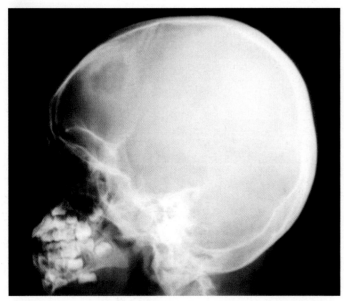

Fig. 23.11: Histiocytosis—Radiograph of skull (Lat view) shows well defined lytic lesion with beveled margins in frontal lobe

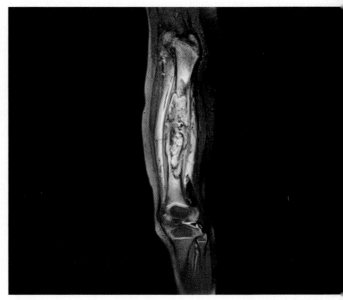

Fig. 23.13: Histiocytosis – MRI of femur shows large heterogeneous signal intensity lesion in diaphysis with cortical destruction, soft tissue and periosteal reaction

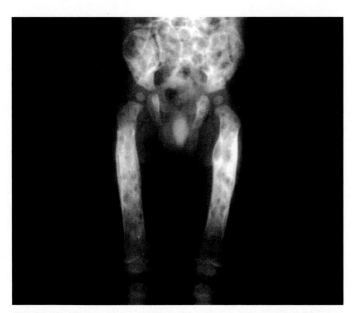

Fig. 23.12: Histiocytosis—Radiograph of the pelvis and upper femora shows multiple well defined and ill-defined lesions with associated periosteal reaction in both femora

located in the medulla of the diaphysis and metaphysis and rarely involves the cortex and epiphysis. Multiple lesions occur in about 25 percent of cases.[15] Pain is most common presenting problem with local tenderness and palpable mass. Histologically, the tumors are composed of Langerhans histiocytes containing their characteristic cleaved nuclei, and electron microscopy reveals Birbeck granules in the cytoplasm adjacent to the cell membrane. Radiographic appearance is variable. The lesion in calvarium typically appears as well defined lytic lesion with scalloped/ beveled borders (Fig. 23.11). Sometimes, a button sequestrum

may be seen in the lesion. Most of the lesions in long bones appear as lytic lesion with well defined borders, however some of the lesions are permeative and associated with periosteal new bone formation (Fig. 23.12). The later findings suggest aggressive behavior. MRI is a very sensitive but non-specific method of detecting eosinophilic granuloma. The lesion can be hypointense or hyperintense on T1 and hyperintense on T2W images associated with extensive marrow and soft tissue edema. Occasionally, there is cortical disruption with adjacent soft tissue seen on MRI (Fig. 23.13). The natural history of isolated lesion is gradual healing.[16] Treatment depends upon the site, location and multiplicity of lesion.

GIANT CELL TUMOR

Giant cell tumors are very rare in children under 15 years of age and commonly seen in girls.[17] Radiographically, these tumors are well defined, eccentric lytic lesions usually located around the knee. The lesion usually shows nonsclerotic margin, cortical thinning without matrix calcification (Fig. 23.14). GCT is located in the metaphysis and do not cross the open physis, but may extend to the subchondral bone if the physis is closed. On MRI the lesion shows generalized hypointensity on T2-weighted images. This T2 hypointensity may result from the tumor cellularity, or from recurrent hemorrhage within the lesion. The solid portions of GCT enhance diffusely after gadolinium administration. Secondary, ABC formation can be seen in about 14 percent of GCT.[17]

TUMOR LIKE LESIONS

Simple Bone Cyst

A bone cyst is a fluid filled lesion with fibrous lining. It occurs in metaphysis of long bones and adjacent to physis in children

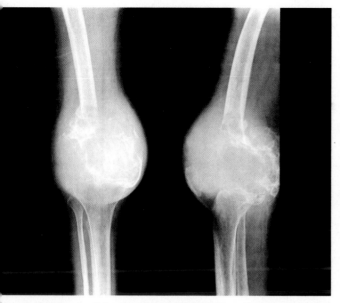

Fig. 23.14: Giant cell tumor—Radiograph of knee (AP and Lat view) show large grossly expansile lytic lesion in lower end of femur, extending up to subchondral region

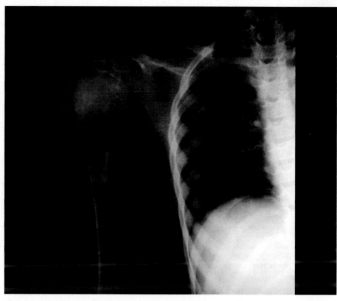

Fig. 23.16: Aneurysmal bone cyst—Radiograph of shoulder joint shows multiloculated expansile lytic lesion, involving upper end of humerus

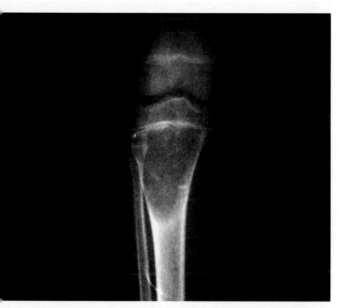

Fig. 23.15: Bone cyst—Radiograph of knee joint show mildly expansile lytic lesion in metaphysis of tibia with thinning of cortex

and young adults. Common locations are proximal humerus and femur.[18] Calcaneum and ileum are less common sites. On plain radiograph, the lesion appears as moderately expansile, well marginated with or without sclerosis (Fig. 23.15). The cortex may be thinned out and may lead to pathological fracture. "Fallen fragment" sign may be seen, when there is piece of bone which migrates into the cavity and settles at the base. CT and MRI can confirm the cystic nature of the lesion. The fluid contents are usually of low intensity on T1-weighted images and hyperintensity on T2-weighted images. However, hemorrhage into the cyst can alter the signal characteristics of the lesion.[5,18]

Aneurysmal Bone Cyst

Aneurysmal bone cyst is solitary, expansile radiolucent lesion and generally located in metaphysis of long bones. Other sites are dorsolumbar spine, small bones of hand, feet and pelvis. Pathologically, the lesion contains multiples cystic spaces containing various stages of blood. Radiologically, the lesion appears as expansile, lytic sharply circumscribed with thin cortex. The characteristic features are its ballooned out appearance and trabeculated appearance (Fig. 23.16). CT may demonstrate fluid-fluid level and thin rim of bone overlying the lesion. MRI shows the various stages of blood products which appear as layers of different signal intensity on both T1 and T2W images[18] (Figs 23.17A and B). The differential diagnosis includes giant cell tumor, osteoblastoma, chondroblastoma, osteosarcoma and simple bone cyst.

Pseudotumor of Hemophilia

Hemophilia is a bleeding disorder that occurs in males. Repetitive hemorrhage occurs close to muscle attachments without significant history of trauma. The common locations are iliopsoas and gastrocnemius muscles. Sometimes there is intraosseous or subperiosteal hemorrhage, which can cause pressure erosion of bone. Plain X-ray shows pressure erosion/destruction of bone associated with large soft tissue component (Fig. 23.18A). Calcification within soft tissue hematoma may be seen. MRI shows variable heterogeneous signal, in form of various stages of blood products (Fig. 23.18B).

SOFT TISSUE TUMORS

The diagnosis of soft tissue tumors in children can be challenging due to broad spectrum of developmental anomalies, neoplasms, inflammatory conditions and pseudotumors. Ultrasonography

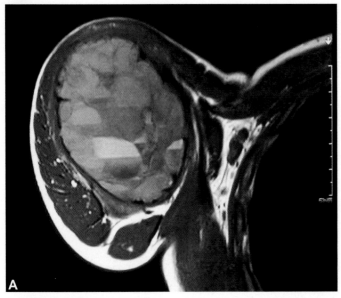
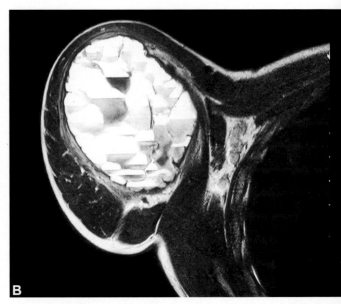

Figs 23.17A and B: Aneurysmal bone cyst—MRI of the same patient, axial T1 and T2W images (A and B) shows well defined multiloculated expansile lesion with fluid-fluid/hemorrhage levels

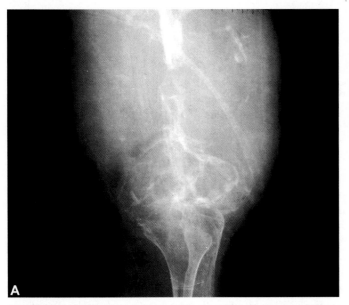
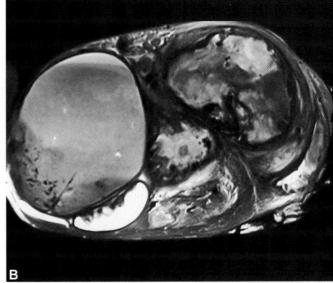

Figs 23.18A and B: Pseudotumor of hemophilia—Radiograph of lower end of femur: (A) Shows lytic destruction of femur associated with large soft tissue component and bony spicules. MRI of the same patient, fat sat T2WI image (B) Shows large soft tissue with various stages of blood components

(USG) and magnetic resonance imaging (MRI) are extremely useful in the characterization of these tumors. However, an accurate diagnosis can only be made by correlating with the patient's age, clinical history and physical examination. Ultrasound is usually the modality of choice for the small and superficial soft tissue masses. It has the advantages of relatively low cost, portability, lack of radiation, no need for sedation, and widespread availability. Gray scale imaging should be performed with the highest frequency transducer available. Color Doppler should be performed to demonstrate the presence of vessels within the lesion.

Due to its multiplanar imaging capabilities, high tissue contrast resolution, and lack of radiation, MR imaging is the modality of choice for the evaluation of large and deep masses or for those cases in which US is not adequate. Magnetic resonance imaging (MRI) should include the entire tumor so as to demonstrate its margins. MR images of soft tissue tumors have low specificity, are only occasionally helpful in differentiating between benign and malignant masses with certainty. Some MR imaging criteria have been postulated as indicators of malignancy, particularly in adults. These include size (>5 to 6 cm), absence of low signal on T2-weighted images, signal heterogeneity or

T1-weighted images, early contrast enhancement, peripheral or heterogeneous enhancement, rapid initial enhancement followed by a plateau or a washout phase, and invasion of adjacent bone, neurovascular bundles, or both.[19]

Vascular Lesions

Vascular lesions are the commonest cause of soft tissue masses in children. Mulliken and Glowacki,[20] divided them in two groups based on the findings on physical examination, clinical evolution, histology, and cellular kinetics: Hemangiomas and vascular malformations. Hemangiomas are neoplastic lesions, whereas vascular malformations are errors of vascular morphogenesis. Categorization of a lesion into one of these two groups has significant implications for a patient's management and prognosis.

Hemangioma

Hemangiomas are considered to be true neoplasms and they account for 7 to 10 percent of all benign soft tissue tumors.[20] Hemangiomas may be localized or diffuse and are histogically benign. Capillary (usually cutaneous), cavernous, venous and mixed types of hemangiomas have been described and classified according to the apparent origin of their vascular channels. Hemangiomas also contain variable amounts of nonvascular tissue and other elements, including fat, smooth muscle, fibrous tissue, myxoid stroma and hemosiderin.

USG, CT, MRI and radiolabelled red cell scintigraphy, can facilitate preoperative diagnosis. Radiographs are important for detecting associated osseous abnormality, and the finding of calcified phleboliths on radiographs or CT images is an indication of a hemangioma (Figs 23.19A and B). Ultrasound shows hemangioma as a well defined mass of variable echogenicity.[21] Color Doppler may show high flow pattern in proliferative phase however vascularity decreases in involuting phase. On T1-weighted MRI images, hemangiomas are either isointense or when they contain sufficient fat, hyperintense to muscle. On T2-weighted images, the lesions are well defined and markedly hyperintense with serpiginous high signal zones, that correlate with torturous vascular channels interlaced with lower intensity fibrous or fatty tissue. Phleboliths are hypointense on both T1 and T2-weighted sequences.

Hemangiopericytoma is a rare soft tissue tumor of low but unpredictable malignant potential that is believed to arise from vascular endothelial pericytes. These tumors are usually located in the thigh or the pelvic retroperitoneum but can arise in any part of the body. Approximately, 10 percent of hemangiopericytomas occur during childhood, and about one-third of these are congenital.[22] Congenital hemangiopericytoma can exhibit rapid initial growth, but spontaneous regression has also been reported. Microscopically, these tumors show endothelial proliferation with some similarity to hemangioma. Calcifications may be detected radiographically or by CT, and the tumors are well circumscribed. There may be partial destruction of adjacent bone. Hemangiopericytomas are very vascular lesions and show marked enhancement and frequently, central necrosis on contrast enhanced CT images.

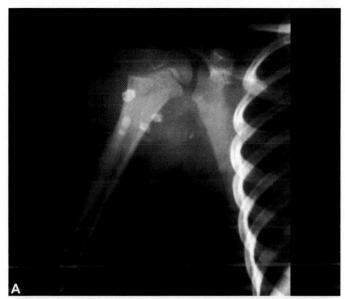

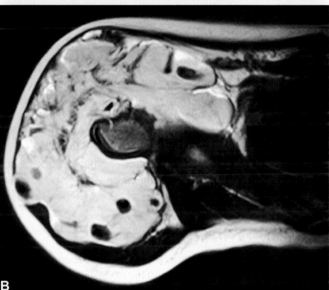

Figs 23.19A and B: Hemangioma – Radiograph of shoulder joint (A) shows large soft tissue around the joint with phleboliths. MRI of same patient (B) shows large lobulated soft tissue with multiple phleboliths

Like most soft tissue sarcomas, hemangiopericytomas are isointense to muscle on T1-weighted images and exhibit high signal intensity on T2-weighted and STIR images and they enhance moderately with gadolinium.

Vascular Malformations

Vascular malformations occur due to errors in vascular development that are always present at birth. Based on the main vascular channel present within the lesion, they are classified as arteriovenous, venous, lymphatic, capillary, or mixed. Arterio-venous malformations are high-flow vascular malformations characterized by direct communication between the arterial and venous systems without an intervening capillary bed. These lesions may be detected at birth (40% of cases) and grow commensurately with the child.[23] On US, they appear as multiple dilated tortuous channels diffusely involving subcutaneous soft tissues, which may not be apparent on gray scale but are easily demonstrated with color Doppler evaluation. These lesions have a high vascular density, and spectral Doppler analysis reveals high velocity in the arteries, but well-defined mass is usually not seen.[21] On MR imaging, they appear as enlarged vascular channels associated with dilated feeding and draining vessels and without an associated well-defined mass. The high-flow vessels appear as signal void foci on spin echo images or as high signal intensity on flow-enhanced gradient-echo images.

Venous malformations are characterized by the presence of anomalous ectatic venous channels. They may be small and localized or extensive. On US, venous malformations are usually of heterogeneous echogenicity, more commonly hypoechoic in comparison with the adjacent subcutaneous tissues phleboliths, may be present in 16 percent of cases. Doppler US usually detects slow venous flow within these lesions, although absence of flow is not uncommon which may reflect very slow flow or thrombosis. On MR imaging, they may appear as dilated tortuous veins or more often as lobulated masses, comprised of multiple locules reflecting dilated venous spaces separated by thin interstitial septa. They are iso- to hypointense to muscle on T1-weighted images, hyperintense on T2-weighted images, and show patchy enhancement after the administration of intravenous gadolinium.[24]

Lymphangioma usually visible at birth, is more frequent in the head and neck but also seen in the trunk, extremities, and in viscera. It may present clinically as, soft, smooth, translucent masses. On US, the macrocystic lymphatic malformations appear as well-defined, multicystic lesions. On MR imaging, the macrocystic lymphatic malformations appear as clearly defined cysts usually of low signal intensity on T1-weighted images and high signal intensity on T2-weighted images, often with fluid-fluid levels. Postcontrast images show only septal enhancement without enhancement of the cystic spaces. This is a helpful feature in the differentiation from venous malformations.[24]

FIBROBLASTIC/MYOFIBROBLASTIC TUMORS

Fibroblastic/myofibroblastic tumors comprise a large number of mesenchymal tumors with both fibroblastic and myofibroblastic features. Common lesions of this group are described here.

Nodular Fasciitis

Nodular fasciitis is an idiopathic, self-limited focal fibrous proliferation, usually confined to the subcutaneous tissues. Common locations include the upper extremities and trunk. On US, nodular fasciitis is a well-defined lesion with, homogeneous/heterogeneous echotexture. The MR imaging appearance is variable, although more commonly, it appears as a fascia-based lesion of homogeneous isointense or slightly hyperintense to muscle on T1-weighted images, hyperintense on T2-weighted images, and homogeneous enhancement after gadolinium administration.[25]

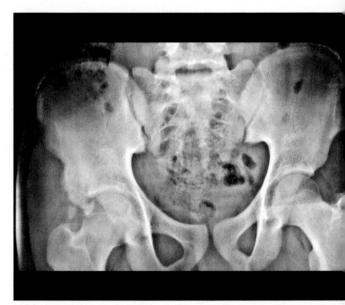

Fig. 23.20: Myositis ossificans – Radiograph of pelvis shows soft tissue ossification adjacent to superior aspect of right acetabulum

Myositis Ossificans

Myositis ossificans is a localized, self-limited, reparativ hypercellular lesion, composed of reactive hypercellular fibrou tissue and bone. In most cases, a clear history of trauma i obtained. It often occurs in an area exposed to trauma, mor commonly in the thighs and arms. Plain X-ray can shov heterogeneous calcification, adjacent to bony attachmen (Fig. 23.20). CT is the modality of choice for the evaluation o myositis ossificans. The appearance of the lesion changes wit time. In the first 2 weeks after trauma, it appears as a noncalcifie hypodense mass, with edema of surrounding soft tissues Curvilinear peripheral calcification becomes evident after 4 t 6 weeks, with progressive internal ossification over the nex several weeks and months.[26]

Myofibroma/Myofibromatosis

Solitary myofibroma is a common, benign fibrous tumo commonly seen in children < 2 years of age. It may present as solitary nodule in the subcutaneous tissues or muscle or a multiple nodules involving soft tissues and bone. The multicentri presentation is known as myofibromatosis. The natural history o myofibromatosis is spontaneous regression; however, a hig mortality is reported in multicentric cases with visceral involve ment. On US, myofibromas have varied appearances but are ofte well marginated with an anechoic center, reflecting centra necrosis, which can be traversed by thick septa.[27] On MR imaging myofibromas appear as nodules of low signal intensity on T1 weighted images and a more variable appearance on T2-weighte images.

Fibromatosis

Fibromatosis is a benign proliferation of fibroblasts an myofibroblasts with a marked production of collagen. It i

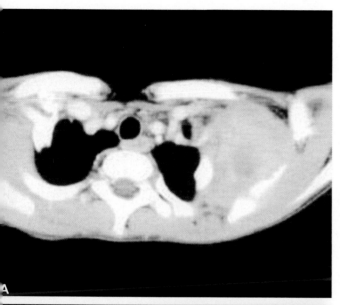

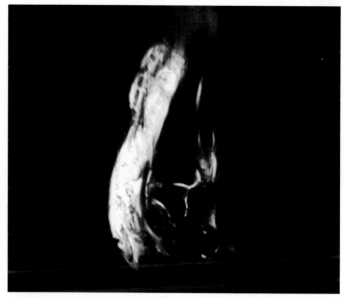

Fig. 23.22: Plexiform Neurofibroma – MRI of leg shows large lobulated heterogeneous signal intensity lesion involving skin and deep soft tissue of leg.

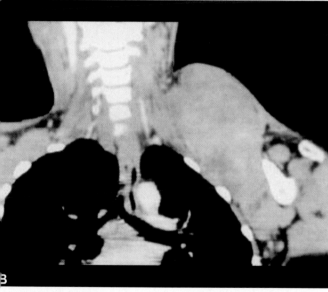

Figs 23.21A and B: Fibromatosis – CT scan axial section (A) and coronal reformation (B) shows large soft tissue mass in the lower part of neck extending into axilla with erosion of adjacent scapula

characterized by infiltrative growth and a propensity for local recurrence. These tumors are variably echogenic on ultrasound and their borders may be smooth or irregular. CT scan is useful to show extent of soft tissue and bony erosion (Figs 23.21A and B). On MR images, their appearance is also variable with a signal that is isointense or slightly hyperintense when compared with that of muscle on T1-weighted images and either intermediate between muscles and fat or high signal on T2-weighted images.[28]

Neurogenic Tumor

Most common neurogenic tumor arising from peripheral nerves in children is neurofibroma. Three types of neurofibroma has been described, localized, diffuse and plexiform type.[29] Localized neurofibroma are usually well defined, encapsulated soft tissue

masses less than 5 cm in diameter. They are isointense to muscle on T1 and heterogeneous signal on T2-weighted images and may show target pattern.[29] Plexiform neurofibroma is a diffuse mass involving multiple fascicles of nerve. These lesions can be deep, superficial or combination of both, depending upon the location of tumor. Superficial types of lesions are more common, diffuse and asymmetric in distribution and extend to skin surface (Fig. 23.22).

Adipocytic Tumor

Common adipocytic tumors are lipoma, lipoblastoma, and lipomatosis of nerve in the pediatric age group. Liposarcoma, which is the most common type of soft tissue sarcoma in adults is rare in children.

Lipoma

Lipoma is the most common adipocytic tumor in children, it is often found in the upper back, neck, proximal extremities, and abdomen. Lipomas are usually subcutaneous, although deep ones are not rare, and these will more often require imaging. On US, lipomas have a variable appearance, with about two thirds of cases demonstrating homogeneous echogenicity and 60 percent with well-defined margins. The echogenicity is varied with hypoechoic, isoechoic, hyperechoic, and mixed echogenicity patterns reported.[30] On MR imaging, lipomas have similar signal characteristics compared with subcutaneous fat, characterized by high signal intensity on T1-weighted images and low signal intensity on fat-suppressed images (Fig. 23.23).

Lipoblastoma

Lipoblastoma is a tumor composed of mature adipocytes and lipoblasts in various stages of development. It represents up to 30 percent of adipocytic tumors in children.[31] It occurs primarily

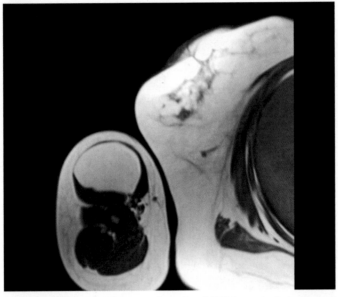

Fig. 23.23: Lipoma – MRI, axial section (T1W image) of shows well defined lesion in anterior compartment of arm with similar signal intensity of subcutaneous fat

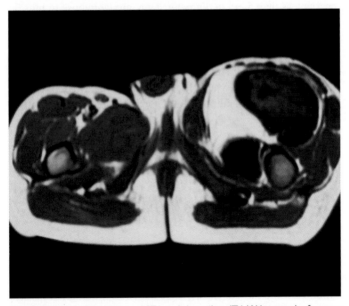

Fig. 23.24: Lipoblastoma – MRI, axial section (T1 W images) of upper thigh, shows large soft tissue mass in left upper thigh with signal intensity of fat as well as soft tissue

in children < 3 years of age and commonly manifests as a painless, progressively growing mass. On US, lipoblastoma usually appears as a homogeneous, hyperechoic mass, although mixed echogenicity and fluid-filled spaces have also been reported. On MR imaging, the appearance reflects the amount of mature adipose tissue relative to lipoblasts and myxocollagenous stromal tissue. They can appear similar to lipoma. When the myxoid component is large the MR signal is heterogeneous and shows contrast enhancement. This imaging appearance is indistinguishable from liposarcoma (Fig. 23.24).[32]

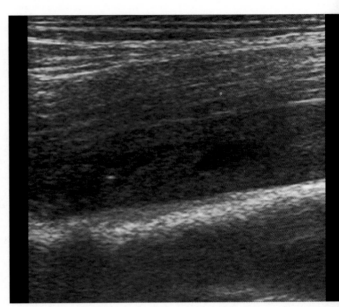

Fig. 23.25: Hematoma – Ultrasound image shows ill-defined heterogeneous echotexture lesion with in the deep muscles of thigh suggestive of hematoma

Pseudotumors

Pseudotumors are non-neoplastic lesions and can present as soft tissue mass. These include hematoma, fat necrosis, inflammatory lesions and periarticular cysts.

Fat Necrosis

It is self-limiting entity and presents as small non-tender subcutaneous nodule. The causes of fat necrosis include cold exposure, trauma, injection, autoimmune disorders and vasculitis. Common locations include the soft tissues overlying bone prominences in the shoulders, back, buttocks, thighs, and cheeks. Imaging findings on ultrasound is quite variable, however predominantly it is a hyperechoic nodule with fuzzy margins. Fat necrosis appears as linear shaped abnormal signal in subcutaneous tissue which is usually hypointense on T1 and hypo/hyperintense on T2-weighted images.[33]

Hematoma

Imaging of hematoma is usually not required, however, it may be indicated in very symptomatic cases, in children without clear history of trauma and in bleeding disorders to know extent of involvement. The imaging appearance of hematoma depends on the age of blood. Ultrasound is the initial investigation of choice. In acute stage, hematoma is hyperechoic however it becomes anechoic/heterogeneous in few days (Fig. 23.25). MRI is useful and it can show hyperintensity on T1-weighted images, hypointense on T2-weighted images and blooming on GRE sequences.[34]

Inflammatory Lesions

Cellulitis occasionally presents as soft tissue mass. Ultrasound shows increased echogenecity of subcutaneous fat. On MRI cellulitis appears as illdefined T1 hypointense and T2 hyperintense

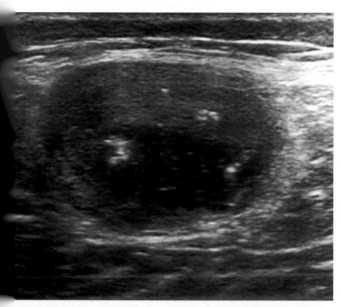

23.26: Abscess—Ultrasound image shows well defined collection ubcutaneous soft tissue with internal echoes suggestive of abscess

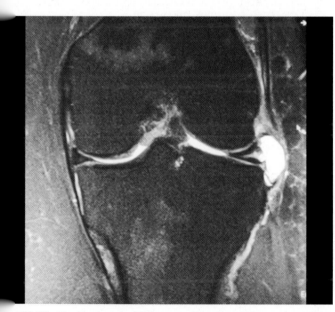

23.27: Meniscal cyst—MRI, coronal section of knee shows tear meniscus with large adjacent fluid collection communicating with suggestive of meniscal cyst

a seen in subcutaneous tissue. Sometimes, aggressive infection ds to abscess formation in soft tissue. On ultrasound, abscess ears as hypoechoic fluid collection (Fig. 23.26). MRI shows, ll defined T1 hypointense and T2 hyperintense lesion with ipheral enhancement on postcontrast images.[35]

riarticular Cysts

ese include ganglion, synovial cyst and meniscal cyst. Ganglion ystic lesion which has fibrous capsule and composed of coid material. Imaging (USG and MRI) shows typical features cyst, however, sometimes internal echoes and septae can be

seen.[36] Synovial cyst is lined by synovial cells. Synovial cyst may communicate with joint space. Typical example of synovial cyst is popliteal cyst. Collection of fluid in the meniscus or parameniscal tissue is called meniscal cyst (Fig. 23.27). It is associated with meniscus tear. MR imaging shows well defined cyst/fluid collection in continuity with meniscus tear.[37]

CONCLUSION

A wide spectrum of benign bone and soft tissue tumor and conditions is seen in children. It is imperative for the radiologist to be aware of entire gamut of imaging findings, so as to avoid unwarranted biopsies and surgeries in these children. Plain radiograph continue to be first line imaging modality of choice and is the cornerstone in diagnosis of pediatric benign bone tumors. MR imaging has emerged to become an integral part of diagnostic algorithm of these lesions, owing to its excellent soft tissue resolution, multiplanar capabilities and nonionizing nature.

REFERENCES

1. Fletcher BD. Benign and malignant bone tumor. In Caffey's Pediatric Diagnostic Imaging Volume 2, Mosby, Elsevier, Philadelphia, 2004.
2. Biermann JS: Musculoskeletal neoplasms in children. In: Orthopaedic knowledge update. Sponseller PD, Shaughnessy JW, (Eds): Rosemont, IL: American Academy of Orthopaedic Surgeons 2002; 51-61.
3. Giudici MA, Moser RP, Kransdorf MJ. Cartilaginous bone tumor. Radiol Clin of North Am 1993; 31:237-59.
4. Mirra JM, Picci P, Gold RH. Bone tumors: Clinical, radiologic and pathologic correlation. Philadelphea, Lea and Fabiger, 1989.
5. Steven S, Srinivas K, Javicr B. MR imaging of tumors and tumor like lesions of upper extremity. Magn. Reson imaging Clin of N America 2004; 12:349-59.
6. Holtz P, Sundaram M. Enchondroma. Orthopedics 1995; 18:509-10.
7. Mermelstein LE, Friedlaender GE, Katz LD. Chondroblastoma. Orthopedics 1997; 20:67-71.
8. McGrory BJ, Inwards CY, Mcleod RA, et al. Chondromyxoid fibroma. Orthopadedics 1995; 18(3):307-10.
9. Bloem JL, Kroon HM. Osseous lesions. Radiol clin of North America 1993; 31(2):261-65.
10. Assoun J, Riichardi G, Railhac JJ, et al. Osteoid osteoma: MR Imaging versus CT Radiology 1994; 191:217-36.
11. Bruners P, Penzkofer T, Günther RW, Mahnken A. Percutaneous radiofrequency ablation of osteoid osteomas: Technique and results. Rofo 2009; 181(8):740-7.
12. Moulton JS, Bvaley SE, Biedel JS. Bone and soft tissue tumors. In clinical Magnetic resonance imaging (2nd edn) 1996; 2042-77.
13. Lucas E, Sundaram M, Boccini T. Polyostotic fibrous dysplasia. Orthopaedics 1995; 18(3):311-3.
14. Zeanah WR, Hudson TM. Springfield DS. Computed tomography of ossifying fibroma of the tibia. J Comput Assist Tomogr 1983; 7:688-91.
15. Marin C, Warrier RP. Langerhan's cell histiocytosis. Orthop Clin of North Am 1996; 27(3):615-23.
16. Copley L, Dormans JP. Benign pediatric bone tumors. Evaluation and treatment. Pediatr Clin North Am 1996; 43:949-66.
17. Murphey MD, Nomikos GC, Flemming DJ, et al. Imaging of giant cell tumor and giant cell reparative granuloma of bone: Radiologic-pathologic correlation. Radiographics 2001; 21:1283–309.

18. Conway WF, Hayes CW. Miscellaneous lesions of bone. Radiol Clin of North Am 1993; 31(2):339-58.

19. Brisse H, Orbach D, Klijanienko J, Fre´neaux P, Neuenschwander S. Imaging and diagnostic strategy of soft tissue tumors in children. Eur Radiol 2006; 16(5):1147-64.

20. Mulliken JB, Glowacki J. Hemangiomas and vascular malformations in infants and children: A classification based on endothelial characteristics. Plast Reconstr Surg 1982; 69(3):412-22.

21. Paltiel HJ, Burrows PE, Kozakewich HPW, Zurakowski D, Mulliken JB. Soft-tissue vascular anomalies: Utility of US for diagnosis. Radiology 2000; 214(3):747-54.

22. Auguste LJ. Razack MS, Sako K. Hemangiopericytoma. J Surg Oncol 1982; 20:260-4.

23. Frieden I, Enjolras O, Esterly N. Vascular birthmarks, other abnormalities of blood vessels and lymphatics. In: Schachner LA, Hansen RC, eds. Pediatric Dermatology. 3rd edn. New York, NY: Mosby 2003; 833-62.

24. Konez O, Burrows PE. Magnetic resonance of vascular anomalies. Magn Reson Imaging Clin N Am 2002; 10(2):363-88.

25. Leung LYJ, Shu SJ, Chan ACL, Chan MK, Chan CHS. Nodular fasciitis: MRI appearance and literature review. Skeletal Radiol 2002; 31(1):9-13.

26. Siegel MJ. Magnetic resonance imaging of musculoskeletal soft tissue masses. Radiol Clin North Am 2001; 39(4):701-20.

27. Koujok K, Ruiz RE, Hernandez RJ. Myofibromatosis: Imaging characteristics. Pediatr Radiol 2005; 35(4):374-80.

28. Lee JC, Thomas JM, Phillips S, Fisher C, Moskovic E. Aggressive fibromatosis: MRI features with pathologic correlation. AJR Am J Roentgenol 2006; 186(1):247-54.

29. Stull MA, Moser RP, Kransdorf MJ, et al. Magnetic resonance appearance of peripheral nerve sheath tumors. Skeletal Radiol 1991; 20:9-14.

30. Fornage BD, Tassin GB. Sonographic appearances of superficial soft tissue lipomas. J Clin Ultrasound 1991; 19(4):215-20.

31. Miller GG, Yanchar NL, Magee JF, Blair GK. Lipoblastoma and liposarcoma in children: An analysis of 9 cases and a review of the literature. Can J Surg 1998; 41(6):455-8.

32. Murphey MD, Carroll JF, Flemming DJ, Pope TL, Gannon FH, Kransdorf MJ. From the archives of the AFIP: Benign musculo-skeletal lipomatous lesions. Radiographics 2004; 24(5):1433-66.

33. Tsai TS, Evans HA, Donnelly LF, Bisset GS III, Emery KH. Fat necrosis after trauma: A benign cause of palpable lumps in children. AJR Am J Roentgenol 1997; 169(6):1623-6.

34. Bush CH. The magnetic resonance imaging of musculoskeletal hemorrhage. Skeletal Radiol 2000; 29(1):1-9.

35. Faingold R, Oudjhane K, Armstrong DC, Albuquerque PAB. Magnetic resonance imaging of congenital, inflammatory, and infectious soft-tissue lesions in children. Top Magn Reson Imaging 2002; 13(4):241-61.

36. Seymour R, Lloyd DCF. Sonographic appearances of meniscal cysts. J Clin Ultrasound 1998; 26(1):15-20.

37. McCarthy CL, McNally EG. The MRI appearance of cystic lesions around the knee. Skeletal Radiol 2004; 33(4):187-209.

CHAPTER 24

Pediatric Malignant Bone and Soft Tissue Tumors

Manisha Jana, Ashu Seith Bhalla, Deep N Srivastava

INTRODUCTION

Malignant bone tumors account for about 6 percent of all childhood malignancies;[1,2] though malignant soft tissue tumors are rare in childhood. The most common malignant bone tumors include osteosarcoma and Ewing's sarcoma, while rhabdomyosarcoma is the commonest pediatric malignant soft tissue tumor.[3,4] Most of the tumors affect the appendicular skeleton and result in significant morbidity and mortality. Table 24.1 shows age distribution of these tumors.

IMAGING MODALITIES

Plain Radiographs

Radiographs are the primary imaging modality in cases of bone tumors, and often a specific diagnosis can be made on plain radiographs alone depending on location of the lesion (Table 24.2). The appearance of the lesion and the patient age remain important considerations for diagnosis. Most of the pediatric malignant bone tumors involve the metaphysis, however, Ewing's sarcoma and lymphoma have a propensity to involve diaphysis. The pattern of bone destruction is a pointer towards the aggressiveness of the lesion. Most malignant bone tumors present radiographically with a permeative lytic or moth-eaten pattern of bone destruction (Fig. 24.1).

In cases of pediatric soft tissue tumors, plain radiographs are often of limited importance. Clinical examination can often prove useful in evaluating small superficial lesions (e.g. lipoma), but for proper assessment of extent of most soft tissue tumors, radiologic evaluation is imperative.

Sonography

Ultrasonography is useful for characterization of some lesions especially for superficial lesions.[5] Doppler can help in the assessment of vascularity of lesion and also for guided biopsies and in monitoring tumor response to chemotherapy.

Computed Tomography (CT)

Among the cross sectional imaging, role of CT has considerably reduced after the introduction of MRI. However, CT is superior to MRI in the detection and characterization of matrix mineralization, bone trabeculation and periosteal reaction. CT is also used in the detection of pulmonary metastases.

Magnetic Resonance Imaging (MRI)

The role of magnetic resonance imaging in pediatric bone tumors include accurate assessment of the extent of the lesion, evaluation of skip lesions, neurovascular and articular involvement. T1W spin echo images remain the most important sequence to assess the tumor extent, owing to the contrast between normal hyperintense fatty marrow and hypointense tumor.[6] Inversion recovery sequence

Table 24.1: Age distribution of pediatric bone and soft tissue tumors		
Age	*Bone Tumor*	*Soft Tissue Tumor*
Less than 5 years	- Osteosarcoma - Ewing's sarcoma - Lymphoma	- Rhabdomyosarcoma - Infantile fibrosarcoma - Hemangiopericytoma - Granulocytic sarcoma
More than 5 years	- Osteosarcoma - Ewing's sarcoma - Lymphoma - Malignant fibrous histiocytoma (rare) - Chondrosarcoma (rare)	- Rhabdomyosarcoma - Synovial sarcoma - Granulocytic sarcoma - Hemangiopericytoma

Table 24.2: Common locations of primary malignant bone tumors	
Location	*Tumors*
Metaphysis	- Osteosarcoma - Metastases - Ewing's sarcoma - Lymphoma - Malignant fibrous histiocytoma
Diaphysis	- Ewing's sarcoma - Lymphoma
Epiphysis	- Aggressive giant cell tumor (rare)

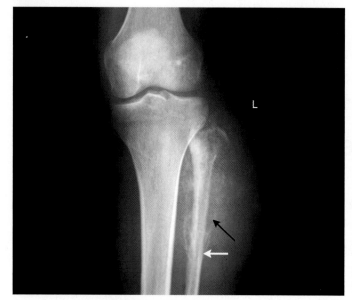

Fig. 24.1: Plain radiograph of the left leg shows permeative lytic destruction, periosteal reaction (white arrow) and Codman triangle (black arrow), typical imaging features of a malignant bone tumor. Histopathology: osteosarcoma

(short tau inversion recovery—STIR) sequence makes the tumor more conspicuous by suppressing normal marrow fat as the hyperintense tumor stands bright. Postcontrast images (after Gadolinium administration) can define the exact extent of the tumor, define viable tumor and the necrotic areas[7] and help in tumor edema differentiation.[8] Peritumoral edema can either be intraosseous or extraosseous and often show high signal on T2 weighted or STIR images. In the bones, edema has poorly defined margin and often difficult to differentiate from the tumor mass. In the soft tissues, edema does not have mass effect and follows muscle and fascial planes.

Most of the malignant bone and soft tissue tumors share common similar imaging features, e.g. they are hypointense on T1W and hyperintense on T2W images.[9-12] However, few lesions show characteristic signal intensities, e.g. fat containing lesions are bright on T1W as well as T2W sequences and fibrous tumors may show hypointense signal on both T1 as well as T2W images. The differentiation of benign from malignant nature of a mass is not possible in most cases on MR imaging; but the useful role of MRI is in tumor staging.

MRI Techniques for Bone and Soft Tissue Tumors

The sequences should include T1W images in coronal or sagittal plane for accurate delineation of tumor extent (Fig. 24.2A) and articular involvement, if any. T2W fat saturated or STIR images is useful for better demonstration of relationship with adjacent muscles, nerves and vascular structures (Fig. 24.2B).

Role of Contrast-enhanced MRI

In primary bone and soft tissue tumors, contrast administration is often not required. However, T1W fat saturated images are helpful in follow-up imaging for detection of recurrence. Dynamic contrast-

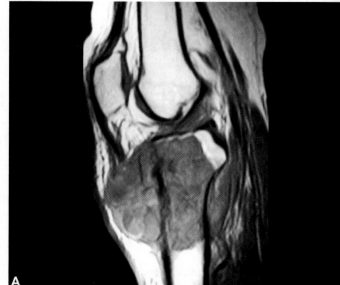

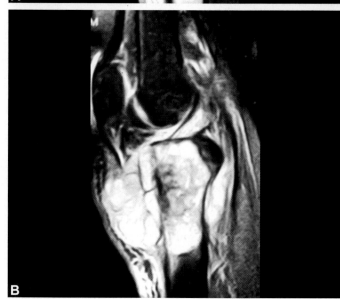

Figs 24.2A and B: Sagittal T1W (A) and T2W (B) MR of a case of osteosarcoma. The tumor is hypointense in contrast to hyperintense fatty marrow on T1W and hyperintense on T2W sequences. The tumor has an extra compartmental extension into the muscle plane (Stage T2)

enhanced MRI is specifically helpful in detecting tumor recurrence,[13] which often shows early contrast enhancement and washout.

Newer MR Imaging Techniques

Diffusion weighted MRI: Diffusion weighted MRI has been used to predict the tumor viability after treatment, and hence, to reflect the response to treatment. After treatment many a times the tumor bulk may not reduce significantly but the apparent diffusion coefficient (ADC) value increases[14] indicating response to treatment.

Dynamic Contrast-enhanced MRI: Dynamic contrast-enhanced MRI is a new addition in the imaging of malignant bone tumors, especially osteosarcoma. It measures the tumor viability by determining the contrast accumulation within the tumor. Dynamic contrast-enhanced MRI assessment of dynamic vector magnitude based on contrast accumulation rate over time and maximal intensity of the tumor) and Kep (measure of the gadolinium exchange between the vascular and the interstitial space) tend to predict the outcome after treatment.[15]

MR spectroscopy: In vivo proton MR spectroscopy is a promising modality in the evaluation of malignant bone and soft tissue tumors. On MR spectroscopy these tumors show choline peak (resonance at 3.2 ppm);[16] which is highly sensitive and specific.

Staging of Malignant Bone and Soft Tissue Tumors

The Enneking system of staging malignant bone and soft tissue tumors[17] (Table 24.3) was based on three criteria: extent of tumor (T1 suggests an intracompartmental tumor, T2 an extra-compartmental spread (Figs 24.2A and B)), presence or absence of metastases (M0 and M1 respectively) and histologic grade of the tumor (low grade G1, high grade G2). Low grade tumors (stage IA or IB; T1G1M0 or T2G1M0) are candidates for wide local excision or limb salvage surgeries. High grade tumor (G2) without metastases are treated with radical surgeries like amputation.

In 1983, AJCC developed another system of staging of bone and soft tissue tumors depending on four criteria: extent of tumor (confined by bone cortex T1; with transcortical extension T2), nodal disease (N0 no nodal disease; N1 regional nodal spread), metastases (absence of metastases M0; presence of metastases M1) and histologic grade of tumor (G1-well differentiated tumor, G2-moderately differentiated, G3-poorly differentiated and G4 undifferentiated). The recent revision in this staging is based on the size of the tumor rather than transcortical extension (T1 tumors being less than 8 cm and T2 more than 8 cm).[18] A new stage T3 has been added to indicate skip matastases. These classification system did not include bone lymphoma or myeloma.

MALIGNANT BONE TUMORS

Osteosarcoma

Osteosarcoma is the most common pediatric malignant bone tumor,[19] usually affecting children in the second decade. Patients with retinoblastoma, Li-fraumeni syndrome, prior radiation therapy are more prone to develop osteosarcoma. The usual clinical presentation is with a painful mass.

Histologic subgroups in osteosarcoma include osteoblastic, chondroblastic, fibroblastic, giant cell rich, telangiectatic or small cell type.[20]

Plain radiographs are usually the first investigation performed. Osteosarcoma in pediatric age groups predominantly involve the metaphyses. On radiographs they present with a permeative lytic destruction with wide zone of transition (Fig. 24.1), blastic lesion (Fig. 24.3) or a mixed pattern. Often there is an associated soft tissue component, 'sunburst' type of periosteal reaction, 'Codman triangle' formation (Fig. 24.1); and an osteoid tumor matrix

	Table 24.3: Enneking staging for primary malignant bone tumors		
Stage	Tumor	Metastases	Histologic grade
IA	T1 (intracompartmental tumor)	M0	G1
IB	T2 (extracompartmental tumor)	M0	G1
IIA	T1	M0	G2
IIB	T2	M0	G2
III	T1 or T2	M1	G1 or G2

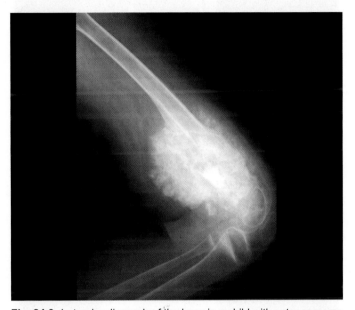

Fig. 24.3: Lateral radiograph of the knee in a child with osteosarcoma of the tibia. The tumor shows dense osteoid matrix mineralization

mineralization (Fig. 24.3). Pathological fractures are more common in a telangiectatic variety.

The work-up of a child with osteosarcoma include computed tomography (CT) of chest (Figs 24.4A to C), ^{99m}Tc MDP bone scan (to detect metastases as it spreads via the bloodstream and about 20 percent may have metastases at presentation)[6] and MRI for the local tumor extent.

MRI tends to show accurate intramedullary extent of the tumor. Tumor mass is usually hypointense on T1W and hyperintense on T2W and STIR images (Fig. 24.5). The rare telangiectatic variety shows blood-fluid levels secondary to intratumoral hemorrhage[3] (Fig. 24.6). Skip lesions within the same bone, may be seen in 15 percent of cases.

Survival and response to chemotherapy depends on the tumor burden which can be measured by tumor size. Histologic response to preoperative neoadjuvant chemotherapy (percent of necrosis) is the strongest predictor of survival.[21-23] Often the tumor size remains unchanged after treatment and it is difficult to determine response based on the size criteria.[15] Newer MR imaging techniques which help in predicting tumor response include diffusion weighted images and dynamic contrast-enhanced MRI. With treatment, the apparent diffusion coefficient (ADC) of the

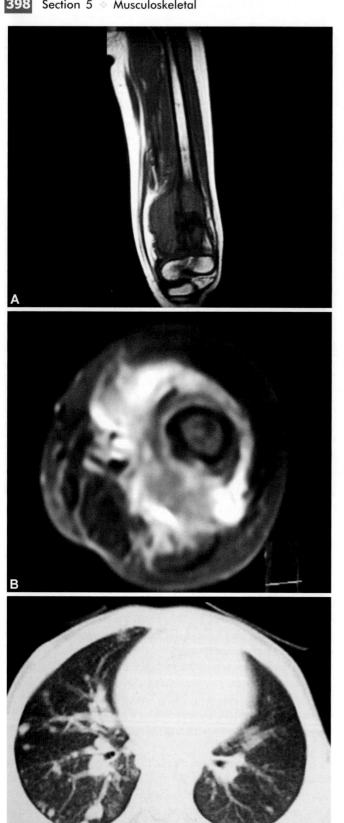

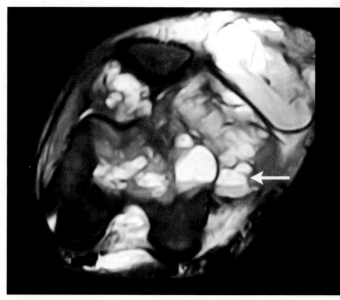

Fig. 24.5: Axial T2W fat saturated MR image in a case of telangiectatic osteosarcoma showing multiple areas of blood-fluid levels (white arrow) suggesting intratumoral hemorrhage

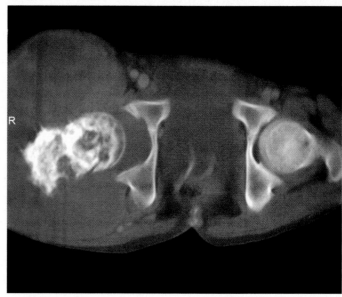

Fig. 24.6: PNET of the right femur. Axial CT scan bone window reconstruction reveals mixed lytic-sclerotic destruction of the right femoral head and neck with adjacent large soft tissue

Figs 24.4A to C: Coronal T1W (A) and axial T2W fat saturated (B) MR of a case of osteosarcoma showing the craniocaudal and axial extent of the marrow involvement. The tumor has extracompartmental extension into the muscle plane (Stage – T2). Axial CT thorax (lung window) (C) of the same patient show multiple lung metastases

tumor mass increases.[14] Dynamic contrast-enhanced MRI assessment of dymanic vector magnitude (based on contrast accumulation rate overtime and maximal intensity of the tumor) and Kep (measure of the gadolinium exchange between the vascular and the interstitial space) tend to predict the outcome after treatment.[15]

Ewing's Sarcoma

Ewing's family of tumors include classic Ewing's sarcoma, primitive neuroectodermal tumor (PNET), Askin tumor (PNET of the chest wall), extraosseous Ewing's tumor and peripheral

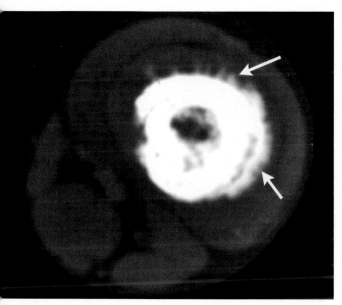

Fig. 24.7: Ewing's sarcoma. Axial CT bone window reconstruction reveals permeative lytic destruction of the femoral diaphysis, with spiculated periosteal reaction (arrows) and associated soft tissue

neuroepithelioma. All these tumors have a common neuroectodermal origin and frequently seen in children.

Classic Ewing's sarcoma is the second most common bone malignancy in children, predominantly seen in the second decade of life. Males and females have equal incidence. Usual clinical presentation is with local pain and swelling; often with constitutional symptoms. Laboratory investigations may show elevated erythrocyte sedimentation rate and leukocytosis; hence the picture often mimics osteomyelitis.

Metadiaphyses of the long bones are the most common site for Ewing's sarcoma. On plain radiographs, the tumor presents as a permeative lytic bone destruction with a wide zone of transition; cortical destruction; onion-peel type of periosteal reaction and often extensive noncalcified soft tissue mass.[24] Saucerisation of the outer cortex may occur due to erosions by tumor growth in the subperiosteal region. In cases of flat bone involvement, the soft tissue component is larger than osseous destruction. CT scan, though not commonly indicated, can define the bony destruction (Fig. 24.7). However, chest CT is done to detect pulmonary metastasis. Radionuclide study is useful in the detection of bone metastasis. The differential diagnosis includes osteomyelitis.

On T1W MRI the mass is isointense to mildly hypointense; on T2W or STIR images it is hyperintense (Figs 24.8A and B) and shows variable contrast enhancement. Skip lesions may be present in 14 percent cases.[24] The soft tissue mass tends to decrease in size and undergo necrosis with treatment. As with osteosarcoma, diffusion weighted MRI and dynamic CE-MRI can predict the response to neoadjuvant chemotherapy or radiotherapy.[23] Positron emission tomography (PET) is also used in monitoring response to therapy and metastatic disease.

PNET of the chest wall (Askin tumor) (Fig. 24.9) usually presents with an intrathoracic extrapulmonary mass having rib involvement

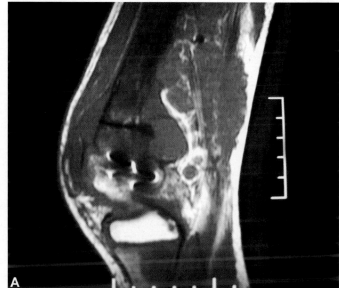

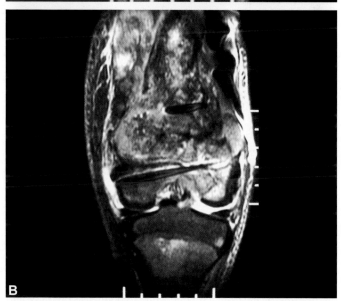

Figs 24.8A and B: Sagittal T1W (A) and Coronal T2W (B) MR of a case of Ewing's sarcoma. The tumor is hypointense on T1 and heterogeneously hyperintense on T2 with diffuse marrow infiltration and extraosseous spread

and extrathoracic component. They are hypointense on T1W and hyperintense on T2W images, showing moderate contrast enhancement. Multiplanar imaging using MRI or CT is helpful in determining the extent of the soft tissue mass.

Chondrosarcoma

Chondrosarcoma is rare in pediatric age group, and should be differentiated from the chondroblastic variety of osteosarcoma. It predominantly involving the long bones of pelvis and shoulder girdle followed by metaphyses of long bones, ribs and spine. The tumors can either be primary or secondary. On radiographs they are usually expansile lytic lesions with variable matrix mineralization (chondroid type). On MR imaging they show low

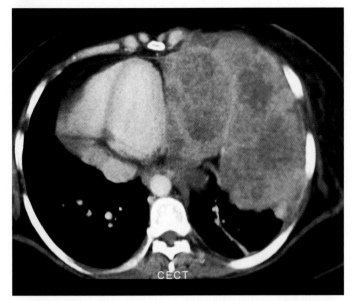

Fig. 24.9: PNET of the left thoracic wall (Askin tumor). Axial image of CECT thorax mediastinal window shows a large heterogeneous mass lesion in the left hemithorax with a small extrathoracic component

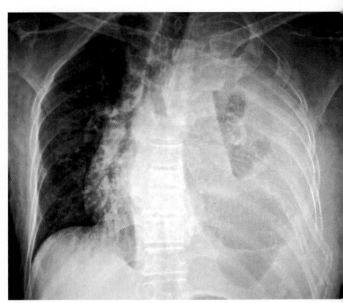

Fig. 24.10A: NHL of the left thoracic wall. Chest radiograph reveals opaque left hemithorax with lytic sclerotic destruction of left 7th and 8th ribs as well as the 8th dorsal vertebral body

signal intensity on T1W images. The signal on T2W images are variable, depending on the matrix. Cartilaginous matrix is bright on T2WI whereas areas of calcification and hemorrhage are hypointense.[25]

Lymphoma

Primary bone lymphoma comprises of 5 percent of all children with lymphoma and most of them are high grade B-cell NHL.[20] Usual locations include the spine and the long bones. On imaging, they commonly show permeative lytic destruction, sometimes with periosteal reaction and commonly associated with soft tissue component. Frank cortical destruction is often not evident, and the lesions are easily missed on radiographs.[26] Hodgkin's disease can cause sclerotic bony lesions and 'ivory' vertebra. MRI reveals the marrow of the affected bone to be hypointense on T1W and hyperintense on T2W images, enhancing after contrast (Figs 24.10A and B).

Secondary bone lymphoma is commoner than primary bone lymphoma, especially in children. The incidence can be as high as 25 percent in children. Secondary skeletal involvement in Hodgkin's disease is usually from contiguous lymph nodal spread, and the lesions are more commonly sclerotic. In secondary involvement by non-Hodgkin's lymphoma, most commonly affected sites are pelvis, spine and skull. The usual presentation is with permeative lytic destruction of bone with cortical destruction.

Metastases

Metastases to bone in pediatric age group commonly occurs from primary tumors like neuroblastoma, Ewing's sarcoma or neuroblastoma. Osseous metastases in osteosarcoma are usually blastic. Metastases from neuroblastoma show a 'sunburst' type of periosteal reaction. When occurring in the calvarium, they often give rise to sutural diastasis secondary to dural deposits.

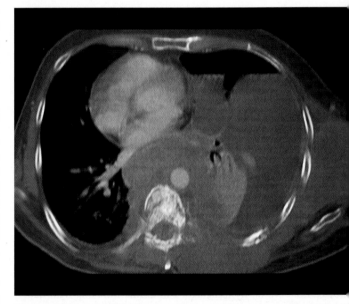

Fig. 24.10B: Axial CECT bone window of the same patient shows permeative lytic sclerotic bone destruction involving the vertebral body posterior element and the posterior ribs having a large soft tissue component in the paraspinal locations and along posterolateral thoracic wall

Malignant Fibrous Histiocytoma

Malignant fibrous histiocytoma occurs very rarely in pediatric age group, and usually affects the adolescents. Most common location includes metaphysis of a long bone. The radiographic findings range from geographic to permeative lytic destruction. Periosteal reaction is uncommon,[27] unlike other malignant tumors. MR features are non-specific.

SOFT TISSUE TUMORS

In the pediatric age group, most of the soft tissue masses are benign; only 1-6 percent being malignant.[28] Rhabdomyosarcoma alone comprises more than half of the pediatric soft tissue sarcomas.[3,4] In the 0-5 years age group, fibrosarcoma is the commonest and in 10-15 years age group, malignant fibrous histiocytoma, synovial sarcoma and rhabdomyosarcoma are common.[29] MR imaging often cannot accurately determine the benignity or malignant nature of a soft tissue mass, but some indicators which favor a benign etiology include younger age group, smaller size of the mass, well circumscribed lesion, subcutaneous or fascial location, homogeneous signal on T2W imaging and no surrounding edema.[30] Sometimes, a malignant soft tissue tumor may have well defined margins with a pseudocapsule and homogeneous in signal intensity on MRI.

The prime important role of imaging in soft tissue tumor is not to provide an accurate diagnosis but to provide information regarding the extent of tumor, extension beyond fascial planes, adjacent bone and neurovascular bundle involvement. Other important role of imaging include response assessment after treatment. Differentiating a residual or recurrent tumor from post-treatment changes is the most challenging part in follow-up imaging. Both can present with high T2W signal intensity. Tumor recurrence is often associated with mass effect and contrast enhancement; whereas post-treatment changes lack these features.[31]

Rhabdomyosarcoma

Rhabdomyosarcoma (Figs 24.11 and 24.12) accounts for 4-5% of all childhood cancers and 10-15 percent of solid tumors in the extremities.[32] The most common locations are the head and neck region, genitourinary tract, the retroperitoneum and the extremities. The histologic subtypes include embryonal, alveolar and the undifferentiated types. The alveolar subtype, which is relatively aggressive, is seen in the extremities. The prognosis of this tumor depends on the size, local invasion, nodal spread and distant metastases. Tumors with a diameter less than 5 cm has better overall prognosis. Extremity tumors, which are usually of alveolar subtype, have a poorer prognosis. Prognosis is better in case of proximal extremity tumors than distal tumors.[33] Complete resection is the treatment of choice and survival in unresectable tumors is poor.

On MR imaging, the tumor is isointense to muscle on T1W and hyperintense on T2W images and shows strong contrast enhancement.[30]

Synovial Sarcoma

Synovial sarcoma (Figs 24.13A and B) is the most common non-rhabdomyosarcomatous soft tissue sarcoma in the children. It is a high grade tumor showing differentiation of tumor cells into spindle cells resembling synoviocytes; and not derived from synovial cells. The usual location of this tumor is in periarticular regions, though it can occur in other places. These tumors commonly present as a painless extremity mass, most commonly around the knee joints. On imaging, they are well defined, lobulated in outline, isointense to muscle on T1W and heterogeneously hyperintense on T2W images, with areas of hemorrhage.[34] Scattered calcification is seen

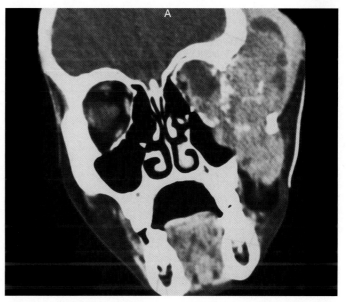

Fig. 24.11: Rhabdomyosarcoma in a child presenting with rapid onset proptosis and facial swelling. CECT orbit coronal reformatted image shows a large heterogeneously enhancing mass lesion causing destruction of the left zygoma and lateral maxillary and orbital wall

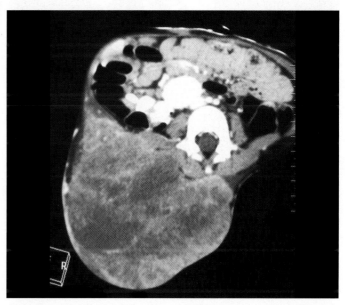

Fig. 24.12: Rhabdomyosarcoma in a child presenting with an enlarging back mass. Axial CECT abdomen shows infiltration of the mass into the paraspinal and posterior abdominal muscles on right side

in as high as one-third of the lesions.[35] Sometimes the lesions are cystic, mimicking a ganglion cyst or Baker's cyst.[28]

Other Non-rhabdomyosarcomatous Tumors

Other non rhabdomyosarcomatous tumors are rare in childhood and include fibrosarcoma, hemangiopericytoma, granulocytic sarcoma, malignant fibrous histiocytoma, epithelioid sarcoma and clear cell sarcoma.

The peak age group affected by infantile fibrosarcoma is below 5 years, specifically in infants or neonates. These are usually large

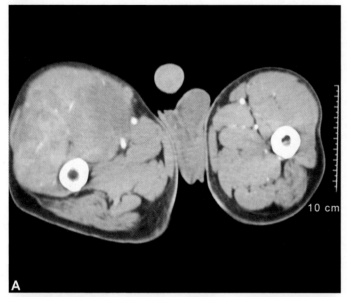

10 cm

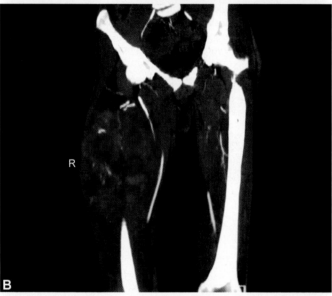

R

Figs 24.13A and B: Synovial sarcoma in a 15-year-old. CECT thigh axial soft tissue window and (A) and (B) Coronal maximum intensity projection (MIP) images show a heterogeneous mass lesion in the extensor compartment, abutting and displacing the right superficial femoral artery

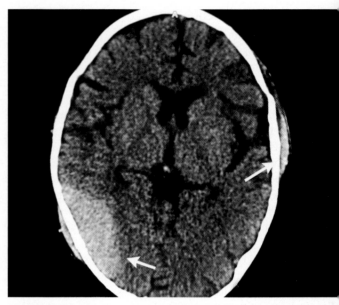

Fig. 24.14: Granulocytic sarcoma in a case of acute myeloid leukemia CECT of head reveals multiple enhancing soft tissue masses (arrows) involving the calvarium

CONCLUSION

Though the pediatric malignant bone tumors account for about 6% of all childhood malignancies, malignant soft tissue tumor are rare in childhood. The role of imaging is to assess the extent of the lesion, thus establishing the accurate stage and determining resectability. Plain radiographs are the most important tool in evaluating bone tumors. MRI offers better assessment of the bone and extraosseous extent and neurovascular involvement, the knowledge of which is crucial for surgery. CT scan of thorax and bone scans are required to determine the presence or absence of metastases.

Soft tissue lesions in childhood are usually benign. The primary role of imaging is to assess the extent in a soft tissue lesion, thus establishing the accurate stage and determining resectability.

REFERENCES

1. Wootton-Gorges SL. MR imaging of primary bone tumors and tumor-like conditions in children. Radiol Clin N Am 2009; 47:957-75.
2. Caudill JSC, Arndt CAS. Diagnosis and management of bone malignancy in adolescence. Adolesc Med 2007; 18:62-78.
3. Arndt CA, Crist WM. Common musculoskeletal tumors of childhood and adolescence. N Engl J Med 1999; 341(5):342-52.
4. Miser JS, Pizzo PA. Soft tissue sarcomas in childhood. Pediatr Clin North Am 1985; 32(3):779-800.
5. Stein-Wexler R. MR imaging of soft tissue masses in children Radiol Clin N Am 2009; 47:977-95.
6. Hoffer FA. Primary skeletal neoplasms: Osteosarcoma and Ewing sarcoma. Top Magn Reson Imaging 2002; 13:231-400.
7. Meyer JS, Nadel HR, Marina N, et al. Imaging guidelines for children with Ewing sarcoma and osteosarcoma: A report from the children's oncology group bone tumor committee. Pediatr Blood Cancer 2008; 51:63-70.

disfiguring masses, but biologic behavior is favorable than their adult counterparts. They rarely metastasize. They are isointense to muscles on T1W images and heterogeneously hyperintense on T2W images.[36] Contrast enhancement is usually heterogeneous. In older children the tumor behaves like those in adults, with a more aggressive course.[4]

Granulocytic sarcoma (also called chloroma) is seen in 5% cases of acute myeloid leukemia and contains primitive precursors of granulocytes. To begin with, they arise in bone marrow and traverses the haversian canals to extraosseous locations. The most common site in head and neck region (Fig. 24.14). They are isointense to muscle one as well as T2W images, showing homogeneous enhancement.[37]

8. Alyas F, James SL, Davies AM, et al. The role of MR imaging in the diagnostic characterization of appendicular bone tumors and tumor-like conditiond. Eur Radiol 2007; 17:2675-86.

9. Berquist TH, Ehman RL, King BF, et al. Value of MR imaging in differentiating benign from malignant soft-tissue masses: Study of 95 lesions. AJR Am J Roentgenol 1990; 155(6):1251-5.

10. Kransdorf MJ, Murphy MD. Radiologic evaluation of soft-tissue masses: A current perspective. AJR Am J Roentgenol 2000; 175(3):575-87.

11. Soler R, Castro JM, Rodriguez E. Value of MR findings in predicting the nature of soft tissue lesions: Benign, malignant or undetermined lesion? Comput Med Imaging Graph 1996; 20(3):163-9.

12. Jelinek J, Kransdorf MJ. MR imaging of soft-tissue masses. Mass like lesions that simulate neoplasma. Magn Reson Imaging Clin N Am 1995; 3(4):727-41.

13. Woude HJ, Bloem JL, Verstraete KL, Taminiau AH, et al. Osteosarcoma and Ewing's sarcoma after neoadjuvant chemotherapy: Value of dynamic MR imaging in detecting viable tumor before surgery. AJR Am J Roentgenol 1995; 165:593-98.

14. Hayashida Y, Yakushiji T, Awai K, et al. Monitoring therapeutic responses of primary bone tumors by diffusion-weighted image: initial results. Eur Radiol 2006; 16:2637-43.

15. McCarville MB. New frontiers in pediatric oncologic imaging. Cancer Imaging 2008; 8:87-92.

16. Wang C-K, Li C-W, Hsieh T-J, Chien S-H, Liu G-C, Tsai K-B. Characterization of bone and soft-tissue tumors with in vivo ^{1}H MR spectroscopy: Initial results. Radiology 2004; 232:599-605.

17. Enneking WF, Spanier SS, Goodman MA. A system for surgical staging of musculoskeletal sarcoma. Clin Orthop 1980; 153:106-20.

18. American Joint Committee on Cancer, Bone. In: Greene FL, Page DL, Fleming ID, et al, (Eds): AJCC Cancer Staging Manual. New York, NY. Springer-Verlag, 2002; 213-19.

19. Longhi A, Errani C, De Paolis M, et al. Primary bone osteosarcoma in the pediatric age: State of the art. Cancer Treat Rev 2006; 32:423-36.

20. Vlychou M, Athanasou N. Radiological and pathological diagnosis of pediatric bone tumours and tumour-like lesions. Pathology 2008; 40(2):196-216.

21. Reddick WE, Wang S, Xiong X, et al. Dynamic magnetic resonance imaging of regional contrast access as an additional prognostic factor in pediatric osteosarcoma. Cancer 2001; 91:2230-7.

22. Bacci G, Ferrari S, Bertoni F, et al. Histologic response of high-grade nonmetastatic osteosarcoma of the extremity to chemotherapy. Clin Orthop Relat Res 2001; 386:186-96.

23. Provisor AJ, Ettinger LJ,Nachman JB, et al. Treatment of nonmetastatic osteosarcoma of the extremity with preoperative and postoperative chemotherapy: A report from the Children's cancer Group. J Clin Oncol 1997; 15:76-84.

24. Peersman B, Vanhoenakcker FM, Heyman S, et al. Ewing's sarcoma: Imaging features. JBR-BTR 2007; 90:368-76.

25. Kaim AH, Hugli R, Bonel HM, et al. Chondroblastoma and clear cell chondrosarcoma: radiological and MRI characteristics with histopathological correlation. Skeletal Radiol 2002; 31:88-95.

26. Krishnan A, Shirkhoda A, Tehrznzadeh J, et al. Primary bone lymphoma: Radiographic-MR imaging correlation. Radiographics 2003; 23:1371-87.

27. Murphey MD, Gross TM, Rosenthal HG. Musculoskeletal malignant fibrous histiocytoma: Radiologic-pathologic correlation. Radiographics 1994; 14:807-26.

28. Bissett GS 3rd. MR imaging of soft-tissue masses in children. Magn Reson Imaging Clin N Am 1996; 4(4):696-719.

29. Kransdorf MJ. Malignant soft-tissue tumors in a large referral population: Distribution of diagnoses by age, sex and location. AJR Am J Roentgenol 1995; 164(1):129-34.

30. Moulton JS, Blebea JS, Dunco DM, et al. MR imaging of soft tissue masses: Diagnostic efficacy and value of distinguishing between benign and malignant lesions. AJR Am J Roentgenol 1995; 164(5):1191-9.

31. Siegel MJ. Magnetic resonance imaging of musculoskeletal soft tissue masses. Radiol Clin North Am 2001; 39(4):701-20.

32. Kim EE, Valenzuela RF, Kumar AJ, et al. Imaging and clinical spectrum of rhabdomyosarcoma in children. Clin Imaning 2000; 24(5):257-62.

33. Tabrizi P, Letts M. Childhood rhabdomyosarcoma of the trunk and extremities. Am J Orthp 1999; 28(8):440-6.

34. Jones BC, Sundaram M, Kransdorf MJ. Synovial sarcoma: MR imaging findings in 34 patients. AJR Am J Roentgenol 1993; 161(4):827-30.

35. Frassica FJ, Khanna JA, McCarthy EF. The role of MR imaging in soft tissue tumor evaluation: Perspective of the orthopaedic oncologist and musculoskeletal pathologist. Magn Reson Imaging Clin N Am 2000; 8(4):915-27.

36. Eich GF, Hoeffel JC, Tschappeler H, et al.Fibrous tumors in children: Imaging features of a heterogeneous group of disorders. Pediatr Radiol 1998; 28(7):500-09.

37. Stein-Wexler R, Wootton-Gorges SL, West DC. Orbital granulocytic sarcoma: An unusual presentation of acute myelocytic leukemia. Pediatr Radiol 2003; 33(2):136-9.

CHAPTER **25**

Congenital Brain Anomalies

N Khandelwal

INTRODUCTION

Congenital malformations of the brain are numerous with over 2000 malformations described so far. Its incidence is reported to be about 1 percent of all live births. About 60 percent of cases have no known etiology while 40 percent may have chromosomal inheritance or acquired cause. Approximately 75 percent of fetal deaths are attributed to these malformations.[1]

Congenital malformations result from abnormal formation of the brain structure during intrauterine development.[2,3] Various classifications have been proposed. Table 25.1 shows the broad subgroups.

Table 25.1: Classification of congenital brain anomalies

I. Disorders of organization
  (Due to arrest of brain development and with normal histogenesis)
  A. Supratentorial
    1. Migrational disorders
      Lissencephaly
      Hemimegalencephaly
      Heterotopias
      Schizencephaly
      Polymicrogyria
    2. Holoprosencephaly
    3. Syndrome of septo-optic dysplasia
    4. Dysgenesis of corpus callosum
    5. Hydranencephaly
  B. Infratentorial anomalies
    1. Dandy-Walker complex
    2. Cerebellar aplasia/ hypoplasia
    3. Chiari malformation
  C. Both intratentorial and supratentorial anomalies
    1. Cephalocele
    2. Arachnoid cyst

II. Disorders of Histogenesis
  (Result from persistent development of abnormal cells in the otherwise normally structured brain)
    1. Neurofibromatosis
    2. Tuberous sclerosis
    3. Sturge-Weber syndrome
    4. Von Hippel-Lindau disease
    5. Ataxia-telangiectasia

* Adapted from Byrd and Charles[2]

DISORDERS OF ORGANIZATION

Supratentorial Malformations

Migrational Disorders

Lissencephaly or smooth brain: In this condition, there i complete or partial absence of sulcation. Complete lack of gyr is termed as agyria and the presence of few, broad and flat gyr is termed as pachygyria. Patient of lissencephaly presents with dysmorphic facies, seizures, mental retardation and microcephaly Sonographic findings include a smooth surfaced cortex withou sulcal or gyral formation. Sonography can only suggest the diagnosis of lissencephaly but the characteristic findings are more readily identifiable on CT or MRI. Based on CT and MRI, three types of lissencephaly have been described:
a. Classic (type I) lissencephaly (4-layer lissencephaly)
b. Cobblestone (type II) lissencephaly (congenital muscula dystrophy) and
c. Lissencephaly not otherwise classified.

Classic lissencephaly is further divided into 3 subcategorie based on associated genetic abnormalities namely:
  i. Deletion of the LIS 1 gene on chromosome 17
  ii. An X-linked lissencephaly and
  iii. An indeterminate subset with neither of the above chromo somal abnormalities.

In classical lissencephaly,[4] the MRI features are that of a abnormal contour and surface of the brain. The cerebral surfac is smooth, devoid of sulci (agyric) or with few areas of pachygyri or with equal areas of pachygyria and agyria. The brain assume a figure of 8 appearance due to the bilateral shallow sylvia fissures. There is marked reduction in the white matter, the gra white matter interface is smooth with loss of cortical white matte distribution[5] (Figs 25.1A and B).

Hemimegalencephaly or unilateral megalencephaly: Thi condition may be idiopathic or may be associated with contralateral somatic hemihypertrophy, linear sebaceous nevu syndrome, neurofibromatosis NF1.[4] The affected cortex i typically dysplastic with broad gyri, shallow sulci and cortica thickening. Gyral pattern may appear grossly normal. It may b associated with lissencephaly or polymicrogyria. There is a indistinct differentiation between the cortex and subcortical whit matter. The ipsilateral lateral ventricle is enlarged with the fronta

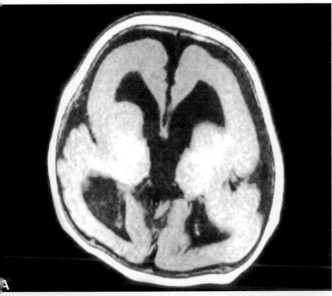

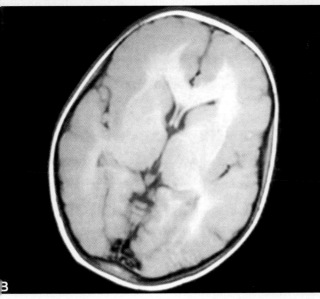

Figs 25.1A and B: Lissencephaly: Short TR axial MR sections in two patients showing the shallow sylvian fissures giving a figure of eight configuration of the cerebral hemispheres. Note the thickened cortex better delineated in B

horn directed anterosuperiorly (Figs 25.2A to C). Rarely brain has a bizarre, hamartomatous appearance.

Heterotopias: Heterotopias are the least severe of all the migrational disorders. The term denotes presence of normal neural tissue at an abnormal location secondary to arrest of neuronal migration along the radial glial fibers.[4] The abnormally located gray matter is isointense with cortical gray matter in all MR imaging sequences and this is a diagnostic feature. Heterotopias are of two types: the common, nodular type (Figs 25.3A and B) is characterized by multiple masses of gray matter which are of variable size. They are commonly located in the subependymal region of the lateral ventricles or in the subcortical white matter. The second type is the uncommon band or lamellar heterotopia

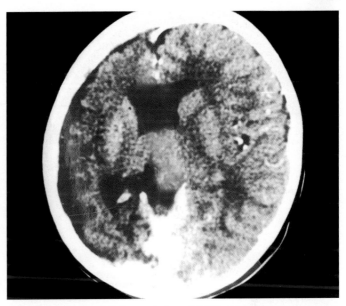

Fig. 25.2A: Hemimegalencephaly: axial CT scan shows overgrowth of the left hemisphere giving asymmetrical appearance of the brain

(double cortex) (Figs 25.3C and D) which appears as a homogeneous gray matter band between the cerebral cortex and the lateral ventricle. It is characteristically surrounded by a zone of white matter. The cortex overlying the heterotopia is nearly always abnormal with pachygyria or polymicrogyria.

Schizencephaly or split brain: It is a form of migrational disorder characterized by abnormal columns of gray matter across the cerebral hemisphere. The basic abnormality is a pial-ependymal seam (gray matter lined cleft) which extends across full thickness of cerebral hemisphere from the ventricular system (ependyma) to the periphery (pial surface) of the brain. These clefts are usually perisylvian but can occur anywhere in the brain. Two types have been described:

- Type I or closed lip schizencephaly is characterized by a gray matter lined pial ependymal seam with both the lips apposed to each other. There is no intervening CSF cavity. The common site of involvement is the roof or lateral borders of lateral ventricle. MR or CT scan will show an outpouching or nipple at the ependymal surface of the cleft in closed lip schizencephaly. MRI demonstrates the full thickness of cleft and the pial-ependymal seam of gray matter (Figs 25.4A and B).

- Type II or open lip schizencephaly in which the pial ependymal seam is widened by a CSF cleft. CT and MRI shows the CSF cleft extending from the ventricular system to the pial surface of brain. The CSF cavity is usually bilateral and symmetric. However, it may be asymmetric or even unilateral. Severe form of open lip schizencephaly presents with massive CSF cavities which communicate with the ventricular system and has an appearance which is a called "basket brain". This congenital malformation has a high association with absence of septum pellucidum, polymicrogyria, septo-optic dysplasia, heterotopia[4] (Figs 25.4C and D).

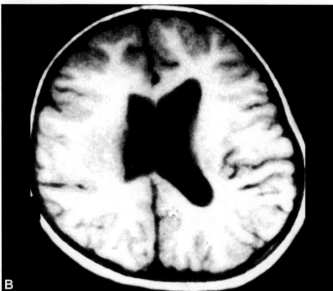

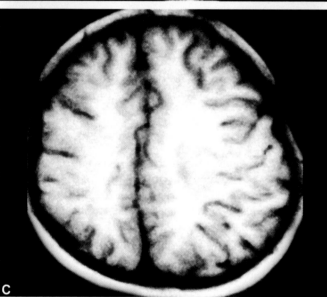

Figs 25.2B and C: Hemimegalencephaly: T1W1 shows unilateral megalencephaly with a larger left hemisphere. Note the larger left lateral ventricle (B) and the prominent sulcation of that hemisphere (C)

Holoprosencephaly

Holoprosencephaly is a congenital malformation characterized by incomplete cleavage and differentiation of the prosencephalon (forebrain) into cerebral hemispheres. Mutation of at least 4 different genetic loci have been identified to be associated with this condition and these are on chromosome 21, 2, 7 and 18. Syndromic association of this condition are encountered in trisomy 13 (Patau's syndrome) and trisomy 18 (Edwards' syndrome). Embryogenesis of holoprosencephaly is postulated to be the lack of mesenchyme in the developing rostral neural tube, as a result of which the telencephalon does not separate from the diencephalon. The telencephalon does not develop in the two hemispheres and there is lack of cortical organization.[6]

There are three types of holoprosencephaly—alobar, semilobar and lobar. Prenatal ultrasound, and postnatal CT or MR can image the confluent ventricles and thalami adequately:

a. Alobar holoprosencephaly is the most severe form of holoprosencephaly. There is no differentiation of the frontal, occipital or temporal lobes. The cerebral hemispheres are fused to form a small flat mass of tissue containing single crescent shaped holoventricle. The flattened cerebrum occupies a small rostral segment of the calvarium. The calvarium is occupied with the large dorsal cyst which communicates with the holoventricle. Thalami may be fused with absence of interhemispheric fissure, falx cerebri and septum pellucidum. The cerebellum and brainstem are relatively normal. This condition is associated with a severely dysmorphic facies, abnormal reflexes and increased tone at birth.

b. Semilobar holoprosencephaly (Fig. 25.5A) is a less severe form of holoprosencephaly. There is partial separation of the cerebral hemispheres with rudimentary temporal and occipital lobes. The frontal lobes are fused. There is a monoventricle with presence of the falx cerebri which is only partially seen posteriorly and suggestion of presence of an interhemispheric fissure. Septum pellucidum is absent and thalami are partially separated. The splenium of the corpus callosum is formed without the genu or body (Fig. 25.5A).

c. Lobar holoprosencephaly (Fig. 25.5B) is the least severe form. Brain appears normal but the frontal horns remain fused with absence of septum pellucidum. Appearance of the frontal horns with angular corners is termed "box-like". Temporal and occipital horns are separated and are of normal size and shape. However, the bodies of the lateral ventricles may be closely apposed. Interhemispheric fissure is formed but is shallow anteriorly. The thalami are separated.

Septo-optic Dysplasia

Septo-optic dysplasia is believed to be a mild form of lobar holoprosencephaly and consists of absence of septum pellucidum with hypoplasia of the optic nerve and optic chiasma and hypoplasia of the hypothalamus. MRI shows these findings with clarity. In addition abnormally squared or flattened frontal horns of the lateral ventricles and an enlarged anterior recess of the third ventricle may be seen. It may be associated with aqueductal stenosis, Chiari II malformation, schizencephaly, and corpus callosum agenesis. In addition, an association of hypothalamus-pituitary dysfunction is seen in two-thirds of the patients with this condition.[7]

Dysgenesis of Corpus Callosum

The corpus callosum is a midline commissure that crosses from one cerebral hemisphere to the other. The corpus callosum develops in the cephalocaudal direction with the genu developing at 2.5 months of gestation followed by the body and splenium. The rostrum is the last to develop. Adult configuration is achieved by 5th month of gestation.[8] In corpus callosum agenesis, genu is usually present but body and splenium are dysgenic.

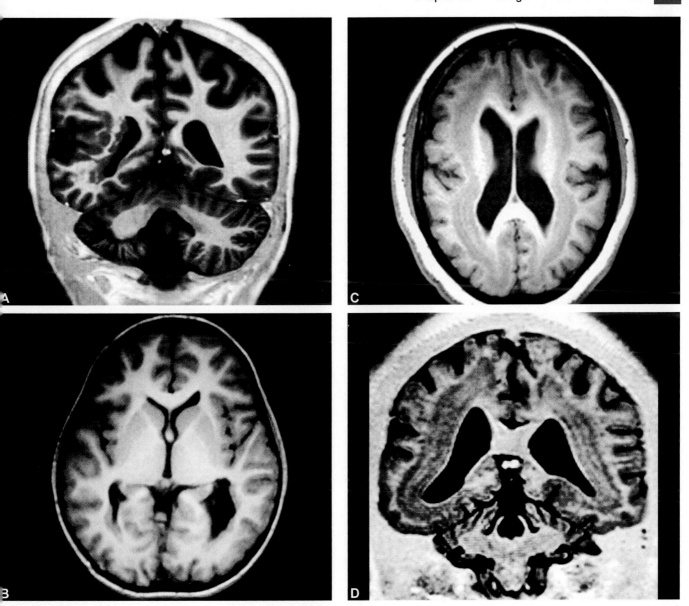

Figs 25.3A and B: Nodular heterotopia: Coronal IR (A) and axial T1W (B) images showing undulating layer of gray matter lining the lateral ventricles

Figs 25.3C and D: Lamellar heterotopia: Axial T1 WI (A) and coronal IR image (B) shows a band of gray matter in the periventricular region which is isointense with the cortex

Diagnostic features on imaging are parallel nonconverging lateral ventricles, dilated occipital horns (colpocephaly) (Fig. 25.6). The third ventricle is widended and is placed between the lateral ventricles. If the dilated third ventricle reaches the interhemispheric fissure it is referred to as dorsal interhemispheric cyst (Fig. 25.6B). Midsagittal MR scan readily demonstrates absence of the corpus callosum. Cingulate sulcus is absent and the gyri appear to radiate from a high riding third ventricle (Fig. 25.6D). Presence of Probst bundle (longitudinally oriented tracts) cause indentation on the medial aspect of the lateral ventricles which appear concave medially on coronal MR sections.[2]

Coexisting congenital malformations are common which include Dandy-Walker complex, arachnoid cyst, cephalocele and colobomas. Aicardi syndrome is association of corpus callosum agenesis, infantile spasms and ocular abnormalities and is especially seen in females.[2,5]

Hydranencephaly

Hydranencephaly is an encephaloclastic porencephaly which results presumably secondary to *in utero* occlusion of either of the internal carotid arteries, or infection such as CMV or due to a genetic cause. This results in infarction, necrosis and destruction of the cerebral cortex. The cerebral hemispheres are replaced by a thin-walled membranous sac which is lined by glial tissue on the inside and leptomeninges on the outside. Diagnosis on ultrasound is easy as the falx cerebri, thalami and cerebellar hemispheres are identified in the presence of the two large fluid-filled sacs.[2]

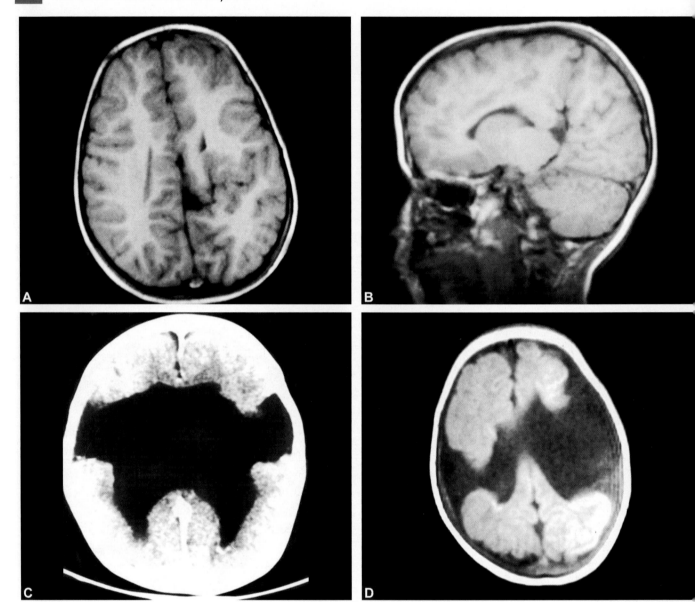

Figs 25.4A to D: Schizencephaly: *Closed lip*: Axial (A) and sagittal (B) T1 W MR sections show deep extension of cerebral sulci reaching up t the ventricle with gray matter lining. *Open lip* : Axial CT (B) and T1 MR (D) sections show bilateral CSF clefts communicating with the latera ventricles

Differential diagnosis includes severe hydrocephalus, in which a rind of remaining cortical mantle can be identified, and alobar holoprosencephaly where absence of falx and presence of fused thalami clinches the diagnosis. CT or MRI may be done when US findings are equivocal (Figs 25.7A and B).

Infratentorial Malformations

Dandy-Walker (DW) complex: This includes Dandy-Walker malformation, Dandy-Walker variant and the mega cisterna magna.[9]

This represents the morphological spectrum of fundamental anomalous cerebellar vermis and adjacent cerebellar hemispheres. The cerebellar vermis is usually hypoplastic with atresia of the outlet of fourth ventricle, resulting in abnormal dilatation of 4th ventricle with expansion of posterior fossa (Fig. 25.8). There i consequently superior displacement of the tentorium and dura sinuses.

Skull radiographs show expansion of posterior cranial foss thinning and ballooning of occipital bone and upward dis placement of lateral sinus groove which indicates elevation c tentorium.

Sonographic features of Dandy-Walker complex includ anechoic posterior fossa cyst, small cerebellar hemisphere: elevated tentorium and hydrocephalus.

CT and MRI are helpful to show the structures in their prop perspective. Multiplanar imaging of MRI is superior to CT f demonstrating the anatomy. Diagnostic criteria of DW comple on CT/MR are as follows:

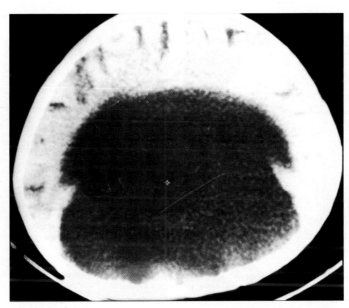

Fig. 25.5A: Semilobar holoprosencephaly: Axial CT section shows a monoventricle with a dorsal cyst and partially formed temporal lobes

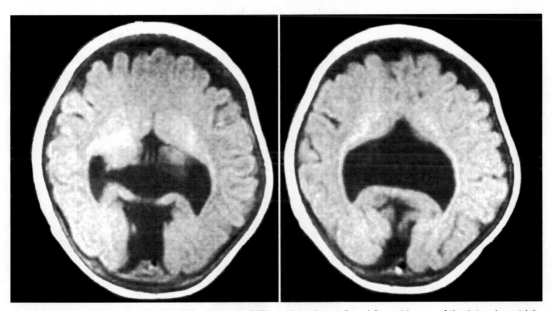

Fig. 25.5B: Lobar holoprocencephaly: Axial short TR sequence MR section shows fused frontal horns of the lateral ventricles. The cerebral hemisphere are well formed however the anterior interhemispheric fissure is partially delineated

a. Dandy-Walker malformation is characterized by absence of or hypoplasia of the cerebellar vermis. There is associated hypoplasia of the cerebellar hemispheres giving a characteristic winged appearance to these hemispheres. The fourth ventricle is enlarged and opens dorsally into a CSF containing cyst. The posterior fossa is enlarged with a high insertion of the tentorium consequently the transverse sinuses are higher in position than normal. Eighty percent of patients have associated hydrocephalus. Associated anomalies include corpus callosum agenesis (20-25%), heterotopias, poly-microgyria, occipital cephaloceles and schizencephaly.[9]

b. In Dandy-Walker variant, there is varying degree of inferior vermian and cerebellar hypoplasia. The retrocerebellar CSF collection communicates with normal or mildly enlarged 4th ventricle via a prominent vallecula. The tentorial position and size of posterior fossa are normal. Coronal images through posterior fossa may show absence of the vermis. The brainstem is usually normal and hydrocephalus is an uncommon association.[7,8]

c. Mega cisterna magna is a large subarachnoid cistern lying posterior to the vermis and can extend all the way up to the straight sinus superiorly and the C1-C2 level inferiorly. It may cause scalloping of the inner table of occipital squama, without any compression of the fourth ventricle. One of the differential diagnosis is a retrocerebellar arachnoid cyst, which is a CSF collection within the layers of arachnoid membrane

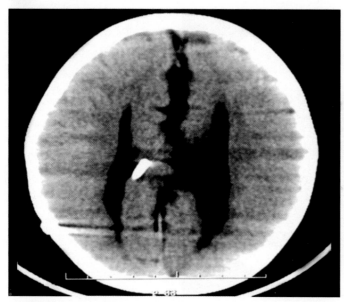

Fig. 25.6A: Corpus collosum agenesis: Axial CT sections show parallel configuration of the lateral ventricles. Absence of the corpus callosum leads to separation of the interhemispheric fissure. A shunt has been placed in the right lateral ventricle

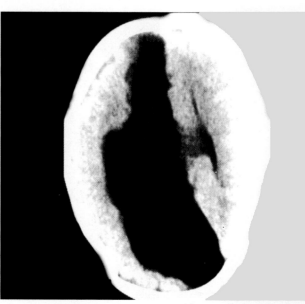

Fig. 25.6B: Corpus callosum agenesis associated with an interhemispheric cyst which extends across the midline

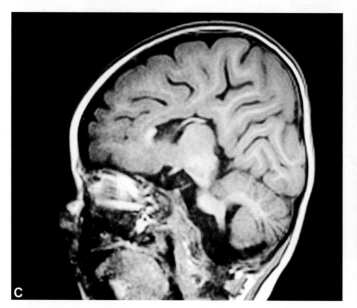

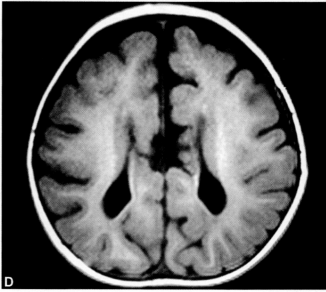

Figs 25.6C and D: Corpus callosum agenesis: T1 W sagittal and axial images depicting partial corpus callosum agenesis with parallel alignment of lateral ventricles (colpocephaly) and radiating pattern of cerebral gyri

and does not communicate fully with the subarachnoid or ventricular spaces. The posterior fossa and ventricular system are normal. The fourth ventricle and vermis may be displaced by the cyst.

The Chiari Malformations

There are four Chiari malformations[10] which represent a spectrum of anomalies of primary neurulation, i.e. those which occur when the brain and upper spine are developing at about 3 to 4 weeks of gestation.

Chiari I malformation (caudal-cerebellar tonsillar ectopia consists of herniation of elongated peg like cerebellar tonsil through the foramen magnum into the upper cervical spinal cana

Chiari's original description of this anomaly included associate hydrocephalus, though it is not mandatory for the diagnosis to b made.[11] Tonsillar descent has been described in four categorie of Chiari I malformation.[4]

1. This malformation can be associated with abnorma intracranial pressure. Intracranial hypotension due to chron CSF leaks or associated with CSF shunts can result in 'saggin

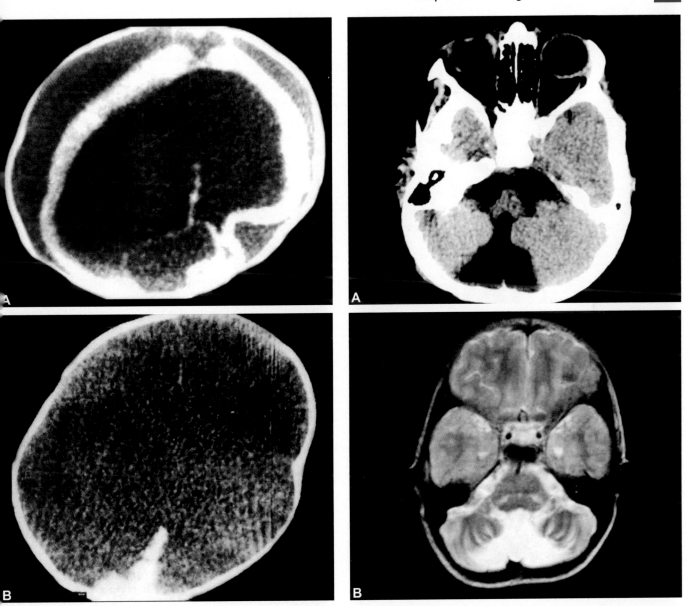

Figs 25.7A and B: Hydranencephaly vs congenital hydrocephalus: Axial CT section (A) shows presence of a preserved cortical mantle with interhemispheric fissure. Bilateral subdural collection favor the diagnosis of hydrocephalus. In hydranencephaly the brain is replaced by a fluid filled sac (B). No cortical mantle is identified

Figs 25.8A and B: Dandy-Walker malformation: Absent vermis with the fourth ventricle communicating directly with a posterior fossa cyst; winged cerebellar hemispheres are characteristic of this malformation

brain'. Raised intracranial tension due to cerebral edema or intracranial masses can push the tonsils downwards.

2. Chiari I malformation can be seen with platybasia or basilar invagination or craniovertebral anomalies such as persistence of proatlas remnants, shortened clivus and C-1 assimilation.

3. Prenatal or postnatal hydrocephalus can result in Chiari 1 malformation, this subset was included in the original description of the malformation.

4. Asymptomatic tonsillar ectopia with no obvious abnormality has been described and may be congenital. The degree of tonsillar descent is of some importance. Descent less than 5 mm below a line from the basion to the opisthion is considered to be of no clinical significance whereas tonsillary

descent more than 6 mm can be associated with clinical symptoms. Correlation between age of the patient and tonsillar descent is also important. Between the age of 5 to 15 years descent of up to 6 mm is not considered pathologic. In older individuals protrusion more than 5 mm below the foramen magnum is invariably associated with an increasing incidence of symptoms. Association of syringomyelia is another important aspect of Chiari I malformation.[12] The incidence reported varies between 25-65 percent. The focus on MR studies which is the mainstay of diagnosis of this condition is to show the degree of tonsillar herniation in midsagittal section, evaluation of the craniovertebral junction, assessment of the lateral ventricles for hydrocephalus and to detect

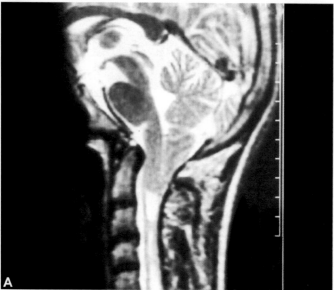

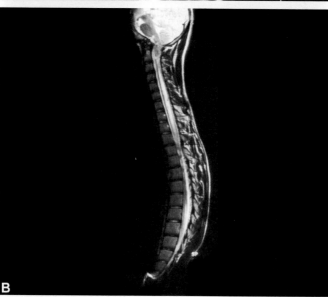

Figs 25.9A and B: Chiari I malformation: Midline sagittal long TR MR section (A) showing herniation of the cerebellar tonsil below the foramen magnum. Sagittal MR section of the whole spine (B) shows presence of the associated syrinx of the cervical and dorsal segments of the spinal cord

presence of syrinx in the upper cervical spine. MR CSF flow studies show increased motion of the tonsil and brainstem and decreased CSF flow to the vallecula[13] (Figs 25.9A and B).

Chiari II malformation is characterized by caudal displacement of the brainstem and inferior part of cerebellum into the upper cervical spinal canal. All patients of Chiari II malformations have a lumbar meningomyelocele. They nearly always develop hydrocephalus after closure of the meningomyelocele for which they are initially imaged when the lesions of the Chiari II malformation are detected.[1] These patients can present with epilepsy (17%), dysphagia, apnoeic spells, shoulder or arm weakness, weak cry or stridor. The hind

brain malformations have been best explained in a theory by McLone and Knepper[14] who have postulated that the basic anomaly is a small posterior fossa into which a normal sized cerebellum develops. Lack of space within the posterior fossa together with a low lying tentorium forces the brainstem and cerebellum through the enlarged foramen magnum.

Sagittal MR scan shows stretching of the pons inferiorly. It is compressed anteroposteriorly. The medulla is pushed inferiorly through the widened foramen. The cervical spinal cord is in turn stretched inferiorly as well. Caudal displacement of the cervical cord is restricted by the dentate ligaments. Therefore, there is kink at the junction of the displaced medulla at the cervicomedullary junction. In severe cases, the cerebellum may wrap around the brainstem. The fourth ventricle is vertically oriented, compressed and displaced inferiorly. The vermis herniates and may be compressed by the superior arch of the C1. The herniated and compressed vermis may degenerate. In severe cases the whole of the cerebellum may atrophy. Beaking of the quadrigeminal plate is probably secondary to the compression by the expanded temporal lobes due to hydrocephalus. Isolation of the fourth ventricle may occur due to aqueductal narrowing and diminished flow through the fourth ventricular outflow foramina. Paradoxically, the fourth ventricle is not dilated, however, the supratentorial ventricles will dilate. In these patients, attempt should be made to look for the presence of syringohydromyelia. Chiari II malformation can be associated with corpus callosum agenesis, enlarged massa intermedia, fenestrated falx cerebri, an abnormal gyral pattern on the medial aspect of the occipital lobe termed as stenogyria.[4]

The Chiari III malformation includes the feature of the Chiari II malformation with a low occipital or high cervical encephalocele. The encephalocele contains occipital lobes, part of the cerebellum and occasionally medulla and pons.

The Chiari IV malformation includes severe cerebellar hypoplasia or absent cerebellum. There is a large posterior fossa CSF space. There is no obstructive hydrocephalus.

Detailed evaluations using current imaging methods have introduced more subtle forms of the malformation, currently named as Chiari 0 and Chiari 1.5 which are characterized by altered CSF flow dynamics.[8]

Supra-and Infratentorial Malformations

Cephalocele is a term given to herniation of intracranial content through defects in the skull.[15] If the herniated contents are leptomeninges and CSF, the cephalocele is termed as a meningocele. When one contains brain tissue, leptomeninges and CSF, it is called a meningoencephalocele. Herniation of meninges, brain and ventricles is termed encephalocysto-meningocele. Herniation of intracranial contents occurring through fracture (growing fracture) or through surgical defect is an acquired cephalocele.

In South-east Asia the commonest cephaloceles encountered in clinical practice are nasal encephaloceles. Occipital (70%) parietal (10%) frontal (9%) and nasopharyngeal (1%) are the commonest types of encephaloceles encountered in North America and Europe.[2]

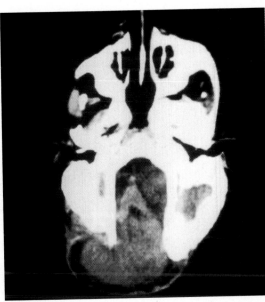 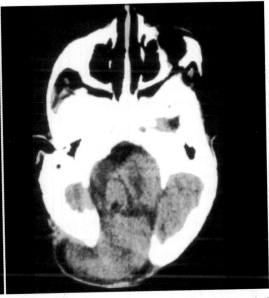

Fig. 25.10A: Occipital encephocele: Axial CT section shows a defect in the occipital bone with protrusion of the right cerebellar hemisphere through the defect

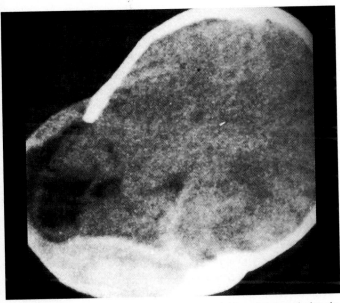

Fig. 25.10B: Parietal cephalocele: A large right parietal cephalocele containing brain matter, CSF and ectatic enhanced dura

On plain radiograph defects in the calvarium associated with cephaloceles appear well defined with sclerotic margins. If the protrusion of the brain content is large, there is a reduction in the craniofacial ratio.

Cross-sectional imaging is necessary to define the contents of the cephalocele. Sonography is a valuable mode of investigation in the prenatal diagnosis of cephaloceles. It can also differentiate whether the cephalocele contains CFS alone or CSF with brain matter. The former appears anechoic and the latter as a complex mass. CT demonstrates the extent of bony defect as well as contents of the cephalocele. MR is the most sensitive and accurate modality to detect and characterise the cephalocele. In addition multiplanar acquisition helps in the assessment of location of the cephelocele. MR venography is useful to assess the position of superior sagittal sinus and torcular herophili as they may herniate into parietal or occipital encephocele.

Frontoethmoidal cephaloceles lie between the nasal and ethmoid bones. They are not associated with neural tube defects.

Nasal encephalocele is formed when there is failure of closure of the dural diverticulum in the prenasal space. This diverticulum connects the superficial ectoderm of the developing nose to the developing brain with the cranium. Thus, there can be a large patent opening through which brain matter can herniate or there can be a sinus tract, i.e. dermal sinus or sequestration of heterotopic or dysplastic glial tissue resulting in the so-called nasal glioma. Thus, these lesions appear as soft tissue masses and CSF collections which appear in continuum with intracranial structures. Absence of the crista galli is a constant feature of a cephalocele, alternatively, it can be split by the presence of a dermal sinus or dermoid in this location. Coronal CT scaning is partially useful in demonstrating the bony defects within location.

Occipital encephalocele originates between foramen magnum and lambda. It contains variable amount of brain matter which is usually gliotic and non-functional. Association with Chiari II and III malformation is common (Fig. 25.10A).

Parietal cephalocele arises between bregma and lambda. Associated anomalies include corpus callosum agenesis, Chiari II malformation and Dandy-Walker complex (Fig. 25.10B). Encephaloceles involving the sphenoid bone are further classified as transsphenoid, transsellar sphenoidal, sphenoethmoidal, sphenomaxillary, spheno-orbital and transethmoidal encephaloceles. These are occult cephalocele with patients presenting with hypertelorism, endocrine dysfunction and mental retardation. They are associated with true clefts of the lip and nose. These cephaloceles protrude through the body of the sphenoid into the nasal cavity or in severe cases, through the palate into the oral cavity. They invariably contain parts of the hypothalamus, pituitary gland and the third ventricle.[16]

DISORDERS OF HISTOGENESIS

"Neurocutaneous syndromes" or "Phakomatoses" constitute a group of congenital malformations which are characterized by cutaneous lesions associated with CNS anomalies.[17]

Prominent amongst these are:
1. Neurofibromatosis/von Recklinghausen's disease.
2. Tuberous sclerosis/Bourneville disease
3. Sturge-Weber syndrome.
4. von Hippel-Lindau disease
5. Ataxia telangiectasia.

Neuroimaging studies are important in the diagnosis of these conditions because based on clinical presentations there are specific diagnostic imaging features in many of the conditions. The diagnosis can almost always be made on MRI because it can differentiate gray and white matter, characterize tumors from hamartomas, show extent of soft tissue lesions through bony defect and to some extent differentiate various vascular anomalies associated with these conditions.[15,16]

Neurofibromatosis

Neurofibromatosis comprises of a group of heterogeneous diseases which have been classified into two groups: Neurofibromatosis 1 (NF 1) and Neurofibromatosis 2 (NF 2).

Neurofibromatosis type 1 (NF 1) accounts for 90 percent of cases of neurofibromatosis with an incidence of 1: 2000 to 3000 live births. This autosomal dominant condition occurs due to mutation on the long arm of chromosome 17. The condition is of variable expression and high penetrance. Inactivation of the tumor repressor gene or NF 1 gene is thought to be the genetic basis of the disease. Diagnosis of NF1 is made when two or more of the following findings are present:[18,19]
- Six or more café-au-lait spots measuring 5 mm or more in largest diameter in pre-pubertal children or 15 mm or more in the post-pubertal period.
- One plexiform neurofibroma or two or more neurofibromas of any type.
- Two or more pigmented hamartomas (Lisch nodules) of the iris.
- Optic nerve glioma
- A distinctive osseous lesion such as dysplasia of the sphenoidal wing.
- Axillary or inguinal freckling
- A first degree relative with NF 1.

Optic pathway glioma is the most common CNS lesion in NF1. It is best imaged by MRI which delineates the entire extent of the lesion from the optic nerve, chiasma, optic tract, optic radiation and the lateral geniculate bodies although latter three structures are rarely involved. It is a low grade pilocytic astrocytoma. On MR scan it appears a fusiform lesion which is hypo to iso-intense on T1WI with variable contrast enhancement. The optic canal is enlarged. Other gliomas associated with NF1 involve the brainstem, tectum and periaqueductal white matter.

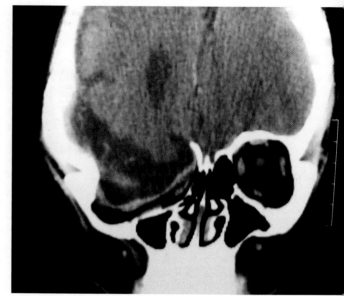

Fig. 25.11: Neurofibromatosis Type 1: Non-contrast coronal CT showing sphenoid wing dysplasia with intraorbital herniation of the dura

Plexiform neurofibroma is a hallmark of NF1. It is an unencapsulated neurofibroma along the path of a major cutaneous nerve, of the scalp and neck. The commonly involved nerve is the first division of the trigeminal nerve. It is invariably associated with dysplasia of the sphenoid bone and bony orbit (Fig. 25. 11A) On CT scan this lesion appears as low attenuating lesion which generally do not enhance. On MR T1WI they are isointense to muscle and show variable enhancement after contrast administration.

Other intracranial lesions include hamartoma, astrocytic proliferation of the retina, intracranial aneurysms, non-aneurysmal vascular ectasias and a progressive cerebral arterial occlusive disease akin to moya-moya pattern.[2]

Skeletal dysplasias that may occur include calvarial defects, hypoplasia of the sphenoid wing, scoliosis, scalloping the posterior aspects of the vertebral bodies with hypoplasia of the pedicles, spinous and lateral processes. Dural dysplasia and lateral/anterior intrathoracic meningoceles are other associated anomalies.[2,16]

Neurofibromatosis type 2 (NF-2) is an autosomal dominant entity which is associated with defect in the chromosome 22. Bilateral acoustic nerve schwannomas are the most consistent and hence diagnostic feature of this condition (Figs 25.11A to 25.12B).

Cutaneous manifestations include neurofibroma and pale café au lait spots. Skin lesions appear in the first decade of life which are followed by development of acoustic neuromas between the age of 10-15 years. Presence of cataracts and skin lesions in a child are valuable clinical indicators of NF-2.

The diagnostic criteria[20] for NF-2 include
1. Bilateral eighth nerve schwannoma
2. A first degree relative with NF-2 and
   a. A unilateral eighth nerve acoustic schwannoma or

b. Two of the following
  • Neurofibroma
  • Meningioma
  • Glioma
  • Schwannoma
  • Juvenile posterior subcapsular opacity or
  • Cerebral calcification
3. Two of the following
  • Unilateral vestibular schwannoma
  • Multiple meningiomas
  • Features listed under 2b above (Except for meningiomas).

Apart from VIIIth nerve schwannoma, the trigeminal nerve, oculomotor nerve, trochlear or the abducens nerve schwannoma are also seen in NF-2. These tend to be isodense to hypodense on CT and shows patchy but significant enhancement after contrast administration.

On MR studies schwannoma appear as well delineated masses which are iso-hyperintense on T2WI. Intense patchy enhancement occurs after gadolinium administration. Other forms of neurofibromatosis have been described. They have been labelled as NF 3 to NF 7. An eighth category NF-NOS includes cases which are atypical and do not fit into the labelled categories.[19,20] Details of these form of neurofibromatosis are beyond the scope of this chapter.

Tuberous sclerosis (TS) is an inherited autosomal dominant condition with a low penetrance. The locus of this condition is identified on two chromosomes. The TSC1 gene is localized to chromosome 9q34 and the TSC2 gene is localized to chromosome 5p13.3 which are associated with hamartoma formations in multiple organ systems.[21] The classical triad of papular facial lesions (adenoma sebaceum), seizure disorder and mental retardation are the hallmark of this disease.[16]

Subependymal hamartomas are the hallmark of tuberous sclerosis. They are located on the ventricular surface of caudate nucleus, immediately posterior to the foramen of Monro and along the frontal and temporal horns of the lateral ventricles. On MR they protrude into the adjacent ventricle. They are hyperintense on T1WI they appear hyper- and hypointense on T2 WI relation to gray and white matter. They show minimal contrast enhancement (Fig. 25.13).

Subependymal giant cell astrocytoma (SGCA) are benign tumors associated with TS usually located at the foramen of Monro in about 15 percent. They are hypo to isointense on T1WI and hyperintense on T2WI and enhance uniformly after contrast administration. Cerebral hamartomas are most characteristic. They are low attenuating on CT and with age become calcified. White matter low attenuating, well defined lesions are highly characteristic lesions of TS. Like NF 2, retinal hamartoma, aneurysm and vascular dysplasia have also been described with tuberous sclerosis.[2,16]

Sturge-Weber syndrome (encephalotrigeminal angiomatosis) is a congenital non-inherited entity. It is a syndrome characterized by angiomatous malformation affecting the skin, eye and brain. The typical lesion is a facial angioma (port wine stain) in the

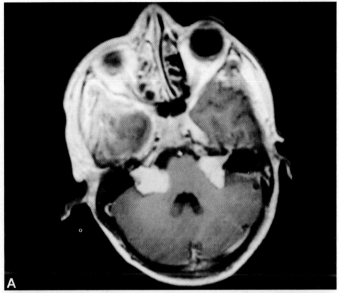

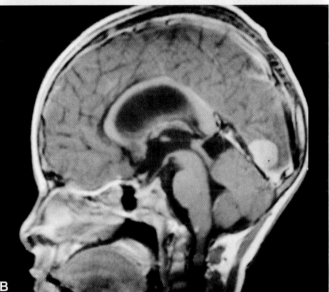

Figs 25.12A and B: Neurofibromatosis Type 2: Contrast enhanced axial T1 section (A) shows enhancing CP angle masses with intracanalicular extension consistent with B/L acoustic schwannomas (A). The enhancing tentorial based lesion is a meningioma (B)

distribution of all the divisions of the trigeminal nerve. It is usually unilateral and there is concomitant involvement of the ipsilateral occipital lobe, parietal lobes, and choroid plexus. Ocular findings of buphthalmos, optic atrophy, iris heterochromia and strabismus may be encountered. Patients may present with hemiparesis, homonymous hemianopia and seizures.

The vascular malformations are low-pressure, slowly-flowing leptomeningeal angiomata. There is a congenital absence of cortical veins, therefore the blood is shunted towards the hypertrophied deep medullary veins and thence to the choroid plexus. The relatively static venous flow leads to hypoxia of the affected cortex which inturn leads to cortical atrophy and dystrophic calcification (Fig. 25.14) which can be demonstrated

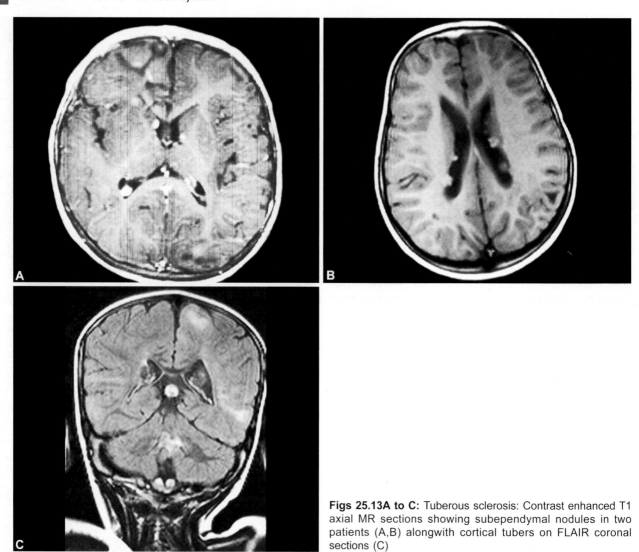

Figs 25.13A to C: Tuberous sclerosis: Contrast enhanced T1 axial MR sections showing subependymal nodules in two patients (A,B) alongwith cortical tubers on FLAIR coronal sections (C)

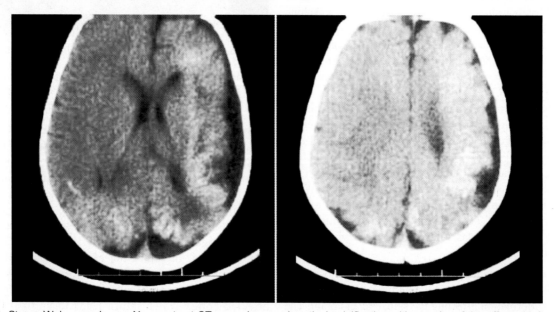

Fig. 25.14: Sturge-Weber syndrome: Non-contrast CT scan shows subcortical calcification with atrophy of the affected left parietal and occipital lobes. Calcification is also present in the right occipital lobe

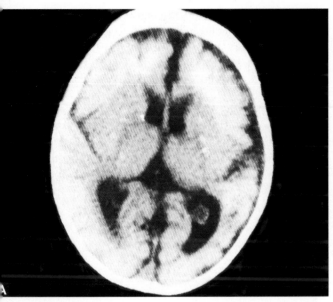
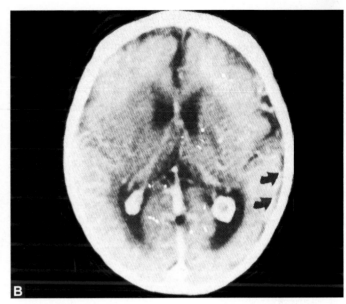

Figs 25.15A and B: Sturge Weber syndrome: A 4-year-old presented with a nevus flammeus on the left half of face. (A) Contrast enhanced CT shows diffuse cortical calcification on both frontal lobes and atrophy of left temporal and occipital lobe. (B) Enhancement of prominent choroid plexus and temporal angioma (curved arrows) can be appreciated

In plain X-ray and CT. The resulting curvilinear calcification is diagnostic of the syndrome. It is commonly seen in the occipital and posterior parietal lobe on the side of the facial angioma. If there is extensive atrophy, there is marked dilatation of the ipsi-ventricle, thickening of the calvarium and prominence of the ipsilateral paranasal sinuses which are obvious on plain radiograph. The ipsilateral choroid plexus is enlarged and may contain cysts and enhance intensely. The pial angiomas can show enhancement on both MR and CT (Fig. 25.15).[22] The abnormal venous channels of the cortex and subependymal location can be identified on angiograms or MRI.

Thus, congenital malformations of the CNS includes a large number of diverse conditions. CT and especially MRI has a very important role to play in characterizing the lesions which help in establishing the diagnosis. MR imaging has been used extensively in recent years to investigate the neuroanatomical basis of congenital brain malformations. Newer techniques like diffusion imaging including diffusion tensor imaging (DTI) and high angular resolution diffusion imaging (HARDI) have helped in fiber tractography and have elucidated the aberrant connectivity underlying a number of congenital brain malformations.[23] They however still remain in the research arena and will take time to come to the clinical field.

REFERENCES

1. Osborn AG. Brain development and congenital malformation. In Osborn AG (Ed): Diagnostic Neuroradiology St Louis: Mosby Year Book 1994; 3-116.
2. Byrd SE, Charles RF. Congenital brain malformations. In Khun JP, Slovis TL, Haller JO (Eds): Caffey's Pediatric Diagnostic Imaging (10th edn). St. louis: Mosby Year Book 2004; 506-29.
3. Barkovich AJ, Kuzhiecky RI, Dobyns WB, et al. A classification scheme for malformations and cortical development. Neuropediatrics 1996; 27:59-63.
4. Abdel Razek AA, Kandell AY, Elsorogy LG, Elmongy A, Basett AA. Disorders of cortical formation: MR imaging features. AJNR Am J Neuroradiol 2009; 30:4-11.
5. Robertson R, Casuso PA, Truwit CL. Disorders of brain development. In Atlas SW (Ed): Magnetic Resonance Imaging of the Brain. Philadelphia: Lippincott Williams and Wilkins 2002; 279-369.
6. Hahn JS, Barnes PD. Neuroimaging advances in holoprosencephaly: Refining the spectrum of the midline malformation. Am J Med Genet C Semin Med Genet 2010; 15:120-32.
7. Morishima A, Aranoff G. Syndrome of septo-optic pituitary dysplasia: The clinical spectrum brain dev 1986; 8:233-35.
8. Paul LK, Brown WS, Adolphs R, Tyszka JM, Richards LJ, Mukherjee P, Sherr EH. Agenesis of the corpus callosum: genetic, developmental and functional aspects of connectivity. Nat Rev Neurosci 2007; 8:287-99.
9. Altman N, Naidich T, Braffman B. Posterior fossa malformation AJNR Am J Neuroradiology 1992; 13:691-724.
10. Vannemreddy P, Nourbakhsh A, Willis B, Guthikonda B. Congenital Chiari malformations. Neurol India 2010; 58(1):6-14.
11. Kollias S, Ball W, Prenger E. Cystic malformations of the posterior fossa, differential diagnosis classified through embryologic analysis. Radiographics 1993; 13:1211-31.
12. Chiari H, Uber Veranderungen des Kleinhirns, des Pons unde der. Medulla oblongata infolge von congenitaler hydrocephalie des Gross hirns Denkschr Kais Akad Wiss Mathnaturew 1896; 63:71-116.
13. Bhaddelia RA, Bogdan AR, Wolpert SM. Analysis of cerebrospinal fluid flow waveforms with gated phase contrast MR velocity measurements. AJNR AM J Neurorad 1995; 10:389-400.
14. McLone DG, Knepper PA. The cause of Chiari II malformaiton. A unified theory. Pediatr Neuroscience 1989; 15:1-12.

15. Naidich T, Altman N, Braffman B, et al. Cephaloceles and related malformations AJNR, Am J Neuroradiology 1992; 13:655-90.

16. Smirniotopoulous JG, Murphy FM. Central nervous system manifestations of the phakomatoses and other inherited syndromes. In Atlas SW (Ed): Magnetic Resonance Imaging of Brain and Spine (3rd edn). Philadelphia: Lippincott Williams and Wilkins 2002; 371-413.

17. Barkovich AJ. The phakomatoses. In: Barkovich AJ. Pediatirc Neuroimaging. 4th edn. Philadelphia: Lippincott Williams and Wilkins 2005; 476–81.

18. Neurofibromatosis, conference statement. National Institutes of Health Consensus Development Conference. Arch Neurol 1988; 45:575-78.

19. Mulvihill JJ. (moderator) Neurofibromatosis I (Recklinghausen disease) and Neurofibromatosis 2 (bilateral acoustic neurofibromatosis) an update. Ann Inter Med 1990; 113:39-52.

20. Ricardi VM. Neurofibromatosis. Neurol Clin 1987; 5:337-49.

21. Orlova KA, Crino PB. The tuberous sclerosis complex. Ann N Acad Sci 2010; 1184:87-105.

22. Stimac GK, Solomon MA, Newton TH. CT and MR of angiomatous malformations of the choroids plexus in patients with Sturge–Weber disease. AJNR, Am J Neuroradiology 1986; 7:623-27.

23. Wahl M, Barkovich AJ, Mukherjee P. Diffusion imaging and tractography of congenital brain malformations. Pediatr Radio 2010; 40:59-67.

CHAPTER 26

Hypoxic-Ischemic Encephalopathy

Atin kumar, Arun Kumar Gupta

Neonatal encephalopathy following birth asphyxia or perinatal hypoxia is referred to as hypoxic-ischemic encephalopathy (HIE).[1]

HIE is a common clinical problem with far reaching consequences. It, therefore, becomes mandatory for the pediatrician and the pediatric radiologist to understand its etiology, pathology, pathophysiological mechanism and imaging features with awareness of the limitations and advantages of each imaging modality.

Exact incidence of HIE is not known but at most centers incidence of perinatal hypoxic-ischemia is between 1.0 to 1.5 percent.[2] Clinically HIE has been graded into mild, moderate and severe grades with prognosis directly related to the severity.[3] Approximately 15 to 20 percent of neonates with hypoxic ischemia would die within the newborn period.[4]

NEUROIMAGING IN INFANTS WITH HIE

Role of neuroimaging in the work up of infants with HIE is two folds:

   i. Imaging of the pathologic lesions and their follow-up.
   ii. Prediction of clinical outcome based on pathologic lesions observed on imaging.

Three important imaging techniques used for examination of the newborn brain are sonography, computed tomography (CT) and magnetic resonance imaging (MRI). Although maturity of the neonatal brain and suspected pathology should dictate the choice of imaging but expertise in conducting and interpreting the images in a particular diagnostic technique, may decide the final selection of an investigation. Sonography, being widely available, possible even at cribside for sick babies, non-ionizing, painless, not requiring sedation or intravenous contrast makes it an ideal screening modality in children. Depending upon the sonographic findings and the clinical status, further imaging protocol may be decided later.

It is a well-established fact that the *pattern of cerebral injury in a newborn infant depends, to a great extent, on the maturity of the brain at the time of insult.* It is generally agreed that the *dividing line between the immature and the mature brain is around 34 weeks.*[5,6]

Therefore, two broad groups, i.e. 'below 34 weeks group – the premature neonate' and 'above 34 weeks group – the term neonate' are discussed separately.

BELOW 34 WEEKS GROUP – THE PREMATURE NEONATE

Preterm neonates are much more prone to HIE than term neonates. It occurs because of increased chances of hypoxic insult due to very low birth weight (<1500 gm),[7,8] hyaline membrane disease, antepartum placental abruption, hypocapnia, twin pregnancy, septicemia, patent ductus arteriosus and also due to poor autoregulatory capacity of the premature brain.[6,9-15]

Imaging features can be subdivided based on severity (and to some extent duration) of injury into two types – severe hypoxia versus mild-to-moderate or partial asphyxia. It must be remembered that features of both severe and partial asphyxia may be seen together in any given patient.

Severe, Total Hypoxia

The most metabolically active regions within the brain in this period, i.e. the deep gray matter including thalami, basal ganglia, hippocampus, cerebellum, dorsal brainstem and corticospinal tracts are the areas of involvement. The thalami, anterior vermis and the dorsal brainstem are the most frequently affected. The basal ganglia and perirolandic cortex myelinate at around 35-36 weeks of gestational age and therefore are less severely and less frequently involved than the thalami.[16]

Cranial ultrasound is the first modality performed in the preterm neonates for screening and diagnosis for HIE. It may be normal in the first 48 hours but may show hyperechogenicity in the basal ganglia and thalami by the third day.[6] CT will similarly show hypodensity within the basal ganglia and thalami with their attenuation values close to that of white matter.

MRI is a sensitive modality to detect the changes of HIE. Diffusion weighted images may show restriction of diffusion within the involved areas, most commonly the thalami, in the first 24 hours. The abnormalities on conventional MRI start appearing in the form of T1 and T2 hyperintensity in the thalami and basal ganglia from 3rd day onwards. The restriction of diffusion reaches peak at around 3-5 days and then starts to 'pseudonormalize' after a week. T2 shortening starts to occur after 1 week in the affected areas. The T1 hyperintense signal may persist into the chronic stage. (Figs 26.1A and B).

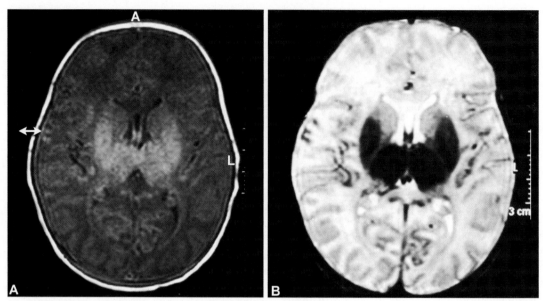

Figs 26.1A and B: Axial MR images of a 9-day-old premature neonate shows the thalami and basal ganglia appearing hyperintense on T1 weighted image (A) and hypointense signal on T2 weighted image (B)

Mild-to-Moderate Hypoxia

This is by far the most common pattern of insult to the premature neonatal brain. The two major pathological lesions observed in this setting are hemorrhage and periventricular leukomalacia (PVL).[5,6]

Hemorrhage

Intracranial hemorrhage (ICH) in premature neonates is directly related to the degree of gestational immaturity. Germinal matrix (GM), the site of initial bleed, is a highly vascular area within the ventricular wall. GM is most prominent and active between 8 and 28 weeks of gestation.[6,17,18] Hemorrhage could be at germinal matrix (GMH), intraventricular (IVH) or parenchymal.[17-21]

Germinal Matrix Hemorrhage (GMH)

Prematurity coupled with respiratory distress syndrome are the two main factors presumed to be responsible for hemorrhage in the immature brain. Following ischemic insult when the ischemic tissue is reperfused, damaged cerebral autoregulation[22-24] associated with sudden rapid rise in cerebral blood flow or perfusion pressure as with handling, suction, artificial ventilation; leads to rupture of fragile weakened blood vessels in the germinal matrix bed.[6,17,18] The germinal matrix involutes by 34 weeks of gestation. The last portion of germinal matrix to involute is the ganglionic eminence located deep to the ependyma in the caudothalamic notch in the groove between the head of caudate nucleus and the thalamus. Hence, it is the most common site for germinal matrix hemorrhage (Figs 26.2 and 26.3). It may also occur in the cerebellum from the germinal zones within the cerebellum and subependymal layer of roof of fourth ventricle.

Intraventricular Hemorrhage (IVH)

IVH results either from rupture of a GMH into the ventricle or from choroid plexus bleeding. Depending upon the amount of

bleeding and alteration in the CSF dynamics, ventricles may o may not show dilatation (Figs 26.4 and 26.5).

Parenchymal Hemorrhage (Periventricular Hemorrhagic Infarction, PVHI)

It is typically unilateral, extensive and always associated wit intraventricular hemorrhage. Unlike hemorrhage occurring in a area of ischemia, periventricular hemorrhagic infarction occu more anteriorly, roughly triangular in shape with apex of the triang in the midline (Figs 26.6 and 26.7). Germinal matrix an intraventricular hemorrhage causes compromise of terminal vei underlying germinal matrix leading on to congestion, thrombos and rupture of medullary veins draining the deep white matte This leads to a hemorrhagic venous infarct in the periventricula parenchyma.[25] PVHI occurs about 24-48 hours after the onset o GMH and IVH. About 15 percent of patients with IVH develo PVHI.[21] On follow-up, such a hemorrhage results in th development of a porencephalic cyst on imaging and hemipleg on clinical examination.

Grading of Intracranial Hemorrhage

Papile et al[19] proposed four grades of severity: Grade (hemorrhage confined to germinal matrix in the subependyma region (SEH or GMH); Grade (II) is associated with IVH bu without ventricular dilatation; Grade (III) IVH is associated wit ventricular dilatation and Grade (IV) bleeding occurs into the brai parenchyma (PVHI). A number of other classifications followe but none has been universally accepted so far due to thei limitations.

Imaging of Intracranial Hemorrhage

Transfontanelle sonography is the most sensitive modality to dete SEH and IVH in the acute stage.[26] SEH is seen as a focal echogen area at the head of caudate nucleus in the most anterior end o

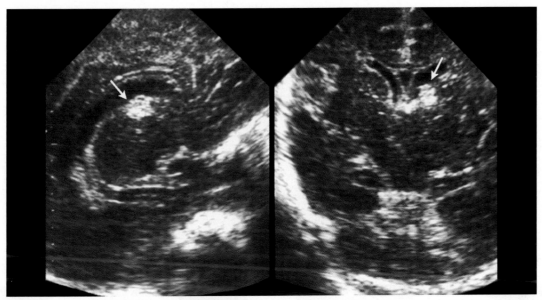

Fig. 26.2: US: Grade II bleed (SEH) on left side (arrow). Note location of bleed at caudothalamic junction in sagittal view

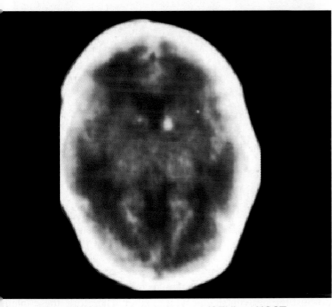

Fig. 26.3: Bilateral grade II bleed (SEH) on NCCT

audothalamic groove.[5,6,26] It is important to document the bnormality in two planes, since normal choroid plexus in the same rea may be mistaken for SEH. Normal choroid plexus tapers as it xtends anteriorly and disappears beyond Foramen of Monro. On he other hand in a GM bleed there is prominent, bulbous nlargement of choroid density which also extends beyond Foramen f Monro (Fig. 26.2). On NCCT head (Fig. 26.3) SEH is visible as focal, high attenuating area. IVH is echogenic on sonography Fig. 26.4) and the organized clot takes the shape of the ventricle vhich later shows dilatation. With time the clot becomes iso and nen hypoechoic. On NCCT IVH is high attenuating initially (Fig. 6.5) becoming iso- and finally hypoattenuating. Periventricular emorrhagic infarction (PVHI) in the acute stage is brightly chogenic, unilateral, clearly defined echodensity (Fig. 26.6) on

sonography[6] with the apex of the triangle pointing towards the ventricle in the midline. Associated IVH is almost always present (Fig. 26.7).

Subarachnoid hemorrhage (SAH) and haemorrhage in the posterior fossa and parieto-occipital area can be easily missed on the sonography. Noncontrast CT (NCCT) head is more sensitive in depicting these bleeds in the acute phase. On MRI both T1WI and even T2WI may miss these bleeds in the acute stage.

On follow up, initially SEH becomes a subependymal cyst (Figs 26.8A and B) which may later disappear completely. IVH cast also resolves with time (Fig. 26.9). Ventriculomegaly may be the only clue of an earlier episode of bleed. Periventricular hemorrhagic infarction evolves into a porencephalic cyst which is usually in communication with the ventricle. With time, visibility of the hemorrhage, both on sonography and CT, decreases but on MRI visibility increases due to the formation of methemoglobin (Fig. 26.10). Also, MRI is more specific for assessing the time of hemorrhage.

Optimum time for sonographic detection of intracranial hemorrhage secondary to HIE is between 4th to 7th day, by end of which 97 percent of hemorrhages will be visible.[26] In order to monitor for the development of hydrocephalus as a complication of IVH, sonography is recommended on the 14th day, and if negative, then at 3rd month.[26]

White Matter Injury of Prematurity/ Periventricular Leukomalacia (PVL)

The term periventricular leukomalacia in literal terms means "white matter softening". A number of theories have been proposed for its pathogenesis. Unlike ICH where prematurity is a clear risk factor; for the development of PVL, a large number of ante or perinatal events have been identified which may result in hypoperfusion to fetal cerebral tissue or injury to oligodendroglial cells, and are thus important causative factors.[27-29] However, besides hypoxic-ischemic insult, other causes like infection,

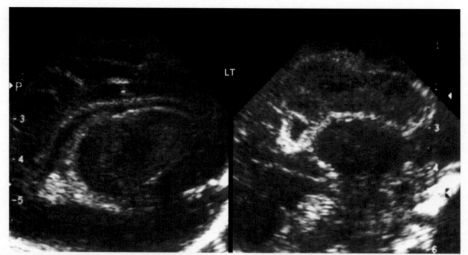

Fig. 26.4: US, Sagittal views: Grade III bleed, IVH with ventriculomegaly. Compare with normal ventricle on opposite side

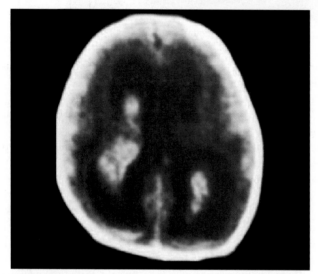

Fig. 26.5: NCCT: Grade III bleed. Note CSF-blood level in dependent parts

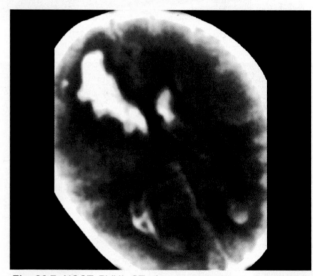

Fig. 26.7: NCCT: PVHI, CT of same patient as in Figure 26.6

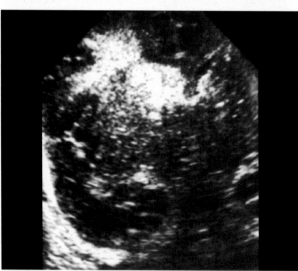

Fig. 26.6: US: PVHI on right side. Note typical appearance of a triangular echodensity extending from apex of frontal horn and associated IVH on same side

metabolic diseases and hydrocephalus also can cause similar injury to the white matter. Also the whole white matter may be involved not just the periventricular white matter. Therefore, these insults are better termed as 'White Matter Injury of Prematurity' rather than PVL.

In a premature neonatal brain, the periventricular area is almost totally perfused by penetrating arteries that extend inward from the surface of the brain (ventriculopetal vessels). Junction of ventriculopetal and the ventriculofugal vessels (watershed area) exists in the periventricular region. In the event of any hypoxic ischemic insult, therefore, this periventricular (watershed) area is at the highest risk. This combined with relative hypovascularity of the periventricular white matter plays a role in the development of PVL. Recently it has been believed that presence of oligo-dendrocyte lineage cells prooligodendrocytes within this area makes them most susceptible to changes of hypoxia-ischemia. These cells mature into oligodendrocytes which are less prone to insult by around 32 weeks of age and hence, there is decreased frequency of PVL after this gestational age.[30,31] Also toxins and

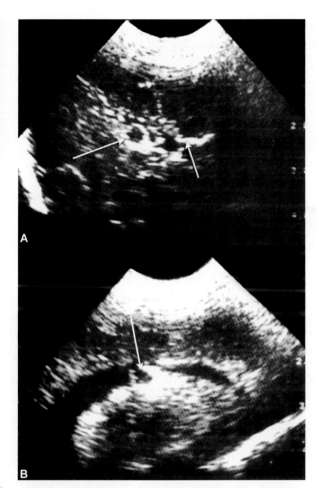

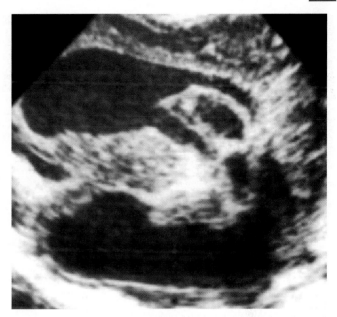

Fig. 26.9: Follow-up of grade III bleed shows a resolving clot and echogenic debris

igs 26.8A and B: Coronal (A) and sagittal (B) transfontanelle onography. SEH (arrow) in the anterior end of right caudothalamic roove with cystic changes. Note that in (A) the normal choroid plexus n the left side (arrow head) may mimick SEH. However, bleed (arrow) slightly more laterally located in the coronal plane and US examination sagittal plane (B) confirms the echodensity to be bleed

excitatory amino acids, especially maternal chorioamnionitis,[32] may play a role in reducing local blood and energy supply and subsequent development of PVL.

Exact incidence of PVL is not clear and would vary depending upon the imaging modality used. Autopsy series report an incidence ranging from 25 percent to 75 percent. On sonography incidence of PVL is reported to vary from 15 percent to 35 percent.[6,33,34]

Pathologically, the temporal sequence of events in the development of PVL are: Coagulation necrosis in the first 24-48 hours followed by cavitation evolving over the next 2-4 weeks (when these cysts can be detected on ultrasound) and after several weeks the cysts collapse and disappear completely with residual

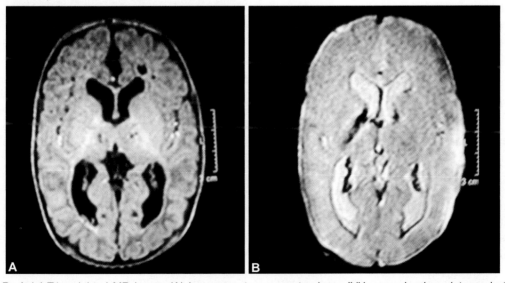

igs 26.10A and B: Axial T1 weighted MR image (A) in a premature neonate shows IVH appearing hyperintense in the occipital horns dependent part). The gradient T2 weighted image (B) is more sensitive in detecting the bleed which is evident as hypointense signal lining the entricular margins, choroid plexus and right caudothalamic groove

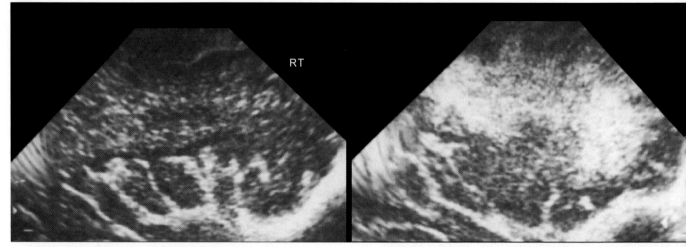

Fig. 26.11: PVL, early: Sagittal US both sides shows marked degree of increased echogenicity on right. Note loss of normal brain architecture on the affected side

white matter atrophy and ventriculomegaly as the only evidence.[6,24] The ventricles have irregular lateral walls and cerebral cortex reaches upto the lateral ventricle wall. PVL may be purely ischemic or at times complicated by blood. Imaging features will therefore vary depending upon the time of imaging in relation to the ischemic insult and whether it is purely ischemic or complicated by hemorrhage.

PVL lesions could be focal or diffuse.[21] Classically, focal PVL lesions are distributed bilaterally, symmetrically, primarily around the trigone areas but may extend also to involve the frontal lobes adjacent to the foramen of Monro.[12,14,35,36] However, lesions may be visible only on one side on imaging and that should not exclude the diagnosis of PVL. Diffuse lesions involve the entire periventricular region.

Clinically, the characteristic neurological abnormality due to PVL is spastic diplegia[26,36] in about 5 to 15 percent. This is because the site of pathological lesions of PVL are located in the periventricular region from where also the corticospinal tracts descend. Tracts of lower limbs are located in the most medial region, i.e; closest to the PVL lesion and are thus first to be affected resulting in diplegia.[24,37] Visual impairment[38,39] and cognitive impairment[40] may occur without spastic diplegia.

Imaging of Early PVL

Ultrasound

Due to hemodynamically unstable state of most of these neonates, a cribside ultrasound (US) in the ICU/nursery is usually the first investigation. Besides portability the other advantages of US are: nonionizing, no i.v contrast or sedation is required and can be repeated frequently without harmful effects. Addition of color Doppler and quantitative analysis[41] to 2 D imaging may improve information content. PVL should be suspected on US studies when increased echogenicity is present in the periventricular regions. On ultrasound (Fig. 26.11) periventricular areas of increased echogenicity is visible within 24-48 hours of ischemic insult. However there are two major potential pitfalls: Firstly, in normal

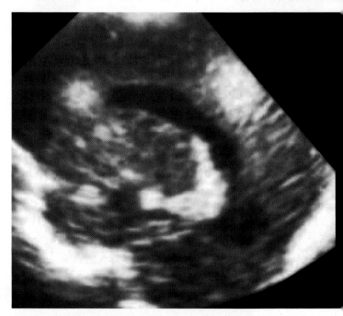

Fig. 26.12: Sagittal US: Focal edema mimicking PVL

new-borns also there is a periventricular increased echogenicity so called 'periventricular blush'.[5,6] Secondly, brain edema also appears bright on US.[42,43] Therefore presence of increased echogenicity in itself is not enough to diagnose PVL. Reliable sign of PVL is the presence of periventricular "flares". The brightness of echogenicity due to PVL 'flare' is more than the normal periventricular echogenicity and approaches or becomes equal to that of adjacent choroid plexus. Also the normal tissue architechture is lost.[6,44,45] However, this limits the capability of US[46-48] since a certain degree of subjective element creeps in especially in milder degrees of abnormality. 'Periventricular flare' should be confirmed and documented in both the coronal and the parasagittal views.

If ischemic PVL is complicated by hemorrhage, then the abnormalities are readily detected by sonography. It is important

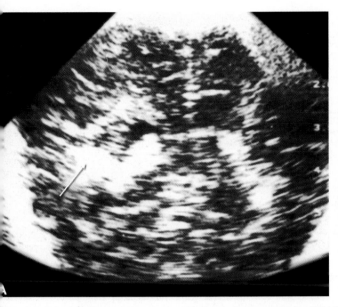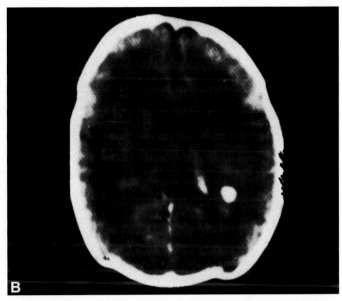

Figs 26.13A and B: Focal parenchymal bleed. On sonography (A) bleed (curved arrow) is again echogenic but "more bright" than edema. CT (B) focal bleed readily diagnosed

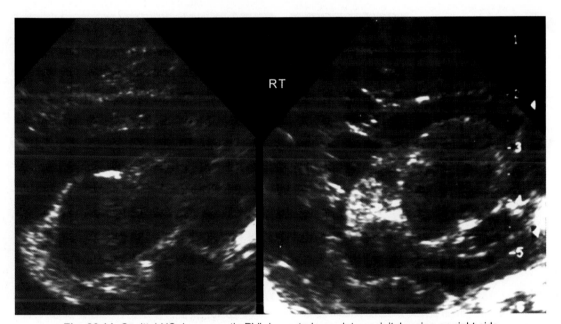

Fig. 26.14: Sagittal US: Large cystic PVL in posterior parieto-occipital region on right side

recognize that both, the edema (Fig. 26.12) as well as the hemorrhage (Figs 26.13A and B), in the brain parenchyma will produce increased echogenicity on ultrasound. Differentiation is possible by observing the *degree of brightness*. In these situations, CT and MRI help to differentiate between the two.

On follow-up, the flares may completely disappear, usually in about half of the patients, within 7-10 days. If however the flares persist beyond 1 week then the term "persistent flares" is used and are considered as grade I PVL.[44] In about 10 percent, the flares may progress to the next pathological stage, i.e. of cavitation, usually within 2-4 weeks. Development of few, small cysts represent milder end of the spectrum of PVL but multiple cysts (Figs 26.14 and 26.15) is an indicator of a poor neurological

prognosis with development of cerebral palsy.[26] Not only the size but also the distribution of cysts is important for predicting the severity of clinical outcome.[49] Thus cysts in the frontoparietal area have a better prognosis as compared to those in the posterior parieto-occipital region. Again ultrasound is superior to CT (Fig. 26.16) for the detection of small cysts of PVL. However, MRI is a superior modality for detection of these cysts (Figs 26.17 and 26.18).

Ultrasound also has been used to grade the PVL. The classification suggested by De Vries[44] is simple to use (Table 26.1). The grading increases with extent and the severity of pathological lesions and is, therefore, directly related to the severity of neurological abnormality.

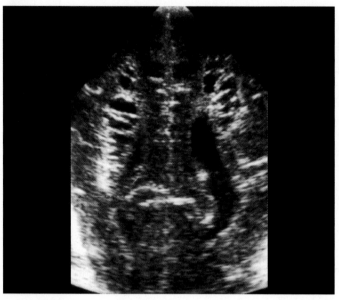

Fig. 26.15: Coronal US: Bilateral extensive cystic PVL

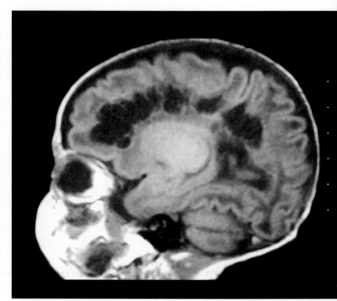

Fig. 26.17: Sagittal T1W MRI shows extensive large cystic PVL

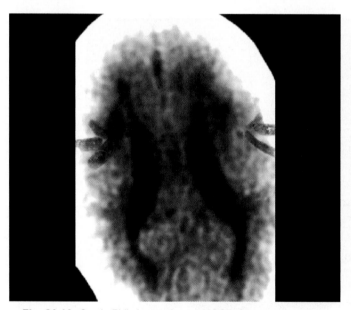

Fig. 26.16: Cystic PVL (arrows) on a NCCT. Same patient as in Figure 26.15. Demonstration on US is easier and better than on CT

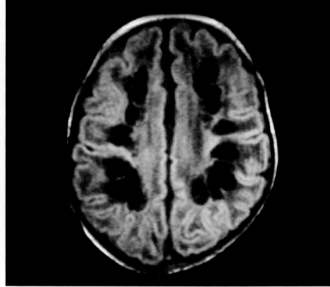

Fig. 26.18: Axial T1W MRI: Extensive bilateral large cystic PVL

Table 26.1: Grading of periventricular leukomalacia (PVL)

Grade of PVL	Description
Grade I	Periventricular echogenic area, persistent for more than seven days
Grade II	Periventricular echogenic areas, evolving into localized small frontoparietal cysts
Grade III	Periventricular echogenic areas evolving into multiple cysts in the parieto-occipital white matter
Grade IV	Echogenic areas in the deep white matter evolving into multiple subcortical cysts (multicystic encephalopathy)

CT

CT has no added advantage over ultrasound and should be avoided because of the associated ionizing radiation exposure. The only exception where CT scores over ultrasound is differentiation of bleed from edema. However, since MRI can also differentiate the two and is generally more sensitive for other findings, it is the next preferred modality after ultrasound.

MRI

The capability of MRI to detect subtle injuries, its superior contrast resolution and its multiplanar potential makes it a far superior

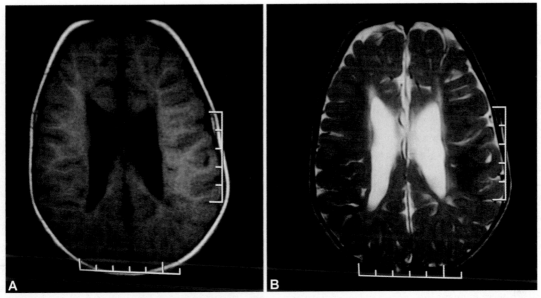

Figs 26.19A and B: End stage PVL. T1 (A) and T2 (B) weighted axial MR images show loss of volume with signal changes in the deep periventricular white matter and ventricular dilatation with irregular marginss

technique to ultrasound for detection of white matter abnormalities. With recent advances in MRI, ventilators and anesthesia equipment hardware, the problems of feasibility of MRI in very sick and premature neonates have been largely overcome.[50]

Early white matter injury appears as foci of T1 hyperintensity in the periventricular white matter by 3-4 days postinsult. These lesions are not evident on T2 weighted images at this time. Instead T2 weighted images show diffuse hyperintense signal within the periventricular white matter. The T1 hyperintense foci subsequently become hypointense on T2 weighted images by 5-6 days. Hemorrhage also gives rise to T2 hypointense lesions but in this case the hypointensity is more marked.

Advances in MRI have made it possible to diagnose early white matter injury. Diffusion weighted imaging (DWI) in a number of studies has been found to be much more accurate than conventional MRI in the acute phase of PVL.[6,46,51,52] Recently further advances have been made and studies using Serial Quantitative Diffusion Tensor MRI[53,54] have reported very high degree of accuracy in diagnosing early white matter injuries. In this technique two parameters are assessed: Apparent diffusion coefficient (ADC) mapping and relative anisotropy of cerebral water. This method has been found so accurate that it is being now a days used for white matter tractography.[55,56]

Imaging of End Stage PVL

After several weeks, usually 3 months onwards, the cysts collapse and completely disappear. Diagnosis on US at this stage is very difficult, if not impossible. A characteristic triad of findings due to white matter collapse is seen both on CT and MRI[5,6,12,14,57] (Fig. 26.19). The triad consists of:

i. Abnormally increased bilateral periventricular white matter signal intensity on a T2W sequence, most commonly in the trigone regions of lateral ventricles. This increased signal intensity corresponds to gliosis and demyelination observed pathologically in late PVL. Important differential diagnosis of similar increased signal intensity includes normal, unmyelinated white matter; myelinoclastic disorders and postradiation or chemotherapeutic administration. However, by careful interpretation of the images in the proper clinical background, one can differentiate each of these conditions from one another and from PVL.

ii. Marked loss of periventricular white matter in the regions of abnormal high signal intensity results in close approximation of the cortical sulci to the ventricles. Many a times, this may be the only clue of an end stage PVL.

iii. Compensatory focal enlargement of the ventricle adjacent to the regions of abnormal high signal intensity with irregular outlines.

On MRI two other findings may also be seen,[6] i.e. observation of delayed myelination and thin, atrophic corpuscallosum particularly in the posterior body and splenium. However, it should always be remembered that all these above late stage signs on imaging may be caused by many different disorders, such as ventriculitis (a common sequel of meningitis in infants), inborn errors of metabolism, hydrocephalus and in utero events.[6] The diagnosis is best made in conjunction with a thorough past medical history.

In addition to PVL, two other distinct type of white matter abnormalities have been described in the premature neonates – punctuate lesions and diffuse excessive high signal (DEHSI).[25,50] These are much better seen on MRI as compared to ultrasound. The punctuate lesions, though more common in premature neonates, may also be seen in term neonates. They are most frequently seen in the corona radiata, posterior periventricular white matter and the optic radiation and rarely in deep gray matter. In some cases they may represent the early and mild end of PVL spectrum. They are seen as T1 hyperintense and T2 hypointense lesions which occasionally show evidence of bleed on gradient sequences and restricted diffusion on DWI. These may regress with time. In contrast, DEHSI refers to diffuse signal changes in deep white matter appearing hypointense on T1 and hyperintense on T2 weighted images. These signal changes are more profound than the normal appearances of unmyelinated white matter in the premature neonatal brain. It may be noted here that even in the normal developing brain there are more distinct zones of high signal intensity on T2 and low on T1 weighted images. These appear in the shape of caps anteriorly in the frontal white matter and arrowheads posteriorly in the peritrigonal white matter.[50] The DEHSI can be differentiated from these by being diffuse. Neonates with DEHSI have been shown to have impaired development in about 50% of the cases with rest leading on to develop normally.[25]

ABOVE 34 WEEKS GROUP—THE TERM NEONATE

Incidence of HIE in term neonates has decreased over the years and is reported to be about 1-2 per 1000 live births.[6,58] Affected neonates may have significant neurologic abnormalities,[24] mental retardation[24] or visual impairment.[59] Hypoxic-ischemic injury in the term neonate usually occurs in association with antepartum risk factors either alone or in combination with intrapartum risk factors. Remaining few cases are associated with intrapartum factors alone or secondary to postnatal complications such as sepsis, shock and respiratory distress.

With the maturity of the infant three important anatomic changes occur:[5,6] (i) involution and regression of the germinal matrix resulting in decreased incidence of intracranial hemorrhage in term neonates in contrast to preterm neonates, (ii) the site susceptible for hypoxic-ischemic injury changes. The watershed zone shifts from the earlier periventricular location in a preterm to a more peripheral location in the subcortical region, and (iii) while earlier the response of the preterm brain to trauma was by liquefaction and resorption of the damaged brain, the mature brain responds to the same trauma by reactive astrogliosis.[6,60]

The pathological lesions and imaging characteristics due to HIE in infants beyond 34 weeks gestation are again dependent on severity and duration of hypoxia and is divided into severe and mild-to-moderate groups.

Severe, Total Hypoxia

Severe hypoxia refers to sudden total loss of oxygenation as may be seen in abruption placenta, prolapsed cord or ruptured uterus. As seen in the preterm neonates, the deep gray matter including putamen, ventrolateral thalamus, hippocampus, dorsal brainstem and lateral geniculate nuclei, are the areas of involvement.[6] In contrast to preterm neonates, the basal ganglia involvement is more severe compared to thalami. The perirolandic cortex may also be affected. The remaining cortex is involved only with more prolonged insults. In this type of injury hypoxia is the predominant component of insult rather than hypotension.

Cranial ultrasound done within the first week has low sensitivity. It may show pattern of diffuse cerebral edema seen as

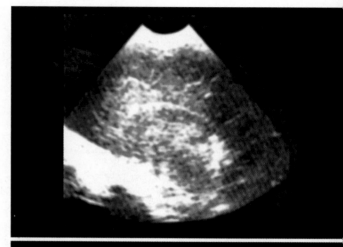

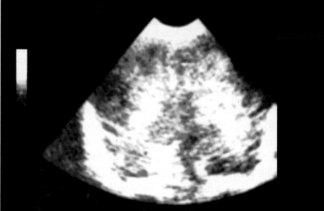

Fig. 26.20: Cerebral edema: On sonography 'a bright brain' with diffuse increase in echogenicity is seen. Lateral ventricles and other landmarks are obliterated

diffuse increased echogenicity of brain with obliterated CSF spaces (Fig. 26.20). Ultrasound done after a week may show increased echogenicity of involved areas of basal ganglia, thalami and brainstem. Follow-up ultrasound shows diffuse cerebral atrophy.

CT is much less sensitive and specific than MRI. CT findings include decrease in the density of basal ganglia, cortex with subsequent loss of gray white matter differentiation (Fig. 26.21). CT may also show evidence of diffuse cerebral edema evident as effacement of sylvian fissures and basal cisterns (Fig. 26.22). It may be seen about 8 hours after insult and peak by 3-4 days.

MRI is the most sensitive modality for evaluation of HIE in the term neonate. Conventional T1 and T2 weighted images in combination with diffusion weighted images (DWI) depict the extent of damage. The conventional images may start showing findings from second day onwards but the abnormalities on these images are best visualized after a week.[6] DWI usually shows the abnormality within the first 24 hours when the conventional images are normal. However the DWI done on the first day, though sensitive, underestimates the extent of injury which is seen to progress on these images to a peak on 3-5 days. The findings then subsequently 'pseudonormalize' by the end of first week. DWI however, can objectively categorize tissue injury based on values

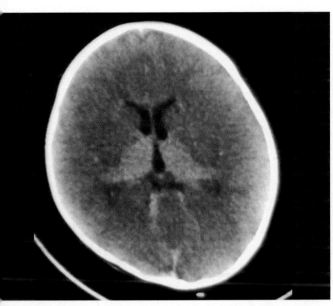

ig. 26.21: Axial CT image in a term neonate with severe hypoxia hows diffuse hypodensity involving the cortical gray matter and basal anglia with loss of gray-white matter differentiation

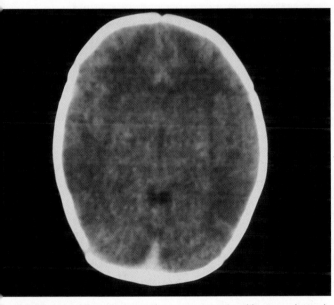

ig. 26.22: Axial CT image in another term neonate with severe hypoxic jury shows diffuse cerebral edema with effacement of sulci, cisterns nd ventricles

f ADC and subsequently predict outcome to a certain extent.[61,62] /IR spectroscopy has been shown to be sensitive modality for etecting hypoxic damage in the early period within first 24 hours ven when the DWI images are normal. Elevated choline, decreased IAA, increased lacatate and increased glutamine-glutamate are een. Lactate elevation seen as a lactate doublet (2 sharp peaks) entred at 1.33 ppm is typically seen due to anaerobic glycosis econdary to mitochondrial dysfunction. It can be detected as early s 4-8 hours after birth but peaks at around 5 days of life.[63] ncreased lactate/NAA ratio observed on first day of life has been

shown to be a very sensitive parameter for injury and may be considered as gold standard. It may be useful in identification of infants who may benefit from early therapeutic intervention.[63-67] Diffusion tensor imaging has also recently shown promise in detecting and timing these lesions by showing decreased FA values in the affected parts of brain which may be seen even after 'pseudonormalization' on DWI.[61]

MRI findings include:

i. T1 hyperintense basal ganglia – Seen in the first 3 days of life. The posterior putamina are the most commonly involved. It should be remembered that mild T1 hyperintensity of the basal ganglia may be seen in normal infants also. Hence, it is important to see for associated findings of HIE.

ii. T1 hyperintense thalami – The signal change is subtle compared to that of the basal ganglia. When abnormal, the thalami show diffuse hyperintense signal on T1 weighted images (Fig. 26.23). This should be differentiated from the focal hyperintense signal seen within the posterolateral part of thalami in normal neonates corresponding to the myelination of ventrolateral thalamic nuclei just medial to the terminal portion of the posterior limb of internal capsule. Both the putamina and thalami appear hyperintense on T2 weighted images in the early period but then progress to develop T2 hypointensity by the 2nd week (Fig. 26.23). The T1 hyperintense signal within the basal ganglia, thalami and also in the perirolandic cortex has been shown to persist for several months.

iii. 'Absent posterior limb' sign – The posterior 50% of the posterior limb of internal capsule (PLIC) normally gets myelinated by 37 weeks of gestational age and is then seen as hyperintense on T1 and hypointense on T2 weighted images. Absence of this normal signal characteristics of the PLIC is a sensitive marker of hypoxia in a term infant (beyond 37 weeks of age). Although, it may be seen on the first day of life, it is usually best evident after 3-4 days. In doubtful cases the signal characteristics of PLIC may be compared with the adjacent posterolateral putamen. In normal neonates, the PLIC appears more hyperintense than the posterolateral putamen on T1 weighted images. Reversal of this pattern is considered very sensitive for hypoxic damage. T2 weighted images showing loss of normal hypointensity in the PLIC may be useful in case of doubt on T1 images especially in the setting of abnormal hyperintense signal within the adjacent basal ganglia and thalami secondary to HII (Fig. 26.24).

iv. Abnormal DWI – Restriction of diffusion may be seen in the basal ganglia, PLIC and thalami in the affected neonates. As stated above, the abnormality may be seen within the first day but usually peaks by about 4-5 days and starts to 'pseudonormalize' by 7-10 days. Initial findings on DWI may underestimate the true extent of injury. Hence, a 'normal' appearing DWI does not exclude insult.

v. Profound global injury – Involving both the cortical gray and subcortical white matter. It is seen much less commonly than the above 4 patterns. On DWI it is seen as the 'white cerebrum' contrast from normal appearing cerebellum. It is usually fatal.

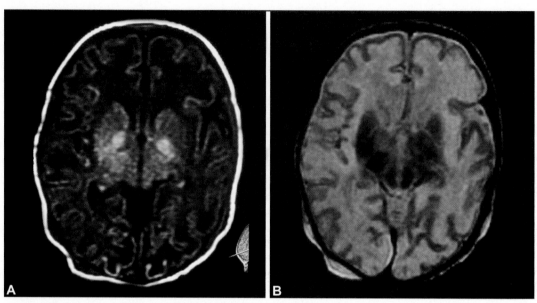

Figs 26.23A and B: Axial T1 (A) and T2 (B) weighted MR images in a 6-day-old term neonate with severe hypoxic injury shows the thalami and basal ganglia appearing hyperintense on T1 and hypointense on T2. Also note the loss of normal T1 hyperintense and T2 hypointense signal within the posterior limb of internal capsule

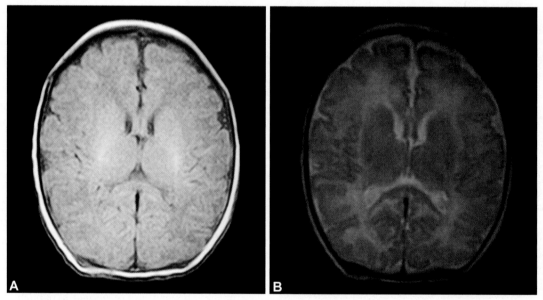

Figs 26.24A and B: A 9-day-old term neonate with severe hypoxic injury shows lack of myelination of posterior limb of internal capsule on T1 weighted (A) and T2 weighted (B) axial MR images

Survivors show multicystic encephalomalacia on follow-up imaging. (Fig. 26.25)

vi. Parasagittal gray and white matter injury – Bilateral cortical and subcortical white matter necrosis in the parasagittal areas extending to involve the parieto-occipital areas of the brain.

Follow-up imaging in these neonates show atrophy of the involved structures with T2 hyperintense signal especially in the posterior putamina, ventrolateral thalami and cortcospinal tracts. Also appreciated is thinning of the corpus callosum in the region of the middle or posterior body, secondary to degeneration of the transcallosal fibres.

Prolonged Partial Hypoxia

Prolonged partial asphyxia refers to a more sustained but incomplete loss of oxygenation as seen in prolonged difficult labor with fetal bradycardia. It is also more common after hypotension, hypoglycemia and infection. Hypotension plays a more major role in this type of insult rather than hypoxia. It results in shunting of blood to the vital brain structures including brainstem, basal ganglia, thalami, hippocampi and cerebellum from the cerebral cortex and white matter which are not so metabolically active. Hence, these above vital brain structures are spared from injury whereas the watershed zones in cortical and subcortical areas get

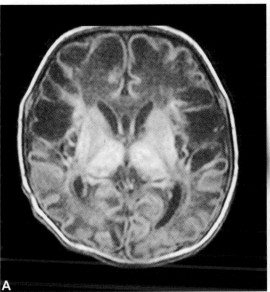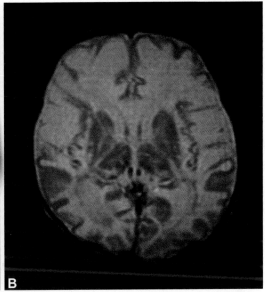

Figs 26.25A and B: T1 (A) and T2 (B) weighted axial MR images of a 18-day-old term neonate with severe hypoxic injury shows diffuse multicystic encephalomalacia involving cortex and subcortical white matter. Also note the persistent signal changes in the basal ganglia and thalami

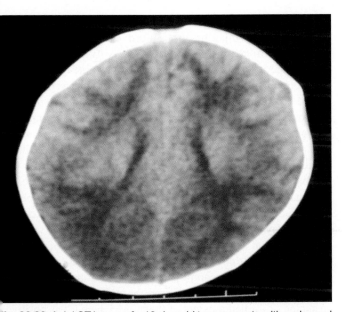

Fig. 26.26: Axial CT image of a 10-day-old term neonate with prolonged partial asphyxia shows hypodensity involving the watershed zones in the frontal and parieto-occipital regions

affected. Abnormalities are earliest seen on DWI (best evident as hypointensity on ADC maps) followed by findings on conventional T1 and T2 weighted images. T2 weighted images show cortical swelling and hyperintense signal within the gray and subcortical white matter with loss of gray-white matter differentiation. The parasaggital watershed zones are the most favored site of involvement but the findings may be diffusely seen in the cerebral hemispheres (Fig. 26.26). Follow-up imaging may show leucomalacia specially in the subcortical areas. This pattern is different from that of a premature neonate where there occurs periventricular leucomalacia.

It is important to remember that any given patient may show imaging features suggestive of both severe and partial prolonged hypoxic insult.

HYPOXIC ISCHEMIC INJURY IN POSTNATAL AGE GROUP

Rapid brain maturation is observed in the postnatal period and the brain becomes almost completed myelinated by 2 years of age. So after 2 years of age the hypoxic injury patterns are similar to those seen in adults. The usual causes for injury in this period are non-accidental trauma, choking, drowning and asphyxiation.

Severe Total Hypoxia

Profound hypoxic ischemic injury in children between 1 and 2 years of age affects the basal ganglia, hippocampi, lateral geniculate body and cerebral cortex in the anterior frontal and parieto-occipital region. The perirolandic cortex and thalami are typically spared in contrast to their involvement seen in the perinatal period.[68] Infants below 1 year of age, however, may show an overlap between these categories and therefore may show involvement of thalami and perirolandic cortex alongwith involvement of basal ganglia, brainstem and other cortical areas. Children above 2 years behave same as adults and basal ganglia, thalami, hippocampi, cerebellum and cortical gray matter gets affected (Fig. 26.27). Cortex may be diffusely involved or may be limited to perirolandic and parieto-occipital regions. Since cranial ultrasound is not feasible after the closure of anterior fontanelle which occurs by about 4 months of age, CT and MRI are the mainstay of imaging in these children.

CT shows features of basal ganglia hypodensity with features of diffuse cerebral edema with relative sparing of perirolandic regions. Few affected children may also show 'reversal sign'

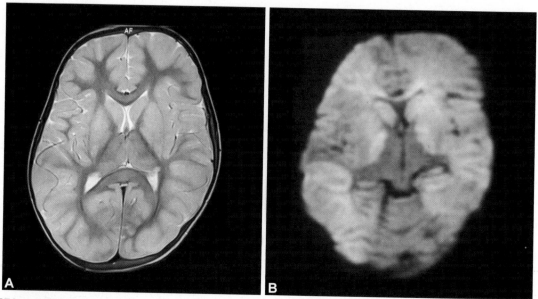

Figs 26.27A and B: Three year old girl with hypoxic injury. Axial T2 weighted (A) MR image shows hyperintense signal changes within the basal ganglia, thalami and the cortical gray matter which show restricted diffusion on the DWI image (B)

defined as white matter appearing hyperdense compared to the gray matter on CT. This results when diffuse edema in the brain leads to elevated intracranial pressure which causes partial venous obstruction and distension of deep medullary veins within the white matter. The 'white cerebellum sign' may also be noted when the supratentorial brain parenchyma shows diffuse hypodensity and the brainstem and cerebellum are spared. This occurs due to redistribution of blood flow to the posterior circulation.

MRI is more sensitive in showing abnormalities in the affected regions which are seen as hyperintense signal changes in the affected regions on T2 weighted images. DWI are most sensitive with abnormal signal detected within 24 hours.

Mild-to-Moderate Hypoxia

The older infants and children below 2 years of age who suffer from mild-to-moderate hypoxia show involvement of cortex and subcortical white matter similar to the pattern seen in the neonates with partial prolonged hypoxia. The watershed zone infarcts are seen with relative sparing of the deep periventricular white matter. The CT and MR features are similar to those described above. On follow-up imaging, T2 weighted MR images may show residual persisting hyperintensity within the involved regions especially within the basal ganglia. T1 weighted images may show gyriform pattern of hyperintensity within the affected cortex representing cortical laminar necrosis.

IMAGING CHOICE FOR EVALUATION OF HYPOXIC-ISCHEMIC INJURY

Neonates with suspected HIE are usually hemodynamically unstable and very sick and therefore a cribside ultrasound in the ICU/nursery is usually the first investigation for screening. Besides portability the other advantages of US are: Nonionizing, no IV contrast or sedation is required and can be repeated frequently

without harmful effects. Addition of color Doppler and quantitative analysis to 2 D imaging may improve information content. However, limitations include low sensitivity and operator dependence. It has good positive predictive value but a negative scan does not rule out injury and in a high risk scenario the neonate should be evaluated with MRI. CT because of radiation exposure and low sensitivity in presence of unmyelinated white matter is not preferred in the neonatal age group. MRI with conventional T1 and T2 weighted images alongwith DWI is the modality of choice for further evaluation. It is also more sensitive than ultrasound for early detection and mild changes specially myelination abnormalities. If MR is negative in the early period, MR spectroscopy may be performed or the MRI can be repeated after 3-4 days.[68]

In postnatal age group especially after 4 months of age when anterior fontanelle closes, cranial ultrasound is no longer feasible. In these children, noncontrast CT can be performed as the first investigation. MR may be required for negative scans with high suspicion or for better extent of the injury where CT is positive.

PREDICTION OF CLINICAL OUTCOME

After imaging, the second most important role of a pediatric radiologist in the work up of infants with HIE is to predict, if possible, the clinical outcome based on imaging findings at an early stage. This is a crucial but difficult situation. A number of workers have used different imaging modalities and have reported various parameters to predict the clinical outcome.

Clinically, it has been observed that decreased rate of head growth during early months in a term neonate correlates closely with the neurological dysfunction and cerebral atrophy at a later stage.

Various studies based on imaging to predict the clinical outcome are as follows:

Ultrasound

Echogenic Thalamus

Normal thalamus and basal ganglia region have medium level echoes on ultrasound. In infants with HIE, characteristic increase in the echogenicity of these tissue has been reported,[69] usually in the second week after the episode of asphyxia. Visualization of this sign predicts poor prognosis and has been reported to be associated with mortality in 1 percent and long-term morbidity in 6 percent.

Cerebral Artery Doppler

Duplex scanning of the cerebral arteries has been studied, both in normal neonates as well as in those affected by perinatal asphyxia.[70,71] Resistive Index (RI), the single most important Doppler parameter, has been used to measure the flow abnormality. Mean RI in normal healthy neonates is 75 and is inversely related to gestational age. With an RI of 60 as the critical level and all cases with values below 60 taken as abnormal, it has been observed that clinical outcome is poor even though 2D sonogram may appear normal. Thus, Doppler scanning of cerebral arteries may provide an easy and a reliable parameter on day 1 of life to predict the clinical outcome in a neonate with HIE.

CT

Reversal Sign

Presence of reversal sign, i.e. diffuse decreased attenuation of the cerebral cortex (Fig. 26.24) with a relative preservation of density in the thalami, brainstem and cerebellum, has been observed to be associated with poor prognosis[72] (Fig. 26.21). Exact mechanism of this sign is not clear although a number of theories have been put forward, e.g. mechanical factor, postischemic hypervascularity, distension of deep medullary veins and high serum glucose level. The sonographic counterpart of reversal sign of CT is echogenic thalamus discussed earlier.

Diffuse Decreased Density

Diffuse low attenuation is a common finding, both in the preterm and term neonates,[6] affected by perinatal asphyxia. However, diffuse low attenuation in preterm (below 34 weeks gestation) has no predictive value because there is very poor correlation with late neurologic sequelae. Reason for it is obvious, i.e. difficulty in differentiating pathological low attenuation from normal immature myelin tissue at this age. On the other hand, diffuse low attenuation in a term neonate is a very important prognostic predictor because it has a good correlation with poor clinical outcome.

MR Imaging

Conventional Sequences

Delayed myelination is one of the hallmark of HIE which can be detected only on MRI. Studies have shown that delayed myelination in a term neonate in the first few days of life suggests significant perinatal asphyxia and hence poor prognosis. With the introduction of Serial Quantitative Tensor MRI technique, assessment for white matter injury has become more reliable and at an early stage.[53-56] Delayed myelination on MRI may, therefore, be used as an early predictor of clinical outcome.

In mature term neonates, abnormal signal intensity within the PLIC has been found to be an excellent predictor of abnormal motor outcome. Asymmetrical involvement predicts hemiplegia and bilateral symmetrical involvement correlates with subsequent development of spastic diplegia or quadriplegia.[73] The severity of basal ganglia and thalamic lesions detected on MRI also has good correlate with severity and nature of cerebral palsy. The involvement of white matter exacerbates cognitive impairment and poor head growth.[74]

In premature neonates, finding of PVHI correlates well with development of hemiplegia in survivors whereas PVL correlates more with spastic diplegia. It has also been observed that most of the neonates with documented PVL on US/CT alongwith DEHSI had neurologic abnormality.[75-77] Also, a general correlation between the neurological impairment and the severity of MR abnormalities was demonstrated. Abnormalities on MRI scan, therefore, can be used not only to predict the neurological deficit but also its severity.

MR-Spectroscopy

MR spectroscopy has proved invaluable to detect early brain injury with good correlation between the degree of abnormality and the clinical outcome. Therefore, MRS may be used as a predictor of prognosis.

CONCLUSION

Hypoxic-ischemic encephalopathy is a relatively common clinical problem in the neonatal period. Pathological changes depend upon the gestational age. Imaging features, therefore, also differ in the preterm and term infants. Depending upon the gestational age and the abnormality suspected, a particular imaging modality is chosen.

Cranial ultrasound remains the first screening modality specially in the premature neonate. However, MRI has a vast potential not only to detect subtle, early, specific abnormalities, but also to predict clinical outcome based on imaging features in the first few days of life. MR spectroscopy has also shown good promise in early detection of changes.

A close cooperation and teamwork is, therefore, required between the neonatologist and the pediatric radiologist to decide the imaging approach appropriate for the gestational age, suspected pathology, imaging facilities available and the expertise, both in performing and interpreting the images, without duplicating the information and keeping the cost-benefit in view.

REFERENCES

1. Singh M. Hypoxic ischemic encephalopathy. In Talukdar B (Ed): Essentials of Pediatric Neurology, New Age International (P) Ltd. Publishers 1997; 95-107.
2. Legido A, Katoseos CD, Mishra OP, et al. Perinatal hypoxic ischemic encephalopathy: Current and future treatments. International Pediatrics 2000; 15:143-51.

3. Teaching files. Perinatal asphyxia (Hypoxic ischaemic encephalopathy). By: Division of Neonatology, Cedars-Sinai Medical center, Los Angeles, California, Webmaster@neonatology.org.

4. Vannucci RC, Perlman JM. Interventions for perinatal hypoxic ischaemic encephalopathy. Pediatrics 1997; 100:1004-1114.

5. Flodmark O. The neonatal Brain-Imaging for prognosis. In Harwood-Nash DC, Pettersson H (Eds): Paediatric Radiology. NICER series on Diagnostic Imaging, Merit Communications 1992; 16-25.

6. Barkovich AJ. Brain and spine injuries. In Barkovich AJ (Ed). Pediatric Neuroimaging (4th edn). Lippincott Williams & Wilkins 2005; 190-290.

7. Horwood LJ, Mogridge N, Darlow BA (Eds). Cognitive, educational and behavioral outcomes at 7 to 8 years in a national very low birthweight cohort. Arch Dis Child Fetal Neonatal 1998; 79:12-20.

8. Emslie HC, Wardle SP, Sims DG, et al (Eds). Increased survival and deteriorating developmental outcome in 23-25 weeks gestation infants, 1990-1994 compared with1984-1989. Arch Dis Child Fetal Neonatal 1998; 78:99-104.

9. Keeney SE, Adecock EW, McArdle CB. Prospective observations of 100 high risk neonates by high field (1.5 Tesla) magnetic resonance imaging of the central nervous system: I. Intraventricular and extracerebral lesions. Pediatrics 1991; 87:421-30.

10. Keeney SE, Adecock EW, McArdle CB. Prospective observations of 100 high risk neonates by high field (1.5 Tesla) magnetic resonance imaging of the central nervous system:II. Lesions associated with hypoxic-ischemic encephalopathy. Pediatrics 1991; 87:431-38.

11. Koeda T, Suganuma I, Kohno Y, et al. MR imaging of spastic diplegia: Comparative study between preterm and term infants. Neuroradiology 1990; 32:187-90.

12. Flodmark O, Roland EH, Hill A, et al. Periventricular leukomalacia: Radiologic diagnosis. Radiology 1987; 162:119-24.

13. Barkovich AJ, Westmark K, Partridge C, et al. Perinatal asphyxia: MR findings in the first 10 days. AJNR 1995; 16:427-38.

14. Flodmark O, Lupton B, Li D, et al. MR imaging of periventricular leukomalacia in childhood. Am J Neuroradiol 1989; 10:111-18.

15. Huppi PS. MR in HIE. Clinical Perinatol 2002; 29(4):827-56.

16. Barkovich AJ, Sargent SK. Profound asphyxia in the premature infant: Imaging findings. Am J Neuroradiol 1995; 16:1837-46.

17. Hambleton G, Wigglesworth JS. Origin of intraventricular hemorrhage in preterm infant. Arch Dis Child 1976; 51:651-60.

18. Wigglesworth JS, Pape KE. An integrated model for hemorrhage and ischemic lesions in the newborn brain. Early Hum Dev 1978; 2:179-99.

19. Papile LA, Brustein J, Koffer H. Incidence and evolution of subependymal and intraventricular hemorrhage: A study of infants with birth weight less than 1500 gm. J Pediatr 1978; 92:529-34.

20. Gould SJ, Howard S, Hope PL, et al. Periventricular intraparenchymal cerebral hemorrhage in preterm infants: Role of venous infarction. J Pathol 1987; 151:197-202.

21. Volpe JJ: Brain injury in premature infant. Neuro-pathology, clinical aspects and pathogenesis. MRDD Res Rev 1997; 3:3-12.

22. Del Toro J, Louis PT, Goddard–Finegold J. Cerebrovascular regulation and neonatal brain injury. Pediatr Neurol 1991; 7:3-12.

23. Hill A. Current concepts of hypoxic-ischemic cerebral injury in the term newborn. Pediatr Neurol 1991; 7:317-25.

24. Volpe JJ. Hypoxic-ischemic encephalopathy: Neuropathology and pathogenesis. In Volpe JJ (Ed): Neurology of the Newborn (3rd edn). Philadelphia: Saunders 1995; 279-313.

25. Rutherford MA, Supramaniam V, Ederies A, Chew A, Bassi L, Groppo M, et al. Magnetic resonance imaging of white matter diseases of prematurity. Neuroradiology 2010; 52:505-21.

26. Maria A, Gupta AK, Paul VK, et al. Germinal matrix Intraventricular hemorrhage of the premature infants and PVL. In Kalra V (Ed): Practical Paediatric Neurology, Arya publication 36-38, 2002. [From DM Dissertation of Maria A at AIIMS Periventricular leukomalacia among the very low birth weight neonates, August 2003].

27. Zupan V, Gonzalez P, Lacaze-Masmonteil T, et al. Periventricular leukomalacia: Risk factors revisited. Dev Med Child Neurol 1996; 38:1061-67.

28. Verma U, Tehani N, Klein S, et al. Obstetric antecedents of intraventricular haemorrhage and periventricular leukomalacia in the low birth weight neonate. Am J Obstet Gynecol 1997; 176:275-81.

29. Nelson K, Ellenberg J. Antecedents of cerebral palsy: Multivariate analysis of risk. N Engl J Med 1986; 315:81-86.

30. Back SA, Luo NL, Borenstein NS, Levine JM, Volpe JJ, Kinney HC. Late oligodendrocyte progenitors coincide with the developmental window of vulnerability for human perinatal white matter injury. J Neurosci 2001; 21:1302-12.

31. Back SA, Han BH, Luo NL, et al. Selective vulnerability of late oligodendrocyte progenitors to hypoxia-ischemia. J Neurosci 2002; 22:455-63.

32. Perlman JM, et al. Bilateral cystic PVL in the premature infants Associated risk factors. Pediatrics 1996; 97:822-27.

33. Hesser U, Katz-Salamon M, Mortensson W, et al. Diagnosis of intracranial lesions in very low birth weight infants by ultrasound Incidence and association with potential risk factors. Acta Pediat Suppl 1997; 419:16-26.

34. Claris O, Besnier S, Lapillonne A, et al. Incidence of ischemic hemorrhagic cerebral lesions in premature infants of gestational age 28 weeks: A prospective ultrasound study. Biol Neonate 1996 70:29-34.

35. McArdle CB, Richardson CJ, Hayden CK, et al. Abnormalities of the neonatal brain: MR Imaging Part II. Hypoxic-Ischemic brain injury. Radiology 1987; 163:395-403.

36. Banker BQ, Larroche JC. Periventricular leukomalacia in infancy A form of neonatal anoxic encephalopathy. Arch Neurol 1962 7:386-410.

37. Weisglas-Kuperus N, Baerts W, Fetter W, et al. Minor neurological dysfunction and quality of movement in relation to neonatal cerebral damage and subsequent development. Dev Med Child Neurol 1994 36:727-35.

38. Pinto-Martin JA, Dobson V, Cnaan A, et al. Vision outcome at age 2 years in a low birth weight population. Pediatr Neurol 1996 14:281-87.

39. Uggetti C, Egitto ME, Fazzi E, et al. Cerebral visual impairment in periventricular leukomalacia: MR correlation. AJNR 1996; 17:979-85.

40. Roth SC, Baudin J, McCormick DC, et al. Relation between ultrasound appearance of the brain of very preterm infants and neurodevelopmental impairment at eight years. Dev Med Child Neurol 1993; 35:755-68.

41. Barr LL, McCullough PJ, Ball WS, et al. Quantitative sonographic feature analysis of clinical infant hypoxia: A pilot study. AJNR 1996; 17:1025-31.

42. Vannucci RC, Christensen MA, Yager JY. Nature, time course and extent of cerebral edema in perinatal hypoxic ischaemic brain damage. Pediatr Neurol 1993; 9:29-34.

43. Grant EG, Schellinger D, Richardson JD, et al. Echogenic periventricular halo: Normal sonographic finding or neonatal cerebral hemorrhage? AJNR 1983; 4:43-46.

44. de Vries LS, Eken P, Dubowitz LMS. The spectrum of leukomalacia using cranial ultrasound. Behav Brain Res 1992; 49:1-6.

45. Perlman JM. Guidelines for cranial ultrasounds in premature infants. In http://neonatal.peds.washington.edu/NICU-WEB/ultrasound.pdf.

46. Debillon, et al. Limitations of ultrasound for diagnosing white matter damage in preterm infants. Archives of Diseases in childhood Fetal & Neonatal 2003; 88:275.

47. Miller, et al. Comparing the diagnosis of white matter injury in premature newborns with serial MR imaging and transfontanel ultrasonography findings. AJNR 2003; 24:1661-69.

48. Inder TE, et al. White matter injury in the premature infants: A comparison between serial cranial sonographic and MR findings at term. AJNR 2003; 24(5):805-09.

49. Graham, et al. Prediction of cerebral palsy in very low birth weight infants: Prospective ultrasound study. Lancet 1987; 2(8559):593-96.

50. Arthur R. Magnetic resonance imaging in preterm infants. Pediatr Radiol 2006; 36:593-607.

51. Bozzao, et al. Diffusion weighted MR imaging in the early diagnosis of PVL. Eur Radiol 2003; 13(7):1571-76.

52. Roelants-van Rijn, et al. Neonatal diffusion weighted MRI: Relation with histopathology or follow-up MR examination. Neuropediatrics 2001; 32(6):286-94.

53. Arzoumanian Y, et al. Diffusion Tensor Brain imaging findings at term equivalent age may predict neurologic abnormalities in low birth weight preterm infants. AJNR 2003; 24:1646-53.

54. Miller, et al. Serial quantitative diffusion tensor MRI of the premature brain – development in newborns with and without injury. J Magn Reson Imaging 2002; 16(6):621-32.

55. Hoon, et al. Diffusion Tensor imaging of PVL shows affected sensory cortex white matter pathways. Neurology 2002; 59(5):752-56.

56. Melhelm ER, et al. Diffusion Tensor MR imaging of the brain and white matter tractography. AJR 2002; 178:3-16.

57. Baker LL, Stevenson DK, Enzmann DR. End stage periventricular leukomalacia: MR evaluation. Radiology 1988; 168:809-15.

58. Hull J, Dodd KL. Falling incidence of hypoxic ischemic encephalopathy in term infants. Br J Obstet Gynecol 1992; 99:386-91.

59. Truwit CL, Barkovich AJ, Koch TK, et al. Cerebral palsy: MR findings in 40 patients. AJNR 1992; 13:67-78.

60. Raybaud C. Destructive lesions of the brain. Neuroradiology 1983; 25:265-91.

61. Rutherford M, Srinivasan L, Dyet L, Ward P, Allsop J, Counsell S, Cowan F. Magnetic resonance imaging in perinatal brain injury: Clinical presentation, lesions and outcome. Pediatr Radiol 2006; 36:582-92.

62. Hunt RW, Neil JJ, Coleman LT, Kean MJ, Inder TE. Apparent diffusion coefficient in the posterior limb of the internal capsule predicts outcome after perinatal asphyxia. Pediatrics. 2004; 114(4):999-1003.

63. De vries LS, Groenendaal F. Patterns of neonatal hypoxic-ischemic brain injury. Neuroradiology 2010; 52:555-66.

64. Hanrahan JD, Sargentoni J, Azzopardi D, et al. Cerebral metabolism within 18 hours of birth asphyxia: A proton magnetic resonance spectroscopy study. Pediatr Res 1996; 39:584-90.

65. Peden CJ, Cowan FM, Bryant DJ, et al. Proton MR spectroscopy of the brain in infants. J Comput Assist Tomogr 1990; 14:886-94.

66. Holshouser BA, Ashwal S, Luh GY, et al. Proton MR spectroscopy after acute central nervous system injury: Outcome prediction in neonates, infants and children. Radiology 1997; 202:487-96.

67. Penrice J, Cady EB, Lorek A, et al. Proton MR spectroscopy of the brain in normal preterm and term infants and early changes after perinatal hypoxic ischemia. Pediatr Res 1996; 40:6-14.

68. Huang BY, Castillo M. Hypoxic-ischemic brain injury: Imaging findings from birth to adulthood. Radiographics 2008; 28:417-39.

69. Connolly B, Kelehan P, Brien NO, et al. The echogenic thalamus in hypoxic-ischemic encephalopathy. Pediatr Radiol 1994; 24:268-71.

70. Seibert JJ, McCowan TC, Chadduck WM, et al. Duplex pulsed Doppler US vs intracranial pressure in the neonate. Clinical and experimental studies. Radiology 1989; 171:155-59.

71. Stark JE, Seibert JJ. Cerebral artery Doppler ultrasonography for prediction of outcome after perinatal asphyxia. J Ultrasound Med 1994; 13:595-600.

72. KimHan B, Towbin RB, DeCourten-Meyers G, et al. Reversal sign on CT: Effect of anoxic/ischaemic cerebral injury in children. AJR 1990; 154:361-68.

73. Rutherford MA, Pennock JM, Counsell SJ, et al. Abnormal magnetic resonance signal in the internal capsule predicts poor neurodevelopmental outcome in infants with hypoxic-ischemic encephalopathy. Pediatrics 1998; 102:323-8.

74. Rutherford M, Biarge MM, Allsop J, Counsell S, Cowan F. MRI of perinatal brain injury. Pediatr Radiol 2010; 40:819-33.

75. Cordes I, Roland EH, Lupton BA, et al. Early prediction of the development of microcephaly after HIE in full term newborn. Pediatrics 1994; 93:703-07.

76. Han, et al. Risk factors for cerebral palsy in preterm. Am J Phy Med Rehab 2002; 81:297-303.

77. van de Bor, et al. Value of cranial ultrasound and MRI in predicting neurodevelopmental outcome in preterm infants. Pediatrics 1992; 90:196-99.

CHAPTER 27

Cranial Sonography

Rashmi Dixit, Veena Chowdhury

Neurosonography is an integral part of neonatal and infant brain imaging while the fontanelles remain open. Current ultrasound equipment allows rapid evaluation of infants in the intensive care nursery with excellent visualization of normal structures and a wide range of pathologies.[1] The advantages of sonography over computed tomography or magnetic resonance imaging include portability, lower cost, lack of ionizing radiation and no need for sedation.[2]

Technique and Normal Anatomy

Neurosonography is most successfully performed in a warm environment, when the baby is quiet or after feeding. For neonates, a 5-7.5 MHz sector transducer and for older infants, a 3-5 MHz transducer provides adequate visualization of the whole brain.[3,4] High frequency (7-10 MHz) sector or curvilinear array probes are excellent for demonstrating the superficial extracerebral spaces and to delineate the sulcal pattern as well as corticomedullary regions in the near field.[5] 3-D ultrasound has also been used to evaluate the infant brain.

The anterior fontanelle is the primary acoustic window and remains open for the first 6-12 months of life.[6] Images are obtained in the coronal and sagittal planes. Additional views may be obtained through the posterior fontanelle, mastoid fontanelle and by transaxial scanning through the squamous temporal bone.[4] The posterior fontanelle and mastoid fontanelle approach can significantly improve the diagnostic utility of neurosonography. The mastoid fontanelle approach improves visualization of the brainstem, cerebellum and subarachnoid cisterns which are suboptimally seen through the anterior fontanelle. Also, small intraventricular hemorrhages may be better visualized through posterior fontanelle. The midline post-fontanelle usually closes by about 3 months of age, whereas mastoid (posterolateral) fontanelle may not fuse until 2 years of age.[7] Important intracranial structures seen on coronal and sagittal sonograms are shown in Figures 27.1A to 27.2B.

Cranial Doppler US: The anterior fontanelle approach for Doppler US provides the most easily accessible view and reveals the best anatomic detail. A combination of coronal scans allows consistent identification of the major intracranial vessels including anterior cerebral artery (A1 segment and distal segment), internal carotid artery and basilar artery. The M1 segment of the middle cerebral artery is not well-demonstrated as the direction of blood flow is nearly perpendicular to the Doppler beam. The internal cerebral veins and the vein of Galen are easily seen on the midsagittal view. The superior sagittal sinus and straight sinus can also be identified.[2]

The temporal approach through the thin squamous portion of the temporal bone provides detailed images of the midbrain and the vessels forming the circle of Willis. The proximal segment of the anterior and middle cerebral arteries and the M1 portion is well seen due to the more favorable Doppler angle. This approach can also be used in older children when the anterior fontanelle is closed.[2,4]

The brain is a low-resistance vascular bed and continuous forward flow should be seen throughout the arteries in systole and diastole. In term infant, RI ranges between 60 to 78 percent.[8,9] It is slightly higher (68 to 88%) in infants less than 34 weeks gestational age.[8] Besides pathological conditions, elevated RI may be seen with increased scanning pressure, high pass filter setting and in the presence of a patent ductus arteriosus. Continued refinement of ultrasound contrast agents allows quantitative cerebral perfusion mapping.[10]

The normal vascular anatomy as seen by CDFI is depicted in (Figs 27.3 to 27.5).

Congenital Brain Anomalies

These may occur at any stage of brain development. Sonography is often the first modality used for an infant with a congenital brain malformation. Many anomalies will be diagnozed, while in others it is useful in directing the patient to MR imaging which is the current standard of reference.

Failure of Neural Tube Closure

The first stage in brain development is neural tube closure in the 1st month of gestation, failure of which caudally causes myelomeningocele and cranially causes anencephaly or encephalocele. A myelomeningocele is very often associated with a Chiari II malformation. Aqueductal stenosis may also develop during neural tube closure in the first trimester. It often causes obstructive hydrocephalus and may lead to severe brain damage.

Infants born with a myelomeningocele require a cranial examination to establish the baseline status of the ventricular system, which frequently enlarges following primary repair of the spinal lesion, due to change in cerebrospinal fluid dynamics.

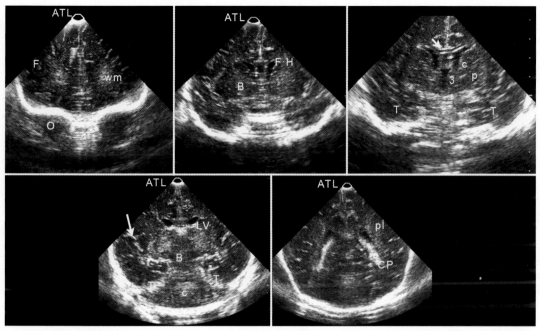

Figs 27.1A to E: Coronal sonograms of a normal infant (A to E). (A) F—frontal lobes, WM — frontal white matter O—orbits (B) FH—frontal horn of lateral ventricle, B—basal ganglia. Arrow points to the cingulate sulcus. (C) c-caudate nucleus, p—putamen, T—temporal lobe, 3—3rd ventricle, arrow points to the corpus callosum. (D) B—brainstem H—hippocampal formation T—tentorium C—cerebellum. Arrow points to the sylvian fissure. (E) pl—parietal lobe, CP—glomus of the choroid plexus. Note that the white matter of the centrum semiovale appears slightly more reflective than the grey matter

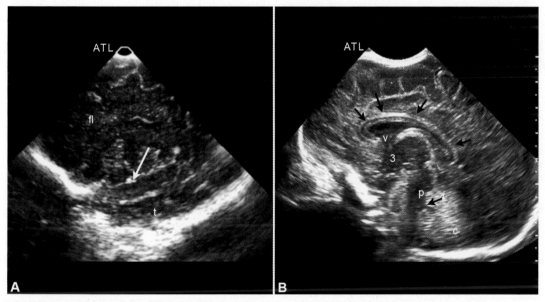

Figs 27.2A and B: (A) parasagittal and (B) midline sagittal scans of a normal infant (A) fl—frontal lobe, t—temporal lobe. Arrow points to the sylvian fissure. (B) V-cavum septum pellucidum and cavum vergae, 3—3rd ventricle, P—pons, 4—fourth ventricle

Chiari II Malformation

Sonographic Appearance

Sagittal sonograms demonstrate a small posterior fossa resulting in displacement of the cerebellar vermis, fourth ventricle and medulla into the cervical canal with a medullary kink. The fourth ventricle is often poorly visualized as it is thin, elongated, compressed and displaced into the upper spinal canal.

The degree of ventricular dilatation is variable at presentation but is usually progressive. The occipital horns and atria are disproportionately dilated compared to the frontal and temporal horns (colpocephaly). On coronal images, there is anterior and inferior pointing of the frontal horns referred to as 'batwing configuration'. The septum pellucidum may be partially or completely absent. The massa intermedia is enlarged and fills a dilated third ventricle. The interhemispheric fissure is often

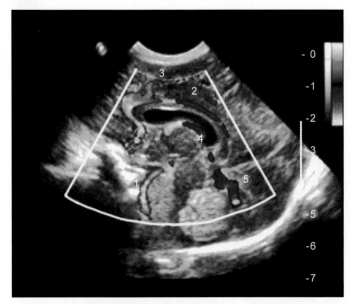

Fig. 27.3: Midline sagittal color Doppler scan showing internal cerebral artery (1), pericallosal artery (2) callosomarginal artery (3) internal cerebral vein (4) straight sinus (5) *(For color version see plate 9)*

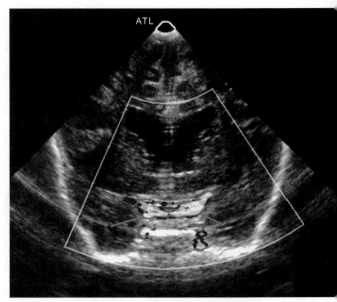

Fig. 27.5: Coronal CDFI scan showing ICA on both sides, arrow point to their bifurcation on both sides *(For color version see plate 9)*

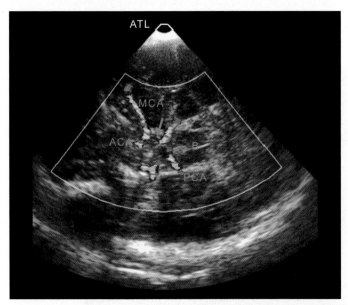

Fig. 27.4: Axial section through the squamous temporal bone showing the vessels of the circle of Willis. Arrow points to the posterior communicating artery *(For color version see plate 9)*

prominent in these patients.[2] Sonography has been a reliable method for follow-up of shunting procedures and evaluation of hydrocephalus in the first year of life,[2] although abnormalities of the Chiari malformation are best appreciated on MRI.

Agenesis of the Corpus Callosum

Corpus callosum forms during the first 8-12 weeks of gestation. Depending on the timing of intrauterine insult, the development can be partially arrested or complete agenesis may occur and is frequently associated with major malformations. The bundles of

Probst that failed to fuse will persist as rounded masses on each side of the midline. The key sonographic findings are widely spaced lateral ventricles which are tiny anteriorly and enlarge posteriorly. The frontal horns are slit like, widely separated with concave medial margins and superolateral peaks. The third ventricle is dilated and high placed and often associated with dorsal cyst (Fig. 27.6). On midline sagittal images, the sulci are arranged radially above the third ventricle.[2,4] It is difficult to diagnose partial agenesis on sonography.

Dandy-Walker (DW) Complex

This includes the Dandy-Walker syndrome and Dandy-Walker variant.

The Dandy-Walker syndrome may be caused by obstruction of the outlet of the fourth ventricle. The fourth ventricle is enlarged and communicates with a large posterior fossa cyst. There is hypoplasia of the cerebellar vermis and cerebellar hemispheres which are displaced anterolaterally. The posterior fossa is large with elevation of tentorium cerebelli, straight sinus and torcular herophili. The brainstem may be compressed or hypoplastic. The cerebral aqueduct may be narrowed or occluded. Generalized obstructive hydrocephalus occurs in 80 percent of patients (Figs 27.7A and B). If corpus callosum is hypogenetic colpocephaly is present. In patients with aqueductal stenosis separate shunts may be required for the supratentorial ventricle and post fossa cyst.

In the DW variant, the posterior fossa is normal in size and although the vermis is small, the cerebellar hemispheres are normal. The fourth ventricle is slightly to moderately enlarged and communicates with the cisterna magna. The differential diagnosis includes a giant cisterna magna and posterior fossa arachnoid cyst (Fig. 27.8) In these conditions, the cerebellar vermis and

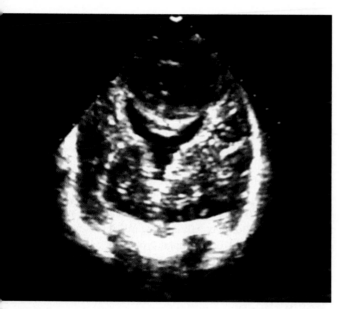

Fig. 27.6: Coronal sonogram showing frontal horns with concave medial borders and sharply angled lateral peaks. The third ventricle is also mildly dilated and slightly high placed, consistent with agenesis of corpus callosum

hemispheres are not hypoplastic and the cyst does not communicate with the fourth ventricle.[11-13]

Disorders of Diverticulation

The second stage of brain development during the 2nd month of gestation is diverticulation into two hemispheres, development of the pineal and pituitary glands as well as optic and olfactory tracts. Malformations include the spectrum from simple absence of the septum pellucidum to alobar holoprosencephaly. Since the face

is formed at the same time, severe midline facial abnormalities are often present.[13]

Holoprosencephaly

A failure of midline cleavage of the prosencephalon causes failure of formation of separate cerebral hemispheres.

The most severe form of holoprosencephaly is ***alobar holoprosencephaly***. On sonography, there is a single horseshoe or crescent shaped monoventricle which communicates with a large dorsal cyst. The thalami are fused and the third ventricle is absent, as are the corpus callosum and interhemispheric fissure. The cortex is thin with sparse convolutional markings and a smooth appearance to the brain surface. The cerebellum and brainstem are often spared. If Doppler is applied, absence of anterior cerebral arteries or occurrence of only a single vessel may be noted. There is absence of internal cerebral veins, the superior sagittal sinus and straight sinus.[3,16]

Semilobar holoprosencephaly is the less severe, variant. The single ventricle persists but there may be separate occipital and temporal horns. Portions of the septum pellucidum and corpus callosum may be present posteriorly. The thalami are partially fused along the floor of the malformed third ventricle.

Lobar holoprosencephaly is the least severe form. There is nearly complete separation of the hemispheres with development of the falx and interhemispheric fissure but the anteroinferior portion is incomplete and the frontal lobes are fused. The septum pellucidum is absent. The anterior horns of the lateral ventricles are fused and square shaped but occipital horns are separated. The third ventricle is usually present, separating the thalami and the splenium and body of corpus callosum are often present with absence of the genu and rostrum.

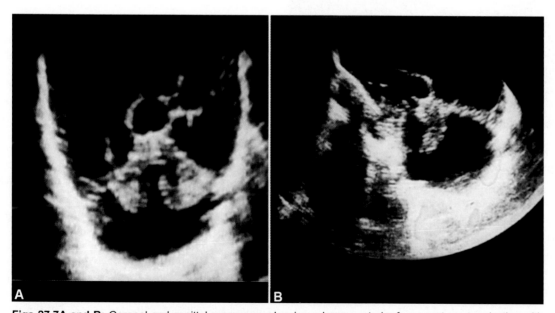

Figs 27.7A and B: Coronal and sagittal sonograms showing a large posterior fossa cyst communicating with the fourth ventricle with hypoplastic vermis and cerebellar hemispheres which are displaced anterolaterally. Marked generalized hydrocephalus is present

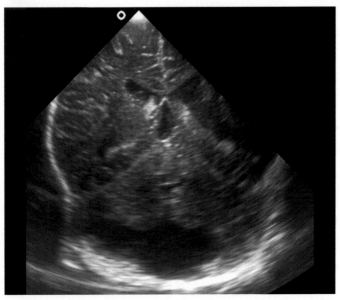

Fig 27.8: Coronal sonogram through the anterior fontanelle shows a large cyst in the posterior fossa not communicating with the fourth ventricle with normal cerebellum – Giant Gisterna Magna

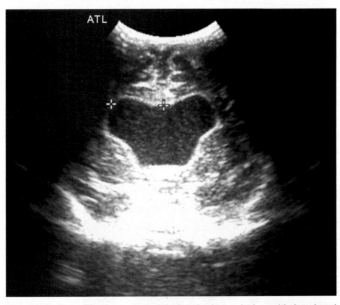

Fig. 27.9: Coronal sonogram showing hydrocephalus with low level echoes within the ventricular system due to ventriculitis. Note the absence of septum pellucidum due to secondary destruction

Pellucidal Agenesis and Dysgenesis

Absence of septum pellucidum is often associated with other malformations such as holoprosencephaly, septo-optic dysplasia, callosal agenesis, Chiari II malformation, etc. Secondary destruction is more common than primary agenesis and may occur following trauma, inflammation or ventricular obstruction[15] (Fig. 27.9).

Disorders of sulcation and migration occur during the 3rd to 6th month of gestation. These result when the neuronal cells fail to migrate to the cortex such that the cortex becomes too thick and/or too smooth or heterotopic nodules of grey matter are left in unusual places. Neuronal migration anomalies are best evaluated by MR imaging.

Schizencephaly

Schizencephaly is a developmental defect resulting in a brain cleft lined by grey matter, which is an asymmetric process resulting in a single or bilateral cleft extending from the surface of the brain to the ventricular system. The asymmetry suggests that in some patients, schizencephaly may represent an early insult during brain development. The lesions have been divided into two groups based on fused or separated lips of the clefts.[16] Type I represents the closed lip schizencephaly and type II represents the open lip schizencephaly. The open lipped type may be easily diagnosed by ultrasound where an echofree cavity extends from the surface of the brain to fuse with the lateral wall of the lateral ventricle.[4]

Lissencephaly

In lissencephaly, the cerebral sulci and gyri fail to develop fully with a thick smooth four cell layered cortex resembling an hourglass in the coronal plane. In type I lissencephaly, microcephaly, facial dysmorphism and severe mental retardation are the rule. On ultrasound, the cerebral cortex resembles that of a 24 week fetus with no cerebral sulci, nearly absent operculization of the insula giving a figure of 8 appearance. Type II lissencephaly typically presents with macrocephaly, secondary to obstructive hydrocephalus. Ultrasound may help to identify the agyric cortex despite severe ventricular dilatation which may be difficult to identify on CT scanning.[4]

Disorders of Histogenesis may result in tumours, arteriovenous malformations or cysts, but they are uncommon in infancy.

Tuberous Sclerosis

CNS manifestations of tuberous sclerosis include hamartomas of the periphery of the brain parenchyma and benign subependymal tubers. Subependymal nodules are seen on sonography as small focal highly reflective nodules in the wall of the lateral ventricle. Echogenic lesions in the brain parenchyma represent peripheral hamartomas.[15]

Sturge-Weber Syndrome

Serpiginous echodensities due to leptomeningeal angiomatosis may be identified in the brain periphery associated with decreased cortical volume of the involved hemisphere, i.e. cortical hemiatrophy. Usually the choroid plexus is enlarged due to the presence of angiomas within the structure.

Vascular Malformations

The most common intracranial vascular malformation presenting in the neonatal period is the vein of Galen malformation. Sonographic hallmark of the lesion is a midline echofree or mixed echogenicity, pulsatile mass that blooms with color when Doppler modalities are applied. CDFI may be helpful in distinguishing the

wo most common types.[17] The choroidal type is characterized
by multiple abnormal feeding vessels arising in the midbrain with
venous drainage via the aneurysmally dilated vein of Galen and
straight sinus. The infundibular type consists of an arteriovenous
fistula with one or few arterial feeders draining directly into the
vein of Galen.

Spectral Doppler imaging typically shows arterialization of
venous flow and increased flow velocities with reduced pulsatility
of arterial feeders. Whether embolization or surgery is planned,
intraprocedural neurosonography is useful in evaluating
completeness of therapy. Patients are generally monitored post
treatment with Doppler sonography.[15]

DESTRUCTIVE BRAIN LESIONS

Porencephalic Cyst

A porencephalic cyst is an area of normally developed brain that
has been damaged and heals with a lining of gliotic white matter.
The resultant lesion usually communicates with the ventricles. On
sonography, an anechoic cavity communicating with the
ventricular system is seen. The term should ideally be restricted
to true *in utero* causes of cystic brain damage[4] (Fig. 27.10).

Focal or diffuse brain damage in neonates can result in areas
of cystic encephalomalacia. These typically do not communicate
with the ventricular system[2,4] (Fig. 27.11).

Hydranencephaly

Occlusion of the supraclinoid internal carotid arteries between the
12th and 26th weeks of gestation, results in destruction of the
formed cerebral hemispheres. A fluid filled membranous sac fills
the calvarium but the falx is present, differentiating this condition
from holoprosencephaly. Variable amounts of frontal and occipital
lobes may be preserved. The thalami, basal ganglia, midbrain and
posterior fossa contents are essentially normal. On CDFI flow in
the internal carotid arteries is absent.[2,4] It can be difficult to
differentiate hydranencephaly from severe hydrocephalus but a
thin rim of cortex should be visualized by sonography in
hydrocephalus.[18-20] Macrocephaly is usual although the head may
be normal or even small in size.

HYDROCEPHALUS

Hydrocephalus is an excessive accumulation of CSF in the
ventricular system, subarachnoid spaces overlying the brain or a
combination of both. It results when there is an imbalance between
its production and absorption or an obstruction to the free flow
of CSF.[21] Hydrocephalus may be considered to be
communicating, i.e. extraventricular obstruction to CSF flow or
non-communicating, i.e. intraventricular obstruction to CSF flow,
upto the level of the outlet foramina of the fourth ventricle. Rarely,
excessive production of CSF may result in hydrocephalus.

Sonography is the preferred modality for the initial evaluation
of an infant with suspected hydrocephalus. Often, hydrocephalus
can be diagnosed *in utero* by 15 weeks of gestation. The size of
the atrium and glomus remain constant in second and third
trimester. *In utero*, an upper limit of 10 mm for the ventricular

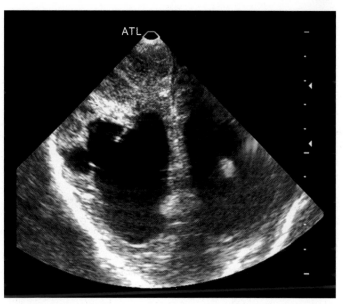

Fig. 27.10: Coronal sonogram showing dilated lateral ventricles with
a porencephalic cyst communicating with the left lateral ventricle

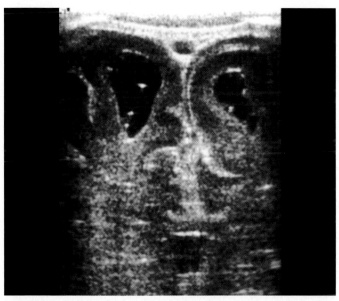

Fig. 27.11: Coronal sonogram showing well defined anechoic areas
representing cystic encephalomalacia in both frontal lobes

atrium has been established. On neonatal sonography, the
ventricular system is well defined with separation of the walls in
preterm infants, whereas in the full term and older infant the
ventricles are less distended and ventricular walls are often
apposed. Measurements taken in the coronal section at the level
of foramen of Monro are the most reproducible[4] (Fig. 27.12).
Reported values range from 9-13 mm for term infants.[4] In preterm
infants, lateral ventricular width varies from 6-12 mm while lateral
ventricular ratio ranges from 20.9 to 26.4 percent with a steady
decline with increasing age.[22-24]

Some authors have described measurement of anterior horn
width—measured between the medial wall and floor of the frontal

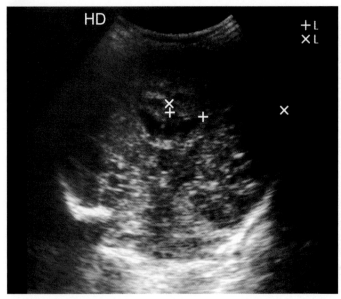

Fig. 27.12: Coronal section at the level of foramen of Monro. The calipers show the points for measurement of lateral ventricles and hemispheric measurement for VH ratio

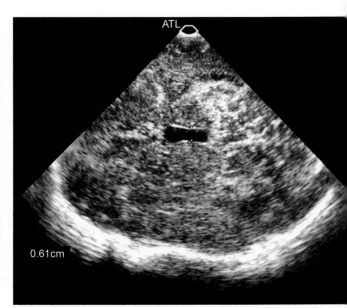

Fig. 27.14: Axial section through the squamous temporal bone demonstrating the third ventricle

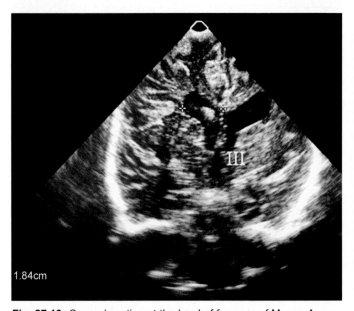

Fig. 27.13: Coronal section at the level of foramen of Monro. Arrows mark the points for measurement of anterior horn width

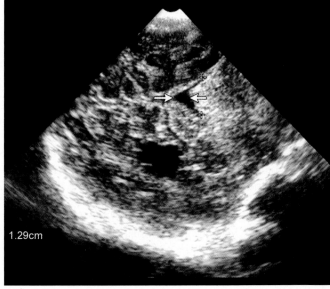

Fig. 27.15: Sonogram through the posterolateral fontanelle showing the triangular fourth ventricle. Calipers mark the position for measurement of width and arrows mark the position for the length

horn at the widest point in coronal section (Fig. 27.13). In normal preterm and term infants, anterior horn width of < 3 mm has been described.[25,26] Qualitative assessment of ventricular size is often used in practice. The most useful signs are progressive rounding and bulging of the superolateral angles of the frontal horns and dilatation of occipital horns.

Sonographic criteria for the enlargement of third and fourth ventricles on transfontanelle scans are not well established. Third ventricular width of 0-2.6 mm on axial scans (Fig. 27.14) and fourth ventricle width of 3.3-7.4 mm and length of 2.6–6.9 mm

on scans through the asterion (Fig. 27.15) have been described in preterm neonates < 33 weeks GA.[25] The presence of rounded fourth ventricle with no recognized cisterna is suggestive of noncommunicating dilation, whereas a triangular fourth ventricle with wide cisterna magna indicates a communicating dilatation.

CDFI techniques may also be helpful in evaluating CSF flow dynamics in these infants. Particulate matter and microbubble formation in CSF passing through the aqueduct, results in flow related color encoded jets. CSF flow produces a highly characteristic sinusoidal spectral Doppler waveform, indicative of

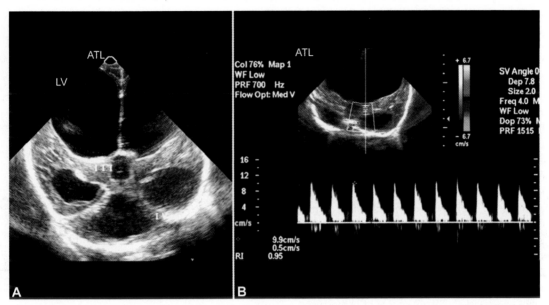

Figs 27.16A and B: (A) Coronal sonogram showing generalized dilatation of the ventricular system. (B) CDFI of the same patient showing markedly elevated RI in the MCA s/o increased ICP *(For color version see plate 9)*

cyclical to and fro motion of CSF within the ventricular system.[4] Examination of the ventricular system during cranial and abdominal compression may induce movement of CSF detectable with color flow or Doppler scanning.[27]

The effect of hydrocephalus on cerebral circulation can be evaluated and the resistive index correlated linearly with the intracranial pressure (ICP) in hydrocephalus, which is more important than the anatomic assessment of ventricular size alone. As the intracranial pressure rises, arterial flow tends to be more affected during diastole than during systole resulting in an increased pulsatility of flow. Increasing RI correlates well with elevation in ICP (Figs 27.16A and B). The resistive index decreases after ventriculoperitoneal shunting or tapping.[28,29] Doppler examination of the anterior or middle cerebral artery during fontanelle compression may be useful in the early identification of infants with abnormal intracranial compliance prior to the development of increased ICP as shown by elevated base line RI.[30] In normal infants, CSF or blood flow can be readily displaced compensating for the small increase in volume caused by compression of anterior fontanelle resulting in no increase in ICP. In infants with hydrocephalus, however, this manoeuvre results in transient increased intra-cranial pressure and an acute increase in arterial pulsatility.[30,31]

Sonography is also useful in determining the level of obstruction. Evaluation of the entire ventricular system should be done so that the level at which there is a transition from a large to small ventricle can be identified.[25] Dilatation of the lateral and third ventricles indicates an obstruction at the aqueductal level, most often secondary to intraventricular hemorrhage or infection or sometimes congenital, often an X-linked recessive trait. Regional flow imaging with color Doppler has been investigated as a method to exclude obstructive hydrocephalus.[27] Free passage of CSF through the ventricles and out into the basal cistern confirms the diagnosis of communicating hydrocephalus.[4]

Sonography is ideal for following ventricular size in infants who are on treatment for hydrocephalus, displaying the position of the shunt tube and size of the ventricles. Following successful shunting, a fall in the arterial RI has also been demonstrated.

Another important type of hydrocephalus in infancy is the so called **benign communicating hydrocephalus** which has also been described as **benign external hydrocephalus** of infancy or chronic subdural hygromas of infancy. It is characterized by an enlargement of the subarachnoid spaces greater than 5 mm overlying the cerebral hemispheres, particularly over the frontal and temporal convexities. There is associated mild or moderate ventricular dilatation. The condition usually presents in the first year of life, the infant presenting with a large head .It is generally a self limiting process that resolves without treatment by two years of age. The etiology is probably transient immaturity of the arachnoid granulations or villi.[32] In the past, excess fluid overlying the hemispheres has been misconstrued as being subdural hygromas of indeterminate aetiology. However, both ultrasound and MRI can demonstrate that the excess fluid is actually in the subarachnoid space dipping into the sulci. This condition is also termed as **BESS syndrome** (Benign Enlargement of Subarachnoid Space). Follow-up imaging is not required but serial head circumference measurements should be obtained. The condition is not entirely benign, as it predisposes to extra-axial hemorrhage after minor head trauma, and transient minor developmental delay occurs in a minority of cases during the period of most rapid head growth at 5-12 months of age.

The differential diagnosis of benign enlargement of the extra-axial fluid spaces includes cerebral atrophy (widened sulci, small or normal head circumference, proportionate ventricular enlargement), subdural collections (arachnoid neomembranes, echogenic fluid, displacement of bridging cortical veins within the subarachnoid space away from skull toward the brain), meningitis (thickened leptomeninges, echogenic fluid), communicating hydrocephalus (larger ventricles), etc.

INTRACRANIAL HEMORRHAGE

One of the most important roles of cranial ultrasound in infancy is the investigation of intra-cranial hemorrhage in the newborn. The patterns and etiology of hemorrhage are different in premature and term infants.

The germinal matrix is the most common site of origin of intracranial hemorrhage in the **preterm infant**. It occurs in 20-45 percent of preterm low birth weight neonates.[33-35] The aetiological factors associated with hemorrhage and hypoxic/ischaemic encephalopathy overlap to a considerable degree. Hemorrhage probably arises due to varying cerebral blood flow in the delicate and immature vessels of the highly vascular germinal matrix.[36] These vessels are particularly vulnerable between 25 and 28 weeks of gestation and become less vulnerable as blood flow is shifted towards the cortex by 32-34 weeks.[37] Veins of the germinal matrix are the likely source of hemorrhage.

The classification/grading[38] of germinal matrix hemorrhage (GMH) most widely used is:

Grade I   Subependymal hemorrhage.
Grade II   Intraventricular extension without hydrocephalus.
Grade III Intraventricular hemorrhage with hydrocephalus
Grade IV   Intraventricular hemorrhage with deep intraparenchymal hemorrhage with or without hydrocephalus.

Sonography is the most effective method for detecting this hemorrhage in the newborn period and for follow-up in subsequent weeks. Most hemorrhages (90%) occur in the first 7 days of life, only one-third occur in the first 24 hours. The recommended time for US screening in preterm infants (<33wks) is around 7-10 days to detect GMH and evolving hemorrhage followed by a late scan at one month to detect cystic changes of PVL and hydrocephalus.[35]

Grade I

These are small hemorrhages confined to the subependymal or germinal matrix area between the lateral ventricle and head of caudate nucleus or the caudothalamic groove[39] (Fig. 27.17). They may be unilateral or bilateral. In the acute stage, this appears as a moderately or highly reflective area in the inferolateral wall of the frontal horn superficially resembling the choroid plexus but in a site where the choroid is absent, i.e. anterior to foramen of Monro. As the hematoma ages it liquefies, becomes sonolucent and subsequently may resolve completely or persist as a subependymal cyst or as a linear echo.[2,4] (Fig. 27.18) The neurological outcome of these children does not differ significantly from preterm infants with normal cranial ultrasound.

Abnormal hyperechogenicity of the subependymal germinal matrix is not always hemorrhagic. Nonhemorrhagic germinal matrix hyperechogenicity has been reported as an isolated finding or in association with cerebral infection CMV, rubella), extracerebral infection (especially rotavirus gastroenteritis), etc.

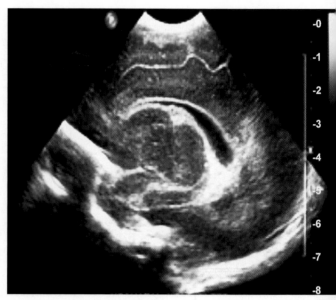

Fig. 27.17: Sagittal sonogram showing a small hyperechoic area i the caudothalamic groove with no evidence of hydrocephalus consister with grade I periventricular hemorrhage

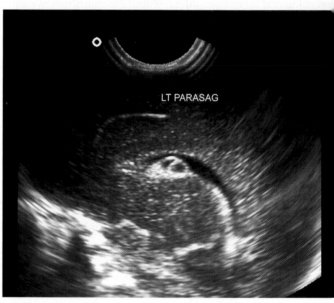

Fig. 27.18: Sagittal scan (of the same patient as in Fig. 27.17) after week shows liquefaction of the hematoma with formation c subependymal cysts

The location is the same as with germinal matrix hemorrhage bu the timing, appearance, and evolution are different.

Nonhemorrhagic germinal matrix hyperechogenicity is see primarily in near-term and term neonates, is teardrop shaped an bilaterally symmetric whereas germinal matrix hemorrhage occur in premature infants predominantly in the first 2 weeks of life an tends to be round and asymmetric or unilateral. Also nonhemorrhagic germinal matrix hyperechogenicity persists o evolves by germinolysis into subependymal pseudocysts wit gliotic walls lacking hemosiderin, whereas germinal matri:

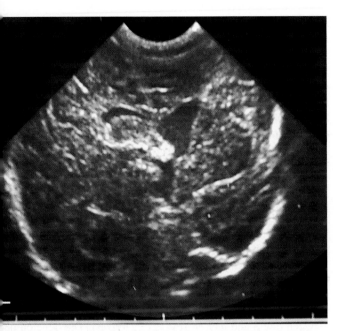

g. 27.19: Intraventricular clot in the left lateral ventricle extending to e 3rd ventricle with only minimal prominence of the ventricular system well seen on this coronal scan, suggesting grade 2 hemorrhage

morrhage liquefies and resolves by resorption, occasionally with emosiderin-lined subependymal pseudocysts as residua.[40]

rade II

his is an intraventricular hemorrhage with minimal or no gnificant ventriculomegaly at presentation. Before the blood has otted it is difficult to visualize in the ventricles, but subsequently can be seen as hyperechoic material that fills a portion or whole f the ventricular system.[2,4] The clots may just produce an hogenic irregular outline/thickening of the choroid plexus ig. 27.19A). Small clots tend to settle in the dependent occipital

horns in the supine infant and are difficult to detect through the anterior fontanelle approach. Use of posterior fontanelle or axial views may improve detection of IVH in normal sized ventricles.[41] If blood extends into the cisterna magna, there is an increased risk of post hemorrhagic hydrocephalus.[35] The incidence of neurological deficits is marginally higher in this group.[42,43]

Grade III

Large intraventricular hemorrhages result in significant ventricular dilatation at presentation. Large highly reflective areas fill the ventricular system producing a 'cast like' appearance. A chemical ventriculitis as a response to blood in the CSF typically produces thickening of the ependymal lining of the ventricle. Hydrocephalus occurs due to expansion of the ventricle by the blood along with impairment of CSF resorption at the level of arachnoid granulations. (Fig. 27.20A and B) Hydrocephalus should be monitored by serial ultrasound scans. In most cases the hydrocephalus may resolve and approximately 34 percent of very low birth infants require shunting.[35,39] The clinical outcome with varying degrees of permanent neurological impairment is significantly worse in this group.[44]

Grade IV

This consists of simultaneous intraventricular and intraparenchymal cerebral hemorrhage (Fig. 27.21). It is usually located in the frontal or parietal lobes because it often extends from the germinal matrix. It has been suggested that the culprit may be venous ischemia complicated by hemorrhage. CDFI may be used to show initial displacement and gradual encasement and obstruction of the terminal veins by an enlarging germinal matrix hemorrhage. This finding may be useful for early prediction of infants at risk for worsening intracranial hemorrhage.[45,46] The neurological sequelae in this group are usually severe and tend to be developmental delay and poor tone as opposed to spastic

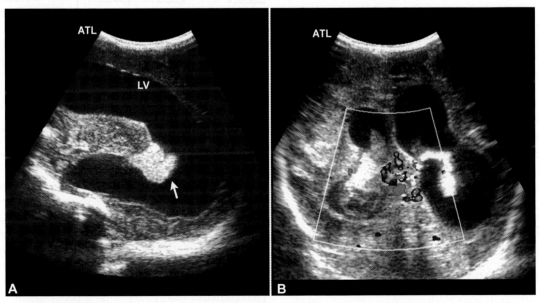

Figs 27.20A and B: Sagittal and coronal sonograms showing a grossly dilated lateral ventricles with enlarged and echogenic choroid plexus appearing avascular on CDFI consistent with haemorrhage

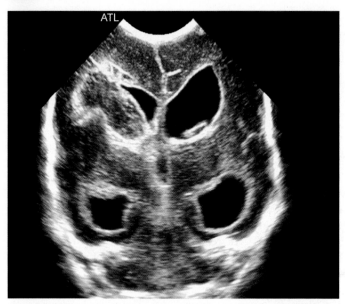

Fig. 27.21: Coronal sonogram showing marked dilatation of both lateral ventricles with intraventricular hemorrhage and deep parenchymal hemorrhage (grade IV) on the left side and intraventricular hemorrhage (grade III) on the right. The ependyma appears echogenic due to chemical ventriculitis

diplegia or quadriplegia in patient with ischemia in the same region.

Subarachnoid hemorrhage may also occur in preterm newborns and is usually difficult to identify on ultrasound due to normal variation in the appearance of subarachnoid cisterns. It may be seen as widening of sylvian fissures with increased reflectivity.

Hemorrhage in the **term newborn** may occur due to birth trauma and subdural hemorrhage is the most commonly encountered lesion due to falcine or tentorial laceration, while extradural hemorrhage is uncommon. Acute SDH appears as a highly reflective linear or elliptical collection that compresses the brain parenchyma. Transcranial scanning may be useful to demonstrate this lesion. Cerebellar hemorrhage is a reported complication of traumatic delivery in full term neonates, in ECMO or with coagulopathy. Posterior fossa hemorrhages are more difficult to demonstrate by the anterior fontanelle approach and the mastoid fontanelle scanning is now routinely used. Subarachnoid hemorrhage may occur in neonates who have experienced asphyxia or trauma and may be the only hemorrhage in full term infants not at risk for GMH.[2,4] Intraventricular hemorrhage has also been reported in term infants probably arising from the choroid plexus or germinal matrix.[35,47,48]

HYPOXIC OR ISCHEMIC ENCEPHALOPATHY

The pattern of involvement differs in the preterm and term neonate and also varies with the degree of hypoxia.

Mild to Moderate Hypotension in the Preterm Neonate

The most common location for injury to the premature brain is the periventricular white matter the periventricular white matter,

since this is the water shed area in the preterm infant, resulting in periventricular leucomalacia or **PVL**.

PVL is an ischemic lesion, that occurs in the peri-ventricular white matter and centrum semiovale in the preterm infant. In the premature infant, these areas are the most vulnerable to hypoperfusion and ischemia. The areas of infarction vary in size and severity.[2,4] There may be mild involvement with resulting gliosis or more severe involvement with resulting cystic changes. Areas of necrosis and infarction may be complicated by superimposed hemorrhage. The white matter in the region of the posterior trigone and adjacent to the frontal horns of the lateral ventricles is most commonly affected.[49]

Diagnosis of PVL may be made during the neonatal period with sonography, although the diagnosis is easier to miss than subependymal hemorrhage because there may be only subtle increase in echogenicity in the first week of life. These areas are more echogenic than the choroid in the acute phase but when they resolve, they may be mistaken for the normal periventricular echogenic blush. Cystic changes may develop later, usually between day 8 and day 28 (Fig. 27.22A to E). The development of macrocysts is a rarity nowadays. Bilateral involvement is common. The loss of periventricular white matter and coalescent cysts which may communicate with the ventricle results in characteristic irregular outline of the ventricle. The recognition of cysts is important because their presence is associated with adverse clinical outcome.

Early Doppler studies may demonstrate increased mean velocities and lower RI of lenticulostriate vessels in preterm infants who develop PVL.[50,51]

Severe Hypotension in the Preterm Neonate

The thalami, brainstem, and cerebellum in the immature brain have high metabolic activity and hence are more susceptible to injury in severe hypotension. This manifests as hyperechogenicity of the injured brain at US imaging. Coexisting periventricular white matter injury and germinal matrix hemorrhage may be present.[52] (Fig. 27.23)

Recent studies suggest that cerebellar infarction and hemorrhage in the preterm infant may not be as rare as once thought. Due to echogenicity of cerebellum, areas of infarction and hemorrhage can be easily missed on ultrasound. Transmastoid scanning may improve the sensitivity of sonographic identification.[36]

Certain normal variants must be kept in mind before interpreting the ultrasound scans as abnormal.

A periventricular echogenic halo or blush, parallels the posterior margin of the lateral ventricles in virtually all neonates, most prominently in premature neonates, and arises from the anisotropic effect of the vascular plexus and radial fibers coursing from the subependyma to the cortex. This is homogeneous, symmetric, and of lower echogenicity compared with the choroid plexus, lacks cysts, and is less conspicuous when viewed from the posterior fontanelle. These features help to distinguish the periventricular halo or blush from periventricular leukomalacia or hemorrhage. A striated pattern of the corona radiata and echogenic stripes external to the periventricular white matter

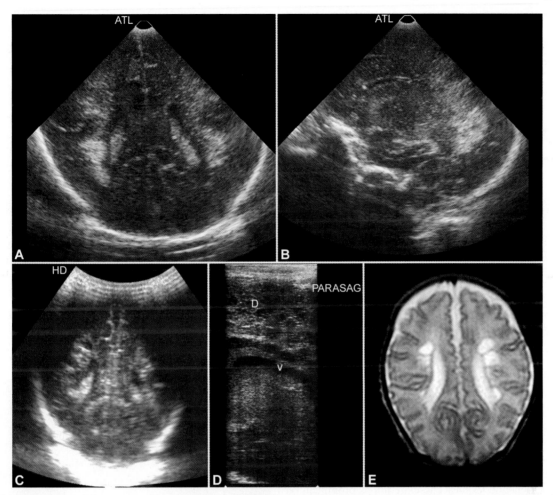

Figs 27.22A to E: Serial cranial sonograms in a preterm neonate with birth asphyxia reveal periventricular areas of increased echogenicity most marked in the peritrigonal region on the initial coronal and sagittal scans (A and B). Subsequent coronal and high resolution sagittal scans reveal partial resolution of the abnormal echogenicity with development of multiple small periventricular cysts. Axial T_2W MR image (E) of the same child depicts the multiple periventricular cysts - consistent with cystic P.V.L.

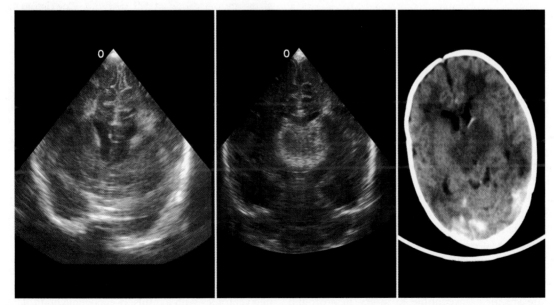

Figs 27.23A to C: Coronal sonograms (A and B) showing abnormal bilateral periventricular echogenicity and markedly increased thalami echogenicity in a neonate with severe asphyxia. The axial CT section of the same shows both the thalami to be hypodense due to hypoxic injury. Note the presence of post-fossa hemorrhages as well (not seen US Scan through anterior fontanelle)

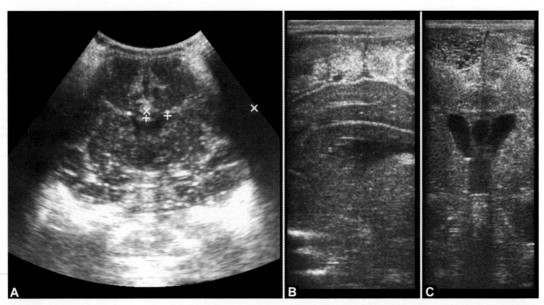

Figs 27.24A to C: Routine coronal scan (A) of a term neonate with birth asphyxia appears unremarkable, however subsequent high resolutio sagittal scan (B) shows marked increase in cortical and subcortical echogenicity. A coronal high resolution scan at a later date demonstrate multiple sub cortical cysts

paralleling the ventricles can be seen for the first few weeks of postnatal life in very preterm neonates, i.e. less than 28 weeks gestational age. These findings are likely due to the anisotropic effect of layers of migrating cells along radial glia fibers. Foci of increased echogenicity in the thalami are visible in one to two-thirds of neonates (more often in preterm neonates) on para-sagittal images through the posterior fontanelle and can mimic hemorrhagic or ischemic lesions. These are not as prominent on images through the anterior fontanelle, suggesting that these are due to the anisotropic effect of fibers from the posterior limb and genu of the internal capsule along the lateral margin of the thalamus or intrathalamic nuclear groups. However, diffuse hyperechogenicity of the basal ganglia and thalami may serve as a marker for brain injury.[40]

Sonography is less useful in evaluation of the term brain that has suffered anoxic-ischemic damage than premature brain because abnormalities are more often peripheral and not central and associated hemorrhage is less often present. Though the pattern of injury may vary with the severity of hypoxia ,diffuse or focal lesions may occur anywhere in the brain parenchyma.[35,53]

Mild to Moderate Hypoxia: The primary locations of ischemic injury in the term neonatal brain are the intervascular watershed zones between the anterior and middle cerebral arteries and between the middle and posterior cerebral arteries or the border zone . The brain parenchyma appears echogenic in the distribution of the injury and there may be either accentuation or loss of grey-white matter interface, depending on the severity of injury. Subsequently, cystic changes develop. (Fig. 27.24)

Severe Hypoxia: The metabolically active tissues in the brain of the term neonate are most susceptible to injury in profound hypotension and include the lateral thalami, posterior putamina,

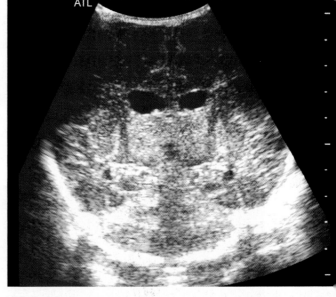

Fig. 27.25: Coronal sonogram showing increased echogenicity bilateral thalami and basal ganglia in a term neonate with severe bir asphyxia

hippocampi, brainstem, corticospinal tracts, and the sensorimot cortex (perirolandic).[52] The thalami show diffuse increase echogenicity (Fig. 27.25). Subsequently, cystic changes ma develop.

Diffuse cerebral edema, is a common result of hypoxic ischem events in full-term infants. Initially, the brain edema causes sl like ventricles with a diffusely echogenic brain. This echogenici may cause silhouetting of the sulci, so that the sulci seem isappear. The brain develops a diffusely reflective and featureless ppearance due to a combination of edema and ischemic damage.

Doppler evaluation of severely asphyxiated infants has emonstrated earlier and at times, more focal abnormalities than n gray scale alone. Doppler studies may be helpful, showing low esistance indices (< 0.6) in the anterior and middle cerebral artery omplexes with increased diastolic flow in the first 48 hours of sphyxia insult. This correlates with adverse neurological utcome. As cerebral edema worsens, cerebrovascular resistance icreases resulting in dampening of diastolic blood flow velocities. everal investigators have used Doppler, either to classify brain lema or to predict outcome. Some studies have shown that loss f diastolic flow, retrograde diastolic flow, and no detectable flow the cerebral arteries did not all have a lethal outcome. Those ith only loss or reversal of diastolic flow may survive with rompt and effective treatment.[35]

xtracorporeal Membrane Oxygenation (ECMO)

CMO is commonly used to treat term infants with respiratory isufficiency. The infants are continuously heparinized during the rocedure and are at risk for intracranial hemorrhage. Baseline inograms are performed prior to ECMO and patients with evere-anoxaeic ischemic injury, large infarcts or intraventricular emorrhage greater than grade 2 are not ECMO candidates. Daily ltrasounds are performed and any hemorrhage greater than grade is cause for discontinuing ECMO. Since haemorrhages ccurring while the patients are anti-coagulated are less echogenic lan hemorrhages in babies with normal clotting factors, a high idex of suspicion should be maintained to notice any mass effect it seen on the previous day's neurosonogram.[15]

ost-traumatic Injury

ubdural and epidural hematomas can be a difficult diagnosis on inography and they present as unilateral or bilateral hypoechoic uid collections. Imaging through the post fontanelle or foramen lagnum may be needed for posterior fossa collection.[2,4]

itracranial Infection

oth prenatal and postnatal infections are a significant cause of lorbidity and mortality in infants. Diagnosis is almost always ispected on clinical grounds, the role of imaging being to support le clinical diagnosis and reveal complications of infection.

The most frequent congenital infections are caused by the **ORCH** complex. The resultant pathology including irenchymal necrosis, vasculitis and gliosis are similar in all these, lough the severity and extent of disease may vary.

Cytomegalovirus (CMV) infection is the most common ongenital infection. Calcifications occur in a characteristic eriventricular location, when these are surrounded by a ypoechoic ring like zone, the ultrasound finding is characteristic f CMV.[15] Calcifications may also occur in the basal ganglia, ortex or subcortical region. Mineralizing vasculopathy is isualized as branching calcification (Fig. 27.26). Intracranial ilcification is also seen in toxoplasmosis, which is the second lost common congenital infection, with a predilection for basal

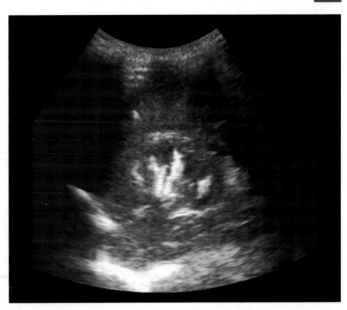

Fig. 27.26: Sagittal sonogram showing branching linear echogenicities in the basal ganglia consistent with mineralizing vasculopathy

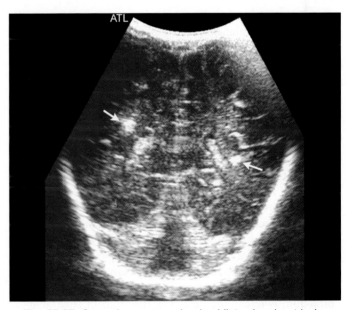

Fig. 27.27: Coronal sonogram showing bilateral periventricular echogenicities representing calcification in a case of CMV

ganglia, but more scattered calcification and periventricular calcification is also often seen (Fig. 27.27).

Herpes simplex type 2 is common in the neonate, resulting in diffuse encephalitis with loss of grey white matter differentiation.

NEONATAL AND ACQUIRED INFECTIONS

Pyogenic Meningitis

Group B streptococci and *E. coli* are the most common bacterial organisms in the neonatal period and *H. influenzae* in infants (more than 3 months of age).

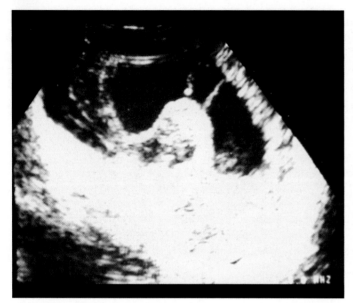

Fig. 27.28: Sagittal sonogram showing dilated lateral ventricle with multiple septations consistent with ventriculitis

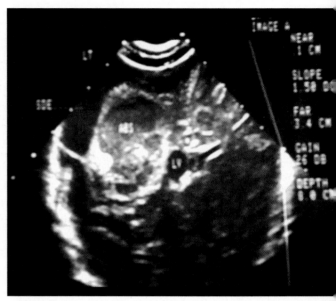

Fig. 27.29: Coronal sonogram showing a large round to oval lesic with hyperechoic walls and internal debris and mass effect s/o absces in the left frontal lobe. A large subdural effusion is also present on th same side

Sonography may be normal in uncomplicated cases. It demonstrates increased reflectivity of the cerebral sulci, secondary to leptomeningeal inflammation and pus.[54,55]

Cerebral vasculitis and thrombophlebitis may produce areas of *cerebritis* or *infarction* which are seen as echogenic areas in a segmental or gyral distribution.

Venous sinus thrombosis may also occur and can be detected using CDFI.[2] This may be associated with more complex patterns of brain injury, including venous ischemia and hemorrhage.

Extra-axial fluid collections are frequent findings in bacterial meningitis, especially *H. influenzae* infection. Subdural and subarachnoid collections may be echofree or may have low level echoes, the more reflective the collection, the more likely it is to represent empyema. CDFI may help to separate subdural and subarachnoid collections. Vessels on the surface of the brain are compressed onto the surface of the brain in subdural fluid collection, whereas they traverse the fluid in subarachnoid collection, this is known as the 'cortical vein sign'.

Mild to moderate *ventriculomegaly* may occur as an early or late sonographic feature. In the acute stage, it probably represents a form of normal pressure hydrocephalus and is usually reversible. At a later date, it may occur due to obstruction to CSF flow at strategic points.

Involvement of the choroid plexus and spread to the ventricular system results in *ventriculitis* and hydrocephalus. The ventricular margins become more reflective, indicating generalized ependymitis. Particulate debris may be seen floating in the ventricles. Subsequently, septations and band adhesions appear resulting in complex multicompartmentalized hydrocephalus which is frequently resistant to effective shunting (Fig. 27.28)

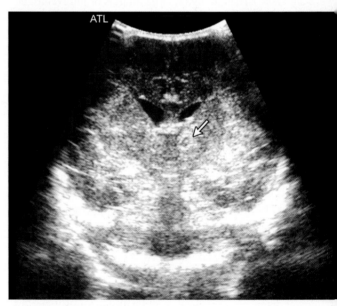

Fig. 27.30: Coronal sonogram in a patient with CSF findings s tubercular meningitis shows a small round hypoechoic granuloma wi echogenic wall in the right thalamic region

Abscess formation may occur in an area previously showir altered echogenicity due to cerebritis/infarction. This is seen well marginated lesion with an echogenic rim and hypoecho center. It may be associated with mass effect (Fig. 27.29).

Tubercular Meningitis

Sonography in tubercular meningitis (TBM) may show echogen sulci as in pyogenic meningitis. TBM can also result in basal occasionally parenchymal calcification and communicatir

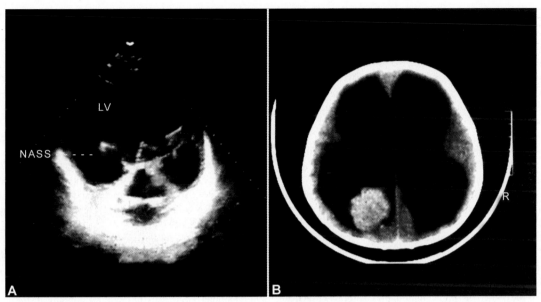

Figs 27.31A and B: (A) Sonogram showing a mass in the left lateral ventricle with hydrocephalus. (B) CECT of the same patient showing an intensely enhancing intraventricular mass consistent with choroid plexus papilloma

drocephalus.[56,57] Aqueductal block and infarcts have been more equently observed in TBM than pyogenic meningitis. ranulomas may also be seen[58] (Fig. 27.30).

eoplasms and Cysts

eoplasms in the infant brain are rare and of all the tumors tected in the pediatric age group on CT, only about 4 percent esent during the first year of life. The majority of the brain mors under 1 year of age are supratentorial and therefore cessible by ultrasound (Figs 27.31A and B). The ultrasound ppearance is variable and non-specific and further evaluation is quired to characterize these lesion. The major use of ultrasound in intraoperative localization of tumors.

ysts

esides parencephalic cysts, the other commonly encountered ysts include arachnoid cysts, choroid plexus cysts and bependymal cysts.

rachnoid cysts are the most common true cysts of the brain, but ey account for only 1 percent of all space occupying lesions in ildren. They are located in the anterior middle cranial fossa, prasellar region, posterior fossa, quadrigeminal region, cerebral nvexities and interhemispheric fissure in decreasing order of equency. The cysts are seen as anechoic areas with discrete alls. Lesions abutting the ventricular system may cause ostructive hydrocephalus (Fig. 27.32).

horoid plexus cysts are common and usually incidental findings. hey range in size from less than 4 to 7 mm and are usually nilateral and left greater than right.

bependymal cysts are usually the sequelae of germinal matrix morrhage. They may also occur following infection, as a part cerebrohepatorenal syndrome or as an isolated finding.

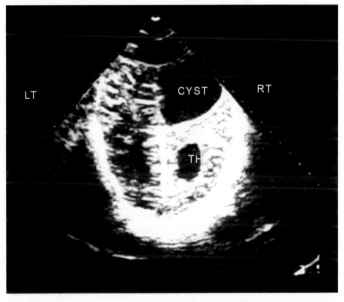

Fig. 27.32: Sonogram showing a large cyst in the right temporoparietal region with displacement of the cerebral hemisphere—arachnoid cyst

Although MR imaging is considered the gold standard for imaging the brain at all ages, some neonates may be too sick to be transported to the MR facility and hence have to rely on information obtained from neurosonography. Further, despite availability, one may not be able to get an MR examination done immediately or at the most appropriate time. Hence, neurosonography continues to be the initial or sometimes the only examination in many neonates and infants. Thus, it is important to be aware of the normal anatomy and imaging appearances of various pathological conditions in order to be able to reach an appropriate diagnosis.

REFERENCES

1. DiPietro MA, Faix RG, Donn SM. Procedural hazards of neonatal ultrasonography. J Clin Ultrasound 1984; 14:361-6.

2. Kaske TI, Rumack CM, Harlow CL. Neonatal and Infant brain imaging in Diagnostic Ultrasound. In Rumack CM, Wilson SR, Charboneau JW (Eds): (2nd ed) Mosby 1998; 1443-1501.

3. Shuman WP, Rogers JV, Mack IA, et al. Real time sonographic sector scanning of the neonatal cranium: Technique and normal anatomy. AJR 1981; 137:821-8.

4. Jaspan T. The neonatal brain, in Clinical Ultrasound a Comprehensive Test. In Meire H, Cosgrove D, Dewbury K, Farrant P (Eds): (2nd ed) 2001; 1055-6.

5. Veyrae C, Couture A, B and C. Pericerebral fluid collections and ultrasound diagnosis. Pediatr Radiol 1990; 20:236-40.

6. Dewbury KC, Bales RI. The value of transfontanellar ultrasound in infants. Br J Radiol 1981; 54:1044-52.

7. DI Salvo DN. A new view of the neonatal brain. Clinical utility of supplemental neurologic ultrasound windows. Radiographics 2001; 21:943-58.

8. Chadduck WM, Seibert JJ. Intracranial duplex Doppler: Practical uses in pediatric neurology and neurosurgery. J Child Neurol 1989; 4:577.

9. Allison JW, Faddis LA, Kinder DL, et al. Intracranial resistive index (RI) values in normal term infants during first day of life. Pediatr Radiol 2000; 30(9):618-20.

10. Taylor GA, Barnewolt CE, Duning PS. Excitotoxin induced cerebral hyperemia in newborn piglets: Regional cerebral blood flow mapping with contrast enhanced power Doppler US. Radiology 1998; 208:73.

11. Taylor GA, Sanders RC. Dandy-Walker syndrome. Recognition by Sonography. AJNR 1983; 1203-6.

12. Estroff JA, Pavad RB, Barnes PD, et al. Posterior fossa arachnoid cyst: An in utero mimicker of Dandy-Walker Malformation. J Ultrasound Med 1995; 14:787-90.

13. Kollias SS, Ball WAS Jr. Congenital malformations of the brain. In Bale Jr (Ed): Pediatric Neuroradiology Philadelphia: Lippincott-Raven 1997; 110.

14. Yakovlev PI. Pathoarchitectonic studies of cerebral malformation III. Arrhinencephalies (holotelencephalies). J Neuropathol Exp Neurol 1959; 18:22.

15. Barr LL. Neonatal cranial ultrasound. Radiol Clin of North Am 1999; 37(6).

16. Yakovlev PI, Wadsworth RC. Schizencephalies: A study of congenital clefts in the cerebral mantle I clefts with fused lips. J Neuropathol Exp Neurol 1947; 5:116.

17. Tessler FN, Dion J, Vinuela F, et al. Cranial arteriovenous malformations in neonates color Doppler imaging with angiographic correlation. AJR 1989; 153:1027-30.

18. Pretorius DH, Russ PD, Rumack CM, et al. Diagnosis of brain neuropathology in utero. In Naidich, Quencer RM (Eds): Clinical Neurosonography Berlin: Springer-Verlag, 1987.

19. Dublin AB, French BN. Diagnostic image evaluation of hydrencephaly and pictorally similar entities with emphasis on computed tomography. Radiology 1980; 137:81-91.

20. Diebler C, Dulac D. Pediatric Neurology and Neuroradiology, Berlin: Springer-Verlag 1987.

21. Carey CM, Tullous MW, Walker ML. Hydrocephalus etiology, pathologic effects, diagnosis and natural history. In Cheek WR (Ed): Pediatric Neurosurgery, (3rd ed) Philadelphia: WB Saunders 199 189-201.

22. Chowdhury V, Gulati P, Arora S, et al. Cranial Sonography preterm infants. Indian Pediatrics 1992; 2.

23. Sauerberi EE, Digney M, Harrison PB, et al. Ultrasonic evaluati of neonatal intracranial hemorrhage and its complication Radiology 1981; 139:677-85.

24. Levine MI. Measurement of growth of lateral ventricles in preter infants with real time ultrasound. Arch Dis Childhood 1981; 56:90 4.

25. Davies MW, Swaminathan M, Churang SL, et al. Reference rang for linear dimensions of the intra-cranial ventricles in preter neonates. Arch Dis Child fetal Neonatal Ed 2000; 82:F218-23.

26. Perry RNW et al. Ventricular size in newborn infants. J Ultrasour Med 1985; 4:475-7.

27. Winkler P. Color encoded echographic flow imaging and spectr analysis of cerebrospinal fluid (CSF) in infants Part II CS dynamics. Pediatr Radiol 1992; 22:31-42.

28. Seibert JJ, Mc Cowan TC, Chadduck WM, et al. Duplex pulse Doppler US versus intracranial pressure in the neonate: Clinic and experimental studies. Radiology 1989; 171:155-59.

29. Bada HS, Miller JE, Menke JA, et al. Intracerebral pressure ar cerebral arterial pulsatile flow measurements in neonat intraventricular hemorrhage. J Pediatr 1982; 100:291-96.

30. Taylor GA, Phillips MD, Ichord RN, et al. Intracranial complianc in infants evaluation with Dopper US. Radiology 1994; 191:78 91.

31. Taylor GA, Madsen JR. Neonatal hydrocephalus Hemodynam response to fontanelle compression-correlation with intracrani pressure and need for shunt placement. Radiology 1996; 201:68 9.

32. Wolpert EM, Barnes PD. Clinical principles in pediatr neuroradiology. In MRI in Pediatric Neuroradiology. Philadelph Mosby Year book 1992;41-80.

33. Very low birth weight outcomes of the National Institute of Chi Health and human development neonatal network. Pediatrics 199 67:587-9.

34. Volpe JJ. Neurology of the Newborn. Philadelphia: WB Saunde 1987.

35. Rumack CM, Drose JA – Neonatal and Infant Brain Imaging Diagnostic ultrasound 3rd Ed. Rumack Wilson Charbonea Johnson(Eds) Mosby 2005; 1623 -1702.

36. Hambleton G, Wigglesworth JS. Origin of intraventricul hemorrhage in the preterm infant. Arch Dis Child 1976; 51:651-

37. Dykes F, Lazzara A, Ahmann I, et al. Intraventricular hemorrha in newborn infant. Arch Dis Child 1974; 49:722-8.

38. Papile IA, Burstein J, Burstein R, et al. Incidence and evaluation subependymal and intraventricular hemorrhage study of infants wi birth weights less than 1500 gm. J Pediatr 1978; 92:529-34.

39. Kirks DR, Bowic JD. Cranial ultrasonography of neonat periventricular/intraventricular hemorrhage who, why, how ar when? Pediatr Radiol 1986; 16:114-9.

40. Guillerman RP. Infant Craniospinal Ultrasonography: Beyor Hemorrhage and Hydrocephalus Semin Ultrasound CT MI 2010;31:71-85.

41. Babcock DS. Sonography of the brain in infants role in evaluati neurologic abnormalities. AJR 1995; 165:417-23.

42. Cooke RW. Early and late cranial ultrasonographic appearances and outcome in very low birth weight infants. Arch Dis Child 1987; 62:931-7.

43. Trounce JQ, Ratter N, Levene MI. Periventricular leucomalacia and intraventricular hemorrhage in preterm neonate. Arch Dis Child 1986; 61:1196-1202.

44. Volpe JJ. Intracranial hemorrhage: Periventricular-intraventricular hemorrhage of the premature infant. In Volpe JJ (Ed): Neuro-Radiology of the Newborn (2nd ed). Philadelphia: WB Saunders 1987; 311-61.

45. Volpe JJ. Current concepts of brain injury in the premature infant. AJR 1989; 153:243-51.

46. Taylor GA. Effect of germinal matrix hemorrhage on terminal vein position and patency. Pediatr Radiol 1995; 25:537-40.

47. Bergman I, Bauer RE, Barmada MA, et al. Intracerebral hemorrhage in the full term neonatal infant. Pediatrics 1985; 75:486-96.

48. Chadha V, Mathur NB, Khaniju CM, et al. Peri-ventricular hemorrhage in term germinal matrix. Indian Pediatrics 1991; 28.

49. De Rinck J, Chatter AS, Richardson GPJ. Pathogenesis and evaluation of periventricular leucomalacia in infancy. Arch. Neurol 1973; 27: 229-36.

50. Blankenberg F, Loh N, Norbash A, et al. Impaired cerebral autoregulation after hypoxic ischemic injury in extremely low risk weight neonates detection with power anal pulsed wave Doppler US. Radiology 1997; 205:563.

51. Bulas DI, Vezine GL. Preterm anoxic injury Radiologic evaluation. Radiol Clin N Am 1999; 27(6).

52. Chao CP, Zaleski CG, Patton AC. Neonatal Hypoxic Ischemic Encephalopathy. Multimodality Imaging Findings Radiographics 2006; 26;5159-72.

53. Daneman A, Epalman M, Blaser S, Jarrin JR. Imaging of the brain in full term neonates, does sonography still plays a role. Pediatric Radiol 2006; 36:636-646.

54. Han BK, Babcock DS, Mc Adams L. Bacterial meningitis in infants sonographic findings. Radiology 1985; 154:645-50.

55. Chowdhury V, Gulati P, Sachdev A, et al. Pyogenic meningitis sonographic evaluation. Indian Pediatrics 1991; 26.

56. Das KM, Padmini P, Sachdeva S, et al. Sonographic evaluation of intracranial abnormalities in neonates and infants. IJR 1(42):193-8.

57. Ganishan S, Dhawan SK, Mukherjee S, et al. Ultrasound in infectious meningitis. IJR 1988; 42(1):199-202.

58. Chowdhury V, Gulati P, Sachdev A, et al. Sonography in pyogenic and tubercular meningitis: A comparative study. Ind J Radiol Imagin 1991; 1(Aug):7-10.

CHAPTER 28

Inflammatory Diseases of the Brain

V Gupta, N Khandelwal, P Singh

INTRODUCTION

Role of imaging in CNS infections is supportive and helps to diagnose the involvement of the meninges, brain parenchyma and CSF spaces. The various imaging modalities available are computerized tomography (CT), conventional MRI pulse sequences and newer modalities like diffusion weighted imaging, MR spectroscopy, magnetization transfer imaging.

INVESTIGATIVE MODALITIES

CT is often the first modality of investigation in CNS infection because patient often presents with nonspecific signs and symptoms such as fever or seizures. CT can depict the late parenchymal changes in supratentorial lesions and complications such as hydrocephalus very well. The specific role of CT comes in evaluation for calcifications such as in congenital TORCH infections and calcifications in parenchymal granuloma. However, the CT findings in the early stage of infection are much non-specific, evaluation of meningeal, cisternal, and posterior fossa parenchymal lesions becomes difficult with contrast CT alone.

MRI plays a complementary role to the CT but is now the procedure of choice, because of lack of bony artifacts especially when visualizing the posterior fossa, has inherently excellent contrast resolution. MR is clearly superior to CT for demonstrating small lesions, white matter and meningeal pathologies. DWI is helpful in demonstrating complications of infections including early ischemia and infarction. Advances in MRI include proton spectroscopy which provides an *in vivo* assessment of the biochemical changes within inflammatory lesions and the surrounding brain.[1]

BACTERIAL INFECTIONS

The most common form of CNS infection is meningitis. Organisms can reach the meninges by five routes: (a) direct hematogenous spread, (b) passage through the choroid plexus, (c) rupture of superficial cortical abscesses, (d) penetrating trauma and contiguous spread from the infected sinuses and middle ear. Except for rare occasions, the diagnosis of meningitis is made from clinical signs and symptoms and the results of lumbar puncture. Imaging in meningitis is not performed routinely other than to ensure the absence of hydrocephalus or abscess formation before a lumbar puncture is performed. Neuroimaging is indicated if the clinical diagnosis is unclear, if the meningitis is associated with persistent seizures or focal neurological deficit.[1] On cross sectional imaging thickened meninges showing continuou abnormal enhancement after contrast administration clinches th diagnosis of meningitis.[2] Contrast-enhanced MR is more sensitiv imaging modality than contrast-enhanced CT in this regar (Figs 28.1A and B). Other imaging findings include inflammator exudates in non-ventricular CSF spaces, which are typically see in granulomatous and fungal infections especially at the bas cisterns that can be hypo-, iso-, or hyperdense on CT and ma show variable enhancement.

Once the meningeal infection is established, neurologica sequelae can be caused by number of mechanisms. These includ hydrocephalus, arteritis of penetrating cortical vessels, brai abscess formation, subdural effusion, subdural empyema ventriculitis and venous thrombosis.

Hydrocephalus is demonstrated by all imaging modalitie including ultrasound in the neonate. However, MR is mos effective in localizing the level of obstruction.[3]

Subdural effusions are commonly encountered in meningiti due to *H. influenzae*. Unlike empyemas they are sterile flui collections over the frontal and temporal lobes. They are usuall not surgically treated as they regress along with the meningiti On CT scan they appear isodense to CSF and may be slightl hyperintense to CSF on MR[4] (Fig. 28.2A).

Subdural empyema (Fig. 28.2B) are associated wit *Pneumococcus meningitis*. The reported incidence is 20 percen of all intracranial bacterial infections.[4] The cause of empyema i spread of infection from the paranasal sinuses, middle ea calvarial osteomyelitis, infection following shunt placement o craniotomy or contamination of effusions. They are commonl located over the frontal lobes or close to the source of infectio from the paranasal sinuses or middle ear.[5,6] On imaging studie empyemas are seen as widening of extracerebral spaces whic appear as hypo-isodense crescentric or lentiform collectio adjacent to the inner table (Fig. 28.2B). On contrast administratio (especially on CT) a thin curvilinear rim of enhancement i present demarcating the empyema. Mass effect may be evider with effacement of sulci, compression of ventricles and midlin shift. In infants, transfontanelle sonography using 7-10 MH transducer will show empyemas as hyperechoic collections ofte with fibrinous strands and a thick hyperechoic inner membran Sterile effusion on the contrary appear anechoic.[6] On MR, ther

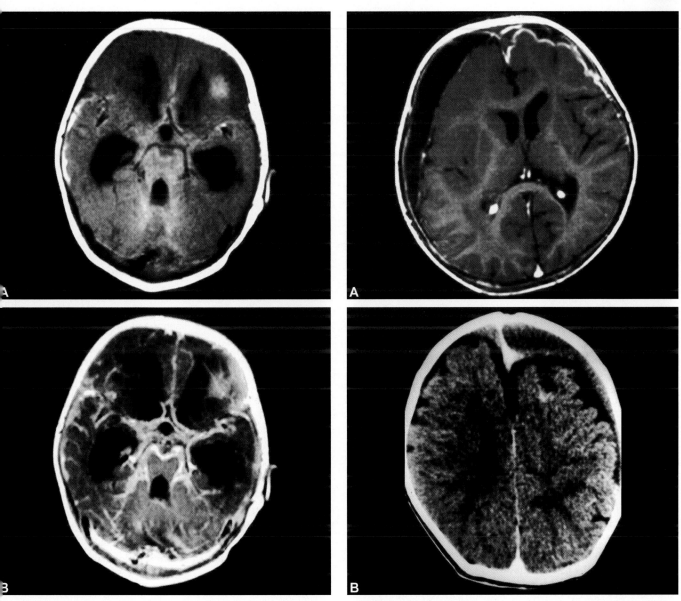

Figs 28.1A and B: Meningitis: Non-contrast and contrast-enhanced short T1 MR sections showing intense leptomeningial enhancement in case of meningitis

Figs 28.2A and B: Sequelae of meningitis: (A) subdural effusions in a patients of *Hemophilus influenzae* meningitis. Effusion appears as extracerebral collection over the frontal lobes which are isointense to CSF. Note leptomeningeal enhancement over the left frontal lobe. (B) Subdural empyema appears as a extracerebral collection which is of higher density than ventricular CSF in this CT scan section

re no signal characteristics which can distinguish empyema from on-purulent collections, because they appear hyperintense to CSF n both T1 and T2 weighted images. It is important to remember hat any extraxial collection associated with sinusitis, otitis or rbital cellulitis indicates presence of empyema. Empyemas re generally unilateral, however reactive effusion due to *. influenzae* are usually bilateral.[6]

Ventriculitis (Figs 28.3A and B) is the term for inflammation f the ependymal lining of one or more ventricles. The cause of entriculitis is due to possible retrograde spread of infections from he basal cisterns or due to a rupture of a periventricular abscess. nother possible source is via the choroid plexus. In neonates ranial sonography can demonstrate hyperechoic CSF or a

proteinaceous debris in the dependent ventricle. On contrast-enhanced MR/CT, the ependymal lining of the ventricle shows intense enhancement which is pathognomonic of ventriculitis.[1,4]

Venous thrombosis can affect deep veins, cortical veins and dural venous sinuses as a complication of meningitis. Sinus thrombosis can be diagnosed on CECT as empty delta sign which is a triangle of decreased density in the posterior segment of the affected sinus.[4,7] On MR acute thrombus is seen as hyperintense structure on T1WI. Other than in the subacute phase thrombi, are difficult to image on MR.[1,4] MR venography by phase contrast technique is particularly useful in detecting venous thrombosis.[4]

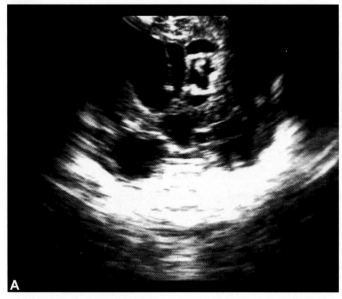 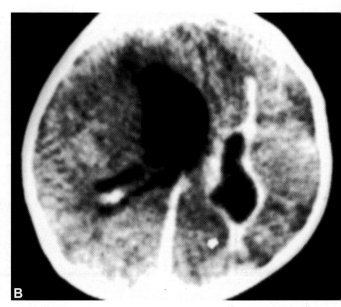

Figs 28.3A and B: Ventriculitis on ultrasound: (A) and CT scan (B) on ultrasound there is increased echogenicity around the left lateral ventricle with internal septations. Ependymal enhancement on CT is the hallmark for diagnosis of ventriculitis

Arteritis occurs when the meningitis process spreads into perivascular space. Arteritis manifests as arterial infarcts which are seen as sharply demarcated areas corresponding to arterial territories on CT or MRI.[4]

Brain Abscess

It implies encapsulated pus within the brain parenchyma, usually secondary to acute pyogenic infection. Cerebral abscess is usually secondary to either trauma or paranasal sinus infection and an equal proportion is idiopathic. Other rare causes are post surgical wound infection and septicemia. Most often brain abscess is solitary, but can be multiple in approximately 11-14 percent of cases and are usually secondary to cyanotic heart disease or middle ear infections. Infratentorial abscesses alone, or in association with supratentorial abscesses are invariably otogenic in origin (Figs 28.4A and B). Overall frontal and parietal lobes are the commonest sites for abscess formation. Cross-sectional imaging helps in the diagnosis, localization and in detecting complications of cerebral abscesses.

Abscesses Evolve in Four Stages

Stage I early cerebritis stage consists of an inflammatory infiltrate of polymorphonuclear cells, lymphocytes plasma cells. Considerable edema is present around this infiltrate.

Stage II late cerebritis stage: This is a stage when focal necrosis of the brain becomes better defined. Encapsulation begins as vessels proliferate around the necrotic area with increasing deposition of reticulin inflammatory cells and minimal amount of collagen.

Stage III early capsule formation is characterized by walling off the necrotic area by increasing deposition of collagen and reticulin. The capsule is better delineated than stage II. The surrounding edema tends to regress with partial resolution of the cerebritis.

Stage IV late capsule formation is a stage when the encapsulation of the abscess by collagen deposition is complete. The abscess is well defined and smaller than stage III. The wall is better delineated and thicker towards the cortex than medially towards the ventricles, possibly due to the increased vascularity of the gray matter. These four stages evolve within 7 to 14 days.[1,7]

The imaging features mirror the evolutionary stages of abscess formation (Figs 28.5A to C).

On non-contrast CT scan abscess appear hypodense with a barely discernable hyperdense wall. On contrast administration the capsule or the wall of the abscess enhances and measure 5 mm or less in thickness. There is surrounding edema.[7]

On MR all four stages can be recognized.[1,8] Stage I is heterogeneous on T1 and T2WI with patchy enhancement after contrast injection. In stage II the abscess wall can be recognized as a hyperintense rim on T1WI. On T2WI the rim is hypointense. Contents of the abscess are heterogeneous on both sequences. Abscess wall is shown to be thicker in stage II than stages III and IV. The abscess wall enhances intensely in this stage. Contents of the abscess may also show enhancement. In stage III the abscess wall will be hyperintense on both T1 and T2 weighted sequences. Contents of the abscess are uniformly hypointense on T1 weighted images and hyperintense on T2 weighted images, abscess wall will enhance after contrast administration and enhance. Stage IV abscesses show isointense walls on T1WI which are hypointense on T2WI. Contents of the abscess are iso hypointense on T1WI and hyperintense on T2WI; abscess wall enhance after contrast administration. Changes in the signal intensities in the wall of the abscess is believed to be reflecting the decreasing free water in the collageneous tissue.[8]

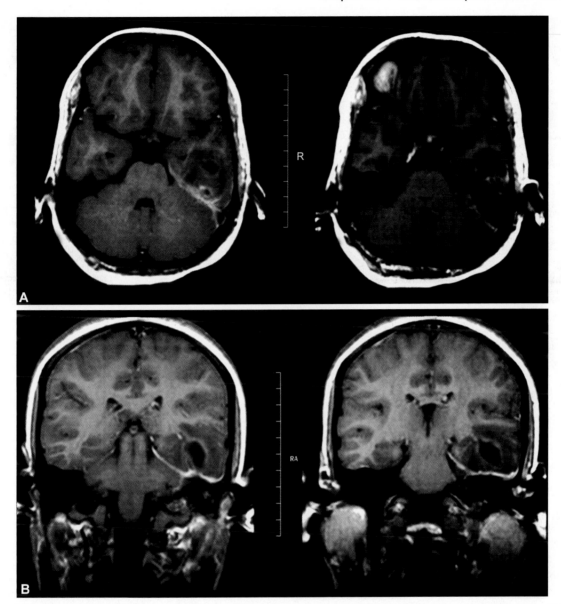

Figs 28.4A and B: Otogenic brain abscess: axial and coronal contrast-enhanced T1 WI showing enhancement within the middle ear cavity, there is enhancement of the leptomeninges over the petrous temporal bone. An ill-defined mixed intensity mass with peripheral rim enhancing lesion is present in the overlying temporal lobe which is suggestive of an evolving brain abscess

Role of protron MR spectroscopy lies in differentiation of abscesses from tumors.[9-12] Tumors show presence of choline, creatinine and NAA peaks whereas abscess show lipid peaks or amino acids together with a lactate peak. Attempts have been made recently to categorize MR spectral patterns with respect to underlying etiologic agents.[13] In this study, differentiation of anaerobic, aerobic or sterile brain abscess was attempted based on significant quantitative differences between lactate levels and ratios of lactate and amino acid peaks.

Complications of brain abscess include extension of the abscess into the ventricular system leading to ventriculitis; and subarachnoid spaces leading to purulent leptomeningitis. Daughter abscesses may develop when due to poorly developed capsule; abscess ruptures into the adjacent parenchyma.

CRANIAL TUBERCULOSIS

Central nervous system involvement occurs in 2-5 percent of all TB patients and in up to 15 percent of AIDS patients. Coexistent pulmonary TB is often seen in 25-83 percent of cases of CNS TB. Adult TB is most often a post primary infection whereas most cases in children are due to primary infection.[14] Intracranial tuberculosis manifests in three forms, viz. isolated meningeal involvement, isolated parenchymal form and compound parenchymal/meningeal lesions.

Tuberculous Meningitis

TB meningitis is the most common form of presentation of CNS tuberculosis in children in India. The cause of tuberculous meningitis is thought to be rupture of a subependymal or subpial

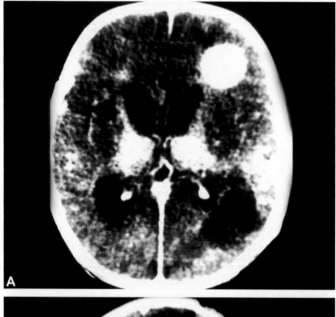

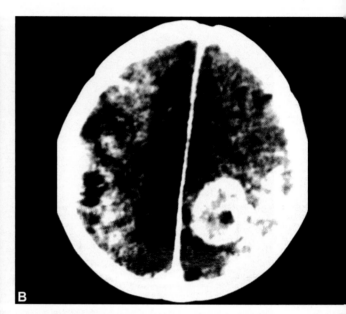

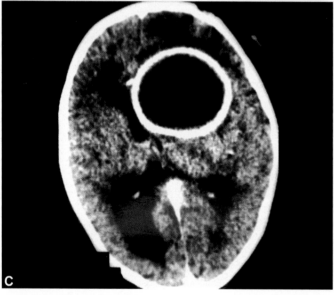

Figs 28.5A to C: Stages of abscess formation. Axial CT sections from different patients show (A) An area of cerebritis in the left frontal lobe which appears as area of focal enhancement (B) Stage of encapsulation and liquefaction. The lesion here shows a central hypodensity which is the area of liquefaction and (C) Formation of an abscess which appears as well defined hypodense area with rim enhancement

focus (Rich focus) from an earlier hematogeneous dissemination into the CSF space.[14] Incidence of tuberculous meningitis (TBM) is directly proportional to the prevalence of endemic tuberculosis. The diagnostic criteria of TBM on imaging are:[15]

1. Enhancing basal exudates
2. Progressive hydrocephalus, and
3. Infarction in the striate cortex.

Basal Exudates

In tuberculous meningitis, there is a thick, gelatinous exudate around the brainstem, extending into the basal cisterns and into the sylvian fissures. Non-contrast CT scan or T1W MR images show these exudates as isodense (isointense) or hypodense (hypointense) areas in the basal cisterns.[1] Intense enhancement occurs after intravenous contrast administration (see Figs 28.1A and B). Exudates can be easily overlooked on T2W MR images because they will appear hyperintense similar to CSF and cannot

be thus distinguished.[14] The degree of involvement of meninges over the convexities and in the depth of sulci are better appreciated on MR than on CT. Meningeal enhancement can extend over the cerebral hemispheres. Bhargava et al[16] have graded the exudates as mild (+), moderate (++), and severe (+++). In mild grade, the cisterns are obliterated but do not enhance; in moderate grade, increased attenuations are seen outlining the obliterated cistern and in severe grade, there are copious and dense exudates with increased attenuation filling and enlarging the cisterns. In their study this grading had a prognostic significance. Patients with severe degree of exudates had a longer duration of illness and carried a higher incidence of morbidity and mortality. Severe grade of exudates were seen to occur mostly in children.

Hydrocephalus

Communicating hydrocephalus is most commenly observed due to obstruction of flow of CSF by the exudates in the basal cistern

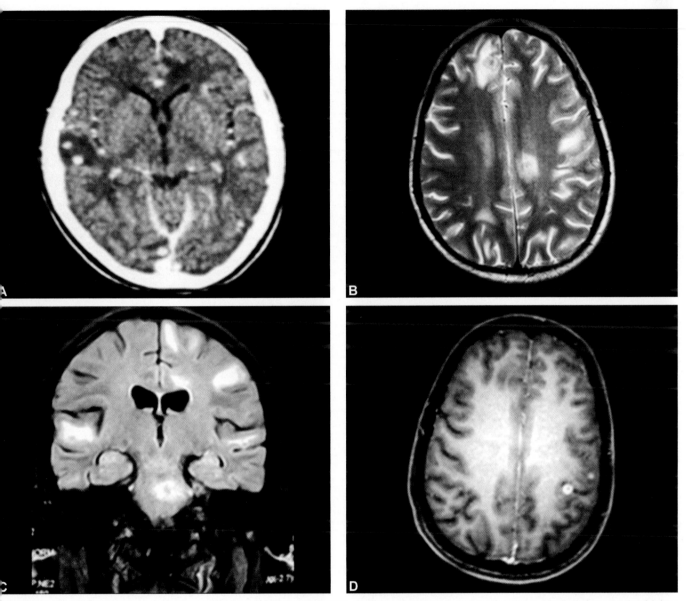

Figs 28.6A to D: Tuberculous granuloma with no caseation (A) NCCT showing non-caseating granulomata in bilateral frontoparietal lobes showing nodular homogeneous enhancement. (B) T2W axial image (C) FLAIR coronal image and (D) T1 postcontrast image showing T2 hypointense lesions with perilesional edema showing nodular homogeneous post contrast enhancement in left parietal lobe

e.g. suprasellar cisterns, cistern ambiens) and over the cerebral convexities. Uncommonly obstruction of the aqueduct by exudates results in noncommunicating hydrocephalus. Presence of hydrocephalus may precede the obliteration of basal cisterns by several weeks and is frequently associated with poor prognosis specially in children. Presence of periventricular ooze suggests high pressure hydrocephalus. The progress of hydrocephalus can be followed up by sequential CT scans, The incidence of hydrocephalus increases with the duration of disease.[16-18]

Infarction

Inflammatory changes in arteries and veins result in formation of thrombi which in turn cause multiple infarcts. The middle cerebral artery territory is the most common area where infarcts due to

meningeal tuberculosis occur. Involvement of the perforating vessels arising from circle of Willis is common and it results in infarcts of the basal ganglia. The area supplied by the medial striate and thalamoperforating arteries are specially affected in tuberculous meningitis and are termed as the medial TB zone as opposed to the area supplied by the lateral striate, anterior choroidal and thalamogeniculate arteries which is termed the lateral ischemic stroke zone.[18-20] Infarcts appear as low density regions on CT and as areas of prolonged T1 and T2 relaxation time on MR. Apart from the regions described above, infarcts can also occur in the cerebral cortex due to involvement of cortical vessels but these are less comment.

Detection of ischemic infarcts by MR is significantly higher as compared with CT. MRI also helps in differentiating cerebritis

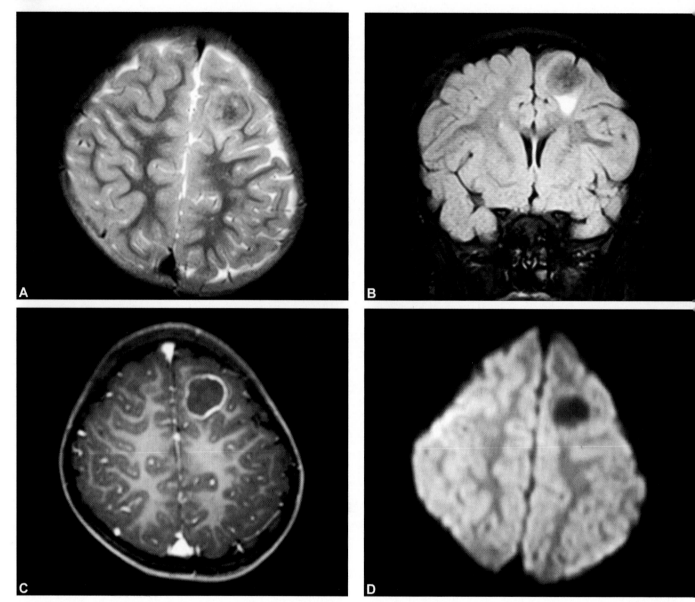

Figs 28.7A to D: Tuberculous granuloma with solid caseation: (A-C) T2, FLAIR hypointense lesion in left high frontal lobe (A,B), (C) This lesion shows peripheral post contrast enhancement. (D) The solid portion of the lesion shows no diffusion restriction on DW image

from infarction because on diffusion weighted imaging (DWI) infarction will appear bright with matching area of decreased signal on apparent diffusion coefficient map. It is important to note that early cerebritis and infarction both appear as areas of increased signal intensity on conventional MR sequences, however, cerebritis will, in time, evolve into an abscess and arterial infarction will confirm to distinct topographical lesion corresponding to arterial territories.[2] In addition, a large number of these infarcts are hemorrhagic in nature on MR, finding which has not been well documented on CT scans. MR angiography may be an useful modality in follow-up of patients with vasculitis secondary to TB meningitis. The findings are similar to those seen on autopsy or conventional angiogram and consist of a triad of narrowing of the arteries at the base of the brain, narrowed or

occluded small or medium sized arteries associated with earl draining veins and wide sweep of pericallosal arteries secondar to hydrocephalus.[18-20]

Parenchymal Tuberculous Granulomas

Tuberculous granuloma (tuberculoma) is the most common forr of parenchymal lesion.[15] Granulomas of tuberculosis occur a all ages. These may be solitary or more commonly multipl (Figs 20.8 and 20.9A to C). Infratentorial lesions are mor common in children.[21,22] Parenchymal tuberculomas appear a multiple conglomerate punctate or ring enhancing lesions at th junction of gray and white matter.

On CT scan tuberculomas appear as low or high density rin lesions which are rounded or lobulated and enhance after contra

Table 28.1: MR features of intracraniotuberculoma			
Lesion	T1WI	T2WI	Post-contrast T1WI
Non-caseating granuloma	Hypointense	Hyperintense	Homogeneous nodular enhancement
Caseating granuloma with solid center	Hypo to isointense core	Iso to hypointense core with striking hypointense rim	Contrast enhancement of rim
Caseating granuloma with central liquefaction	Hypointense	Hyperintense with hypointense rims	Contrast enhancement of rim (resembling abscess)

administration. The walls of these ring lesions are irregular and of varying thickness. There is moderate to marked perilesional edema frequently seen with parenchymal tuberculomas.[23,24]

MR features of individual tuberculomas are dependent on whether the lesion is non-caseating, caseating with a solid center or caseating with a liquid center[24] (Table 28.1).

The non-caseating granuloma is hypointense on T1WI and hyperintense on T2WI. On contrast administration the lesion usually shows homogeneous nodular enhancement (Figs 28.6A to D). The caseating granuloma with a solid center (Figs 28.7A to D) appears hypointense to isointense on T1 weighted images and isointense to hypointense on T2 weighted images. The wall of the caseating TB granuloma often has a striking hypointense rim on T2WI which enhances on administration of gadolinium. *In vivo* proton MR spectroscopy has shown presence of lipids in caseating granulomas which characterizes this lesion.

Caseating granulomas with central liquefaction of caseous material appears hypointense on T1WI and hyperintense on T2WI with a peripheral hypointense rim on T2WI (Figs 28.8A to C). Enhancement of the rim occurs after gadolinium administration as in the granulomas with a solid center and are indistinguishable from pyogenic abscess on the imaging characteristics.

Differential diagnosis of parenchymal tuberculoma includes cysticercosis, pyogenic and fungal lesions and foci of primary or metastatic neoplasia. Ring enhancing lesions on CT in patients presenting with epilepsy present a diagnostic dilemma since granulomas of cysticercus and tuberculosis both have similar morphological appearances.

Rajshekhar et al[25] have reported that it is possible to distinguish between solitary cysticercus granuloma and tuberculous granuloma in patients presenting with seizures on the basis of clinical signs and radiological (CT) findings. In patients with tuberculoma there is evidence of raised intracranial tension with progressive neurological deficit. On CT scanning the size of ring enhancing lesion is usually larger than 20 mm. Some of these may show irregular outlines, most of them cause midline shift. In contrast to this, neurocysticercus granuloma are less than 20 mm in size, rounded or oval in outline and appear as disks or rings. There is no significant mass effect. These findings based on the size and shape of lesions in their study had a specificity of 100 percent and 96 percent respectively. They have also stressed the role of repeat CT scans after 8-12 weeks of anticonvulsant therapy to rule out enlarging lesions which could be due to different etiologies. They advocated that all lesions larger than 20 mm should be biopsied to reach definitive diagnosis.

In recent times, MR spectroscopy has been used with some success in distinguishing tuberculomas from pyogenic abscesses. Intracranial tuberculomas on protron MRS primarily show peaks from lipids at 0.9.1.3, 2.0 and 2.9 ppm (Figs 28.9A to F).[26] The major difference between spectra of tuberculomas and pyogenic abscess is that although lipid and lactate peaks are found in both conditions, an increased amino acid peak (choline peak) is found only in pyogenic abscesses (Figs 28.10A to C).[27]

Compound Parenchymal and Meningeal Tuberculosis

Meningeal and meningocerebral forms of tuberculous pathology of the brain can coexist and in one series they are the least common of all presentations.[23]

Rare presentation of intracranial tuberculosis includes tuberculous abscess and miliary tuberculosis. In general, true abscess formation is uncommon in CNS tuberculosis. Tuberculous abscess may be found more frequently in adults and immuno-compromised patients.[21] Children are less commonly affected. Tuberculous abscess as opposed to tubercular granuloma is composed of pus teeming with tubercular bacilli which are few or absent in the latter. Tuberculous abscess is thin walled (Fig. 28.9). Walls are smooth and regular in thickness and indistinguishable from pyogenic abscesses on CT and MR although tuberculous abscesses are often multiloculated. Response to chemotherapy is variable as TB abscesses may not resolve and may have to be treated surgically.[28-30]

Miliary tuberculomas in the brain may be a feature of generalized miliary tuberculosis and the primary focus may be found in the lung or elsewhere. They are distributed in the cortical –white matter junction and in the distribution of the perforating vessels. They appear on CT as small round homogeneously enhancing lesions in the supra- and infratentorial compartments. On MR they appear as high intensity foci throughout the brain on T2WI. There is associated tuberculous meningitis. Their appearance may rarely precede the onset of meningitis. If treatment is successful the lesions may disappear. Paradoxical response to treatment may occur with the lesions increasing in size and new lesions appearing during the course of therapy.[31,32]

NEUROCYSTICERCOSIS

Pediatric neurocysticercosis should be considered an endemic disease in the third world countries. It assumes significance in the wake of its presentation in the form of one of the most common cause of focal epilepsy. The disease is transmitted by encysted

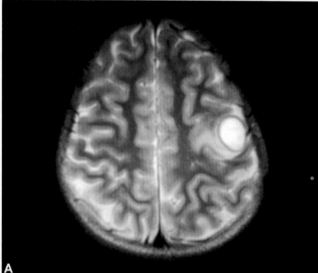

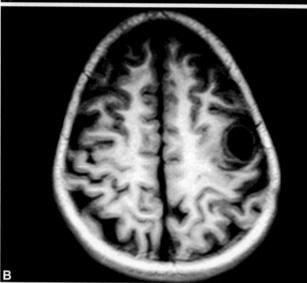

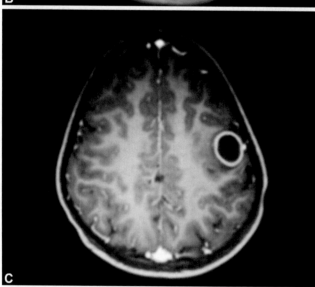

Figs 28.8A to C: Tuberculous granuloma with liquid caseation: (A and B) T1 isointense and T2 hyperintense lesion in left high frontal lobe (C) This lesion shows peripheral post contrast enhancement

form of *Taenia solium*. To become clinically manifested two host are needed to complete its life cycle. Humans are an intermedia host, acquiring the organism by accidental ingestion of tapeworm eggs from fecal contaminated substances. The eggs hatch in the small intestine, burrow into the mucosa, and penetrate the venule mature larvae, or cysticerci, develop after 60 to 70 days.[33]

Clinical Features and Pathology

The expression of the disease is variable, although seizures have been reported in as high as 92 percent of patients. Headaches an focal neurological deficits are also common. Pathologically, fou forms of cysticercosis have been described: (a) parenchyma cysticerci, (b) leptomeningitis, (c) intraventricular cysticerci (racemose cysts.[1]

Parenchymal cysticerci are categorized according to Escoba four pathological stages.[34]

Vesicular stage: The larva is seen as a small marginal nodul projecting into a small marginal nodule projecting into a sma cyst containing clear fluid. The parasites are viable and elicit litt or no inflammatory response in the surrounding tissue.On imagin a clearly marginated cyst with cyst fluid similar to the CSF signa intensity. A discrete, eccentrically placed scolex is seen. N contrast enhancement is seen in the cyst wall (Figs 28.11A and B

Colloidal vesicular stage: As the larva begins to degenerate an the scolex shows signs of hyaline degeneration, the cyst shrink in size, cyst fluid becomes turbid and cyst wall becomes thic with presence of surrounding inflammatory reaction. The cyst i slightly hyperintense on T1 weighted images and markedl hyperintense on T2 weighted images. There is associated contra enhancement of cyst wall and perilesional edema.

Granular nodular stage: The cyst undergoes retraction and th scolex is transformed into a coarse mineralized granule an surrounding edema regresses gradually. The cyst may be seen a a nodular or a thick small ring-like enhancement. Occasionall a target or bull eye appearance is seen with the calcified scole in the center of the mass.

Nodular calcified stage: By this stage the granulomatous lesio has contracted to a fraction of its initial size. On NCCT scans small calcified nodule without mass effect or enhancement i typical (Fig. 28.12).

Leptomeningitic Form

It is seen on CT and MR scans as soft tissue filling the basa cisterns. After intravenous contrast administration, as with othe granulomatous meningitides, there is marked enhancement of th subarachnoid space in the involved areas.The enhancemen charecteristics of these granulomata are similar to those o parenchymal granulomata. Hydrcephalus and vasculitis ar common with leptomeningitic form.[35]

Intraventricular Form

They are important to identify because affected patients can di from acute intraventricular obstruction. They are most commonl seen in fourth ventricle followed by lateral ventricle and thir

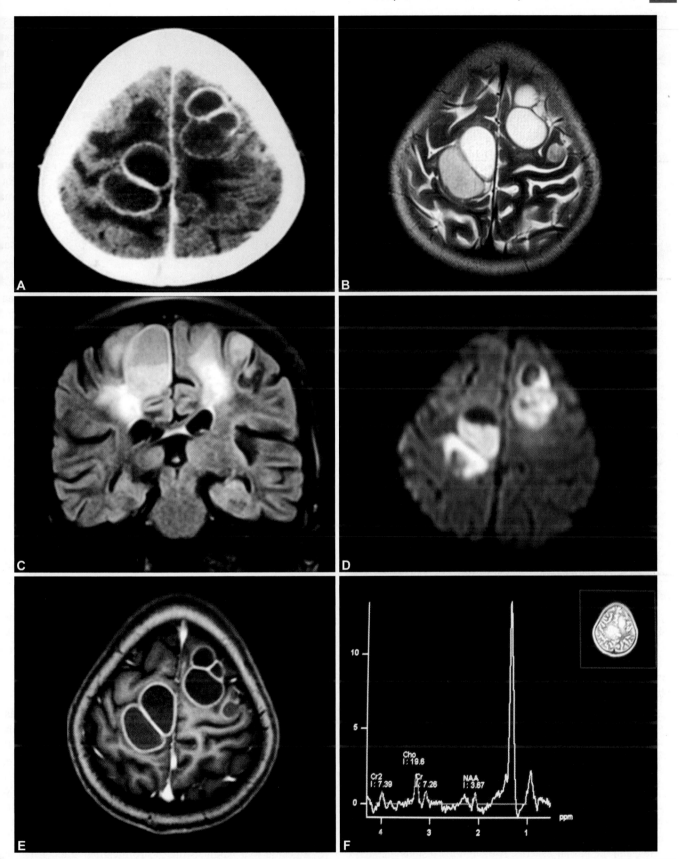

Figs 28.9A to F: An 11-year-old child with multiple tubercular abscesses on antitubercular therapy: (A) CECT, (B) T2W1, (C) FLAIR, (D) DWI, (E) CEMR images showing multiple conglomerate ring enhancing lesions in bilateral high frontoparietal lobes. Few of these lesions are showing restriction on DWI suggestive of partially treated lesions. Single voxel MR spectroscopy done at TE = 30 showing lipid peak at 1.3 ppm (F)

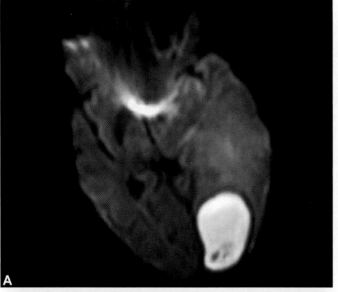

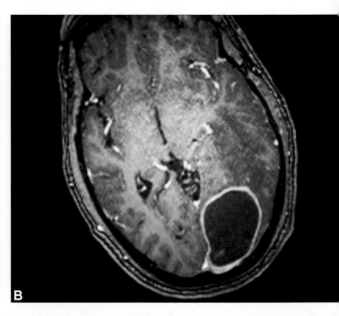

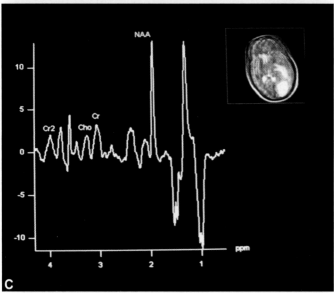

Figs 28.10A to C: The DW image shows restriction in the cavity of the lesion (A). Pyogenic abscess in left occipital lobe (B). Single voxel MR spectroscopy of pyogenic abscess at TE 30 shows lipid lactate peak at 1.3 ppm and presence of acetate (2.3 ppm) and succinate (2.5 ppm) peaks (C)

ventricle and can migrate from one ventricle from another ventricle and can be trapped in aqueduct of sylvius to cause acute hydrocephalus. The MR imaging is superior to CT in imaging of these lesions. T1 weighted images 3 mm or less in thickness optimize detection of the scolex (Figs 28.13A and B). The use of steady state sequences such as constructive interference in steady state can also be useful in finding intraventricular or cisternal cystic lesions. Sagittal and coronal plane images allow better appreciation of fourth ventricular lesions.[34]

Racemose Cysts (Subarachnoid Form)

These are multilobular, nonviable (therefore lacking scolex) cysts located in the subarachnoid space. They are most commonly seen in the cerebellopontine angle, the suprasellar region, the sylvian fissures, and the basilar cisterns. Although the lesions are sterile these lesions can grow by proliferation of cyst wall. On CT scans, large cystic lesions are seen which may enhance after contrast

administration. On MRI, multiple cysts of varying size, clustered together like grapes are seen in the involved cisterns (Figs 28.14A to D). A combination of large cyst/cysts, multilobulation of a cyst lack of mural nodule within the cyst, cisternal location and leptomeningeal enhancement on MRI strongly suggests that the lesion is caused by racemose cysticercus especially in endemic areas. A chronic leptomeningitis and arteritis may accompany these cysts.[1,34]

HYDATID DISEASE

Hydatid disease is caused by *Echinococcus granulosus* and less frequently by *Echinococcus multilocularis*. Human infection occurs by contact with definite host dog or by drinking or eating contaminated water or vegetables.

Ingested ova hatch in the gastrointestinal tract. Liberated embryos can then spread to virtually every organ or tissue via the portal and systemic circulation. They subsequently develop in

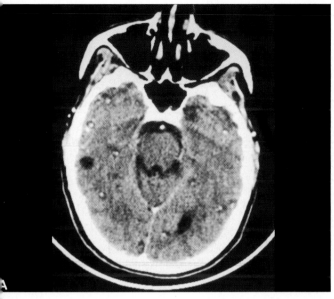
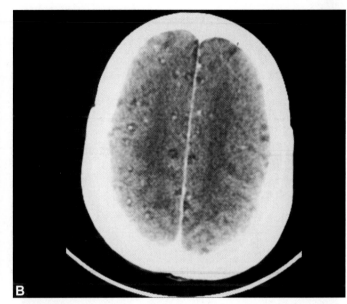

Figs 28.11A and B: Diffuse intraparenchymal neurocysticercosis: (A and B) CECT axial sections showing multiple cystic attenuation lesions seen in bilateral cerebral hemispheres. These lesions are not associated either with perilesional edema or enhancement suggestive of vesicular stage of NCC. The scolices are seen as eccentric hyperdense foci within the cysts

cystic larva termed as hydatid cyst. CNS involvement occurs in percent of cases as compared to liver (65-75%) and lung 15-20%). The cysts are usually unilocular, solitary and located n parietal lobes.[36]

CT shows presence of a thin walled spherical CSF density cyst n the parietal area. Calcification of the wall is rare and enhancement is uncommon. The MR T2W sequence shows a typical thin ow signal intensity rim surrounding a high signal intensity lesion Figs 28.15A and B).

VIRAL ENCEPHALITIS

ncephalitis is defined as generalized and diffuse inflammatory isease of the brain with parenchymal infiltration of inflammatory ells either due to direct invasion (usually viral infections) or due o immune-mediated hypersensitivity process. Although a large umber of viruses may effect the brain, all exhibit two common athological processes—neuronal degeneration and inflammation. naging is required for early detection and accurate diagnosis ecause some patients may present with atypical clinical features nd laboratory findings. MRI is widely accepted as a sensitive echnique for the diagnosis of encephalitis and is very useful for etecting early changes.[37]

Herpes Simplex Encephalitis (HSE)

HSE is the most common among sporadic encephalitis. HSV-1 auses 95 percent of all herpetic encephalitis. Herpes simplex irus type 2 is the cause of neonatal herpes encephalitis. Initial HSV-1 infection occurs in oronasopharynx through contact via nfected secretions. Later it invades along the cranial nerves olfactory, trigeminal nerves). HSV-1 reactivation occurs may ccur spontaneously or be precipitated by various factors like ocal trauma, immunosuppression. The pathological hallmark of HSV encephalitis is hemorrhagic necrotizing encephalitis which

results in severe edema and massive tissue necrosis. HSV-1 disease has a predilection for the limbic system and the lesions are localized to the temporal lobes, the insular cortex, subfrontal areas and the cingulate gyrus. HSV-1 encephalitis has a characteristic sequential bilaterality, i.e. initial lesions are unilateral but are followed by less severe contralateral disease. Changes appear earlier on MR than on CT. The findings include gyral edema in the involved regions which are better appreciated on T2WI and FLAIR sequences (Figs 28.16A and B). Contrast administration shows enhancement of the affected cortex and surrounding leptomeninges.

As the disease progresses T1 and T2 shortening develop secondary to hemorrhage and calcification.[38,39]

Herpes simplex virus-2 encephalitis is seen in neonates is acquired from infection in maternal genital tract. The virus destroys the brain leaving the pial glial membrane, ependyma and choroid plexus. Sonography of affected neonates show diffuse hyperechogenicity of the brain without ventricular compression. As the disease progresses, the ventricles dilate and the encephalomalacic brain shows increasing hyperechogenicity. On MR, the lesions are nonspecific with shortened T1 and T2 relaxation times in all sequences which persists for weeks or months. The changes are most marked in cortical gray matter.[38,39]

Japanese Encephalitis

Japanese B encephalitis (JE) is a major health problem in Southeast Asian countries. The JE virus belongs to the mosquitoborne flavivirus group and has an established endemicity, with frequent seasonal epidemics. The subclinical infections by JE virus outnumber the clinically overt disease. When clinically apparent, JE manifests as acute fulminant neurologic disease with fever, rapid development of focal neurologic signs, and unconsciousness, often resulting in death. Pathologic changes in the

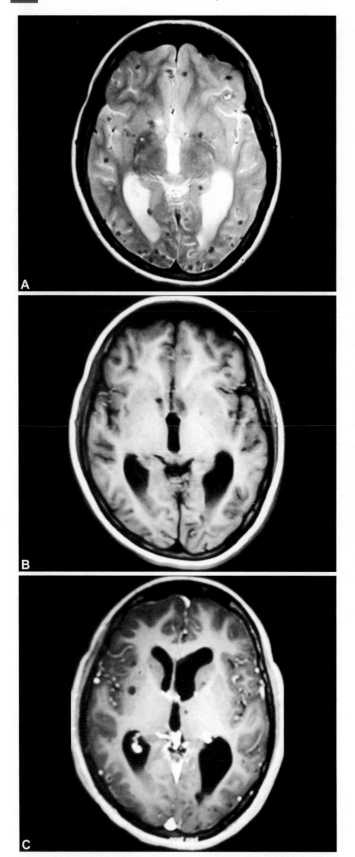

Figs 28.12A to C: Calcified nodular stage of neurocysticercosis: (A to C) Multiple well defined lesions that are hypointense on both T1 and T2W images with no definitive post contrast enhancement

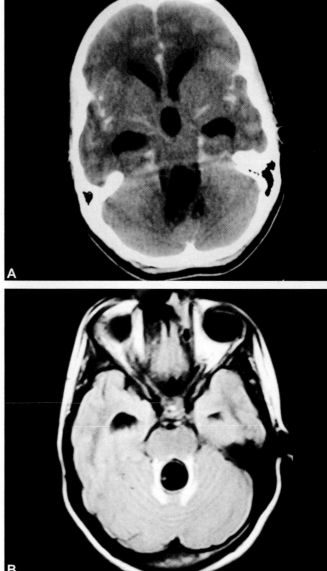

Figs 28.13A and B: Intraventricular neurocysticercosis: (A) CECT image reveals presence of dilated supratentorial ventricular system and cystic lesion in fourth ventricle having enhancing eccentric nodular focus. (B) FLAIR image delineates the scolex in the cystic lesion

brains of acute JE patients are characterized by glial nodules and circumscribed necrolytic foci. These involve the thalami, substantia nigra (SN), corpus striatum, cerebral cortex, brain stem and cerebellum.

The imaging findings on CT and MR imaging reflect the pathologic changes. The most consistent finding in JE is bilateral thalamic lesions with or without hemorrhagic changes on MR imaging (Figs 28.17A and B). Hemorrhage in the thalami and basal ganglia is reported but is not a usual feature of JE. Although thalamic, SN, and basal ganglia lesions are characteristic of JE temporal lobe involvement involving hippocampus sparing rest of temporal lobe may also be seen. This and the concurrent involvement of the thalami, SN, and basal ganglia allow

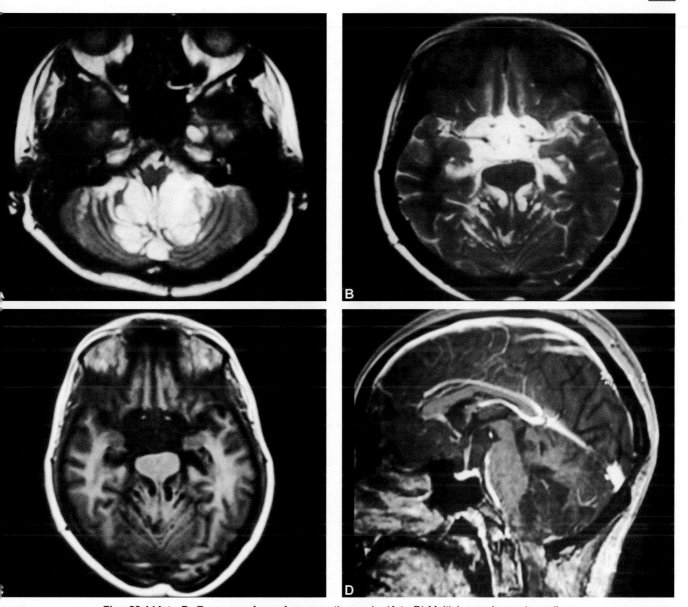

Figs 28.14A to D: Racemose form of neurocysticercosis: (A to D) Multiple conglomerate cystic signal intensity lesions in bilateral sylvian fissures and basal cisterns

fferentiation from HSE.[40,41] Diagnosis of JE is confirmed by owing a four-fold rise in the antibody titer in a paired sample.

ost varicella encephalitis occurs in <0.1 percent of children with past history of chickenpox. Darling et al[42] have shown that aricella Zoster Virus (VZV) encephalitis takes two forms:) Bilateral, symmetric, hypodense, nonenhancing basal ganglia sions on CT and nonenhancing low intensity lesion on T1WI d high signal intensity on T2WI on MRI, (2) Diffuse, multiple ay and white matter lesions of similar imaging characteristics.[42]

bacute sclerosing panencephalitis (SSPE) is a slow progressive fection by measles virus (Morbilli virus genus). The condition anifests after a latent period of 3-9 years after measles infection. oys are affected more than girls. MRI is more sensitive in tection of the lesion and in assessing the extent of the disease.

In the early stages the lesion is usually located in the gray matter and subcortical white matter of the parietal and temporal lobes (Figs 28.18A to C). It is asymmetrical and bilateral. As the disease progresses, high signal intensity in the centrum semiovale and periventricular white matter is observed. In the final stages of the disease, diffuse cortical atrophy develops with T2 prolongation in the brainstem. Basal ganglia involvement is seen in 20-35 percent of affected patients.[43]

Acute disseminated encephalomyelitis (ADEM) is a delayed sequelae of viral encephalitis. It can occur following vaccination. It is a rare disease and has been reported as a sequelae with measles, varicella, smallpox, infectious mononucleosis, herpes zoster, mumps or influenza. Subcortical demyelination at gray-white matter junction is the hallmark of ADEM. It appears as areas

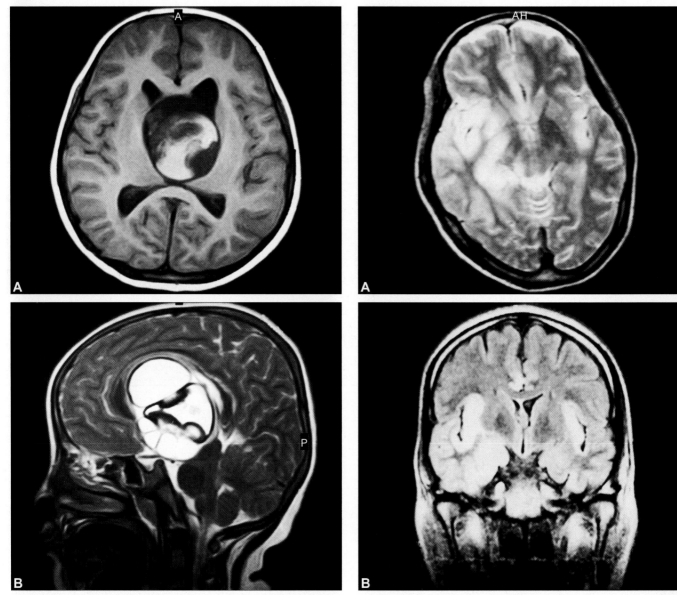

Figs 28.15A and B: Suprasellar hydatid cyst: (A) T1 axial and (B) T2 sagittal images showing a large cystic lesion in suprasellar location with surrounding T2 hypointense rim T2 hypointense membranes within it

Figs 28.16A and B: Herpes encephalitis: (A) T2W image and (B) FLAIR image showing hyperintensities involving bilateral medial tempora lobes, bilateral insular cortex and cingulate gyri

of hyperintensity on T2WI in the periventricular white matter, centrum semiovale and corona radiata. The lesions are not surrounded by oedema, are sharply demarcated and do not show mass effect. Contrast enhancement is variable. Involvement of spinal cord, cerebellum and brainstem may be present together with lesions in the deep cerebral nuclei mainly the thalamus, globus pallidii and putamina in about 50 percent of affected patients.[1]

DWI in Encephalitis

The MR appearance on DWI may be related to pathologic changes that occur following viral invasion. In the acute stage there are areas of congestion, perivascular cuffing and thrombus formation pathologically. These changes are responsible for the

cytotoxic edema that leads to restricted diffusion and low ADC changes that may not be picked up on conventional MR puls sequences (Figs 28.19A to D and 28.20A to D). In the late acu and early subacute stages, the components of vasculitis an perivascular cuffing diminish, so the proportion of diffusio restriction decreases and ADC starts to increase. At this stage du to vasogenic edema the number and extent of the lesion will b more marked in T2 and FLAIR images.[44]

CONGENITAL INFECTIONS

Infections of the fetal nervous system differ from those of olde children and adults in that the age of the fetus at the time of insu is more important than the nature of insult. In general, infectio during the first trimesters will result in congenital malformatio

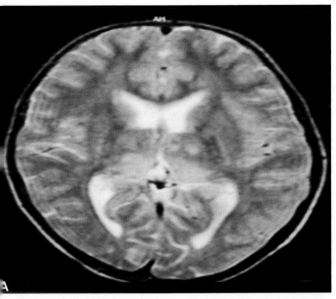

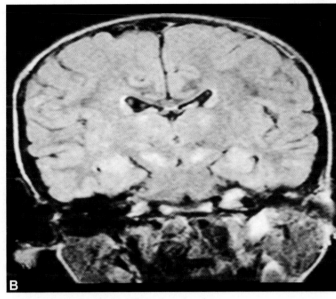

Figs 28.17A and B: Japanese encephalitis: (A) T2W image and (B) FLAIR image showing hyperintensities involving bilateral thalami and substantia nigra

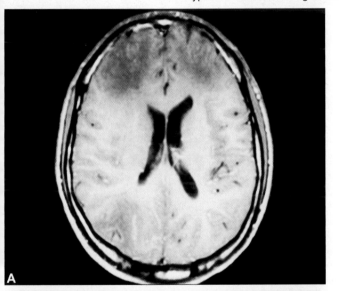

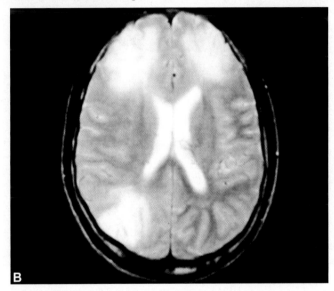

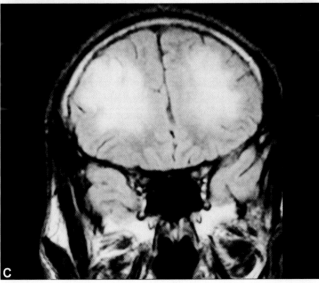

Figs 28.18A to C: Subacute sclerosing panencephalitis: (A to C) T1 hypointense and T2 and FLAIR hyperintense lesions are seen in bilateral frontal and parietooccipital lobe white matter

whereas those that occur during the third trimester are manifested as destructive lesions.[1,45]

The transmission of infection is by two modes. Bacteria travel through the amniotic fluid whereas toxoplasmosis, syphilis and viruses usually pass through the placental circulation.

Cytomegalovirus

Congenital cytomegalovirus disease is the most common cause of CNS infection in neonates. It results from vertical transmission of the cytomegalovirus from the mother to the fetus transplacentally. It can cause hematologic, neurologic and developmental signs symptoms.

Patients presumably infected during the first half of the second trimester, have lissencephaly with a thin cortex, hypoplastic

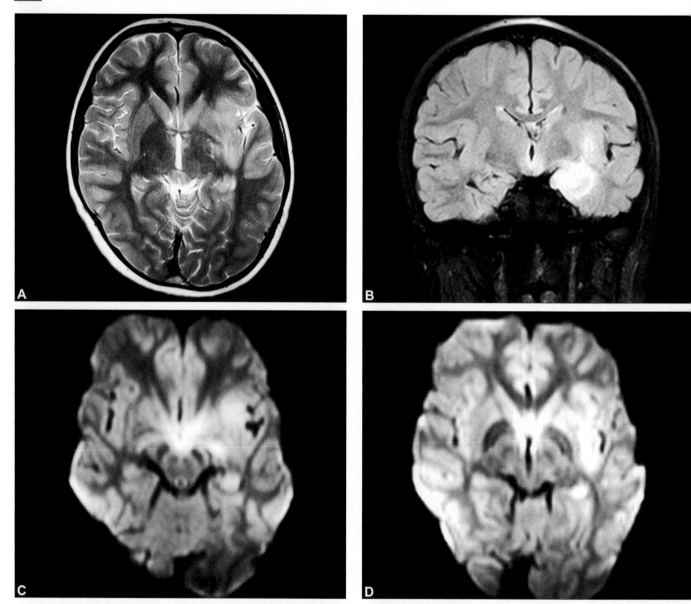

Figs 28.19A to D: DWI in Herpes encephalitis:Unilateral involvement in early stages on T2W and FLAIR images (A-B) of HSV encephalitis showing diffusion restriction (C-D) in the left medial temporal lobe and insular cortex

cerebellum, delayed myelination, marked ventriculomegaly and significant periventricular calcification. Those infected in the middle of second trimester have more typical polymicrogyria, less ventricular dilatation. Patients infected near the end of gestation or in early post natal period have normal gyral pattern, and damaged periventricular or subcortical whitematter with scattered periventricular calcification (Figs 28.21A to E). When the findings of dystrophic calcifications, cortical malformations, myelination delay and cerebellar hypoplasia are present in a child with developmental delay or seizures, a diagnosis of congenital CMV is considered.[1]

Toxoplasmosis

It is the second most common cause of congenital CNS infections. The infection may be generalized or localized to the central

nervous system. The CNS findings are choroiretinitis hydrocephalus and seizure activity. The findings on cross sectional imaging may be similar to those in CMV infection. Dystrophic calcifications located in basal ganglia, periventricular region and cerebral cortex are seen. Microcephaly, large ventricles, and hydrocephalus can be seen. Absence of cortical and gyral malformations can be differentiating feature from CMV infection.

Neonatal Herpes Simplex Encephalitis

Herpes simplex virus-2 encephalitis is seen in neonates is acquired from infection in maternal genital tract. The virus destroys the brain leaving the pial glial membrane, ependyma and choroid plexus. Sonography of affected neonates show diffuse hyper echogenicity of the brain without ventricular compression. On MR for the first two days, the lesions are patchy, widespread areas of

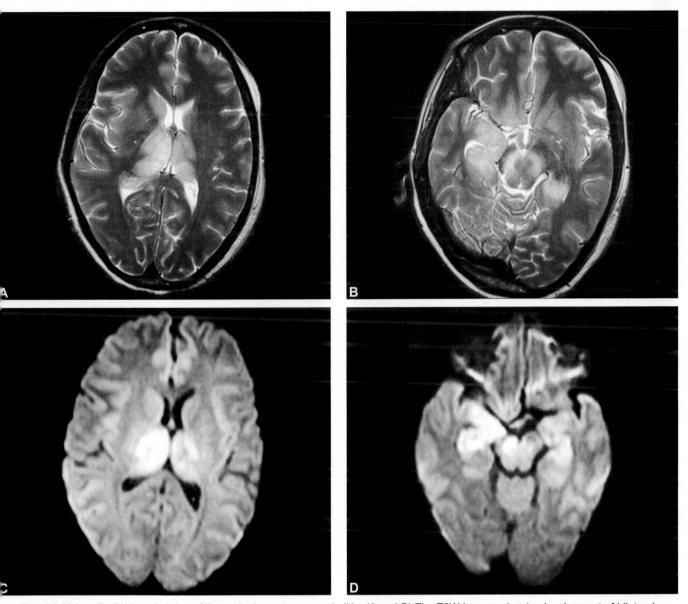

Figs 28.20A to D: DWI on 3rd day of illness in Japanese encephalitis: (A and B) The T2W images showing involvement of bilateral hippocampi, substantia nigra and bilateral thalami. (C and D) The diffusion weighted images showing restriction in the involved areas

rolonged T1 and T2 relaxation times in white matter, with estriction on DWI. Later the changes are seen in cortical gray natter. As the disease progresses, cortex shows thinning, the entricles dilate and the encephalomalacia changes are seen in vhite matter and gyral or punctuate calcifications are seen.

Rubella

Congenital rubella is transplacentally transmitted infection. Risk f fetal damage is highest during the first trimester and decreases ubsequently. Infection results in microcephalic brain with cortical nd basal ganglia calcifications. CT show hypodensity through ut the white matter together with calcification in periventricular egion, basal ganglia and cortex. On MR multifocal bright lesions vill be seen on T2WI with delay in myelination. Predilection of

the virus for vascular endothelium may cause thrombosis or hemorrhagic infarction.

Congenital HIV Infection

HIV infection is a significant public health problem because of large number of HIV infected women who are having children. Nearly 80 percent of all childhood HIV infections are maternally transmitted, although only one third of HIV positive mothers pass on the infection. CNS manifestations are primarily of two types: Progressive encephalopathy and static encephalopathy. Neuro-imaging studies reveal meningoencephalitis, atrophy and calcific vasculopathy. HIV encephalitis results in diffuse cerebral atrophy (90% cases) and calcification of basal ganglia and subcortical white matter (33% cases). Calcification is seen in those infected

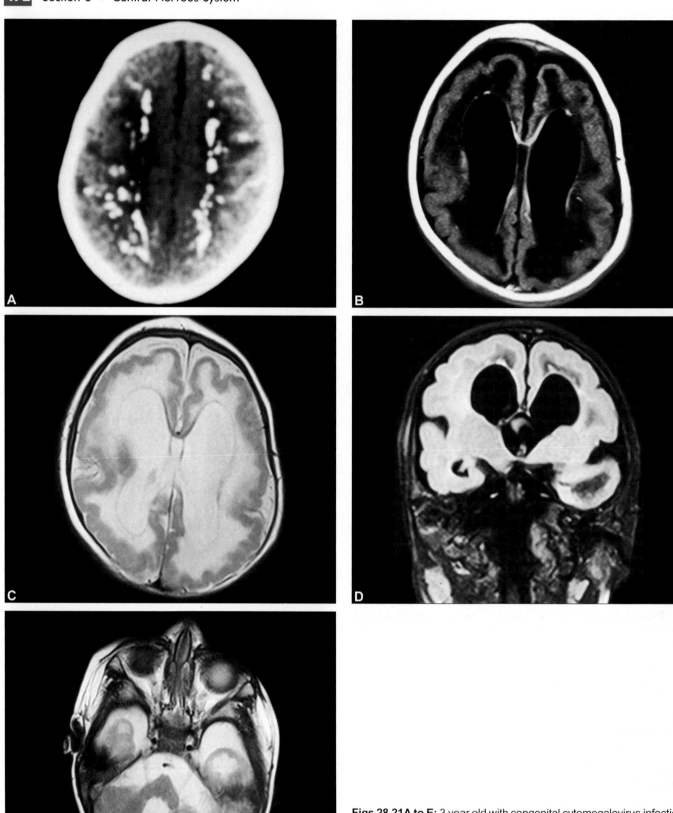

Figs 28.21A to E: 3 year old with congenital cytomegalovirus infection (A) NCCT image showing multiple periventricular calcifications. (B) T1 weighted image showing ventricular dilatation, periventricular hyperintensities and presence of thickened cortex with loss of sulcation in bilateral frontal regions (C and D) T2W and FLAIR images showing hyperintensities in bilateral cerebral white matter (E) T2 W image showing cerebellar dysgenesis

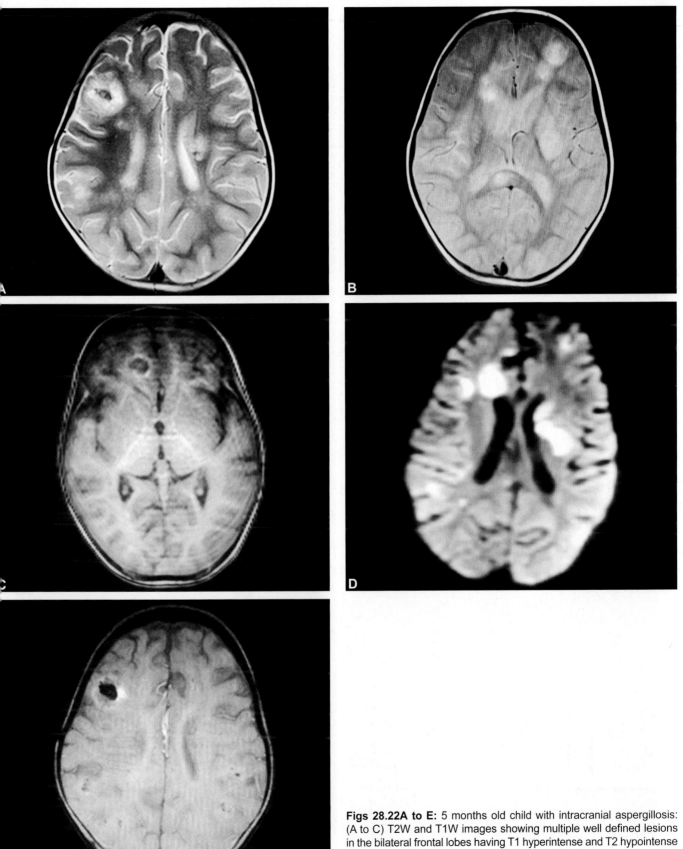

Figs 28.22A to E: 5 months old child with intracranial aspergillosis: (A to C) T2W and T1W images showing multiple well defined lesions in the bilateral frontal lobes having T1 hyperintense and T2 hypointense wall (D) DWI images show presence of diffusion restriction in the periphery of the lesions. (E) Susceptibility weighted imaging shows blooming of the wall of the lesions

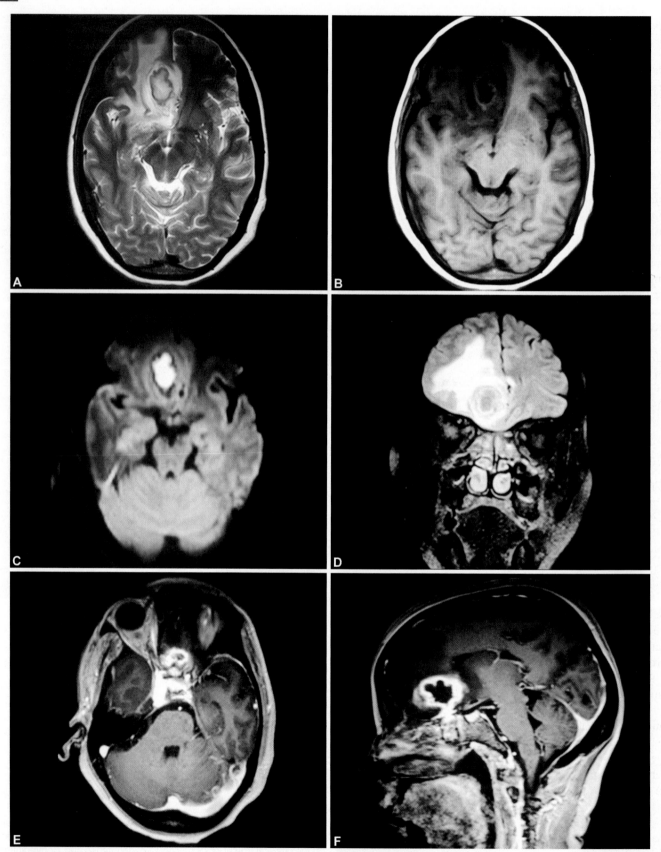

Figs 28.23A to F: Fungal sinusitis with intracranial involvement: (A to C) Heterogenous lesion with T2 hypointense rim and T1 isointense rim with central diffusion restriction. (D to F) The FLAIR image show hyperintense contents in the ethmoid sinuses with enhancement of the sinus contents, bilateral cavernous sinuses, and wall of the frontal abscess

a utero and hence usually never seen below 1 year of age. HIV asculopathy can result in infarcts.[46-48]

In contrast to adults, opportunistic infections and tumors are elatively rare (15% of cases), the most common neoplasm being ymphoma reported with 5 percent incidence and CMV and PML re more common opportunistic infections. Proton MR pectroscopy has been used in pediatric patients. The NAA/Cr atio is normal in static disease and significantly lower in rogressive encephalopathy patients.[49,50]

FUNGAL INFECTIONS

ungal infections are uncommon in children. Fungal infection can e classified in two broad categories: (i) those occurring in atients with lowered resistance as in diabetes, leukemia, ymphoma and in children on long-term cytotoxic, immuno-uppressive or antibiotic therapy, and (ii) those due to pathogenic ungi infecting immunocompetent children. The former infections re generally due to aspergillus, Candida and mucormycosis pecies and the latter are due to Cryptococcus histoplasmosis and lastomyces species.[1]

Fungal infections of the central nervous system (CNS) are eing increasingly diagnosed both in immunocompromised and nmunocompetent individuals. Sinocranial aspergillosis is more equently described from countries with temperate climates, more ften in otherwise immunocompetent individuals. Certain clinical yndromes are specific for certain fungal infections. The inocerebral form is the most common presenting syndrome with ygomycosis and skull-base syndromes are often the presenting linical syndromes in patients with sinocranial aspergillosis. ubacute and chronic meningitis in patients with HIV infection s more likely to be due to cryptococcal infection.

Aspergillosis

spergillus is saprophytic opportunistic ubiquitous fungi found n soil, plants. Aspergillus fumigatus is the most common human athogen.[51]

CNS aspergillosis is a rare condition. The infection reaches ne brain directly from the nasal sinuses or is hematogeneous from ne lungs and gastrointestinal tract. Three pathological nanifestations can occur with aspergillosis: infarction, abscess ormation and meningitis.[52]

The most distinct imaging characteristics at computed omography or MR imaging are multiple lesions with infarction r hemorrhage in a random distribution due to the angioinvasive ature of the fungus. Aspergillus abscesses are usually hypointense n T1W images but areas of high signal intensity may be seen ue to presence of iron, manganese, or methemoglobin. lemorrhage occurs in approximately 25 percent of cases and ontrast enhancement is usually minimal or absent. On T2W nages peripheral low signal areas may be seen which correspond o areas of hemorrhages (Figs 28.22A to E). On diffusion weighted nages most lesions show peripheral areas of high signal intensity uggestive of restriction of diffusion that are interspersed with ark foci which can be due to susceptibility artifact due to emorrhagic or iron products.[52,53]

Mucormycosis

Mucormycosis is a life-threatening opportunistic fungal infection caused by one of the members of the mucoraceae family. Rhizopus oryzae is the most common cause of infection.

When spores are converted into the hyphae, they become invasive, involve blood vessels and disseminate hematogenously or may spread through the paranasal sinuses into the brain and orbits. Diabetes comprise at least 70 percent of the reported cases. Infections can also be seen in patients of anemia, leukemia, uremia and severe burns and in those receiving steroid or chemotherapy. The rhinocerebral form is the most common infection. The organism may spread directly through the cribriform plate, via retrograde proliferation along vessels or through the superior orbital fissure or optic canal. Isolated CNS mucormycosis, a focal intracerebral infection, is rare and is most commonly seen in drug abusers.

Findings on CT and MR images include opacification of paranasal sinuses with absence of air fluid levels (Figs 28.23A to F). The finding of bony erosion of the sinuses is strongly suggestive of the diagnosis in the appropriate clinical setting. Sinus contents may have variable MR imaging charecteristics, from hypointensity to hyperintensity on T2WI. Intracranial findings include infarcts related to vascular thrombosis, mycotic emboli and fungal abscesses.[51,54]

CONCLUSION

Inflammatory diseases of the brain encompasses numerous causes. CT and MRI are the two main imaging modalities. Majority of lesions can be characterized for a specific disease based on imaging features along with clinical and biochemical information.

REFERENCES

1. Barkovich AJ. Infections of the nervous system. In Benkovich AJ (Ed). Pediatric Neuroimaging (4th edn). Lippincott Williams and Wilkins 2005; 801-5.
2. Smirniotopoulos JG, Murphy FM, Rushing EJ, Rees JH, Schroeder JW. Patterns of Contrast Enhancement in the Brain and Meninges. Radiographics 2007; 27(2):525-51.
3. Friede RL. Developmental Neuropathology (2nd edn). Berlin. Springer-Verlag, 1989.
4. Raybaud C, Girard N, Sevely A, et al. Neuroradiologic pediatrique (1). In Raybaud C. Girard N, Sevely A, et al (Eds): Radiodiagnostic-Neuroradiologic-Cppariel Locomotor Paris: Elsevier Science 1996; 26.
5. Moseley IF, Kendall BE. Radiology of intracranial empyema with special reference to computed tomography. Neuroradiol 1984; 26:333-45.
6. Courville CB. Subdural empyema secondary to purulent frontal sinusitis. Arch Otolaryngol 1944; 39:211-30.
7. Enzmann DR. Britt RH, Placone R. Staging of human brain abscess by computed tomography. Radiology 1983; 146:703-8.
8. Haimes AB, Zimmerman RD, Mrogello S, et al. MR imaging of brain abscesses. Am J Neuroradiol 1989; 10:279-91.
9. Kim SH, Chang KH, Song IC, et al. Brain abscess and brain tumor discrimination with in vivo H-1 MR spectroscopy. Radiology 1997; 204:239-44.

10. Marmer-Perez 1. Moreno A, Alonso J, et al. Diagnosis of brain abscess by magnetic resonance spectroscopy. J Neuro Surg 1997; 86:708-13.

11. Venkatesh SK, Gupta RK, Pal L, et al. Spectroscopic increase in choline signal is a non-specific marker for differentiation of infective /inflammatory from neoplastic lesions of the brain. J Magn Reson Imaging 2001; 14:8-15.

12. Luthra G, Parihar A, Nath K, Jaiswal S, Prasad KN, Husain N, Husain M, Singh S, Behari S, Gupta RK. Comparative evaluation of fungal, tubercular, and pyogenic brain abscesses with conventional and diffusion MR imaging and proton MR spectroscopy. AJNR Am J Neuroradiol 2007; 28:1332-8.

13. Garg M, Gupta RK, Husain M, et al. Brain abscess, etiologic categorization with in vivo protron MR spectroscopy. Radiology 2002; 230:519-27.

14. Morgado C, Ruivo N. Imaging meningoencephalic tuberculosis. European J of Radiology 2005; 55:188-92.

15. Wallace RC. Brutons EM, Beret FF, et al. Intracranial tuberculosis in children CT appearance and clinical outcome. Pediatr Radiol 1991; 21:241-6.

16. Bhargav S, Gupta AK, Tandon PN. Tuberculous meningitis-A CT study. BJR 1982; 55:189-96.

17. Fischbein N, Dillon W, Barkovich A (Eds). Tuberculosis. In:Teaching atlas of brain imaging. Thieme 2000; 165-8.

18. Bonafe A, Manelfe C. Gomea MC, et al. Tuberculous meningitis, contribution of computerize tomography to its diagnosis and prognosis. J Neuroradiol 1988; 12:302.

19. Hsuh EY, Chi a LG, Shen We. Location of cerebral infarctions in tuberculous meningitis. Neuroradiol 1992; 34:197.

20. Reid H, Fallon RJ. Bacterial infections. In Adams JH Duchen L (Eds). Greenfields Neuropathology (5th edn). New York: Oxford University Press 1992; 317-42.

21. Bhargava, Tandon PN. Intracranial tuberculomas: A CT study. Br J Radiol 1980; 53:935-45.

22. Welchman JM. CT of intracranial tuberculomata. Clin Radiol 1979; 30:567-79.

23. Jinkins JR. CT of intracranial tuberculosis. Neuroradiology 1991; 33:126-35.

24. Jinkins JR. Gupta R, Chang KH, et al. MR imaging of CNS tuberculosis. In Goodman Pc. Jinkins JR (Eds): Imaging of Tuberculosis and Craniospinal Tuberculosis. Radiological column of North America 1995; 33:771-89.

25. Rajshekhar V, Haran RPO, Prakash GS, et al. Differentiating solitary small cysticercus granulomas and tuberculomas in patients with epilepsy. J Neurosurg 1993; 78:402-7.

26. Gupta RK, Vatsal DK, Husain N, Chawla S, Prasad KN, Roy R, Kumar R, Jha D, Husain M. Differentiation of tuberculous from pyogenic brain abscesses with in vivo proton MR spectroscopy and magnetization transfer MR imaging. AJNR Am J Neuroradiol 2001; 22:1503-9.

27. Tyson G, Newman P, Strachan WE. Tuberculous brain abscess. Surg Neurol 1978; 10,323-5.

28. Whitener DR. Tuberculous brain abscess. Report of a case and review of the literature. Arch Neurol 1978; 35:148-55.

29. Wouters EF, Hupperts RM, Vreeling FW, et al. Successful treatment of tuberculous brain abscess. J Neurol 1985; 232:118-28.

30. Yang PJ, Reger KM, Seeger JF, Carmody RF, Iacono RP. Brain abscess: An atypical CT appearance of CNS tuberculosis. AJNR 1987; 8:919-20.

31. Withman RR, Johnson RH, Roberts DL. Diagnosis of miliary tuberculosis by cerebral computed tomography. Arch Intern Me 1979; 139:479-80.

32. Gee GT, Bazan C III, Jinkins JR. Miliary tuberculosis involvin the brain: MR findings. AJR 1992; 159:1075-6.

33. Osborn A (Ed). Infections of the brain and its things. In Diagnosti Neuroradiology. New York: Mosby Year Book 1994; 673-715.

34. Suss RA, Maravilla KR, Thompson J. MR imaging of intracrani cysticercosis: Comparison with CT and anatomopathologic feature AJNR 1986; 7:235-42.

35. Suh D, Chang K, Han M, et al. Unusual MR manifestations c neurocysticercosis. Neuroradiology 1989; 31:396-402.

36. Gupta S, Desai K, Goel A. Intracranial hydatid cyst: A report c five cases and review of literature. Neurol India 1999; 47:214-7.

37. Koelfen W, Freund M, Guckel F, et al. MRI of encephalitis i children: Comparison of CT and MRI in the acute stage with long term follow up. Neuroradiology 1996; 38:73-9.

38. Demaerel P, Wilms G, Robberecht W, et al. MRI of herpes simple encephalitis. Neuroradiology 1992; 34:490-3.

39. Tien R, Felsberg G, Osumi A. Herpes virus infections of the CNS MR findings. Am J Roentgenol 1993; 161:167-76.

40. Kumar S, Misra UK, Kalita J, et al. MRI in Japanese encephaliti Neuroradiology 1997; 39:180-4.

41. Shoji H, Kida H, Hino H, et al. Magnetic resonance imaging finding in Japanese encephalitis. White matter lesions. J Neuroimagin 1994; 4:206-11.

42. Darling CR, Larsen MB, Byrd SE, et al. MR and CT imagin patterns in post varicella encephalitis. Pediat Radiol 1995; 25:241-4

43. Brismar J, Gascon GG, Yon Steyern KV, et al. Subacute sclerosin panencephalitis. Neurology 1996; 47:1278-83.

44. Kiroglu Y, Yunten N, Kitis O, et al. Diffusion-weighted MR imagin of viral encephalitis. Neuroradiology 2006; 48:875-80.

45. Barkovich AJ, Girard N. Fetal brain infections. Childs Nerv Sy 2003; 19:501-7.

46. Kauffman WM, Sivit CJ, Fitz CR, Rakusan TA, Herzog K, Chandr RS. CT and MR evaluation of intracranial involvement in pediatr HIV infection: A clinical-imaging correlation. AJNR Am Neuroradiol 1992; 13:949-57.

47. Spreer J, Enenkel-Stoodt S, Funk M, Fiedler A, de Simone A, Hacke H Neuroradiological findings in perinatally HIV-infected childre Rofo 1994; 161:106-12.

48. States LJ, Zimmerman RA, Rutstein RM. Imaging of pediatr central nervous system HIV infection. Neuroimaging Clin N Ar 1997; 7:321-39.

49. Lu D, Parlakis SG, Frank Y, et al. Proton MR spectroscopy of th basal ganglia in healthy children and children with AIDS. Radiolog 1996; 199:423-8.

50. Paralakis SG, Lu D, Frank Y, et al. Magnetic resonance spectroscop in childhood AIDS encephalopathy. Pediatr Neurol 1995;12:277-82

51. Jain KK, Mittal SK, Kumar S, Gupta RK. Imaging features of centra nervous system fungal infection. Neurology India 2007; 55:241-50

52. Tempkin AD, Sobonya RE, Seeger JF, et al. Cerebral Aspergillosi Radiologic and Pathologic Findings. Radiographics 2006 26:1239-42.

53. Almutairi BM, Nguyen TB, Fansen GH, et al. Invasive Aspergillos of Brain: Radiologic – Pathologic Correlation. Radiographics 200 29:375-9.

54. Smith AB, Rushing JR. Central nervous system infections associate with Human Immunodeficiency Virus infection: Radiologi Pathologic Correlation. Radiographics 2008; 28:2033-58.

CHAPTER 29

Pediatric Brain Tumors

Shailesh B Gaikwad, Ajay Garg

INTRODUCTION

Fifteen to twenty percent of all intracranial tumors occur in children under 15 years of age, with the peak occurrence between 5 and 8 years of age. Only 1-2 percent of all brain tumors occur in children under 2 years of age.[1]

In neonates, brain tumors are uncommon and represent congenital tumors. They are most common in the supratentorial region than infratentorial region. Common primary brain tumors in the neonatal period are teratomas, embryonal tumors and congenital glioblastoma multiforme. In children between the ages of 2 and 10 years, primary brain tumors are generally more benign and 70 percent of these are infratentorial in location.[2]

Most frequent supratentorial tumors in the cerebral hemispheres are astrocytic tumors (50%), embryonal tumors (15%) and ependymomas (15%). In the suprasellar region, 75 percent of tumors are craniopharyngiomas. Common tumors in the infratentorial region in the pediatric population are pilocytic astrocytoma, medulloblastoma, and ependymoma and brainstem glioma.

CLASSIFICATION OF CHILDHOOD TUMORS BASED ON TOPOGRAPHY[3]

The location of the tumor is a useful tool in the differential diagnosis and narrowing the list of possible tumors.

1. *Cerebellum*
   - Medulloblastoma
   - Pilocytic astrocytoma
   - Atypical teratoid/rhabdoid
   - Hemangioblastoma
2. *Brainstem*
   - Diffuse astrocytoma
   - Pilocytic astrocytoma
   - Anaplastic astrocytoma
   - Glioblastoma multiforme (GBM)
3. *Fourth ventricle*
   - Ependymoma
   - Medulloblastoma
   - Pilocytic astrocytoma
   - Choroid plexus papilloma
4. *Cerebellopontine angle*
   - Ependymoma
   - Choroid plexus papilloma
   - Astrocytoma
5. *Cerebral hemispheres*
   - Diffuse astrocytoma
   - Pilocytic astrocytoma
   - Anaplastic astrocytoma
   - Glioblastoma multiforme (GBM)
   - Pleomorphic xanthoastrocytoma
   - Primitive neuroectodermal tumor (PNET)
   - Ganglion cell tumors
   - Ependymoma
   - Oligodendroglial tumors
   - Atypical teratoid/rhabdoid
6. *Lateral ventricle*
   - Ependymoma
   - Choroid plexus papilloma (CPP)
   - Astrocytoma
   - Subependymal giant cell astrocytoma (SEGA)
   - Primitive neuroectodermal tumor (PNET)
7. *Third ventricle*
   - Ependymoma
   - Astrocytoma
   - Choroid plexus papilloma
8. *Pineal region*
   - Pineal cell tumor
   - Germ cell tumors
   - Glial tumors
9. *Sellar region*
   - Craniopharyngioma
   - Germ cell tumors
   - Pilocytic astrocytoma
   - Hamartoma

POSTERIOR FOSSA TUMORS

Medulloblastoma

Medulloblastoma (MB) is a malignant primitive neuroectodermal tumor and is the most common posterior fossa tumor in children, accounting for one-third of childhood pediatric tumors.[4] About three-quarters of MBs occurs in children 5-15 years old. Although much less common, the disease may also occur in adults, usually in the 3rd and 4th decades of life.

MBs are usually midline tumors and the most common site (80%) is in the region of the vermis and inferior medullary velum. A less frequent location, encountered in older patients, is the

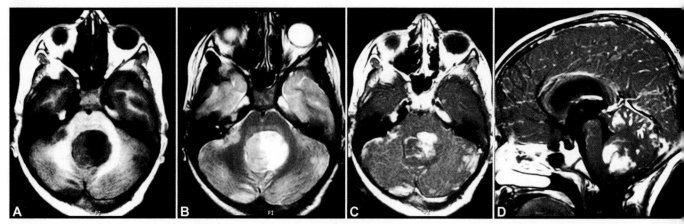

Figs 29.1A to D: *Medulloblastoma.* Axial images show a vermian mass which is iso-hyperintense on T1WI (A) and iso-hypointense on T2W (B). Post gadolinium axial (C) and sagittal (D) T1WI shows patchy enhancement within the mass and enhancement of the leptomeninge deposits in right cerebellopontine angle cistern and cerebellar sulci

cerebellar hemisphere. Approximately 80 percent of patients with MB present with features of raised intracranial pressure and the most common symptoms include headache, nausea and vomiting. Cerebrospinal fluid seeding occurs in 10-30 percent of patients with MB.

Surgical resection, radiation therapy, and chemotherapy have substantially lowered the mortality associated with this tumor and a 5-year survival rate is now about 50-65 percent. However, dissemination at the time of diagnosis and recurrence remain major obstacles in achieving a cure.

Pathology

Medulloblastomas have long been classified into two chief histological variants, "classical" and "desmoplastic.[5] In classic MBs, densely packed cells in diffuse sheets have hyperchromatic, round or carrot shaped nuclei and scanty, ill-defined cytoplasm. In desmoplastic MBs, more often are found in adolescents or young adults, a nodular architecture is seen.

Imaging

MB is a well-circumscribed mass, centered near the midline and filling the fourth ventricle. Midline extension through the foramen of Magendie into the cisterna magna may occur, while lateral extension is uncommon. The tumor has characteristic hyper-attenuation on unenhanced CT scans that reflects the hyper-cellularity and high nuclear-cytoplasmic ratio of the tumor cells.[4] MB show moderate to strong homogenous enhancement on contrast administration. Cystic and necrotic degeneration is most commonly found in adult MBs. Calcification is seen in 20 percent of cases.

On MR imaging, these tumors are hypo- to isointense on T1WI and iso- to hypo-intense on T2WI (Figs 29.1A and B). Cysts, hemorrhage, necrosis and clump-like calcification are responsible for the signal heterogeneity on T2WI.[4] Enhancement after contrast administration is intermediate to strong (Figs 29.1C and D). Evidence of leptomeningeal metastatic spread is present in 33 percent of all cases at the time of diagnosis and is well evaluated with contrast-enhanced MR imaging of the brain and

the spine (Figs 29.1C and D).[4] Diffusion-weighted MRI in M shows a marked increase in the signal intensity reflecting the dens nature of the tumor, which restricts the extracellular diffusion c water protons, and the high nuclear-to-cytoplasm ratio of thes neoplastic cells, which limits intracellular motion.[6]

Combination of high density on NCCT and isointense-lo signal on T1WI is believed to be highly suggestive of MB an this may help to differentiate it from other posterior fossa tumors

Pilocytic Astrocytoma (PA)

Pilocytic astrocytomas are benign tumors of CNS (WHC Grade I) and are of specific histologic type. They usually preser in first two decades of life. They often arise from the cerebellun hypothalamus, optic nerve, optic chiasm, brainstem and les commonly from cerebral hemispheres. Classically, cerebella astrocytoma manifests with waxing and waning headache. Trunca ataxia, dysdiadochokinesia are other cerebellar signs. They hav an excellent prognosis with 90 percent of patients having 25 year survival rate.

Pathology

Grossly, the pilocytic astrocytoma is usually sharply circums cribed, with a very narrow zone of microscopic infiltration. Th tumor is partially cystic, often with a mural nodule supplied b capillaries that lack a complete blood-brain barrier (BBB). It ha open tight junction in the endothelial cells with fenestration an therefore differs from low-grade astrocytomas. This fact and lac of BBB is the cause of both intense enhancement, as well as th source of production of the proteinaceous fluid that accumulate in the "cyst" of the tumor.

Imaging

Classically cerebellar PA present as a cystic mass with a enhancing mural nodule.[8] MR appearance is variable and nor specific. Solid portion is hypointense on T1WI and hyperintens on T2WI. MR with contrast shows enhancement of the soli component (Figs 29.2A to D). Presence of fluid-fluid levels an waveforms from fluid pulsations are pathognomonic for cysti

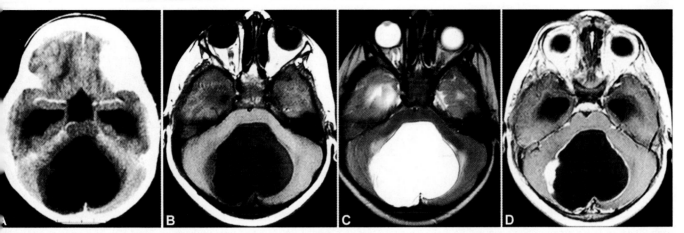

gs 29.2A to D: *Pilocytic astrocytoma.* NCCT (A) shows a cystic lesion in the vermis. A solid nodule of the tumour that is of lower attenuation an surrounding cerebellum is located within right lateral aspect of tumour. The cyst is hypointense on T1WI (B) and hyperintense on T2WI (C) d nodule shows intense enhancement after gadolinium administration (D)

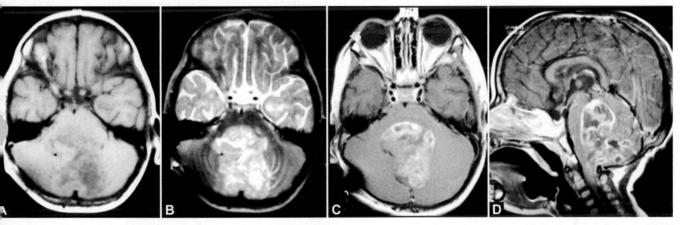

gs 29.3A to D: *Ependymoma.* Axial T1WI (A) and T2WI (B) show a heterogeneous mass filling the fourth ventricle. Post gadolinium axial (C) d sagittal (D) T1WI demonstrate heterogeneous enhancement. The tumour is creeping through foramen of Magendie and reaching upper rvical canal

asses on MR. Other features of PA include the absence of companying edema.[8] Hemorrhage and intratumoral calcification rare.

pendymoma

pendymomas are common tumors in children, comprising) percent of pediatric CNS neoplasms and 15 percent of sterior fossa tumors. The peak age at presentation is 1-5 years, ith a smaller peak occurring in the fourth decade. Common esenting symptoms include nausea, vomiting, disequilibrium, d headaches, while common presenting signs include ataxia and stagmus.

athology

pendymomas are glial tumors arising from the cuboidal or lumnar cells lining the ventricles and central canal. In the sterior fossa, they arise from the floor of the fourth ventricle ith a tendency to fill it or track along its lateral recesses into e cerebellopontine angle. Subtypes of ependymoma include llular, papillary, and myxopapillary forms. Typical gross

pathology shows a lobulated mass, often with a cystic component. Histologic findings include perivascular pseudorosettes with ependymal cells organized around blood vessels. Less commonly, true rosettes are seen.

Imaging

On NCCT ependymoma is iso-to hyperdense, with moderate enhancement after intravenous contrast.[9] Small intratumoral cyst and multifocal punctate calcification is common. Up to 45 percent of posterior fossa ependymomas contain calcifications. On MRI the typical appearance of posterior fossa ependymoma is a heterogeneous mass filling the fourth ventricle and causing obstructive hydrocephalus. MR signal characteristics of ependymoma are non-specific and vary from hypointense lesion on T1WI, to hyperintense on T2WI (cysts, necrotic areas) with low intensity areas (calcification, hemorrhage) within the tumor mass (Figs 29.3A and B). Enhancement after administration of gadolinium is heterogeneous (Figs 29.3C and D). CSF seeding is found in small percentage of the cases. The distinguishing imaging feature for these tumors is their morphologic plasticity. These tumors have

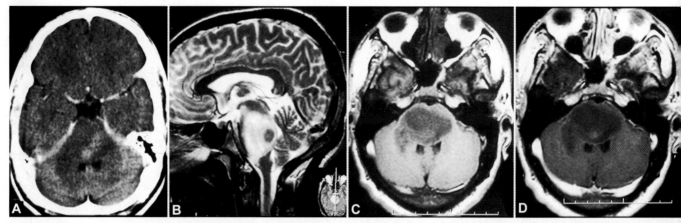

Figs 29.4A to D: *Diffuse pontine glioma.* CECT (A), sagittal T2WI (B), axial T1WI (C) and post gadolinium T1WI (D). The pons is expanded Diffuse pontine glioma flattens fourth ventricle, envelops basilar artery, extends into right cerebellum and shows patchy enhancement

a tendency to conform to the ventricles that they are associated with and may indeed herniate through the ventricular foramina. An ependymoma may squeeze through foramen of Luschka into the cerebellopontine angle cistern.[9]

Brainstem Gliomas

Brainstem gliomas account for 10-20 percent of pediatric CNS tumors, and 75 percent of these occur before the age of 20 years. The majority (85%) are composed of high-grade fibrillary gliomas, which arise predominantly in the pons and less frequently in the medulla. There is no sex predilection, and children between 3 and 10 years of age are commonly affected. Multiple cranial nerve palsies, pyramidal tract signs, ataxia and nystagmus are the usual presentation. Pontine gliomas have the worst prognosis.

Pathology

Brainstem gliomas can be divided into the diffusely infiltrative glioma and focal glioma.[10] On pathologic study, diffuse gliomas are infiltrative astrocytomas of varying grade, whereas the focal gliomas are frequently pilocytic astrocytomas. The former has a tendency for anaplasia, necrosis and hemorrhage. Except in tectal gliomas, hydrocephalus is uncommon in brainstem gliomas.

Imaging

Before the advent of MR imaging, radiographic diagnosis of diffuse glioma was based solely on indirect signs of subtle enlargement or morphologic distortion of brainstem on CT (i.e. flattening of ventral aspect of fourth ventricle or reduction of the diameter of prepontine cistern).[11] Contrast enhancement could be patchy, irregular, homogeneous or absent. CP angle cistern widening may be seen due to an exophytic component producing extra-axial effect.

MR imaging is useful for diagnosis and localization of the tumor. Diffuse glioma appears as poorly defined regions of low intensity on T1WI and high intensity on T2WI. Intratumoral heterogeneity is occasionally present, but cysts are not common. The signal changes may extend into the cerebellum and/or adjacent brainstem. The basilar artery is often engulfed by the

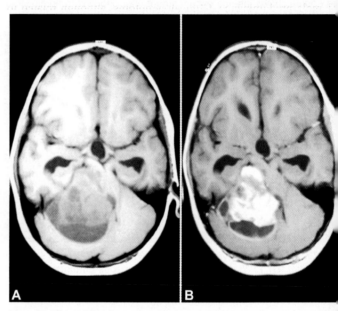

Figs 29.5A and B: *Dorsally exophytic brainstem glioma.* Axial T1W (A) shows a large tumour originating from posterolateral aspect pons. The tumour is heterogeneous with cystic areas and shows heter geneous enhancement (B)

anterior extension of the tumor. An undulating ventral border of the brainstem on sagittal image may be an indirect clue to the presence of the mass lesion. Contrast enhancement has bee reported in approximately one-half of the cases and is often foc and nodular (Figs 29.4A to D).

Pilocytic brainstem gliomas are often well circumscribed ar sometimes markedly exophytic. Exophytic component is readi identified on MR, due to its multiplanar imaging capability. Th dorsally exophytic lesions are grossly multicystic and ofte enhance intensely (Figs 29.5A and B). The presence enhancement has not been correlated reliably with type or grad of malignancy.

Differential diagnosis includes encephalitis, tuberculom resolving hematoma, and vascular malformation.[11] MR can easi

fferentiate vascular malformation and resolving hematoma from
ainstem tumor by demonstrating blood and blood breakdown
oducts exquisitely.

typical Teratoid/Rhabdoid Tumor

alignant rhabdoid tumor (MRT) is an extremely rare and highly
alignant neoplasm of undetermined histogenesis. The term
habdoid" was used due to the similarity of these tumors to
abdomyosarcoma under light microscopy. The tumor may arise
any site within the central nervous system, but 56 percent are
cated in the cerebellum and 17 percent are located in the
erebrum.[12] The hypothesis that the tumor is derived from the
eningothelial cells may account for this predisposition to occur
the cerebellum where there are abundant meningothelial
foldings. The average age of presentation with primary MRT
the brain is 24.5 months (range 1 month to 12 years),[12] with a
1 male predominance. Clinical symptoms, although related to
e location of the tumor, are often non-specific and include
thargy, vomiting, failure to thrive, visual disturbances, and head-
t. One-third of the patients have CNS dissemination of tumor
presentation. MRT has a strong tendency for subarachnoid
ssemination.

athology

IRT shows diffuse growth with areas of an alveolar or trabecular
rangement and an angiocentric pattern, with infiltration along
e blood vessels.[13] All tumors, by definition, contain a population
rhabdoid cells and two-thirds contain fields that, taken in
olation, would be classical primitive neuroectodermal tumors
NETs).

naging

he imaging features are non-specific. Lesions are commonly
rge at presentation, with moderate-to-marked surrounding
lema. On CT, these tumors are solid or mixed lesions.[14] The
lid portion is hyperdense on NCCT. Areas of necrosis, cyst
rmation, hemorrhage and calcification may occur with various
tterns of enhancement (Fig. 29.6).[13] On MR, MRT are
pointense on T1WI, isointense on PD and iso-hypo on T2WI
ith inhomogeneous enhancement. Meningeal enhancement and
inal tumor seeding are common and hence the spine should also
imaged.

emangioblastoma

lthough hemangioblastoma occurs in young and middle aged
lults, less than 20 percent occur in children. Approximately
percent are associated with von Hippel-Lindau disease (retinal
tachment multiple cysts or tumors of kidney, lung, pancreas,
er and rhabdomyomas of the heart). The tumors are usually
cated in the cerebellum (83-86%). Other sites include spinal
rd (3-13%), medulla (2-5%) and cerebrum (1.5%).[15]

athology

assically, hemangioblastoma are well-circumscribed, cystic
mors with a mural nodule (60%), but may also be solid (40%).

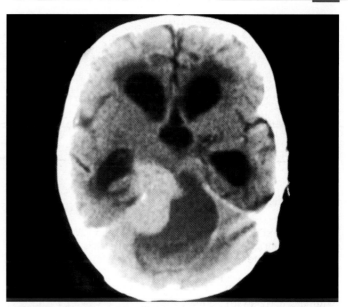

Fig. 29.6: *Atypical rhabdoid tumour.* CECT demonstrate a mixed density lesion in the vermis. The solid part of the tumour is densely enhancing

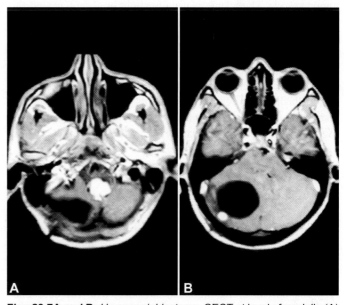

Figs 29.7A and B: *Haemangioblastoma.* CECT at level of medulla (A) and pons (B) show a solid enhancing tumour in dorsal medulla and cyst with a mural nodule in the right cerebellar hemisphere

Imaging

On NCCT, hemangioblastoma usually appears as a well-
marginated, cystic lesion with a mural nodule.[9] The cystic lesion
appears hypodense, while the mural nodule is isodense with the
brain parenchyma. The mural nodule abuts the pial surface and
show strong homogeneous contrast enhancement. Solid
hemangioblastomas appear hyperdense on NCCT and show strong
homogeneous enhancement (Fig. 29.7).

On MRI the cystic component of hemangioblastoma is either
iso- or slightly hyperintense relative to CSF on T1-weighted image
and hyperintense on T2-weighted image.[16] The nodule appears

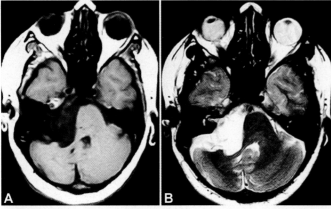

Figs 29.8A and B: *Epidermoid.* Axial T1WI (A) and T2WI (B) show an extra-axial right cerebellopontine angle mass which is hypointense on T1 and hyperintense on T2WI. The mass shows little internal heterogeneity

hypointense on T1WI and hyperintense on T2WI and enhances intensely after injection of gadolinium contrast material. Flow voids within and at the periphery of the tumor represent abnormal tumor vessels. The edema is usually slight or absent around this intra-axial tumor. On diffusion-weighted images, cystic portion of the tumor appears to be hypointense, reflecting increased diffusion properties of the cyst content. As on enhanced CT the solid portion of tumor shows marked enhancement.

The vascular component of the tumor shows homogeneous tumor blush at angiography. In patients with von Hippel-Lindau disease, the incidence of spinal hemangioblastoma is extremely high; therefore, it is mandatory to image the spine in these patients.

Epidermoid and Dermoid

Epidermoid and dermoid are generally considered congenital/developmental masses rather than neoplastic, arising from ectodermal heterotopia. Both cysts are lined with stratified squamous epithelium, with dermoids having additional mesodermal elements such as hair, sebaceous and sweat glands.

Epidermoids are slightly more common than dermoids. They typically spread along the basal surfaces, with the cerebellopontine angles being the most common location, followed by parasellar sites. Epidermoids on CT appear as hypodense masses with irregular borders and have contrast enhancement rarely. Dense epidermoids have also been reported and calcification is occasionally seen. On MR, they have low signal on T1- and of increased signal on T2WI.[17] Occasionally, epidermoids are hyperintense on T1WI and then they need to be differentiated from the dermoid and lipoma. Chemical shift artifact is absent in epidermoids and also a fat saturation pulse sequence will suppress the high signal of dermoid and lipomas, but not of epidermoids. A lobulated mass with linear heterogeneities within the mass differentiates epidermoid from arachnoid cyst (Figs 29.8A and B). Diffusion-weighted imaging will show arachnoid cyst having diffusion characteristic of fluid, while epidermoids have diffusion characteristic of a solid lesion (similar to brain tissue).[18]

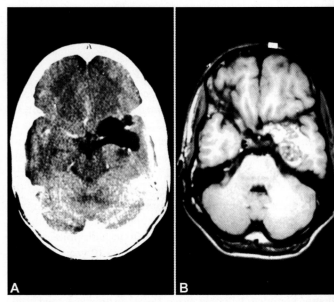

Figs 29.9A and B: *Parasellar dermoid.* CT scan shows a hypointense mass in left parasellar lesion (A) which is heterogeneously hyperintense on T1WI (B)

Magnetization transfer techniques will show significant transfer of magnetization from solid matrix of the tumor to adjacent free water but cysts show no magnetization transfer. Epidermoids are hyperintense on FLAIR while arachnoid cyst signal gets suppressed (iso-intense to CSF).

Dermoids are midline lesions, occurring in the parasellar, frontobasal region or posterior fossa (vermis or fourth ventricle). Dermoids on CT are essentially fat density, extra-axial midline masses that do not enhance on contrast administration. They may be associated with bone defect in nasofrontal or occipital region that indicate the presence of a dermal sinus tract. CT is essential for detection of the calvarial defect, while MR delineates the tumor better. Tumor is hyperintense on both T1- and T2WI (Figs 29.9A and B). Chemical shift artifact is present similar to lipomas. However, dermoids are less lobulated than lipomas, and displace blood vessels and neural structures, in contrast to encasement of these structures by the lipomas.

SUPRATENTORIAL TUMORS

Tumors in supratentorial region are more common than infratentorial region in children below 2 years and those older than 10 years of age.

Cerebral Astrocytoma

Cerebral astrocytomas constitute approximately 30 percent of supratentorial tumors in children. Males and females are equally affected, with a slight peak at 8 years of age.

Pathology

In the supratentorial compartment, pilocytic astrocytomas often arise from hypothalamus, optic nerve, optic chiasm and less commonly in cerebral hemispheres.

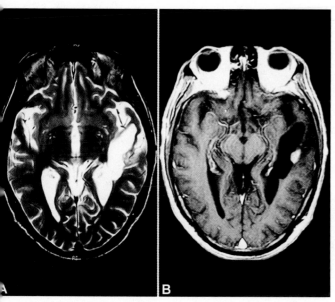

Figs 29.10A and B: *Supratentorial pilocytic astrocytoma.* Axial T2 WI (A) shows a well-defined cystic lesion in the left temporal lobe which is hyperintense with an isointense mural nodule on its lateral aspect. The mural nodule is showing dense enhancement on gadolinium administration (B)

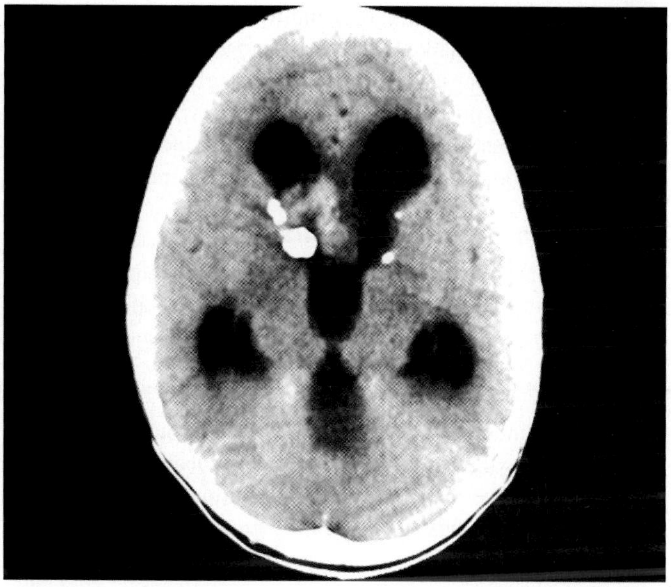

Fig. 29.11: *Subependymal giant cell astrocytoma in patient with tuberous sclerosis.* CECT shows heterogeneous intraventricular mass near foramen of Monro with calcified subependymal nodules

Imaging

Imaging features are similar to the infratentorial astrocytoma. MR reveals deeply located hemispheric mass, which is hypointense and hyperintense on T1WI and T2W images respectively. Low-grade astrocytoma is homogeneous, well circumscribed with no associated hemorrhage or edema (Figs 29.10A and B). High-grade tumors are heterogeneous due to necrosis, intratumoral hemorrhage and vascularity.

Subependymal Giant Cell Astrocytoma

Subependymal giant cell astrocytoma (SEGA) occurs in 6-16 percent of patients with tuberous sclerosis and affects the region near the foramen of Monro eventually causing hydrocephalus.[19] This tumor is also known as "Ventricular tumor of tuberous sclerosis". The peak age of occurrence is 8-18 years.

Imaging

CT shows hypo to isodense mass in the region of foramen of Monro. Hydrocephalus and focal calcification is common (Fig. 29.11). Associated stigmata of tuberous sclerosis include presence of cortical tubers, calcified subependymal nodules and white matter lesions. On MRI, SEGAs show mixed signal intensities on T1- and T2WI. Most of them are isointense on T1- and hyperintense on T2WI.[19] Presence of subependymal nodules and also small multiple cortical hamartomas are easily identified on MR. Contrast enhancement is common with these tumors on both CT and MRI.

Ganglioglioma

Gangliogliomas are composed of neoplastic ganglion cells and glial cells in variable proportions. These tumors account for 1–4

percent of all pediatric neoplasms of CNS. Most (80%) occur in patients younger than 30 years with a peak age of incidence between 10 and 20 years. The temporal lobe (38%) is most commonly affected, followed by the parietal lobe (30%) and the frontal lobe (18%). Numerous other locations have been reported, including the brainstem, cerebellum, pineal region, spinal cord, optic nerve, optic chiasm, and ventricles. Gangliogliomas of the temporal lobe are commonly associated with the clinical presentation of medically refractory partial complex seizures. These tumors are the most common cause (40%) of chronic temporal lobe epilepsy.[20]

Imaging

NCCT reveals hypoattenuation mass (38%), mixed attenuation mass (32%), isoattenuating mass (15%) or hyperattenuating mass (15%). Calcification is seen in 30 percent of lesions.[21] Remodelling of the skull may be seen if the neoplasm is located within the peripheral brain. Occasionally, the neoplasm may be completely undetectable on CT. The enhancement is seen in 16–80 percent of gangliogliomas.[21]

The MR imaging appearance of gangliogliomas is also variable and nonspecific.[20,21] In general, the lesions are hypointense to isointense relative to gray matter on T1 and hyperintense relative to gray matter on T2 images. The solid-appearing components have an even more variable presentation at imaging. Some tumors may manifest as a hyperintense mass on T1WI. They commonly have at least some regions of high signal intensity on T2WI. Not all gangliogliomas are truly cystic despite a cyst like appearance, and the term *cystic* should be reserved for those that demonstrate a fluid-fluid level or pulsation artifact on MR images. Enhancement following intravenous administration of gadolinium contrast material is highly variable, ranging from nonenhancing to ring like to intense homogeneity.

Suggested imaging features for ganglioglioma include temporal lobe or posterior fossa location, involvement of both gray and white matter, combination of well-defined cystic and ill-defined solid components, calcification and enhancing nodule(s).

Supratentorial Ependymoma

Between 20 percent and 40 percent of childhood ependymomas are located in the supratentorial region. Male predominance is seen with a peak incidence between the ages of 1 and 5 years.

Pathology

Histology is similar to infratentorial lesions. About 60 percent of the lesions are extraventricular and therefore subarachnoid seeding is uncommon. The incidence of cystic component in the supratentorial ependymomas is significantly greater than infratentorial ependymomas.

Imaging

The diagnosis of ependymoma should be considered in the presence of juxtaventricular hemispheric mass with focal calcification, cystic necrosis and heterogeneous enhancement (Fig. 29.12). MR reveals heterogeneous mass due to presence of calcification, necrosis and intratumoral hemorrhage.[11] High-grade astrocytoma and PNET should be considered in the differential diagnosis.

Primitive Neuroectodermal Tumor (PNET)

Primitive neuroectodermal tumors (PNETs) are malignant embroynal tumors occurring most commonly in the cerebellum of young individuals. The neoplasm is composed of primitive poorly differentiated neuroepithelial cells that appear as small blue cells, regardless of the location of the tumor or the type of focal cellular differentiation. The multipotential nature of the PNET cell is well-documented by morphologic evidence of ependymal, oligodendroglial, melanocytic, mesenchymal and photoreceptor differentiation. The most common location is the cerebellar vermis, where such tumors have long been known as medulloblastoma. PNETs constitute up to 25 percent of CNS tumors in children and have a high rate of proliferation and a tendency to metastasise throughout the leptomeninges. Medulloblastomas make up 85 percent of this group of tumors. Supratentorial PNETs are highly malignant tumors that have a much worse prognosis than medulloblastomas and include pineoblastomas, retinoblastoma, ependymoblastoma, cerebral neuroblastomas, ganglioneuroblastomas and medulloepithelioma. They are also recorded in the spinal cord and occasionally in brainstem. They account for less than 5 percent of supratentorial neoplasms in children. Children under 5 years of age are commonly affected.

Pathology

Supratentorial PNET most frequently occur in deep cerebral white matter and usually quite large at the time of presentation. Grossly, they have sharp margins with necrotic areas and foci of

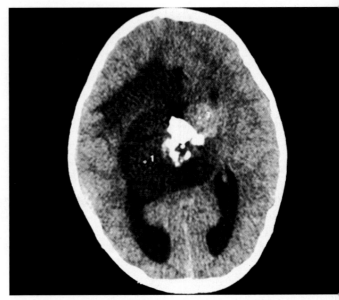

Fig. 29.12: *Supratentorial ependymoma.* CECT shows a juxta ventricular heterogeneous cystic and solid mass with areas c calcification and perilesional oedema

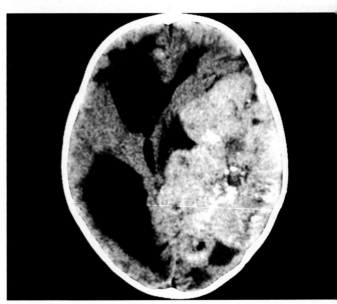

Fig. 29.13: *Primitive neuroectodermal tumour.* CECT shows a larg hemispheric mass with foci of calcification

calcification. Subarachnoid seeding and distant metastases ar frequent.

Imaging

The tumor is hyperdense to the normal brain on NCCT. Foc calcification, necrosis and hemorrhage have been reported i 10 percent of cases. Enhancement may be homogeneou heterogeneous or ring like (Fig. 29.13). MR reveals a well-define mass varying in signal intensity from homogeneous t heterogeneous.[22] Enhancement is variable. Presence of a larg

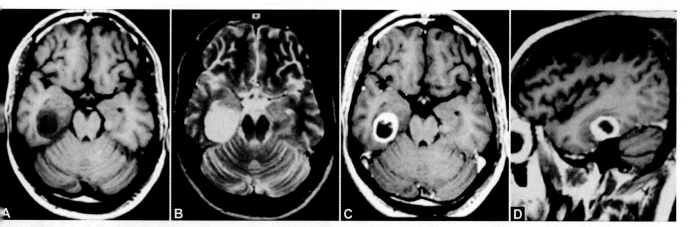

Figs 29.14A to D: *Dysembryoplastic neuroepithelial tumours.* Axial T1W image (A) showing a predominantly cystic hypointense lesion in right medial temporal lobe. The lesion is heterogeneously hyperintense on T2WI (B) and shows thick ring enhancement (C and D)

mass with well-defined margins and markedly heterogeneous signal in a young child is highly suggestive of PNET.

Oligodendroglioma

Oligodendrogliomas are rare in children. They are typically slow growing hemispheric tumors with a propensity to involve the cortex. CT typically demonstrates a peripherally located hypodense tumor, however, intraventricular oligodendrogliomas have a tendency toward hyperdensity. Calcifications (40-90%), cysts (20%) and calvarial erosions (17%) have been identified on CT. MRI better delineates the tumor extent. The tumor usually is hypointense on T1WI and hyperintense or heterogeneous on T2WI. Distinguishing imaging features of oligodendrogliomas include gray and white matter involvement, the presence of calcification, and signal heterogeneity on MRI.[11]

Dysembryoplastic Neuroepithelial Tumors (DNETs)

Dysembryoplastic neuroepithelial tumors (DNETs) are benign lesions affecting young people and are clinically characterized by drug-resistant partial seizures and normal neurologic examination.[23] The temporal lobe is the most common site (62%), followed by the frontal lobe (31%) and parieto-occipital lobe (9%).[23] They may also arise within the caudate nucleus, cerebellum, or pons. Since cortical dysplasia is commonly seen with these tumors, perhaps they represent the tumoral form of cortical dysplasia or neoplastic transformation of a dysplastic area. These are stable and benign lesions.

Neuroimaging typically shows a predominantly cortical based well-demarcated lesion with gyral or nodular configuration. At CT, the tumor manifests as a hypodense mass that may occasionally have areas of calcification.[23] Remodelling of the adjacent inner table of the skull may also be seen.[23] They are hypointense on T1, hyperintense on T2WI and homogeneous in 57 percent of cases (Figs 29.14A to D). Edema and mass effect on midline structures are lacking, although they may be observed in cases of hemorrhagic complications. Some lesions may appear as an enlarged gyrus, producing a soap bubble appearance at the cortical

margin. Sometimes DNETs show a multicystic appearance more commonly than do gangliogliomas. About one-third of DNETs enhance following intravenous administration of contrast material, which is typically focal and punctate.[23] Distinguishing features of DNET include a thick nodular or gyral configuration with little or no white matter extension is rarely seen in other glial tumors.[23]

Desmoplastic Infantile Ganglioglioma

Desmoplastic infantile ganglioglioma (DIG) is a voluminous, mixed ganglion and glial cell tumor (WHO grade I) with extensive desmoplasia and cyst formation.[24] Typically the tumor is superficially located in frontal and parietal lobes. Growth into the subarachnoid space and adjacent meninges is uniformly present in these tumors. Barring isolated case reports, almost all cases have occurred in children less than 18 months of age.

The most striking imaging feature of DIG is its relatively large size. CT reveals a large tumor with formation of a large hypodense cyst and a hyperdense solid component, which enhances intensely. On MR, signal characteristics of the solid component have been variably reported as hypo-, iso- or hyperintense relative to gray matter. The cystic component has low T1 and high T2 signal. The solid component enhances markedly and typically is adjacent to the meninges.[25]

Differential diagnosis includes PNET, ependymoma and astrocytoma. DIG should be suggested in infants presenting as a large superficial cerebral mass with large cystic component and enhancing solid component adjacent to meninges. Its identification is important since it has a significantly better prognosis and different considerations relative to other infantile brain tumors.

SELLAR AND SUPRASELLAR TUMORS

Chiasmatic/Hypothalamic Gliomas

Gliomas of the hypothalamus and optic pathways represent 5 percent of pediatric brain tumors with 60 percent involving the optic chiasm and hypothalamus.[26] They represent 25-30 percent of pediatric neoplasm of suprasellar region. The vast majority are slow growing pilocytic astrocytomas, although malignant gliomas and in particular glioblastoma multiforme may occur, especially in adults. About 20 to 50 percent of these patients, have clinical evidence or family history of neurofibromatosis type I (NF1). It is almost impossible to determine the exact site of origin, since both hypothalamus and chiasm are involved regardless of origin. The mean age of presentation is 5 years. Patients usually present with visual symptoms, headaches and endocrine abnormalities.

Imaging

MR is examination of choice. The lesions tend to be solid with microcyst formation. They are usually iso- or hypointense on T1-WI, hyperintense on T2-WI and demonstrate enhancement with contrast. The sella is usually normal.

Craniopharyngioma

Craniopharyngiomas are complex epithelial tumors arising from remnants of Rathke's pouch. They most commonly arise in the suprasellar region (90%) and account for up to 10 percent of pediatric brain tumors. More than half of all craniopharyngiomas occur in children and young adults. A second, smaller peak occurs in middle-aged adults. Patients may present clinically with headaches, visual disturbances, and hypothalamic and pituitary dysfunction. On gross pathology, most craniopharyngiomas are cystic masses with cholesterol-rich fluid and calcifications. Clinicopathologically, two distinct subtypes are recognized: the adamantinous type, which tends to occur in children, and the squamous-papillary variant, which tends to occur in adults.[27]

Imaging

On CT, craniopharyngiomas can be cystic, mixed cystic and solid, or solid, and exhibit enhancement of more solid portions. Nodular or rim calcification is found in about 90 percent of cases (Figs 29.15A and B). Attenuation of the cystic component is variable but is often slightly higher than CSF. The imaging characteristics of craniopharyngiomas on MRI are variable, reflecting wide range of components histologically composing these tumors. High signal intensity on T1-WI and T2-WI is seen in cysts with high cholesterol content or/and subacute hemorrhage. Cysts containing large amount of keratin are hypointense on T1-WI. Heterogeneous enhancement of the solid component has been noted on contrast-enhanced images. Encasement of vessels, a lobulated shape, presence of hyperintense cysts and recurrence favor adamantinous type of craniopharyngioma. A round shape, presence of hypointense cysts and predominantly solid appearance is seen with squamous-papillary tumors.

Despite benign histopathologic features, craniopharyngiomas are locally invasive, with projections of tumor extending into the adjacent brain. Hence, total resection of this tumor is often difficult and local recurrence at the primary site or in the contiguous brain may ensue, usually within 5 years.

Hypothalamic Hamartoma

The lesion consists of mature neuronal ganglionic tissue projecting from the hypothalamus down into the suprasellar cistern. It is usually attached to the mamillary bodies or tuber cinereum.[28]

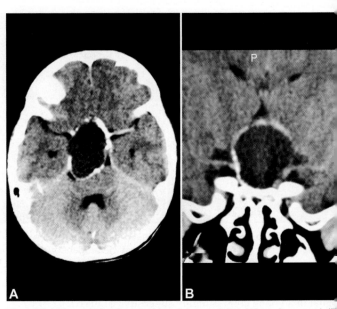

Figs 29.15A and B: *Craniopharyngioma.* Axial (A) and coronal (B) contrast enhanced CT through sella demonstrates a sellar and suprasellar cystic mass with calcifications at its margins and peripheral enhancement

There is a definite male predilection. Presenting symptoms include precocious puberty, gelastic seizures, developmental delay and hyperactivity. It usually measures 1 to 2 cm in diameter.

Imaging

On CT, hamartoma is a round or ovoid isodense mass that projects into the suprasellar or interpeduncular cistern. On MR, T1WI demonstrates a slightly hypointense mass in the suprasellar cistern which abuts against the floor of the hypothalamus. The mass is generally isointense to adjacent gray matter and does not show enhancement after gadolinium administration (Figs 29.16A and B). T2WI demonstrates the mass to be isointense to adjacent gray matter and may contain patchy regions of slightly higher signal intensity.[28] The higher intensity areas may represent the gliotic areas seen histologically. These imaging findings are fairly characteristic and are helpful in differentiating the hypothalamic hamartoma from the more common suprasellar lesions such as craniopharyngioma and hypothalamic/opticochiasmatic glioma seen in children.

Pituitary Adenomas

Pituitary adenomas represent less than 3 percent of all pediatric intracranial tumors. In childhood, they are usually seen in adolescent males and are commonly macroadenomas, in particular prolactinomas and they tend to be hemorrhagic.[29] Adenomas measuring 10 mm or less are referred to as microadenomas and these tumors do not have suprasellar extension. Most microadenomas enhance less rapidly than surrounding normal pituitary tissue and therefore are seen as hypodense or hypointense areas on contrast-enhanced CT and MR studies, respectively. Macroadenomas are more common than microadenomas and enhance uniformly and intensely.

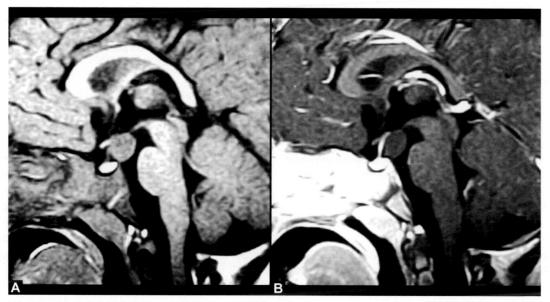

Figs 29.16A and B: *Hypothalamic hamartoma.* T1WI sagittal image at the level of hypothalamus show a 1 cm mass in the suprasellar cistern abutting against floor of third ventricle. The mass is isointense to gray matter and do not show any enhancement after gadolinium administration (B)

Arachnoid Cyst

Arachnoid cysts are congenital lesions of the arachnoid membrane lined by specialized cells that contain enzymes for secretory activity. Therefore, true arachnoid cysts expand by accumulation of CSF secreted by these cells. On the other hand, leptomeningeal cysts are caused by trauma or inflammation and represent merely loculation of cerebrospinal fluid surrounded by arachnoid scarring. Common locations are sylvian fissure, suprasellar, quadrigeminal, CP angle and posterior infratentorial midline cisterns, interhemispheric fissure, cerebral convexity and anterior infratentorial midline cisterns. Small arachnoid cysts are usually asymptomatic. Large midline lesions cause hydrocephalus. Sylvian fissure cysts are commonly associated with seizures and headache.

Imaging

Arachnoid cysts on CT and MR are well-defined homogeneous unilocular masses that are similar to CSF density on all imaging modalities and pulse sequences (Fig. 29.17).[28] Large suprasellar cysts may cause hydrocephalus by obstructing the foramen of Monro. FLAIR is particularly useful in arachnoid cysts, because the signal should be completely suppressed if the contents represent CSF.[28] Pulsation artifacts may occasionally be seen within the large cysts and are revealed as focal streaks of hypointensity on T2WI.[28] Subdural and intracystic hemorrhages may complicate middle cranial fossa cysts, either following trauma or spontaneously.

PINEAL REGION MASSES

Germ cell tumors are the most common neoplasms of pineal gland that comprise about 3 to 8 percent of pediatric brain tumors.

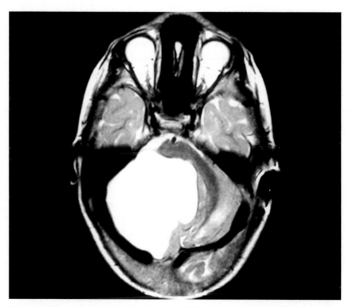

Fig. 29.17: *Arachnoid cyst.* Axial T2WI shows a well-defined extra-axial cyst in right cerebellopontine angle which is isointense to the CSF

Germinomas

Germinomas are the most common germ cell tumors and also are the most common pineal mass. Pineal region accounts for more than 50 percent of germinomas. Suprasellar/hypothalamic region and basal ganglia are the other common sites for germinoma (35%). Synchronous pineal and suprasellar lesions occur in 6-12 percent of germinomas and are considered diagnostic.[30] Primary suprasellar germinomas have no sexual predilection, in contrast to pineal germinomas, which show a male predominance. Hydrocephalus and Parinaud syndrome are the common presentations of pineal germinoma. Subarachnoid seeding is frequent.

Imaging

Pineal germinomas are well-circumscribed relatively homogeneous lesions that are not separable from the pineal body itself. These are hyperdense on NCCT. Germinomas are typically low intensity (i.e. isointense to gray matter) on T2WI.[11] Intratumoral hemorrhage may be seen in these lesions. Germinomas and their metastases enhance markedly and homogeneously after IV contrast administration. Pineal germinomas do not calcify nor do they contain cysts, features that differ from those described for germinomas arising in basal ganglion.

Teratomas

The second most common pineal germ cell tumors are teratomas. They exclusively affect males, and present in the first decade. Symptoms are similar to those of germinoma.

Pathology

Pineal teratomas are extremely heterogeneous masses with irregular and lobulated margins and are non-invasive in nature.

Imaging

On CT, these lesions are heterogeneous due to presence of fat, calcification, bone, hemorrhage, and cystic or necrotic areas. MR reveals a mass with variegated appearance. Both CT and MRI show heterogeneous or ring-like enhancement. Pineal teratomas may rupture either during surgery or spontaneously causing chemical meningitis. Malignant teratomas tend to invade surrounding structures such as tectum, the brainstem and the splenium of corpus callosum.

Other Germ Cell Tumors

Choriocarcinoma, embryonal cell carcinoma, and endodermal sinus tumors are highly malignant tumors of pineal gland. Choriocarcinomas have a tendency to bleed, a feature which differentiates it from other pineal tumors on imaging. Serologic and CSF analysis for tumor markers can aid in specificity of preoperative diagnosis.

Pineal Parenchymal Tumors

Pineal parenchymal tumors account for less than 15 percent of all pineal region tumors. There are 2 types of tumors—pineocytomas and pineoblastomas. Both tumors arise from neuroepithelial cells of the gland itself.

Pineoblastomas appear predominantly in male infants and may be rarely associated with bilateral retinoblastomas. On MRI the tumors show a heterogeneous pattern which is isointense to gray matter on T1-WI and iso-hypointense to gray matter on T2WI due to cellularity of the tumor.[31] They exhibit intense enhancement.

Pineocytomas appear between 18-50 years of age and almost exclusively in females. On CT they appear as slightly hyperdense mass with a noticeable amount of calcification. On MRI the tumors appear homogeneous with high signal on T2WI and low

to isointense signal on T1WI reflecting high amount of cytoplasm.[31] The tumors exhibit significant contrast enhancement and for large tumors heterogeneity is observed.

Pineal Cysts

Cystic lesions of the pineal gland are found in 21 to 41 percent of autopsy series and between 1.4 to 4.3 percent of cranial MR studies and are usually incidental. Pineal cyst development, small changes in cyst size, and cyst involution can all be seen on serial MR imaging without the development of specific symptoms. These lesions may, however, become clinically important for two reasons: first, pineal cysts may enlarge over time (because of either increased cyst fluid or intracystic hemorrhage) and become symptomatic. Second, benign-appearing cysts of the pineal gland may represent malignant or pre-malignant conditions. Rarely pineocytomas may present as purely cystic tumors, or tumors may develop on the pineal cyst wall. The cysts are isointense to CSF on T1WI and slightly hyperintense with respect to CSF on T2WI.[32] Hemorrhage within the pineal cyst is rare and appears hyperintense on both T1WI and T2WI. On contrast study, a rim of normal pineal gland enhances around the cysts. Typical pineal cysts found incidentally on MR imaging may be followed clinically without further imaging.

EXTRAPARENCHYMAL TUMORS

Choroid Plexus Tumors

Choroid plexus papillomas (CPPs) and carcinomas originate from choroid plexus epithelium. They constitute 5 percent of supratentorial pediatric tumors and less than 1 percent of all primary intracranial neoplasms. CPPs are most frequent in the first year of life, and usually present with hydrocephalus. Choroids plexus carcinomas (CPCs) make up 30-40 percent of choroid plexus tumors and occur mostly during first 5 years of life. Focal neurologic deficit resulting from adjacent brain invasion is the frequent presentation of CPC. Male predominance is observed for both the tumors. Hydrocephalus frequently occurs with CPPs as a result of either the overproduction of CSF and/or occurrence of blockage in the subarachnoid cisterns or intraventricular pathways.

Pathology

In children, 80 percent of CPPs arise in the lateral ventricles; 16 percent in the fourth ventricle and 4 percent in the third ventricle. Fourth ventricle is the commonest site of adult CPP. Papillomas are very irregularly lobulated masses projecting into and enlarging the ventricular cavity. Foci of small hemorrhages and calcification may be found. Anaplastic papillomas frequently invade the brain and are difficult to differentiate from carcinomas. Metastasis through CSF pathways is common for both anaplastic papilloma and carcinomas.

Imaging

On NCCT, they are hyperdense or isodense relative to cortex, frequently contain prominent calcifications and display intense

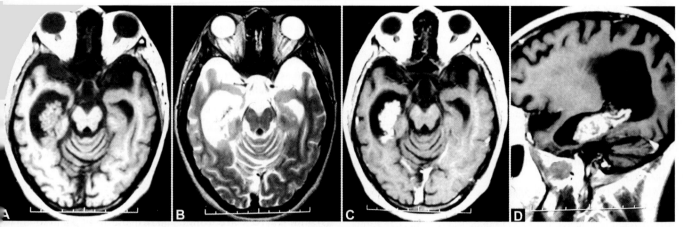

Figs 29.18A to D: *Choroid plexus papilloma.* Axial T1 (A) and T2WI (B) show a lobulated intraventricular mass in the temporal horn of right lateral ventricle. The mass is isointense to gray matter on T1WI (C) and hypointense on T2WI (D). The mass shows intense enhancement following gadolinium administration

enhancement after IV contrast administration. On T1W MRI tumor usually have a lobulated margin and is iso- to slightly hypointense to gray matter. Areas of hypointensity within the tumor may represent calcifications or flow-voids. On T2WI the tumor may show a very heterogeneous hyperintensity due to presence of calcifications, flow-voids and iron from old hemorrhages.[33] Gadolinium administration will demonstrate enhancement throughout the tumor that may be heterogeneous in its pattern depending on degree of tumor calcification, vascularity and cystic changes (Figs 29.18A to D).

Anaplastic papillomas invade the ependyma and grow into the surrounding white matter, producing vasogenic oedema. They are more irregular in outline and closely resemble CPC.

Compared to papillomas, CPCs are much more aggressive, irregular in contour, are of mixed density on non-contrast study and show variable enhancement. Cysts and hemorrhage are frequent. They almost always grow through the ventricular wall into the brain with associated oedema. Carcinomas are more heterogeneous on both T1WI and T2WI and may show evidence of intratumoral hemorrhage. Pathologically, carcinomas resemble PNET and ependymomas.

Meningiomas and Related Tumors

Childhood meningiomas represent 1 to 4.2 percent of central nervous system tumors and 1.5 to 1.8 percent of all intracranial meningiomas. Childhood meningiomas are associated with significant shorter survival due to limitation in surgical intervention, association with neurofibromatosis, increased incidence of sarcomatous change, large size of tumors and inability to use adjuvant radiotherapy and chemotherapy to treat the residual tumors.

Pathology

Pediatric meningeal tumors include meningioma, meningeal fibromas, meningeal sarcomas and meningeal melanomas. Sylvian fissure meningiomas are common, lack a dural attachment and

originate from heterotopic meningeal rests within the brain. Significant percentage of pediatric meningiomas are intraventricular.

Imaging

The tumors are iso-to-hyperdense on non-contrast CT and the solid portion shows diffuse enhancement on contrast injection. Heterogeneity is seen in about 50 percent of cases and is related to cystic changes and intratumoral calcification. A typical CT features should suggest a malignant tumor such as meningeal sarcoma or meningeal PNET. Intraventricular meningiomas originate from choroid plexus.[34]

On MR, meningiomas have well-defined margins, and are isointense on T1WI, and iso-to-hyperintense on T2WI. Areas of cystic necrosis have prolonged T1 and T2 relaxation times. Solid portions show uniform enhancement on infusion of paramagnetic substance. Densely calcified areas may be of very low intensity on precontrast T1W images whereas less densely calcified areas may be iso-to-hyperintense on T2WI. At angiography, meningiomas usually have dual blood supply, meningeal branches from both internal carotid and external carotid arteries may feed the tumor.

Leukemia and Lymphoma

Meningeal and parenchymal metastatic disease from leukemia and lymphoma are extremely uncommon. Meningeal enhancement after contrast administration is found in 5 percent of leukemic patients with CNS symptoms. Granulocytic sarcoma is a solid tumor found in association with systemic leukemia, usually the myelogenous type. It is postulated to arise from neoplastic cells that traverse the calvarial marrow to involve the dura, than pass through the perivenous adventitial tissue to invade the brain parenchyma. On CT granulocytic sarcomas appear iso-to-hyperdense with uniform enhancement on contrast administration. The MR characteristics are variable, but in most cases the lesions are hypo- to-isointense on T1WI and iso-to slightly hyperintense on T2WI. The lesions enhance uniformly and intensely following contrast on both CT and MR.[28]

TUMORS OF THE ORBIT AND NECK

OCULAR TUMORS

Retinoblastoma

Retinoblastoma is the commonest intraorbital malignancy of childhood. Autosomal dominant inheritance is found in 10 percent of cases that are frequently bilateral. Two to 5 percent of patients with bilateral retinoblastoma will eventually develop pineoblastoma, the term trilateral retinoblastomas is then applied. Bilateral lesions are seen in 31 percent and 33 percent are multifocal.

Majority (80%) of retinoblastomas occur in children below 2 years of age. Soft tissue sarcomas subsequently develop in 10 to 15 percent of affected patients. Leukocoria or 'Cats eye reflex' is the usual clinical presentation in early childhood.

Imaging

CT shows a retinal mass with ill-defined margins and commonly associated with calcification (95%). Intracranial extension occurs through scleral lymphatics along the optic nerves. CT is the imaging modality of choice to detect calcification and identification of the tumor. MR is useful for detection of intracranial extension.

Differential diagnosis includes Coats' disease, which is a degenerative proliferative disease of retina. Retinal detachment and subretinal hemorrhage is a common complication of Coats' disease. Larval granulomatosis is caused by Toxocoris canni infection, and has CT appearance similar to Coats' disease. Both conditions lack calcification and therefore, could be differentiated from majority of retinoblastomas containing calcification. Persistent hyperplastic primary vitreous is also associated with leucocoria, retinal detachment and subretinal hemorrhage. Absence of calcification and hypoplastic affected globe are its major differentiating features from retinoblastoma.[35]

RETROBULBAR ORBITAL TUMORS

Vascular Tumors

Orbital hemangiomas and lymphangiomas are hamartomatous malformations. Capillary hemangiomas are the most common vascular masses, which typically present at birth and grow rapidly within first 6 months of life. They stop growing during the second year and subsequently involute over 5-6 years.

CT shows a diffuse, retrobulbar mass with ill-defined margins, present extraconally, intraconally or both. Contrast enhancement is diffuse. MR reveals a mass that is hyperintense to extra-ocular muscles and hypointense to fat on both T1WI and T2WI. Serpiginous flow void areas within the mass helps to differentiate it from malignant masses such as rhabdomyosarcomas. Orbital enlargement is seen frequently.

Lymphangiomas present between the ages of 1 and 15 years. Recurrent hemorrhages within the mass cause recurrent episodic proptosis. On CT lymphangiomas are heterogeneous, ill-defined masses with occasional phleboliths and heterogeneous enhancement. Recent hemorrhage appears hyperdense. On MR, lymphangioma appears as lobulated, multicystic mass, which is hypointense to muscle on T1WI and hyperintense to muscle on T2WI. Fluid-fluid levels, when present, are strongly suggestive of lymphangioma. Heterogeneous enhancement is seen on contrast administration. Cavernous hemangiomas are rare in children. They present as painless proptosis, which does not change with Valsalva maneuver, when compared with orbital varices. Cavernous hemangiomas are intraconal masses that spare the orbital apex and frequently have phleboliths within it. MR shows the mass as isointense on T1WI and hyperintense on T2WI compared to orbital muscles. Homogeneous contrast enhancement is noted on both CT and MR.[36]

Orbital Varices

Orbital varices are venous malformations located in the retrobulbar region. They present in older children or adulthood. Classical presentation is intermittent proptosis, which increases on Valsalva maneuver on lying prone or on bending forward. CT and MR show a mass with curvilinear configuration, phleboliths and dense enhancement after contrast administration. CT is better modality since imaging can be performed during a Valsalva maneuver in short time.[36]

Neuroblastoma

Neuroblastoma is a common tumor of childhood, which involves the CNS either by direct extension, primarily in the spine, or blood-borne metastases. Neuroblastoma metastases commonly involve the orbit and calvarium and rarely the brain. Unenhanced CT scan may show multiple intracranial hyperdense masses, some of which mimic intraparenchymal lesions. Bony spicules are seen radiating centripetally from the calvarium. Splitting the coronal and sagittal sutures is another characteristic finding in neuroblastoma. Coronal images are useful to verify a dural extradural location of these lesions. Primary neuroblastoma originates in the sympathetic chain of upper cervical or skull base portion. On MR, the tumor masses have intensity similar to soft tissue. Enhancement is marked and elevated periosteum also shows enhancement which helps to differentiate it from normal hemopoietic calvarium. Metastatic Ewing's sarcoma and leukemia cannot be differentiated from metastatic neuroblastoma to the skull base.[36]

Plexiform Neurofibroma

Plexiform neurofibroma is seen in the setting of NF1. They diffusely infiltrate the connective tissue and peripheral nerves of the orbit. Proptosis, visual loss, marked facial asymmetry, enlarged orbit and dysplastic adjacent greater sphenoid wing is commonly found. The mass may extend through the superior orbital fissure into the cavernous sinus. The masses are isodense to extraocular muscles on CT. MR is preferred to CT, since cavernous sinus involvement and other manifestation of NF1 can be assessed well even without contrast.[36]

Rhabdomyosarcoma

Rhabdomyosarcoma is a common childhood malignancy, only next to intracranial brain tumors and retinoblastoma. Orbit and asopharynx are commonly involved, followed by paranasal inuses and middle ear, constituting 40 percent of all rabdomyosarcomas. Primary intracranial rhabdomyosarcomas re rare, although cranial involvement is common from extension f extracranial tumors. Rhabdomyosarcomas are classified into tree major groups depending on the site of origin.

. Parameningeal
. Orbital
. Other head and neck locations.

The parameningeal group consists of tumors originating in the iddle nasopharynx, paranasal sinuses and nasal cavity. Prognosis , very poor since tumor in this location commonly invades the kull or spread through the foramina at the skull base.

Orbital rhabdomyosarcoma spread through orbital fissures in ie cranium cavernous sinus and middle cranial fossa. The tumor isodense on NCCT and enhances uniformly after IV contrast. dditionally, the involved foramina are expanded. MR findings onsist of mass that is isointense on T1WI and hyperintense on 2WI as compared to muscle. Uniform enhancement is found ollowing IV contrast. Fat suppression technique with contrast is referred for better delineation of the tumor from fat and muscle.[36]

uvenile Angiofibroma

hese tumors are benign but locally invasive lesions that arise in ie sphenopalatine foramen, nasopharynx or posterior nasal cavity. dolescent boys are commonly affected. Local invasion is quite ommon.

Nasal obstruction and recurrent epistaxis are the frequent linical presentation. Proptosis and cranial neuropathies are seen ith intracranial extension of the tumor. CT shows a soft tissue 1ass in the nasopharynx/pterygopalatine fossa, with well-ircumscribed margins and homogeneous enhancement following V contrast. It produces anterior bowing of posterior maxillary all sinus. Sphenoid sinus extension is quite common.

MR shows a mass that is iso-to hypointense on T1WI and iso-o-hyperintense on T2WI as compared to muscles. Tumor vessels re seen as serpiginous flow void areas. Intense homogeneous nhancement of the tumor is a characteristic finding on IV ontrast. Angiography reveals a very vascular tumor, mainly upplied by external carotid arteries. Endovascular embolisation 1ay be carried out to reduce intraoperative blood loss.[37]

MR SPECTROSCOPY (MRS) IN BRAIN

umor Imaging

1RS is helpful in biochemical tissue characterization of tumors nd differentiating radiation-induced necrosis from recurrent or esidual tumor.

ositron-Emission Tomography (PET) in leuro-oncology

ET is relatively non-invasive modality to study regional cerebral hysiology in patients with brain tumors. PET provides *in vivo* quantitative information about glucose, oxygen metabolism, blood flow, tissue drug uptake and receptor, and the effects of various therapeutic regimens.

Initial reports with 18 *fluorodeoxyglucose (FDG)* PET have suggested the possibility of grading cerebral tumors *in vivo*. High grade neoplasms show large increases in glucose metabolism and low grade neoplasms show hypometabolism.[20]

Thus, combination of PET with anatomic MR imaging or CT enhances the clinical usefulness of PET in neurooncology.

Diffusion Weighted Imaging

- Diffusion weighted imaging derives image contrast from the movement of water molecules in tissues.
- Brownian motion—All molecules at temperatures greater than absolute zero experience random translation driven by their internal thermal energy.
- In the context of diffusion imaging, Brownian motion is also called self-diffusion or intravoxel incoherent motion.
- Thus, normal water motion results in decreased signal intensity, while reduced water motion that is, restricted water diffusion—Results in relatively increased signal.
- In routine clinical imaging, Diffusion weighting can be achieved with TSE, EPI, STE, SSFP and PSIF.
- Highly cellular tumors such as lymphoma, PNET, cellular gliomas have a higher ADC than the normal brain parenchyma.
- Viable tumor shows normal-high SI on DWI (normal-decreased ADC).
- In areas of tumor necrosis, there is low SI on DWI and increased ADC.

Uses in Glioma Evaluation

- Grading of glioma.
- Stereotactic biopsy guidance.
- Distinguishing radiation necrosis from recurrent cancer.
- Determining prognosis and response to treatment.
- Gliomas—Higher grade-Increased angiogenesis-Increased rCBV.
- Mean rCBV ratio (obtained by division by contralateral WM value) is 4.82 in high grade gliomas and 1.83 in low grade gliomas. Proposed cut-off value for rCBV ratio is 2.93 and rCBF ratio is 3.57.
- High cerebral blood volume foci can be found in non-GD enhancing tumors.
- Helps to direct stereotactic biopsy to areas of increased rCBV, which are more aggressive and hence increased chances of malignant tissue retrieval.
- Radiation necrosis versus tumor recurrence are difficult to differentiates.

On Conventional CT and MRI- as BBB breakdown, mass-effect and edema are common to both differentiate on Perfusion MRI-Irradiated areas reveal rCBV decrease in values, whereas rCBV increases in tumor recurrence.

NANOTECHNOLOGY

Imaging and Nanomedicine for Diagnosis and Therapy of CNS Tumors

Neuroimaging techniques have become increasingly important in assessing the biologic and physiological properties of brain tumors and neurologic lesions. Role of newer contrast media such as iron peroxide nanoparticle MR contrast or molecular agents based on therapeutic agents or tumor specific antibodies or agents is presently under evaluation. Superparamagnetic iron peroxide (SPIO) and utrasmall superparamagnetic iron peroxide (USPIO) nanoparticle MR contrast agents are being increasingly used in CNS for charactering particle delivery, monitoring trafficking of particles and cells and visualizing intracerebral tumors. Newer molecular imaging techniques should be integrated into brain tumor management to providing critical information that may significantly improve the survival and care of patients with brain tumors.[38]

Newly codified glial neoplasms of the 2007 WHO classification of tumors of the central nervous system[39]

This new classification system proposed in 2007 has recognized three new entities:

1. Angiocentric glioma (AG)-is a slowly growing cerebral tumor that typically presents with seizures in children and young adults. It is characterized by monomorphous, bipolar tumor cells with typical perivascular growth pattern. The cell of origin of AG is not clear but the ultrastructural evidence points to an ependymal derivation. It is designated WHO grade I and can be completely cured by surgical resection.

2. Polymyxoid Astrocytoma (PMA)-is a solid, circumscribed tumor occurring mainly in the region of hypothalamus of young children. It is composed of monomorphous population of bipolar tumor cells within a rich background of myxoid with a conspicuous angiocentric arrangement. While PMA is considered a more aggressive variant of pilocytic astrocytoma, this relationship awaits further clarification.PMA has been designated WHO grade II.

3. Pituicytoma-The pituicytoma involves the posterior pituitary and or the stalk and affects young adults. It is solid in architecture and composed of spindle cells and presumably derived from pituicytes. Pituicytomas are indolent tumors and designated WHO grade I.

CONCLUSION

CNS is the second most common site of pediatric neoplasm. Infratentorial tumors account for 52 percent, while 48 percent involve the supratentorial region. Aside from the initial recognition and characterization of these lesions, the mechanical effects and structural deformities resulting from intracranial neoplasms are also of great importance. Therefore, the neuroradiologists must be able to appreciate the consequences resulting from the combined effects of tumors and the associated oedema, many of which are potentially life-threatening such as transtentorial herniation. For the optimal interpretation of MRI, it is essential for the neuroradiologists to be particularly familiar with neuro pathology in addition to the requisite mastery of neuroanatom since imaging abnormalities reflect pathologic findings in these lesions.

REFERENCES

1. Miltenburg D, Louw DF, Sutherland GR. Epidemiology c childhood brain tumors. Can J Neurol Sci 1996; 23(2): 118-22.
2. McKinney PA, Parslow RC, Lane SA, et al. Epidemiology c childhood brain tumors in Yorkshire, UK, 1974-95: Geographic distribution and changing patterns of occurrence. Br J Cancer 1998 8(7):974-9.
3. Karkavelas G, Tascos N. Epidemiology, histologic classificatio and clinical course of brain tumors. In Drevelegas A (Ed): Imagin of brain tumors with histological correlation. New York: Springe 2002.
4. Koeller KK, Rushing EJ. From the archives of the AFIF Medulloblastoma: A comprehensive review with radiologic pathologic correlation. Radiographics 2003; 23:1613-37.
5. Giangspero F, Bigner SH, Kleihues P, et al. Medulloblastoma. I Kleihues P, Cavenee WK (Eds): Pathology and Genetics of Tumor of the Nervous System. Lyon: IARC Press 2000; 129-37.
6. Kotsenas AL, Roth TC, Manness WK, et al. Abnormal diffusio weighted MRI in medulloblastoma: Does it reflect small ce histology? Pediatr Radiol 1999; 29:524-26.
7. Tortori-Donati P, Fondelli MP, Rossi A, et al. Medulloblastoma i children: CT and MRI findings. Neuroradiology 1996; 38:352-5⁹
8. Lee YY, Van Tassel P, Bruner JM, et al. Juvenile pilocyti astrocytomas: CT and MR characteristics. AJR Am J Roentgenc 1989; 152(6):1263-70.
9. Tortori-Donati P, Fondelli MP, Cama A, et al. Ependymomas of th posterior cranial fossa: CT and MRI findings. Neuroradiology 1995 37(3):238-43.
10. Fisher PG, Breiter SN, Carson BS, et al. A clinicopathologi reappraisal of brainstem tumor classification. Identification c pilocytic astrocytoma and fibrillary astrocytoma as distinct entitie Cancer 2000; 89(7):1569-76.
11. Atlas SW, Lavi E, Fisher PG. Intraaxial brain tumors. In Atlas S\ (Ed): Magnetic Resonance Imaging of Brain and Spine (3rd edn Philadelphia: Lippincott 2002; 565-693.
12. Rorke LB, Packer R, Biegel J. Central nervous system atypic teratoid/rhabdoid tumors of infancy and childhood. Journal c Neuro-Oncology 1995; 24:21-28.
13. Agranovich AL, Ang LC, Griebel RW. Malignant rhabdoid tumc of the central nervous system with subarachnoid dissemination. Sur Neurol 1992; 37(5):410-4.
14. Zuccoli G, Izzi G, Bachini E, et al. Central nervous system atypic teratoid/rhabdoid tumor of infancy: CT and MR findings. Clinic Imaging 1999; 23:356-60.
15. Ho VB, Smirniotopoulos JG, Murphy FM, et al. Radiologic pathologic correlation: Hemangioblastoma. AJNR Am J Neuroradic 1992; 13(5):1343-52.
16. Lee SR, Sanches J, Mark AS, et al. Posterior foss hemangioblastomas: MR imaging. Radiology 1989; 171(2):463-8 AJNR 1997; 18:77-87.
17. Horowitz BL, Chari MV, James R, et al. MR of intracrani epidermoid tumors: Correlation of in vivo imaging with in vitr 13C spectroscopy. AJNR Am J Neuroradiol 1990; 11(2):299-302

8. Bergui M, Zhong J, Bradac GB, et al. Diffusion-weighted images of intracranial cyst-like lesions. Neuroradiology 2001; 43(10):824-9.

9. Jelinek J, Smirniotopoulos JG, Parisi JE, et al. Lateral ventricular neoplasms of the brain: Differential diagnosis based on clinical, CT, and MR findings. AJNR Am J Neuroradiol 1990; 11(3):567-74.

0. Koeller KK, Henry JM. From the archives of the AFIP: Superficial gliomas: Radiologic-pathologic correlation. Armed Forces Institute of Pathology. Radiographics 2001; 21(6):1533-56.

1. Castillo M, Davis PC, Takei Y, et al. Intracranial ganglioglioma: MR, CT, and clinical findings in 18 patients. AJNR Am J Neuroradiol 1990; 11:109-14 (ganglioma).

2. Davis P, Wichman RD, Takei Y, et al. Primary cerebral neurocytoma: CT and MR findings in 12 cases. AJNR Am J Neuroradiol 1990; 11:115-20.

3. Daumas-Duport C, Scheithauer BW, Chodkiewicz JP, et al. Dysembryoplastic neuroepithelial tumor: A surgically curable tumor of young patients with intractable partial seizures. Report of thirty-nine cases. Neurosurgery 1988; 23(5):545-56.

4. VandenBerg SR, May EE, Rubenstein LJ, et al. Desmoplastic supratentorial neuroepithelial tumors of infancy with divergent differentiation potential ("desmoplastic infantile gangliogliomas"): Report on 11 cases of a distinctive embryonal tumor with favorable prognosis. J Neurosurg 1987; 66:58-71.

5. Fernandez C, Girard N, Paz Paredes A, et al. The usefulness of MR imaging in the diagnosis of dysembryoplastic neuroepithelial tumor in children: A study of 14 cases. AJNR Am J Neuroradiol 2003; 24:829-34.

6. Janss AJ, Grundy R, Cnaan A, et al. Optic pathway and hypothalamic/chiasmatic gliomas in children younger than age 5 years with a 6-year follow-up. Cancer 1995; 75(4):1051-9.

7. Sartoretti-Schefer S, Wichmann W, Aguzzi A, et al. MR differentiation of adamantinous and squamous-papillary craniopharyngiomas. AJNR Am J Neuroradiol 1997; 18(1):77-87.

28. Atlas SW, Lavi E, Goldberg HI. Extraaxial brain tumors. In Atlas SW (Ed): Magnetic Resonance Imaging of Brain and Spine (3rd edn). Philadelphia: Lippincott 2002; 695-772.

29. Poussaint TY, Barnes PD, Anthony DC, et al. Hemorrhagic pituitary adenomas of adolescence. AJNR Am J Neuroradiol 1996; 17(10): 1907-12.

30. Sugiyama K, Uozumi T, Kiya K, et al. Intracranial germ-cell tumor with synchronous lesions in the pineal and suprasellar regions: Report of six cases and review of the literature. Surg Neurol 1992; 38(2):114-20.

31. Zee CS, Segal H, Apuzzo M, et al. MR imaging of pineal region neoplasms. J Comput Tomogr 1993; 15:56-63.

32. Lee DH, Norman D, Newton TH, et al. MR imaging of pineal cysts. J Comput Assist Tomogr 1987; 11(4):586-90.

33. Tomita T, Melone DG, Flannery AM. Choroid plexus papillomas of neonates, infants and children. Pediatr Neurosci 1988; 14:23-30.

34. Hope JKA, Armstrong DA, Babyn PS, et al. Primary meningeal tumors in children-correlation of clinical and CT findings with histologic type and prognosis. Am J Neuroradiol 1992; 13:1353-64.

35. Price HI, Batnitzky S, Danzinger A, et al. The neuroradiology of retinoblastoma. Radiographics 1982; 2(2):7-23.

36. Bilaniuk LT, Zimmerman RA, Newton TH. Magnetic resonance imaging - orbital pathology. In Newton TH, Bilaniuk LT (Eds) Radiology of the Eye and Orbit. Clavadel 1990; 531-84.

37. Lloyd GAS, Phelps PD. Juvenile angiofibroma imaging by MR, CT and conventional techniques. Clin Otolaryngol 1986; 11:247-59.

38. LL Muldoon, PG Tratnyek, PM Jacobs, et al. Imaging and Nanomedicine for diagnosis and therapy in the central nervous system. AJNR Am J Neurorad 2006; 27:715-21.

39. Daniel J Brat, Bernd W Scheithauer, Gregory N Fuller, Tarik Tihan. Brain Pathology Vol 17, issue 3, July 2007; 319-24.

CHAPTER 30

Metabolic Disorders of the Brain

Sapna Singh, Veena Chowdhury

INTRODUCTION

Myelination begins during the fifth fetal month with the myelination of the cranial nerves and proceeds rapidly following the order of phylogenetic development—occurring first in the peripheral nerves then the spinal cord and lastly in the brain.[1] Myelin is composed of a bi-layer of lipids (cholesterol and glycolipids) and large proteins. Although white matter diseases affect the myelin, there are now many studies which reveal that myelin is not the only brain tissue damaged in "demyelinating disease" as the oligodendrocyte is the cell responsible for wrapping the axon concentrically to form the myelin sheath.[2] With the addition of the magnetic resonance imaging (MRI) to the diagnostic armamentarium it is possible to closely follow maturation and myelination of the neonatal and infant brain with a better understanding of the nature of diseases and a more precise histopathologic analysis. Cholesterol (fat) has a short T1 and protein also decreases the T1 value of water. The result is a shortening of T1 and an increased intensity (increased brightness) on a T1 weighted (T1W) MR image. Myelin lipids are hydrophobic, hence, when myelination occurs there is loss of brain water. This results in a decrease in T2 value in white matter and as a result a decreased intensity or darker appearance on T2 weighted (T2W) images. Thus, myelination will be seen as an area of increased intensity (brighter) on T1W images and decreased intensity (darker) on T2W images.[3]

Normal Myelination of the Brain

At birth, as seen on T1W images, myelination is present in the medulla, dorsal midbrain, cerebellar peduncles, posterior limb of internal capsule and ventrolateral thalamus[4] (Figs 30.1A to D). Maturation proceeds from:
1. Central to peripheral
2. Inferior to superior
3. Posterior to anterior

The cerebellum is myelinated at 3 months of age with an adult appearance on T2W images.[5]

The pre- and post-central gyri are myelinated at 1 month and maturation of motor tracts is complete by 3 months.

The pons matures from 3-6 months with maturation proceeding rostrally along the corticospinal tracts, cerebral peduncles through the posterior limb of internal capsule and central portion of the centrum semiovale.[6]

The optic nerves, tracts and radiations into the occipital white matter are myelinated by 3 months[7] and the anterior limb of internal capsule by 2-3 months. The subcortical white matter maturation starts at 3 months in the occipital region and proceeds rostrally to the frontal lobe.

Myelination in the corpus callosum can be a helpful landmark when estimating myelin development. Myelination begins in the splenium posteriorly at 4 months and is complete involving the genu anteriorly at 6 months.

MR Imaging at 1.5 T (Tables 30.1A and B)

Brain maturation occurs in an orderly manner commencing in the brainstem and progressing to the cerebellum and cerebrum. The changes appear at different times with T1 and T2W MR images possibly because of T1 shortening by the components of the developing myelin sheaths. The difference in the maturation rate makes the T1W images more useful in the first 6-8 months and the T2W images thereafter.[8]

Thus, the early primary process of myelination from about 1-6 months is best evaluated using strongly T1W images (short TR/short TE). The T1W image will appear adult like at about 9 months. T2W images are better at depicting the associated changes of water loss that occur with myelination and may be helpful after 6 months of age.

On T1W images the sequential progression of myelination is seen and myelination is identified approximately 2 months earlier than on T2W images.[5,8]

Table 30.1A: Milestones: Normal myelination (1-6 months) (T1W images at 1.5T)		
Cerebellar white matter	-	3 months
Splenium	-	4 months
Genu	-	6 months
Adult	-	9 months

Table 30.1B: Milestones: Normal myelination (T2W images at 1.5T)		
Splenium	-	6 months
Genu	-	8 months
Anterior limb internal capsule	-	11 months
Frontal white matter	-	14 months
Adult pattern	-	18 months

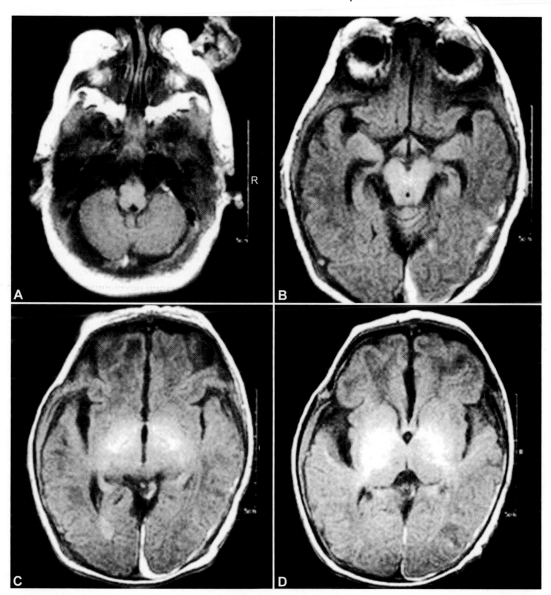

Figs 30.1A to D: Axial T1W MR images in a newborn depicting normal myelination as an area of increased signal intensity (bright) in medulla (A), dorsal midbrain (B), ventrolateral thalamus (C) and in posterior limb of internal capsule (D)

Inversion recovery sequences also give excellent depiction of yelin deposition (Figs 30.2A to D), (Figs 30.3A to D) and may e extremely helpful in selected cases, the additional time needed obtain them makes them less practical than SE sequences in e evaluation of young children.⁵

ray-white Matter Differentiation

2W spin echo pulse sequences can distinguish gray and white atter in infants and demonstrate early progression of yelination.

Although developmentally normal children show a spectrum relative intensities of gray and white matter, their gray-white atter patterns fall into three distinct groups:- infantile, isointense d early adult.⁷ At birth and first 6 to 8 months the "infantile" ttern shows reversal of the normal adult pattern seen on T2W ages, i.e in neonates the white matter is hyperintense to gray

matter. Children between the ages of 8 to 12 month demonstrate the transient "isointense" phase with poor differentiation of gray and white matter. The early "adult" pattern where gray matter has higher intensity than white matter is seen in all children over 12 months and may be seen as early as 10 months of age.

METABOLIC DISORDERS

Metabolic disorders are classically divided into inborn errors of metabolism and acquired metabolic diseases. Acquired metabolic diseases usually occur in specific or suggestive clinical settings, such as kernicterus in neonatal hyperbilirubinemia, hypovitaminoses in malnutrition or neontatal hypoglycemia in premature infants. Toxic encephalopathies are special, exogenous forms of acquired metabolic diseases.

Inborn errors of metabolism represent a vast and complex group of pathologies. The cause is generally a mutation resulting

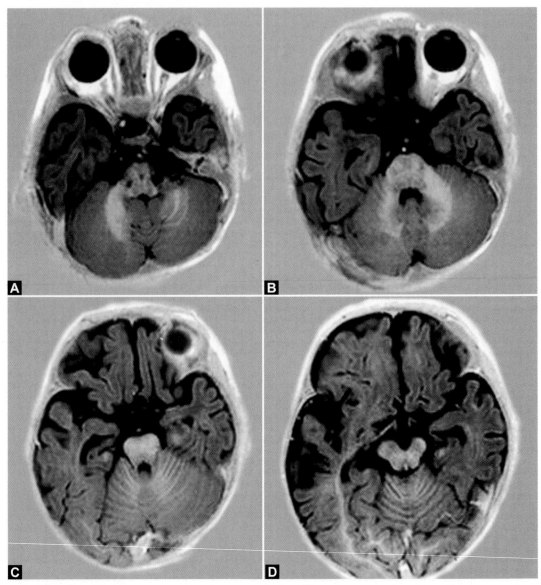

Figs 30.2A to D: Inversion recovery images in a 9-month-old infant showing normal myelin deposition in medulla and inferior cerebellar peduncles (A), pons and middle cerebellar peduncles (B), cerebellum (C) and in midbrain (D)

in a biochemical alteration involving one or more metabolic pathways. The diagnosis of these disorders is often a challenge for all concerned with the care of the affected child. The presenting symptoms are usually non-specific such as seizures, spasticity, ataxia, movement disorder or delay in achieving the developmental milestones. Biochemical tests and genetic analyses are often negative. As a result, at least 60% of children with the inborn errors of metabolism never receive a specific diagnosis despite extensive investigations.[8] Some methods of organizing the metabolic diseases from an imaging perspective are helpful to both the radiologist and the clinician as narrowing the differential diagnosis facilitates the clinical work-up. Many classifications exist, all of them with the aim of facilitating the systematic approach to these diseases.

Classification According to Cellular Organelle Dysfunction

The cellular organelles have distinctly different functions in the metabolism: the mitochondria are involved mainly in energy metabolism, lysosomes in the degradation of macromolecules (lipids, lipoproteins, mucopolysaccharides) and peroxisomes both anabolic and catabolic functions.

Classification of Metabolic Disorders on the Basis of Organelle Disorder[9,10]

Lysosomal Storage Diseases with White Matter Involvement

- Metachromatic leukodystrophy
- Krabbe disease

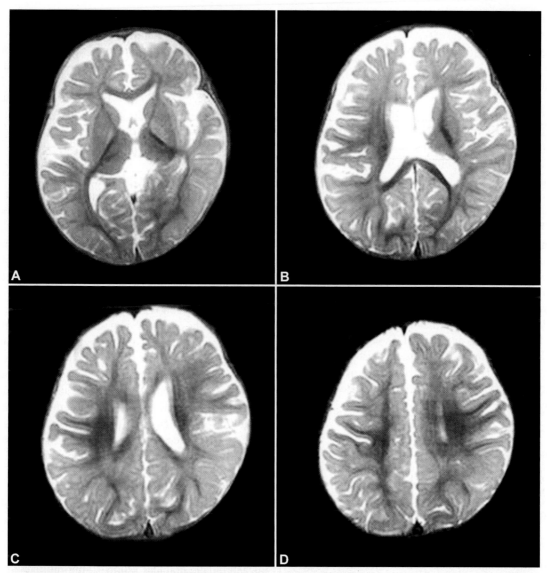

Figs 30.3A to D: Inversion recovery images in a 9-month-old infant showing normal myelin deposition in post and ant. limbs of internal capsule, genu of corpus callosum and optic radiation (A), splenium of corpus (B) and peripheral white matter (occipital and parietal) (C,D)

Niemann-Pick disease
Fabry disease
GM1 gangliosidosis
GM2 gangliosidosis
Mucopolysaccharidosis
Fucosidosis
Wolman disease and cholesterol ester storage disease
Ceroid lipofuscinosis

eroxisomal Disorders

Zellweger syndrome
X-linked adrenoleukodystrophy (ALD)
Neonatal ALD
Pseudoneonatal ALD
Classic Refsum disease

- Hyperpipecolic acidemia
- Cerebrotendinous xanthomatosis
- Abetalipoproteinemia
- Rhizomatic chondrodysplasia calcificans punctata.

Mitochondrial Dysfunction with Leukoencephalopathy

- Leigh disease
- MELAS syndrome
- MERRF syndrome
- Kearns-Sayre syndrome

Disorders of Amino Acid and Organic Acid Metabolism

- Canavan disease

White Matter Disorders with Unknown Metabolic Defect

- Pelizaeus-Merzbacher disease (PMD)
- Alexander disease
- Congenital muscular dystrophy (Fukuyama type)

Classification of Metabolic Disorders According to Brain Substance Involvement

The classification takes into account the dominance of substance involvement, i.e. gray matter, white matter or both within the brain. This is usually best shown by magnetic resonance imaging (MRI).

Leukodystrophies

Dysmyelinating diseases, or leukodystrophies, encompass a wide spectrum of inherited neurodegenerative disorders affecting the integrity of myelin in the brain and peripheral nerves. Diseases that present with white matter abnormalities are referred to as leukodystrophies. Leukodystrophies result from inherited enzyme deficiency that causes abnormal formation, destruction or turnover of myelin. Most of these disorders fall into one of three categories—lysosomal storage diseases, peroxisomal disorders and diseases caused by mitochondrial dysfunction. Each leukodystrophy has distinctive clinical biochemical, pathologic and radiological features.

Poliodystrophies

This group comprises diseases that present with predominantly gray matter abnormalities. Some degree of white matter involvement, however, is often present. Classical disease categories are respiratory chain disorders (so called 'mitochondrial diseases') and organic acidopathies.

Pandystrophies

The majority of the metabolic disorders fall into this category, since exclusive involvement of the gray or white matter structures is rare.

Following the classification according to the cellular organelle dysfunction, the metabolic disorders can be described as:

LYSOSOMAL STORAGE DISORDERS

Metachromatic Leukodystrophy (MLD)

Metachromatic leukodystrophy is the most common of all the familial leukodystrophies. It is an autosomal recessive disorder caused by a deficiency of the lysosomal enzyme arylsulfatase A.[11,12] This enzyme is necessary for the normal metabolism of sulfatides, which are important constituents of myelin sheath. Cerebroside sulfate (galactosyl sulfatide) abnormally accumulates within the white matter resulting in breakdown of the membrane of the myelin sheath, kidneys, gallbladder and other viscera. The accumulation of sulfatides within glial cells and neurons causes the characteristic metachromatic reaction. The name metachromatic is derived from the neuropathologic description of metachromatic staining which consists of a brownish or reddish color compared with the blue color of cell nuclei when staine[d] with cresyl violet or toluidine blue.[13]

Metachromatic leukodystrophy is diagnosed biochemically o[n] the basis of an abnormally low level of arylsulfatase A in urin[e] peripheral blood leukocytes or cultured fibroblasts. Diagnosis ca[n] also be made by sural nerve biopsy. Prenatal diagnosis can b[e] achieved by assaying the activity of the enzyme in culture[d] amniotic fluid cells.

Clinical Features

According to the patient age three patterns of MLD a[re] recognized—the late infantile, juvenile and adult forms.[14] Th[e] most common type is the late infantile variety, which usuall[y] manifests in children between 12 and 18 months of age and [is] characterized by motor signs of peripheral neuropathy followe[d] by deterioration in intellect, speech and coordination. The disea[se] progresses quickly and within 2 years of onset, gait disturbanc[e] quadriplegia, blindness and decerebrate posturing may be see[n.] Disease progression is continuous and death occurs 6 months [to] 4 years after the onset of symptoms.[15] In the less common juveni[le] form, symptoms usually do not develop until 4 years of age. Th[e] clinical picture is similar to the late infantile form except that th[e] child is old enough to manifest behavioral disturbances as we[ll.] There is impaired school performance and emotional lability. Th[e] neurological examination reveals cerebellar incoordinatio[n] pyramidal tract signs and decreased reflexes as in the low[er] extremities. In the uncommon adult form patients tend to prese[nt] with dementia and progress to develop motor signs.

Pathologic Findings

At autopsy the surface of the brain appears atrophic, the whi[te] matter is shrunken and sclerotic and the ventricles are dilate[d.] Changes in the peripheral nerve myelin explain th[e] polyneuropathy noted in MLD. The hallmark of the disease [is] metachromatic granules (20 to 30 mm in diameter) presumab[ly] derivatives of cerebroside sulfate.[16]

Imaging Features

The typical CT appearance of MLD is a symmetrical lucency [of] the white matter, especially prominent in the centrum semiova[le] and in corpus callosum.[17] There is no evidence of inflammati[on] or contrast enhancement and the cortical gray matter is spar[ed] (Figs 30.4A and B).

The characteristic MR features of MLD include symmetr[ic] confluent areas of high signal within the periventricular a[nd] cerebellar white matter on T2W images.[18,19] There is sparing [of] the subcortical U fibers until late in the disease (Figs 30.5A[-] C). *Thus, MLD is a progressive centrifugal white matter diseas[e.]* In the late onset (juvenile and adult forms) there is predomina[nt] involvement of the frontal white matter. In the late infantile for[m] of MLD, the most common type, a posterior (occipita[l] predominance of signal abnormality has been reported wi[th] dorsofrontal progression of disease. Involvement of t[he] corticospinal tracts may also be seen in the late infantile form[s]

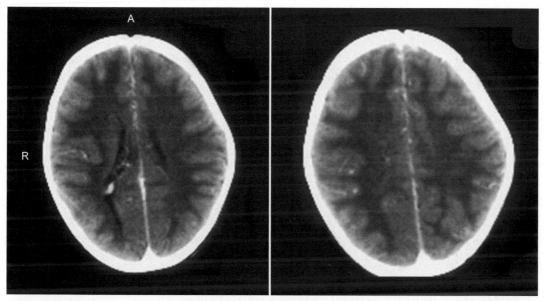

Figs 30.4A and B: CT image in a 2-year-old child showing diffuse white matter hypodensity in periventricular location with relative sparing of the subcortical white matter – Metachromatic leukodystrophy (MLD)

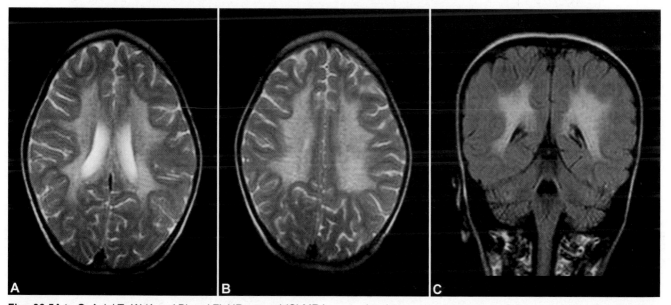

Figs 30.5A to C: Axial T_2 W (A and B) and FLAIR coronal (C) MR images showing a symmetric pattern of high signal intensity in the deep periventricular white matter with relative sparing of the subcortical U fibers. The tigroid pattern of white matter involvement is well seen (B)—Metachromatic leukodystrophy (MLD)

MLD. High signal intensity is seen on the long TR images along the path of corticospinal tracts in the posterior limbs of the internal capsules and brainstem. The corpus callosum is invariably affected and hypointensity may be seen within the thalami on T2W images. The so called tigroid pattern of demyelination with alternating areas of normal white matter within areas of demyelination may also be seen in the infantile form.[12,18] As the disease progresses the signal abnormality becomes more extensive and confluent with associated atrophy The corpus callosum (first the splenium then the anterior portions), the internal capsule and the deep hemispheric white matter are always involved (Figs 30.6A to D).

In later stages, considerable atrophic dilatation of the lateral ventricles is seen. Atrophy may be the only finding in late adult onset cases (Figs 30.7A to C).

Diffusion weighted images usually show signal abnormalities. Moderate hypersignal is seen in the presumed progression zone of the demyelinating process. In the late stages, diffuse hyposignal is seen. The tigroid pattern is also sometimes conspicuous on the diffusion weighted images.[20,21] Proton MR spectroscopy frequently demonstrates abnormality in the metabolic peaks before conventional MR imaging. The spectrum includes decrease NAA, abnormal elevation of choline, myoinositol and lactate peak

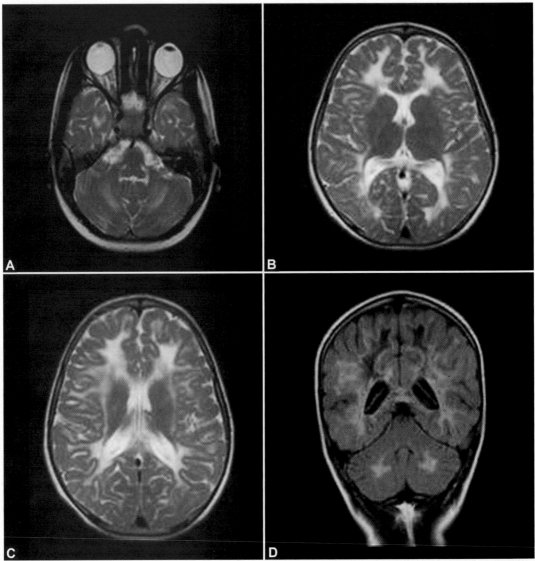

Figs 30.6A to D: Axial T$_2$ W (A to C) and FLAIR coronal (D) MR images showing involvement of the deep periventricular white matter wi[...] relative sparing of the subcortical U fibers. There is involvement of the posterior limbs of internal capsule (B), the cerebellar white matter (A,[...] and the splenium of the corpus callosum (D)—Metachromatic leukodystrophy (MLD)

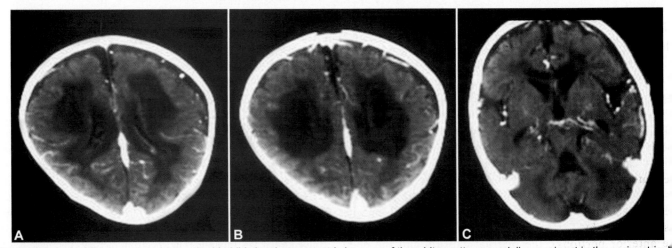

Figs 30.7A to C: CT images in a 14 month-old-child showing symmetric lucency of the white matter especially prominent in the periventricul[...] white matter, centrum semiovale with involvement of cerebellar white matter and corpus callosum. Cerebral atrophy and moderate enlargeme[...] of the ventricles is also seen – Metachromatic leukodystrophy

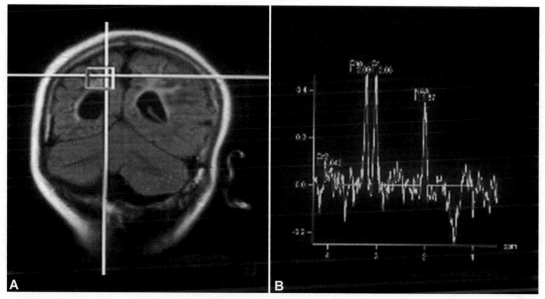

Figs 30.8A and B: Coronal FLAIR images with voxel placement in the hyperintensity in frontal white matter shows abnormal elevation of choline peak – an early finding in MLD

Fig. 30.8). The elevation of myoinositol is highly suggestive of MLD.[22]

Krabbe Disease/Globoid Cell Leukodystrophy (GLD)

Krabbe disease is an autosomal recessive disorder caused by a deficiency of lysosomal enzyme beta galactocerebrosidase, an enzyme that degrades cerebroside, a normal constituent of myelin. As soon as myelination commences and myelin turnover becomes necessary, cerebrosides accumulate in the lysosomes of macrophages within the white matter forming the globoid cells characteristic of the disease.[23] The abnormal accumulation of galactocerebroside and its derivative psychosine to toxic levels kills oligodendroglial cells. The genetic basis for the enzyme defect in Krabbe disease has been traced to a faulty gene on chromosome.[24] The diagnosis is made by demonstrating a deficiency of the enzyme in peripheral blood leukocytes.

Clinical Features

The clinical presentation of the disease varies with the age of onset.[25] In the early onset form, presentation is either before or at the age of 2 years while the late onset form presents after the age of 2 years. The early infantile form of the disease is the most common clinical form and has three phases. By 6 months of age the infant is irritable and hypertonic with spasticity and fever. Development fails to progress and the infant regresses neurologically. The second phase is characterized by rapid deterioration in motor function with chronic opisthotonos and myoclonic jerking accompanied by hyperpyrexia. In the third phase, the child appears decerebrate and has flaccid paralysis that culminates in death by 2 years of age.[26] The late onset forms have variable clinical presentation with a slower progression of disease.[27,28]

In early onset GLD, CSF analysis always demonstrates an abnormally high protein level with a normal cell count. In the late onset form the protein level is not consistently high in CSF. Bone marrow transplantation has been shown to halt/reverse the neurologic manifestation of disease.[29]

Pathologic Findings

The brain is small and weighs only 600 to 800 gm. The white matter is rubbery to firm but the cortex is relatively unaffected. The pathologic hallmark of Krabbe disease is a massive accumulation of large multinucleated cells containing PAS positive material (globoid cells). There is complete myelin destruction with loss of oligodendroglia and marked astrogliosis.

Imaging Features

The CT findings in GLD range from white matter lucency to diffuse cerebral atrophy. The CT findings of hyperdense thalami, caudate nucleus and corona radiata are characteristic but not specific for the disease and have been shown to correspond to fine calcifications at autopsy. The most characteristic MR finding in both early and late onset forms of GLD is high signal intensity on T2W images found along the lengths of the corticospinal tracts. Additional findings in the early onset form include abnormal signal intensity within the cerebellar white matter[30,31] and deep gray nuclei (dentate, basal ganglia, thalamus) with progressive involvement of the parieto-occipital white matter and posterior portion of the corpus callosum[32] (Figs 30.9A to D).

The cerebellar white matter and deep gray nuclei are not involved in the late onset form. Classically, the subcortical U fibers are spared until late in the disease. Enhancement at the border between the white matter and arcuate fibers has been described but is not seen in most cases. The cranial nerves may be affected with evidence of thickened optic nerve seen on MR

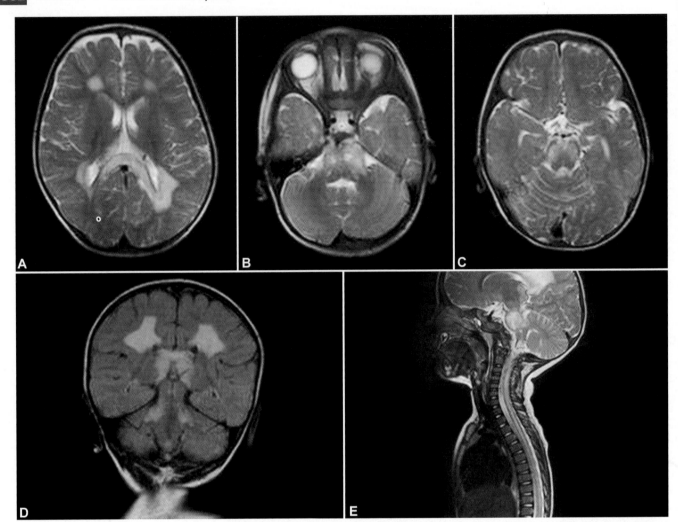

Figs 30.9A to E: Axial T2 W (A to C) and FLAIR coronal MR image (D) showing symmetric areas of white matter hyperintensity predominantly involving the parieto-occipital white matter with some involvement of the frontal white matter with relative sparing of the subcortical U fibers (A D.) Involvement of the splenium (A) and the corticospinal tracts (B,C) is seen. Sagittal T_2 W MR image of the cervicodorsal spine (E) reveals high signal intensity within the spinal cord parenchyma – Late onset Krabbe disease

imaging and at autopsy.[33,34] Optic nerve atrophy has also been described in late onset form.[35] Late onset cases of GLD with primary involvement of the parietal periventricular white matter, splenium of the corpus callosum and corticospinal tracts may appear similar on imaging to adrenoleukodystrophy (ALD) However, auditory pathway involvement is characteristic of ALD and is not seen in GLD.[36] MR imaging of the spine shows diffuse hypersignal within the spinal cord parenchyma (Fig. 30.9E). Nerve root enhancement may also be detected after intravenous contrast injection.[37]

Diffusion weighted images, like MLD, may show prominent hypersignal along the presumed progression zone of the demyelinating process (Figs 30.10A to D). In the late stages, diffuse hyposignal is seen suggesting complete myelin loss.[38] Diffusion tensor derived anisotropy maps are useful as a quantitative evaluation of white matter abnormalities in these patients.[39] DTI scans are being studied as a potential tool for follow-up of patients before and after stem cell transplantation. Perfusion MR techniques have also been used in the evaluation of white matter lesions in Krabbe disease. It shows a decreased intralesional CBV.

Sphingolipidosis

The sphingolipidoses involve abnormal metabolism and accumulation of sphingolipids. Deficiency of hexosaminidase A alone results in GM_2 gangliosidosis, the classic form of which is Tay-Sachs disease. Sandhoff's disease is caused by a deficiency in both hexosaminidase A and B. Clinical findings are identical to that of Tay-Sachs with additional findings of hepatosplenomegaly and bony deformities.[41]

Clinical Features

Onset of symptoms is between 3 and 6 months of age. The initial sign is an excessive startle reflex. A macular cherry red spot

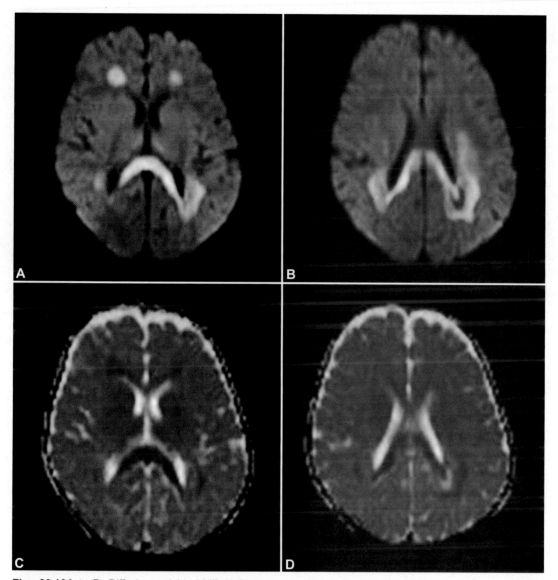

Figs 30.10A to D: Diffusion weighted MR (A,B) images in the same case showing a prominent hypersignal along the progression line of the demyelinating process reflecting the centrifugal gradient and the posteroanterior gradient of the disease process. ADC maps (C,D) reveal a hyposignal suggestive of a restricted pattern of diffusion—Krabbe disease

most always present at this stage and psychomotor regression then begins. Patients are macrocephalic and there is progressive psychomotor retardation, pyramidal and later extrapyramidal (choreoathetosis) signs and generalized tonic clonic seizures.

Imaging Features

The imaging findings in Tay-Sachs and Sandhoff disease are quite similar and the pattern is suggestive. CT examination of the brain shows hyperdensities within the basal ganglia and or thalami due to calcifications. MR imaging is sensitive in demonstrating the widespread white matter changes within the cerebral hemispheres. All the white matter structures are involved except for the corpus callosum, the anterior commissure and the posterior limbs of the internal capsules. The external and extreme capsules, the globi

pallidi and the putamina are all abnormal. The involved basal ganglia structures (putamina, caudate nucleus) are somewhat swollen particularly initially during the disease course. The thalami are spared and show low signal on T_2 weighted images (Figs 30.11A to C). The cerebellar white matter often shows signal abnormalities on the T_2 weighted images, the hyperintensities are less prominent than supratentorially. Typically, no abnormalities are seen within the brainstem and spinal cord. The overall lesion pattern in a macrocephalic infant can be highly suggestive of the disease.

Diffusion weighted images are usually quite unremarkable which suggest a slow demyelinating process. MR spectroscopy shows non-specific alteration, the NAA peak is decreased and the choline peak is increased. No lactate is identified.

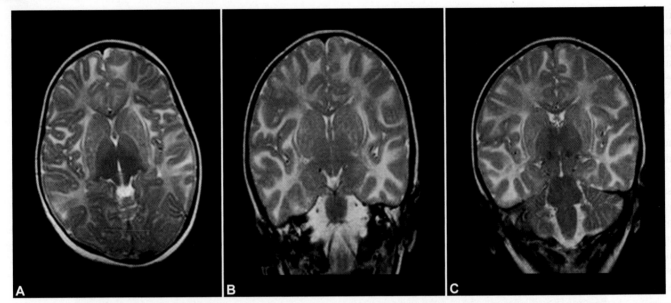

Figs 30.11A to C: T2 W Axial (A) and FLAIR coronal (B,C) MR images showing extensive white matter changes in the supratentorial compartme with relative sparing of the infratentorial compartment. The basal ganglia (the putamina, caudate nucleus), the external and the extrem capsules are all abnormal showing a high signal (A, B). The claustra are well delineated due to the involvement of the external and extrem capsules.(A)The thalami are spared and show low signal on the T2 W images – Tay-Sachs disease

Fabry Disease

This is a X-linked recessive disorder due to deficiency of the lysosomal enzyme-galactosidase A, which results in accumulation of glycosphingolipids in the vascular endothelium, smooth muscles and neurons.

Clinical Features

It typically presents late in childhood but occasionally is not recognized until third or fourth decade of life.[16] Early manifestations include a punctate telangiectatic skin and mucous membrane lesion followed by fever, weight loss and pain in extremities and abdomen. Retinal, corneal and conjunctival abnormalities are present early in the disease. Cardiac disease develops with age and is typically worsened by a systemic hypertension secondary to vascular disease. Patients may eventually present with transient ischemic attacks or strokes secondary to small vessel ischemia and focal infarcts.

Pathologic Findings

Glycosphingolipids accumulate in the vascular endothelium particularly in the small vessels throughout the brain and spinal cord. Storage of lipids is seen within neurons of amygdala, hypothalamus and the brainstem. Focal infarcts are frequently found in the basal ganglia and central white matter.

Imaging Features

Early in the disease small areas of high signal intensity are seen on long TR sequences, most commonly in the basal ganglia and periventricular white matter.[42] The periventricular disease becomes more extensive and confluent with time and associated generalized loss of cerebral volume. Cerebral hemorrhage has also been reported.

Gaucher's Disease

Gaucher's disease includes several autosomal recessive *lip storage diseases* in which there is a deficiency of the lysosom enzyme glucocerebroside.

Clinical Features

Neurologic symptoms include seizures, developmental regressio spasticity, mental deficiency, incoordination and tics.

Imaging

CT and MR findings are similar to those of Fabry disease wi atrophy, infarction and occasional hemorrhage.[43]

Mucopolysaccharidoses (MPS)

In the mucopolysaccharidoses (MPS) impaired degradation of tl various mucopolysaccharides (also known as glycosamin glycons) cause variable combinations of coarse facies, sho stature, bony defects, stiff joints, mental retardation, hepatosplen megaly and corneal clouding. All forms of MPS are autosom recessive except MPS type-II (Hunter syndrome) which X-linked recessive. Imaging studies are usually performed wh hydrocephalous or spinal cord compression is suspected. CT a MR usually reveals delayed myelination, atrophy, varying degre of hydrocephalous and white matter changes.[44] In all types MPS the white matter abnormalities are manifest as sharp defined foci in the corpus callosum and basal ganglia, isointen with CSF on all imaging sequences. These represent enlarg perivascular spaces filled with mucopolysaccharide or CSF. W progression of the disease, the lesions become larger and mc diffuse and resemble a leukodystrophy, reflecting the developme of infarcts and demyelination. The atrophy and white mat changes become more progressive with time. Affected patients a commonly macrocephalic from a combination of hydrocephalous and mucopolysaccharide deposition within the brain, meninges and skull.[45,46] A high incidence of intracranical arachnoid cysts has also been seen. The spines in MPS are usually imaged to determine the site and cause of cord compression which occurs frequently in MPS types IV and VI. The most common location for the cord compression is at the atlantoaxial joint. Atlantoaxial subluxation may occur in these patients as a result of laxity of the transverse ligament in conjunction with hypoplasia of the odontoid.

Magnetic resonance shows a shortened odontoid with a soft tissue mass of variable size with intermediate signal on T_1 and low signal on T_2 W images. The low signal on T_2W images is a combination of unossified fibrocartilage and reactive changes. Another cause of cord compression at the $C_1 - C_2$ level is dural thickening resulting from intradural deposition of collagen and mucopolysaccharides. This is seen as a thickening of the soft tissue proterior to the dens with consequent cord compression.

MR spectroscopy shows a decreased NAA/Choline ratio and elevated glutamate glutamine and myoinositol.

PEROXISOMAL DISORDERS

Peroxisomes are small intracellular organelles that are involved in the oxidation of very long chain and monounsaturated fatty acids. Peroxisomal enzymes are also involved in gluconeogenesis, lysine metabolism and glutaric acid metabolism.

Neuropathologic lesions in the peroxisomal disorders can be divided into three major classes. The first group is characterized by defects in the formation and maintenance of white matter and X-linked adrenoleukodystrophy is the prototype. The second group is associated with migrational disorders and Zellweger syndrome is the classic example. The third group is associated with post developmental neuronal degenerations such as cerebellar atrophy seen in rhizomelic chondrodysplasia punctata.

X-linked Adrenoleukodystrophy (ALD)

X-linked adrenoleukodystrophy is a peroxisomal disorder that affects the white matter of the central nervous system, adrenal cortex and testes.[47] This is the best known and most frequent of the peroxisomal disorders. It is a true leukodystrophy with no involvement of the gray matter structures.

The genetic defect responsible for X-linked ALD is located in Xq28, the terminal segment of the long arm of the X chromosome. X-linked ALD is caused by a deficiency of a single enzyme, acyl CoA synthetase. The deficiency prevents the breakdown of very long chain fatty acids which then accumulate in tissue and plasma.[48] A rare form of ALD, neonatal ALD is an autosomal recessive disorder characterized by multiple enzyme deficiencies. Adrenomyeloneuropathy probably represents a phenotypic adult variant of adrenoleukodystrophy and is characterized by adrenal insufficiency.[49] Typically, the disease has slow progression, with survival into the eighth decade.

Clinical Features

The clinical features of X-linked ALD include the onset of neurologic symptoms between the ages of 5 and 9 years with behavior problems, decreasing mental function, poor school performance, visual and hearing disorders progressing to motor signs and ataxia. The disease progresses to include seizures, spastic quadriplegia with death ensuing within the first few years of onset.[50]

Pathologic Findings

The histologic findings reflect the zones of activity seen on imaging studies. Three zones of demyelination are characteristically seen.[51] The central portion of the lesion reveals absent myelin sheaths and oligodendroglia with glial stranding and scattered astrocytes with no evidence of active disease. The next zone of involvement shows evidence of active inflammation with many macrophages filled with lipid. The outer zone is characterized by active myelin break-down but no inflammatory changes.

Imaging Features

The CT and MR appearance of adrenoleukodystrophy is somewhat specific with symmetric areas of white matter abnormality in the peritrigonal regions and extending across the splenium of the corpus callosum[52,53] (Figs 30.12A and B). Demyelination then spreads outward and cephalad as a confluent lesion until most of the cerebral white matter is affected.[54] The subcortical white matter is relatively spared in the early stage but often becomes involved in the later stages. The progression pattern is thus centrifugal and posteroanterior (Figs 30.13A to C).

The central or inner zone which corresponds to irreversible gliosis and scarring is moderately hypointense on T1W MR imaging and markedly hyperintense at T2W imaging. The intermediate zone corresponding to active inflammation is isointense or slightly hypointense and rapidly enhances after administration of contrast (Figs 30.14A and B). The peripheral or outer zone representing the leading edge of active demyelination appears moderately hyperintense on T2W MR imaging and demonstrates no contrast enhancement.[55,56] Pontomedullary corticospinal tract involvement is a common finding in adrenoleukodystrophy and is uncommon in other leukodystrophies.[57] Atypical case of ALD with unilateral or predominantly frontal lobe involvement may occur.[58]

Diffusion weighted MR images also reveal the three distinct zones in the cerebral hemispheric white matter lesions. The burned out zone is hypointense, the intermediate inflammatory zone is moderately hyperintense and the most peripheral demyelinating zone is very faintly hyperintense (Figs 30.15A to E). Proton MR spectroscopy typically shows a decrease in NAA peak and an increase in the choline peak (Figs 30.16A to D). The spectra may be abnormal before the conventional MR findings and studies have shown the potential of MRS for the prognostic assessment of ALD.[59-61]

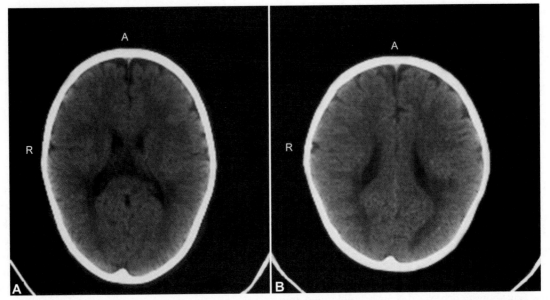

Figs 30.12A and B: CT image in a child showing white matter hypodensity in the parieto-occipital and the peritrigonal areas—X-linked adrenoleukodystrophy

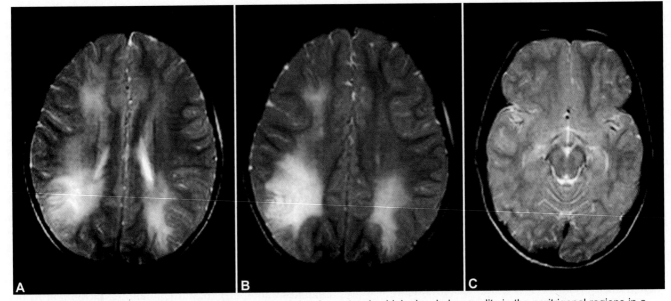

Figs 30.13A to C: Axial T2W (A to C) MR images are showing extensive high signal abnormality in the peritrigonal regions in a bilateral symmetric pattern. Involvement of the corticospinal tracts is also seen (C). – X-linked adrenoleukodystrophy

Adrenomyeloneuropathy

Adrenomyeloneuropathy is not an independent disease entity, it is actually one of the clinical phenotypes of X-linked adrenoleukodystrophy. The age of onset is usually between 20 and 30 years but since both the clinical and the imaging findings are quite different from those in X-linked adrenoleukodystrophy, it is treated as a separate disease entity. Ataxia and paraparesis as well as peripheral neuropathy dominate the neurological presentation, mild cognitive disorder is often present as well. Adrenal insufficiency is a frequent associated clinical finding.

On MR imaging, the lesions are predominantly found within the cerebellum and the brainstem. Both structures are atrophic. The brainstem signal abnormalities are significant but the tegmental structures are relatively spared. The cerebellar white matter is diffusely abnormal. Involvement of the supratentorial white matter is limited mainly to the posterior limbs of the internal capsules and the splenium of the corpus callosum as well as the hemispheric white matter occasionally. Enhancement may also occur within the lesions after intravenous contrast injection. MR of the brain in adrenomyeloneuropathy may even be normal with

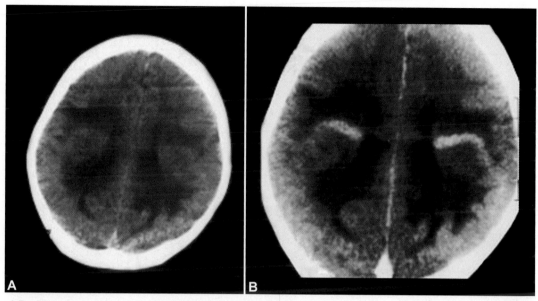

Figs 30.14A and B: CT images showing symmetric areas of hypodensity in the peritrigonal regions extending across the splenium of the corpus callosum. These hypodensities are seen to extend outward and cephalad as a confluent lesion. Contrast enhancement is seen at the site of active inflammation—X-linked adrenoleukodystrophy

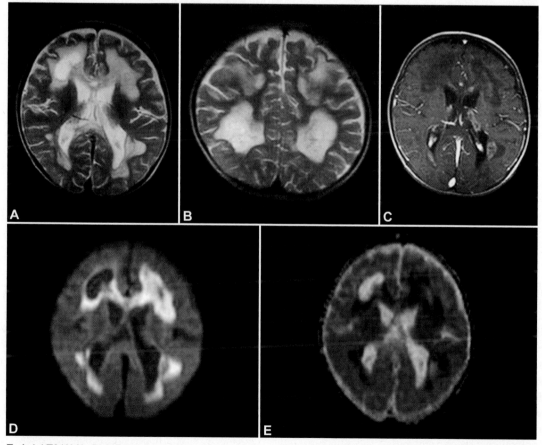

Figs 30.15A to E: Axial T2 W (A, B) MR images showing symmetrical parieto-occipital white matter lesions with sparing of subcortical U fibers. The intermediate zone of inflammation shows enhancement on the post contrast images (C). Diffusion weighted images show isotropically restricted water diffusion within the intermediate zone (D) with faint hyposignal on the apparent diffusion coefficient image (E).—X-linked adrenoleukodystrophy

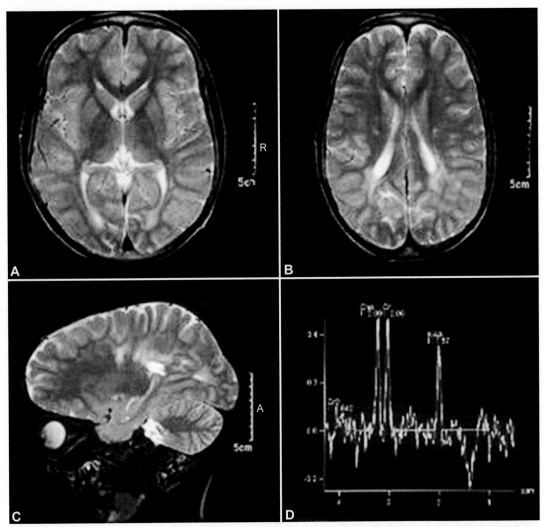

Figs 30.16A to D: MR spectroscopy with voxel placement in the demyelinating zone in the peritrigonal region reveals a decreased NAA and increased choline consistent with increased myelin breakdown—Adrenoleukodystrophy

neurologic involvement confined to the spinal cord and peripheral nerves.[62]

Zellweger Syndrome

Zellweger syndrome or cerebrohepatorenal syndrome, is an autosomal recessive disorder caused by multiple enzyme defects and characterized by liver dysfunction with jaundice, marked mental retardation, weakness, hypotonia and craniofacial dysmorphism.[63] It may lead to death in early childhood. The severity of the disease varies and is determined by the degree of peroxisomal activity.

MR imaging reveals diffuse demyelination with abnormal gyration that is most severe in the perisylvian and perirolandic regions. The pattern of gyral abnormality is similar to that seen in polymicrogyria or pachygyria.[64]

MR hallmarks of the disease are very markedly delayed myelination, brain atrophy, periventricular germinolytic cysts and bilateral symmetrical perisylvian cortical dysplasia

(polymicrogyria) and gray matter heterotopias. The combination of these is pathognomonic of Zellweger syndrome.

Refsum Disease

This rare peroxisomal disorder is transmitted as an autosomal recessive condition and is caused by a deficiency of phytanic acid 2 hydroxylase which causes phytanic acid to accumulate in the myelin.[16] The myelin thus affected has less viability. The infantile form is more severe. The affected children present with severe sensorineural deafness, retinitis pigmentosa, facial dysmorphism hepatomegaly, growth retardation and mental retardation. MR may show diffuse white matter hyperintensity in the brain and in the cerebellum on T2 weighted images. The involvement of the cerebellar white matter is more intense than in other conditions.

Cerebrotendinous Xanthomatosis

In this condition patients are deficient in a liver mitochondrial enzyme required for side chain oxidation of cholesterol to bile

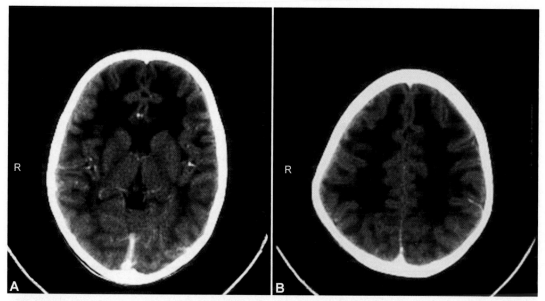

Figs 30.17A and B: CT image in a child with macrocephaly showing diffuse white matter hypodensity with involvement of subcortical white matter – Canavan disease

lts. The patients may show pyramidal and cerebellar signs and may have mental retardation and usually present xanthomas in the chilles tendon, the knees and the elbows. CT may show ecreased density in the cerebellum involving the region of ntate nuclei bilaterally. Hypointensity in the same areas is shown n MRI.[65]

hizomelic Chondrodysplasia Calcificans unctata

his rare autosomal recessive disorder causes short limbs, varfism, abnormal facies, psychomotor retardation, congenital taracts and joint contraction. These patients usually die within e first year of life. The radiographs show finely stippled piphysis. T2 MRI may show periventricular white matter and bcortical changes, particularly in the occipital region.

NCLASSIFIED LEUKODYSTROPHIES

anavan Disease

anavan disease (Canavan-van Bogaert-Bertrand disease) or ongy degeneration of the brain is an autosomal recessive sorder caused by deficient activity of the enzyme. N-etylaspartylase, which results in accumulation of N-acetyl-partic acid in the urine, plasma and brain.[66,67] This is the only own disease with a defect in NAA metabolism.

linical Features

usually manifests in early infancy as hypotonia followed by asticity, cortical, blindness and macrocephaly.[68] Macrocephaly ay not be apparent in the first few months of life but the head larges above the ninetieth percentile within 6 months to 1 year age. Canavan disease is a rapidly progressive illness with a ean survival time of 3 years, although protracted cases do occur. efinite diagnosis usually requires biopsy or autopsy.

Pathologic Findings

Grossly the brain is heavy and soft with markedly increased water content. Canavan disease is characterized at pathologic analysis by extensive vacuolization that initially involves the subcortical white matter, then spreads to deep white matter. Normal myelin is absent and electron microscopy demonstrates increased water content within the glial tissue, described as having the texture of a wet sponge and dysmyelination.[69]

Imaging Features

The CT shows diffusely decreased attenuation of the cerebral and cerebellar white matter (Figs 30.17A and B). The disease has a centripetal progression. The MR imaging findings demonstrate diffusely decreased T1W signal and increased T2W signal within the white matter that corresponds to the CT abnormalities.[70] Typically, there is diffuse symmetric increased signal on T2W images throughout the white matter. Unlike metachromatic leukodystrophy or Krabbe disease the subcortical U fibers also are usually involved. The subcortical white matter appears swollen with broadening of the gyri. **Typically, there is diffuse, symmetric increased signal intensity on the T2-weighted images throughout the white matter with relative sparing of the internal and external capsules and corpus callosum.** The central white matter becomes involved with disease progression. High signal intensity is always seen within the globus pallidus, with frequent involvement of the thalamus and relative sparing of the putamen and caudate nucleus (Figs 30.18A to E). Cerebral and cerebellar atrophy is a late finding.

There is also evidence of restricted diffusion within the abnormal white matter structures (with increased signal on DWI and decreased signal on the ADC maps), likely related to myelin edema or a "gelatinous-like" state of the extracellular space.[71] **On MR spectroscopy there is a characteristic increase in NAA peak**[72] (Fig. 30.19).

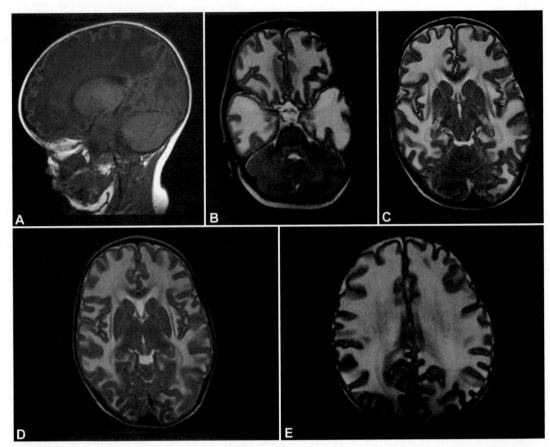

Figs 30.18A to E: Sagittal T1W (A) MR image showing a widespread diffuse low signal throughout the cerebral white matter. Axial T2W (B,C) MR images reveal a high signal intensity in the white matter with extensive involvement of the subcortical U fibers.There is involvement of the cerebellar white matter and the brainstem.(B,C). There is involvement of the globus pallidus with relative sparing of the corpus striatum.(D).The subcortical white matter appears swollen with broadened gyri. (E)—Canavan disease

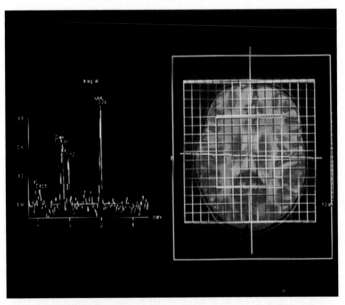

Fig. 30.19: MR showing a characteristic increase in NAA peak—Canavan disease.

Alexander Disease

Alexander disease or fibrinoid leukodystrophy is a rare disorder that occurs sporadically with no known pattern of inheritance.

Pathologic Findings

It is characterized at pathologic analysis by massive deposition of Rosenthal fibers seen as dense eosinophilic, rod like cytoplasmic inclusions found in astrocytes in the subependymal subpial and perivascular regions.[73]

Clinical Features

Three clinical subgroups are recognized. The infantile subgroup is characterized by early onset of macrocephaly, psychomotor retardation with seizures and death occurs within 2-3 years. The diagnosis is made on the basis of a combination of macrocephaly early onset of clinical findings and imaging findings but definit diagnosis usually requires brain biopsy or autopsy.[74]

In the juvenile subgroup, onset of symptoms occurs between 7 and 14 years of age. Progressive bulbar symptoms with spasticity are common. In the adult subgroup, onset of symptom

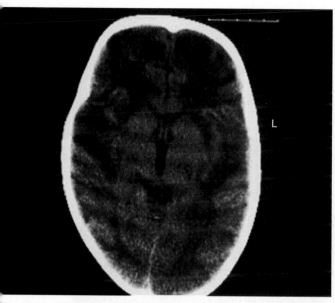

ig. 30.20: CT scan showing bilateral symmetric low density areas ithin the frontal white matter and genu of the corpus callosum – lexander disease

occurs between the 2nd and 7th decade. The symptoms and disease course can be indistinguishable from those of classic multiple sclerosis in the adult subgroup.

Imaging Features

Alexander disease has a predilection for the frontal lobe white matter early in its course (Fig. 30.20). CT demonstrates low attenuation in the deep frontal lobe white matter. The characteristic frontal lobe areas of hyperintensity are seen on T2W MR imaging. The hyperintense areas progress posteriorly to the parietal white matter and internal and external capsules. The subcortical white matter is affected early in the disease course. Large cystic lesions are typically seen in the frontal and temporal regions. Enhancement is often seen near the tips of the frontal horns early in the disease course.[75] Contrast enhancement may also be seen along the ependymal linings of the lateral ventricles, within the basal ganglia or even the dentate nuclei (Figs 30.21A to E). Cystic dilation of the cavum septum pellucidum has been described. The occipital white matter and cerebellum are usually spared, however, involvement should not exclude the diagnosis. With disease progression, cavitation and atrophy of the white

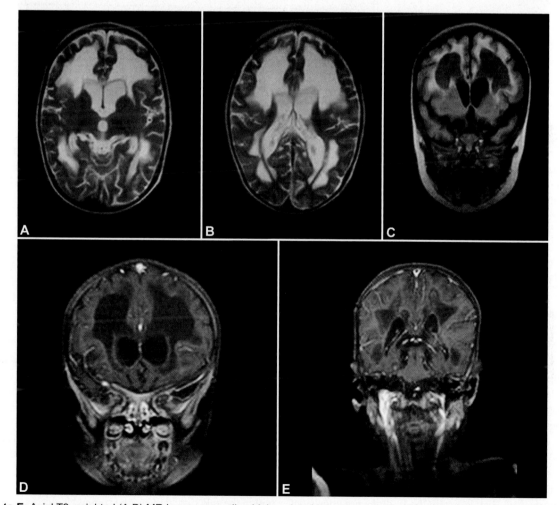

igs 30.21A to E: Axial T2 weighted (A,B) MR images revealing higher signal intensity in the frontal white matter than the parietal and occipital gions.FLAIR coronal (C) image showing involvement of the subcortical U fibers. Post contrast MR images reveal enhancement of the endymal lining of the frontal horns and also of the bodies of lateral ventricles (D,E)—Alexander disease

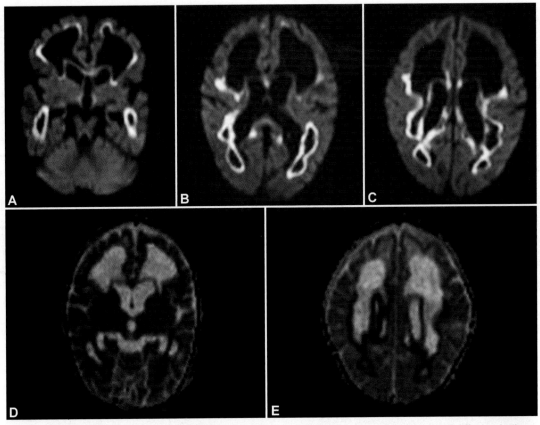

Figs 30.22A to E: Diffusion weighted MR (A to C) images revealing a restricted pattern of diffusion in the areas of signal abnormality with a hyposignal seen on the ADC maps (D,E)—Alexander disease

matter may be seen. Diffusion weighted MR images may reveal a restricted pattern of diffusion (Figs 30.22A to E). When there is diffuse white matter signal abnormality and swelling in a patient with macrocephaly, the differential diagnosis is mainly between Canavan and Alexander diseases. Brain biopsy is usually necessary to establish the diagnosis. MR spectroscopy may show a lactate peak, decreased NAA and elevated myoinositol.

Van der Knaap Disease/Megaloencephalic Leukodystrophy with Subcortical Cysts

This is one of the more recently identified leukodystrophies. It is also called infantile-onset spongiform leukoencephalopathy with a discrepantly mild clinical course or megaloencephalic leukodystrophy with subcortical cysts. The disease has an autosomal recessive inheritance. The onset of the disease is usually during the first year of life but usually it is diagnosed several years later. Patients present with macrocephaly. The initial motor and mental development of the patients is either normal or slightly delayed. The disease is characterized by a slowly progressive course; in particular, ataxia, spasticity, gait disturbances and in the later stage of the disease, mental deterioration and seizures develop. No peripheral neuropathy is detected. Laboratory tests fail to demonstrate any specific metabolic abnormality. Histologically the findings are consistent with vacuolating myelinopathy.

The MR imaging findings are pathognomonic. The brain is diffusely swollen during the early stage of the disease. In the later stages, sulcal and ventricular enlargement may be present. **The white matter disease is always severe and it shows a clear centripetal progression pattern.** The peripheral white matter stuctures of the cerebral hemispheres are the most severely involved, including widespread disappearance of the subcortical U-fibers and the presence of large subcortical cyst formation in the frontoparietal and the temporal regions. *These subcortical cysts are best seen on the FLAIR images* (Figs 30.23A to C). These changes, as well as the initial slight sparing of the periventricular and subcortical white matter in the occipital regions suggest an additional anteroposterior gradient. The deep white matter structures, the corpus callosum and the internal capsules are spared but the external and extreme capsules are involved (Figs 30.24A to E). The cerebellar white matter is involved but much less makedly than the supratentorial white matter structures. Subtle signal changes may be present within the brainstem along the pyramidal tracts. The cortical and deep gray matter structures are normal. No abnormal signal enhancement is seen within the brain parenchyma after intravenous contrast injection.

Diffusion-weighted imaging shows prominent hyposignal within the subcortical cysts and somewhat decreased signal within the affected white matter. No definite hypersignal is seen within

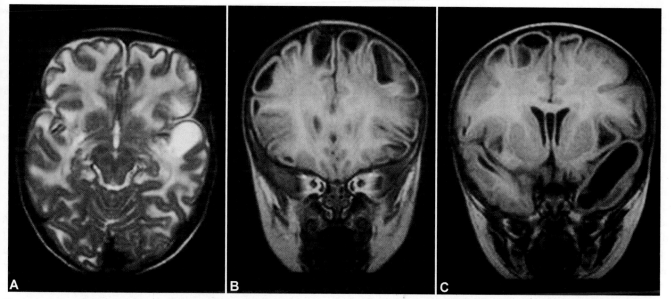

Figs 30.23A to C: Axial T2 W (A) and FLAIR coronal (B,C) MR images showing widespread involvement of the subcortical white matter. Subcortical cyst formation in the frontal and parietal regions is best seen on the FLAIR images (B,C) – Van der Knaap disorder

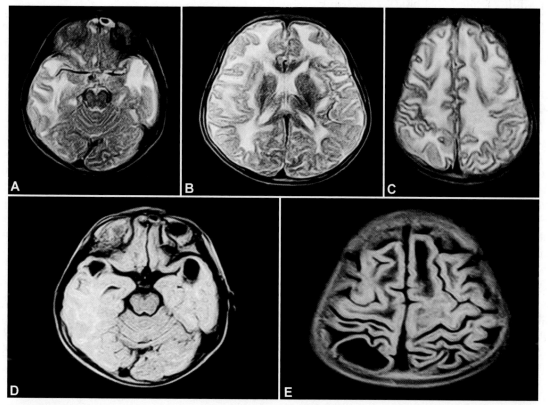

Figs 30.24A to E: Axial T2 W MR images (A to C) revealing extensive white matter changes with diffuse brain swelling with predominant involvement of the subcortical U fibers (B,C) There is a relative sparing of the deep white matter structures, i.e. the corpus callosum and internal capsule (B). Signal changes are present in the brainstem along the pyramidal tracts (A) with relative sparing of the cerebellar white matter. Subcortical cyst formation is best seen on the FLAIR images (D,E) – Van der Knaap disease

the non-affected white matter structures or along the interface between the normal and abnormal areas.

The proton spectroscopic findings are non-specific, the N-acetyl aspartate peak is decreased and the choline peak may be increased but no abnormal metabolites are demonstrated.

Vanishing White Matter Disease/Childhood Ataxia with CNS Hypomyelination

This is a recently described, distinct clinical radiological entity. The disease is typically of childhood onset. Initially, the psychomotor development of the patients is normal. Affected patients present with ataxia, spasticity, gait disturbance but only mildly impaired mental capacities. The clinical manifestation of the disease seems to be preceded by minor head trauma or infection, the same factors are also responsible for episodes of deterioration. During the later stages of the disease optic atrophy and mild epilepsy may develop. The disease is always progressive but the disease course varies. The severe forms lead to death at a relatively young age (2-6 years) but patients with more moderate clinical phenotypes, live up to adulthood. A set of criterion were suggested by Van der Knaap et al to identify children with vanishing white matter disease.[76]

1. Normal or mildly delayed initial psychomotor development.
2. Neurologic deterioration with a chronic progressive and episodic course.
3. Presence of cerebellar ataxia and spasticity with relative preservation of mental function. Optic atrophy and epilepsy may occur.
4. Diffuse symmetric white matter involvement on MRI with all or part of white matter exhibiting a signal intensity similar to CSF.

The MR imaging findings are fairly characteristic. The brain appears to be slightly swollen but some of the gyri are somewhat broadened. The lateral ventricles show mild to moderate dilatation. *The white matter changes are very prominent; the signal properties of the affected myelin are practically identical to those of the CSF both on the T1 and T2 weighted images.* The posterior limbs of the internal capsules are often involved, whereas the anterior limbs are spared. The corpus callosum is also involved, with the exception of the outer rim. The cerebellum is usually slightly atrophic and the cerebellar white matter is mildly abnormal. In the brainstem, the posterior tegmental and the pyramidal tracts also show abnormal hypersignal. The gray matter structures including the basal ganglia are normal. MR spectroscopy of the affected gray matter shows decreased N-acetyl aspartate, normal or slightly increased choline, rather prominent lactate and glucose (at 3.43, 3.80 ppm) peaks.[77] The affected white matter shows decreased NAA, choline and creative peaks.

Aicardi-Goutieres Syndrome

This rare microcephalic disease is also called leukodystrophy with chronic CSF lymphocytosis and calcifications of the basal ganglia. The disease appears in the neonate or in early infancy. It is a relatively rapidly progressive, devastating disease, characterized by delayed development and spasticity leading to death in a fe months or years.

Computed tomography is an essential diagnostic modality i this disease since it almost always demonstrates calcificatio within the basal ganglia and the periventricular white matter. O MRI, the disease presents with an essentially superatentorial an very extensive white matter disease with possible cystic lesior in the temporal and parietal lobes. The internal capsules are som what less affected but are abnormal also. The brainstem and th cerebellar structures are spared.

Pelizaeus-Merzbacher Disease

Pelizaeus-Merzbacher disease, a sudanophilic leukodystrophy, the best example of a hypomyelinating leukoencephalopath PMD has been linked to a severe deficiency of myelin specifi lipids caused by a lack of proteolipid protein (PLP). This myeli specific proteolipid is responsible for oligodendrocyt differentiation and survival.

Pathologic Findings

The brain is usually atrophic particularly severe in the posteri fossa. Histologically, there is a profound lack of myelin. There astrocytosis and lack of oligodendroglia. The residual myel preferentially remains around blood vessels giving rise characteristic "Tigroid" appearance. There is accumulation sudanophilic droplets containing cholesterol and triglycerides the white matter which is the histological hallmark of sudanophi leukodystrophy.[78]

Clinical Features

PMD has traditionally been divided into classic and connat forms[79] Classic PMD begins during late infancy with X-link recessive inheritance. Connatal PMD is a rarer and more seve variant that begins at birth or in early infancy. This form has eith X-linked or autosomal recessive inheritance. Patients with forms of PMD present with clinical signs and symptoms includi abnormal eye movements, nystagmus, extrapyramid hyperkinesias, spasticity and slow psychomotor development.

Imaging Features

CT may demonstrate only atrophy. T2W MR findings reveal nearly total lack of normal myelination with diffuse high sign intensity that extends peripherally to involve the subcortical fibers, along with early involvement of the internal capsule (Fi 30.25A to C). Sometimes, the white matter demonstrates hig signal intensity with small scattered foci of more normal sign intensity—a finding that may reflect the tigroid pattern myelination seen on histology[80] (Fig. 30.26).

Cockayne Syndrome

Cockayne syndrome is another sudanophilic leukodystrophy The affected children may be normal until late in infancy and m live long enough to develop dwarfism. Transmitted as autosomal recessive trait, this syndrome consists of grow retardation, mental retardation, microcephaly, retinopath

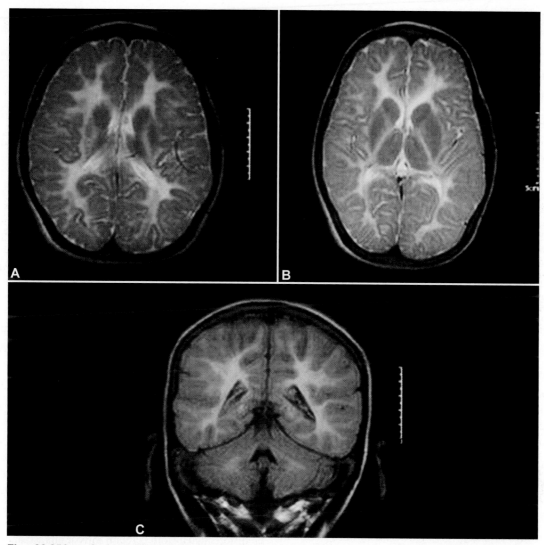

Figs 30.25A to C: Axial T2 W (A,B) and FLAIR coronal (C) MR images demonstrating diffuse high signal intensity within the white matter including the posterior limbs of the internal capsules which should be myelinated at birth – Pelizaeus-Merzbacher disease

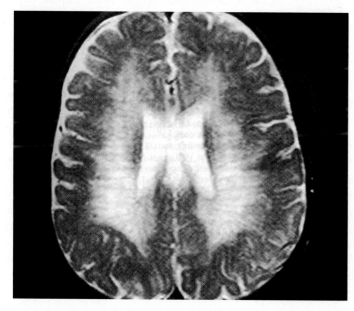

Fig. 30.26: Axial T2 W MR image in an infant with slow psychomotor development with nystagmus and choreoathetoid movements revealing diffuse high signal intensity in the white matter with small scattered foci of more normal signal intensity within – Tigroid pattern of myelination seen in Pelizaeus-Merzbacher disease

Disease	Age of onset	Head size	White matter changes	Gray matter changes	Subcortical involvement
Alexander disease	Less than a year	Large	Usually in frontal region	May show minimal changes	Early
Canavan disease	1-2 years	Large	Diffuse involvement	Cystic changes in gray matter	Early
Metachromatic leukodystrophy	1-2 years, 4-7 years (2nd peak)	Normal	Predominantly deep periventricular white matter	Often normal	Late
Adrenoleukodystrophy	5-10 years	Normal	Primarily occipital and splenium of corpus callosum	Normal	Late
PMD	Late infancy	Normal	Tigroid pattern	Normal	Early

Table 30.2: Distinctive features of various leukodystrophies

cutaneous photosensitivity and ataxia. The pathologic changes are similar to other leukodystrophies. However a significant difference is that small vessels become involved by mural and extramural colloid deposits which frequently contain iron and exhibit striking calcification. The deposits occur chiefly in the basal ganglia, the cerebral white matter and the dentate nuclei of the cerebellum. There is extensive cortical calcification in both hemispheres.

MR Spectroscopy

Proton MR spectroscopy may reveal no abnormal peak consistent with the absence of sclerosis and well-preserved axons. Diffuse or focal reduction in NAA consistent with axonal damage may be seen in more severe cases.[82]

MITOCHONDRIAL DISORDERS/DEFECTS OF THE RESPIRATORY CHAIN

Mitochondrial encephalopathy comprises a heterogeneous group of neuromuscular disorders caused by defect in the oxidative metabolic pathways of energy production, owing to a structural or functional mitochondrial defect. The so-called respiratory chain is a complex multiunit system within the inner membrane of the mitochondria. Multisystem involvement is the rule in the diseases related to defect of the respiratory chain. It is an important clinical diagnostic clue. In respiratory chain deficiencies, practically any organ or tissue in any combination may be involved, the most frequently affected organs are, however, the central nervous system and the muscles (both skeletal and visceral).

Mitochondrial Encephalomyopathy—Lactic Acidosis and Stroke-like Symptoms (MELAS)

Clinical Features

Patients with MELAS syndrome usually appear healthy at birth with normal development, then exhibit delayed growth, episodic vomiting, seizures and recurrent strokes and cortical blindness.[83] The age of onset is typically between 4 and 15 years but early infantile and adult forms have also been reported. No ophthalmoplegia or heart block is seen. These stroke like episodes are the result of a proliferation of dysfunctional mitochondria in the smooth muscle cells or small arteries giving rise to either permanent or reversible deficits. The disease course is progressiv with periodic acute exacerbation. Systemic manifestations of th disease include cardiomyopathy and diabetes (both types 1 and :

Pathologic Findings

At electron microscopy the affected tissue demonstrates a increased number of mitochondria which are enlarged and hav lipoid inclusions. Serum and cerebrospinal fluid lactate levels a usually elevated.

Imaging Features

CT and MR findings of MELAS syndrome have been report as multiple infarct like lesions, calcification of the basal gang and diffuse atrophy.[84,85] CT examination in MELAS frequent reveals basal ganglia calcifications. These infarct like lesions sho low attenuation on CT and elongation of both T1 and T relaxation times on MR images, usually with a bilateral symmetr or asymmetric cortical and subcortical distribution. There is posterior predilection for the lesions. The MELAS syndrome c be differentiated from cerebral infarct of vascular origin becau the lesions are not restricted to a specific vascular territory a angiography reveals no vascular occlusion.[86] During the cour of the disease lesions resolve with clinical improvement residual atrophy while new lesions appear in other regions. Th finding of migrating infarct like lesions in childhood is almc unique to MELAS.[87] Another useful sign is the absence restricted pattern on diffusion weighted MR images whi supports the hypothesis that the lesions are actually not ischemic origin but rather secondary to metabolic crash or ener failure.

There may be generalized cerebral and cerebellar atrophy. T finding of multiple migrating infarct like lesions not limited t specific vascular territory especially in the basal ganglia and t posterior part of the cerebral hemisphere in children sugge MELAS syndrome (Figs 30.27A to D). Muscle biopsy important to confirm the diagnosis. MR spectroscopy may be useful complementry test since a small amount of lactate is oft detected even in apparently normal brain areas. Abnorma decreased FA values have been described in the abnormal bra areas and cervical spinal cord.[88]

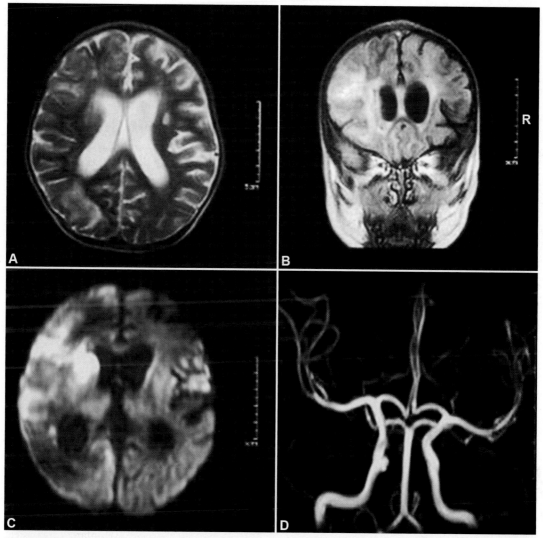

Figs 30.27A to D: Axial T2 W (A) and FLAIR coronal (B) images showing asymmetrical infarct like lesions involving the subcortical white matter and basal ganglia .The lesions are not restricted to any specific vascular territory and show high signal on the ADC maps (C). MR angiography reveals no vascular occlusion (D) —Mitochondrial encephalopathy (MELAS)

yoclonic Epilepsy with Ragged Red Fibers (ERRF)

like MELAS syndrome MERRF causes no strokes leading to rebral infarcts.[89] The patients usually present with myoclonus, axia, weakness and generalized seizures.[90] The patients, have ort stature and cardiac conductive defects.

athologic Findings

uscle biopsy reveals ragged red fibers in skeletal muscles. This ding implies degeneration of granular fibers and a proliferation mitochondria.

aging Features

e CT and MR show cerebral and cerebellar atrophy. MR dings may show hyperintense signal abnormalities in the white tter and deep gray matter (Figs 30.28A to C). CT may show cification of the dentate nucleus and globus pallidus.

Kearns-Sayre Syndrome

First described by Kearns and Sayre, this mitochondrial disorder occurs more frequently in females and is inherited as an autosomal dominant tract.[91]

Clinical Features

It presents as a triad of ophthalmoplegia, retinal pigmentary degeneration and complete heart block. There is short stature and frequently mental deterioration.

Imaging Features

MR findings in Kearns-Sayre syndrome reflect the pathology of spongiform degeneration and reveal high signal intensity on long TR images in the white matter with a predilection for involvement of peripheral U fibers and sparing of the periventricular white matter.[92] Symmetric high signal on T2W images can be seen in basal ganglia. The cerebellar white matter and the dorsal

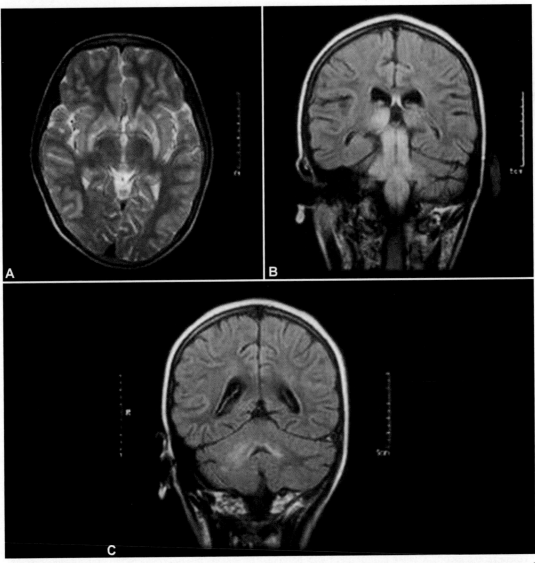

Figs 30.28A to C: Axial T2 W (A) and FLAIR coronal (B,C) MR images in a child showing symmetric areas of hyperintense signal abnormality involving the basal ganglia, brainstem and the cerebellar white matter-Mitochondrial encephalopathy

brainstem may also demonstrate abnormal hyperintensity.[93] Diffuse atrophy is commonly seen involving the cerebrum and cerebellum.

Subacute Necrotizing Encephalomyopathy (Leigh Disease)

Leigh disease, or subacute necrotizing encephalomyopathy is an inherited, progressive, neurodegenerative disease of infancy or early childhood.[94] Affected infants and children typically present with hypotonia and psychomotor deterioration. Ataxia, ophthalmoplegia, ptosis, dystonia and swallowing difficulties inevitably ensue.[95] Acute respiratory failure may occur. Respiratory problems and ocular abnormalities (external ophthalmoplegia, nystagmus, strabismus) are suggestive clinical features.

Pathologic Features

Characteristic pathologic abnormalities include microcyst cavitation, vascular proliferation, neuronal loss and demyelinatio of the midbrain, basal ganglia and cerebellar dentate nuclei a occasionally of the cerebral white matter.[96]

Imaging Features

Typical MR finding in Leigh disease is the remarkab symmetrical involvement, most frequently in the putamen. The lesions are also commonly found in the globus pallidus a the caudate nucleus but never in the absence of putamin abnormalities.[98] Other areas of involvement include t paraventricular white matter, corpus callosum, substantia nig decussation of superior cerebellar peduncles, periaqueduc region, brainstem and the gray matter in the spinal cor

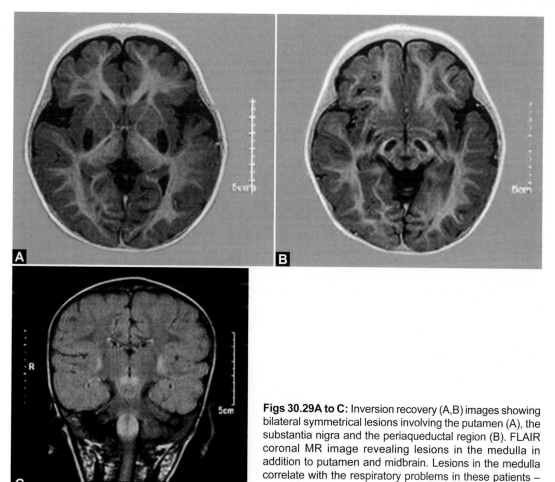

Figs 30.29A to C: Inversion recovery (A,B) images showing bilateral symmetrical lesions involving the putamen (A), the substantia nigra and the periaqueductal region (B). FLAIR coronal MR image revealing lesions in the medulla in addition to putamen and midbrain. Lesions in the medulla correlate with the respiratory problems in these patients – Leigh disease

igs 30.29A to C). Loss of respiratory control in Leigh disease s been found to correlate with lower brainstem lesions articularly situated in the periaqueductal gray matter and icular formation of the medulla oblongata). Upper brainstem nal abnormalities are often transient and the associated piratory difficulties resolve. The dentate nuclei frequently show normalities. White matter lesions in the cerebral hemispheres usually patchy and predominantly subcortical. The important ferential diagnosis is organic acidopathies but the presence of culiar brainstem lesion in Leigh disease usually allows a nfident differentiation.

Proton MR spectroscopy with voxel placement in the basal nglia typically demonstrates an abnormal lactate peak with a crease in NAA/Cr. Diffusion weighted images may show a persignal during the acute metabolic attacks within lesion areas the brainstem, the basal ganglia and the dentate nuclei[100] gs 30.30A to D).

ON

ber's hereditary optic neuroretinopathy (LHON) presents with idly progressive visual loss due to degeneration of the optic ves. The disease typically occurs in young adults. No skeletal scle involvement has been described in this disease. MR

imaging usually shows signal abnormalities within the distal intraorbital optic nerves. Putaminal lesions and scattered white matter lesions within the centrum cerebral hemispheric white matter may also be present. See Table 30.3 for mitochondrial disorders.

Table 30.3: Mitochondrial disorders: Distinguishing clinical features and magnetic resonance findings[16]		
KSS	Ophthalmoplegia Retinal degeneration Heart block CSF protein >100 mg/dL	T2WI: high signal in U fibers, thalami, dorsal brainstem, cerebellar WMT1 WI: high signal in basal ganglia
MERRF	Myoclonus Ataxia Weakness	T2 WI: high signal in deep GM and WM
MELAS	Episodic vomiting Cerebral blindness Hemiparesis, hemianopsia	T2 WI: high signal in subcortical WM, brainstem, basal ganglia, cerebellum infarcts (may not be in vascular territories)
Leigh	Respiratory failure Visual/auditory problems Ataxia, weakness	T2 WI: high signal in bilateral symmetric basal ganglia (particularly putamen), thalami, dorsal brainstem

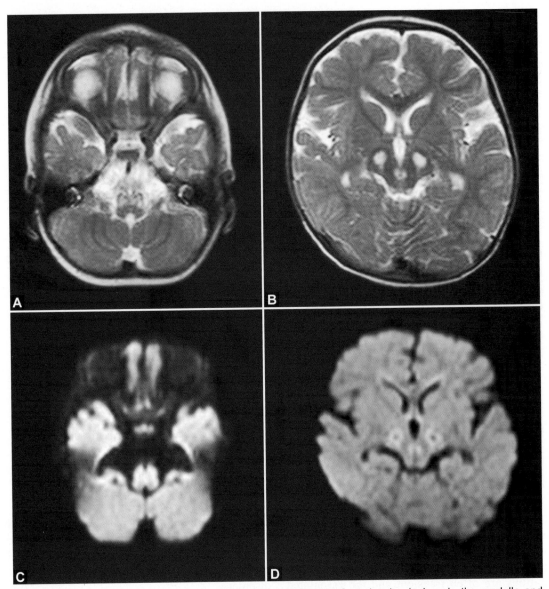

Figs 30.30A to D: Axial T2 W (A,B) images in a 20-month-old infant showing lesions in the medulla and symmetrical lesions in the substantia nigra and the periaqueductal region (B). These lesions reveal a restricted pattern of diffusion seen as hypersignal on the diffusion weighted images (C,D) during the acute metabolic crisis – Leigh disease

DISORDERS OF AMINO ACID METABOLISM/ AMINOACIDOPATHIES

Urea Cycle Defects

The urea cycle is a complex metabolic process, the primary role of which is to convert the toxic ammonia in to non-toxic urea. Urea cycle defects are characterized by autosomal recessive inheritance except ornithine carbamoyl transferase deficiency, which is X-linked. The most common metabolic derangement in each disease entity is hyperammonemia and impairment of the metabolism of various amino acids (alanine, glutamine, citrulline and arginine). Some of the urea cycle defects present in neonates as a devastating metabolic disease of almost immediate postnatal onset. If the disease is of later onset (infantile, juvenile or adult), it may manifest with neurological signs and symptoms of acute or chronic encephalopathy. The urea cycle defects inclu⟨e⟩ carbamyl phosphate deficiency, ornithine transcarbamyla⟨se⟩ deficiency, citrullinemia and argininosuccinic aciduria.⟨?⟩ Hyperammonemia induces brain swelling and Alzheimer Type ⟨II⟩ changes in astrocytes and chronic elevation leads to neuron⟨al⟩ degeneration.

MR imaging findings in neonates with urea cycle defects a⟨re⟩ dominated by the prominent brain swelling and white matter sign⟨al⟩ changes related to vasogenic edema. The myelinated white matt⟨er⟩ is less severely affected than the non-myelinated areas (Fi⟨gs⟩ 30.31A to H). Certain regions of the cerebral cortex and deep gr⟨ey⟩ matter show prolongation of T_1 and T_2 relaxation times on M⟨R,⟩ in particular the insular cortex (posterior more than anterio⟨r),⟩ perirolandic cortex and basal ganglia (particularly the gl⟨obus⟩

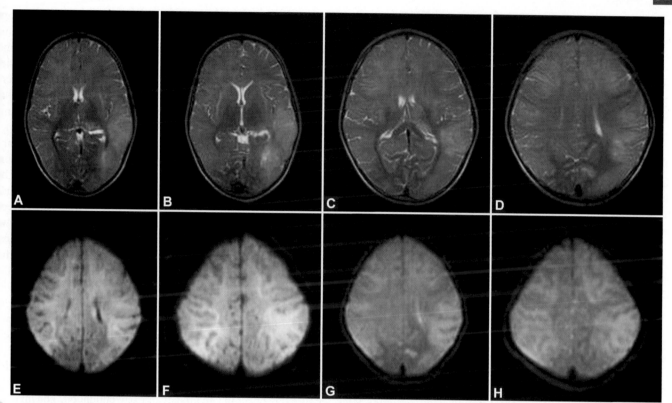

Figs 30.31A to H: Axial T2 W MR images (A to D) in a few months old infant showing a diffuse swelling of the brain. The unmyelinated white matter exhibits an abnormal increased signal intensity. There is a relative sparing of the myelinated optic radiation (B). Diffusion weighted (E,F) images and ADC maps (G,H) do not reveal a restricted pattern consistent with vasogenic edema—Urea cycle disorder

allidi) show early T_2 prolongation and swelling. The differentiation from hypoxic ischemic injury can be made by the predominant globus pallidus and putaminal injury in urea cycle disorders in contrast to the predominant thalamic injury in hypoxic injury. MR spectroscopy reveals a characteristic elevated lactate doublet centred at 1.33 ppm) and glutamate resonance at 2.2 to .6 ppm and at 3.75 ppm. The glutamate and glutamine resonances are best seen with short (20-30 ms) TEs.[102] As the case progresses, atrophy is often severe and may be multicystic.

henylketonuria

lassic Phenylketonuria (PKU) is an autosomal recessive disorder aused by a deficiency in the enzyme phenylalanine hydroxylase hich converts phenylalanine to tyrosine owing to which eurotoxic phenylketones accumulate. Two forms of phenylketo-uria are known. The more frequent "classical" phenylketonuria caused by the deficiency of the phenylalanine hydroxylase izyme. The other, more malignant and rare form is related to the eficiency of the tetrahydrobiopterin coenzyme which is also dispensable in the break down of phenylalanine into tyrosine.

The clinical and imaging manifestations of the two forms of nenylketonuria are different.

linical Features

fants are normal at birth but in the first year of life manifest ith progressive cognitive delay, microcephaly, spasticity,

recurrent eczematous rash and a peculiar musty odour of the urine, skin and hair. Seizures occur in about 25% of untreated patients.

Imaging Findings

Imaging studies show primarily abnormal signal in the white matter that corresponds to the delayed and defective myelination. MR shows T_2 prolongation that is predominantly found in the periventricular white matter in the initial stages.[103] The subcortical white matter is involved later. Diffusion weighted MR images obtained in the acute phase will show a reduced diffusion in the affected white matter due to spongiotic changes of myelin.[104] Proton MR spectroscopy shows the presence of a peak from elevated phenylalanine at 7.37 ppm. The size of the peak is useful for monitoring response to treatment.[105]

Malignant Form of Phenylketonuria

In the malignant form, microcephaly and delayed development are also typical but the disease if not treated, often leads to death in early childhood. Neurologically, the patients present with prominent extrapyramidal signs (infantile Parkinsonism, choreoathetosis) myoclonic and grand mal seizures. Progressive pyramidal and bulbar signs develop in conjunction with severe congnitive deterioration.

In the biopterin-dependent form of phenylketonuria, CT examination shows calcifications at the level of the putamina and/

or the globi pallidi as well as along the cortical-subcortical junction area in the frontal regions somewhat similar to what may be seen in carbonic anhydrase II deficiency.

The MR imaging study shows signal changes within the calcified areas: hyperintense on the T1 and hypointense on the T2 weighted images. White matter lesions may be seen, sometimes, they are diffuse and in other cases focal with cystic degeneration in the parietal-occipital regions.

Maple Syrup Urine Disease (MSUD)

Maple syrup urine disease is a genetically heterogeneous disorder caused by abnormal oxidative decarboxylation of the branched chain amino acids leucine, isoleucine and valine. Four clinical phenotypes are distinguished: the classical, the intermediate, the intermittent and the thiamine responsive. The most severe form is the classical MSUD characterized by early postnatal onset and rapid progressive neurological deterioration leading to death, if untreated.

In the classic type, the infant is normal for about the first week. In the second week, the infant starts to eat poorly, fails to thrive, develops hypotonia, lethargy and vomiting. Urine, sweat and cerumen smell like maple syrup. The disease quickly progresses to coma, seizures and death if untreated.[106] The severity of neurologic sequelae is strongly correlated with the duration of the acute toxic phase in the neonatal period. Conventional MR imaging shows diffuse swelling of the brain. This is mainly due to the vasogenic edema involving the non-myelinated white matter structures. On the other hand, even more prominent signal changes are also present within the myelinated brain areas (posterior brainstem tracts, central cerebellar white matter, posterior limbs of the internal capsules) representing myelin edema secondary to vacuolating myelinopathy.

The **less severe** forms of the disease with higher residual enzymatic activity can present later in childhood with metabolic crisis resulting in lethargy, irritability, vomiting that may progress to stupor or coma. An intermittent form may present later in life as attacks of transient ataxia sometimes accompanied by cerebral edema. Tests during an attack show elevated leucine isoleucine and valine in blood as well as branched chain amino acids in urine. Chronic management relies on dietary restriction of branched chain amino acids.

Imaging Findings

The neonatal form typically presents on the seventh day after birth. The imaging findings may be normal in the first ten days of life. Because classic maple syrup urine disease presents in the neonatal period, it is one of the few metabolic diseases in which transfontanelle sonography may play a role in diagnosis. Cranial sonography may show a symmetric increase in the echogenicity of the periventricular white matter, basal ganglia and thalami.[107] The CT and MR findings are quite characteristic, revealing, profound localized edema seen as increased signal on T$_2$ weighted images in the deep cerebellar white matter, dorsal brainstem, cerebral peduncles, inferior limb of the internal capsule,

perirolandic white matter and the globi pallidi. The region involved correspond to those that are myelinated or myelinatin at the time of birth. Generalized edema of the cerebral hemi spheres may be superimposed on the localized abnormailitie particularly in the first weeks of life. Diffusion imaging is ver useful in the acute stage as areas with MSUD edema (cerebella white matter, dorsal brainstem, cerebral peduncles, costicospina tracts, globi pallidi) show reduced diffusion with ADC value falling to 20 to 30 percent of their normal values. Myelin edem presents with isotropically restricted water diffusion, hence ther is high signal. The vasogenic edema is characterized b isotropically increased water diffusion which causes hyposigna on the diffusion-weighted images. **The sharp contrast betwee the diffusion-weighted imaging signal properties of these tw edema types and the peculiar distribution of the pathologica hypersignal (strictly limited to the myelinated white matte structures) results in a pathognomonic imaging pattern**. Aft the acute phase of the disease has resolved patients are left wi a variable degree of brain damage dependent upon the time initiation of the treatment. Proton MR spectroscopy in the acu phase of illness shows slight reduction of NAA and amino aci peak of leucine, isoleucine and valine at 0.9 ppm on short TE.[1]

The intermittent and intermediate forms of maple syrup uri disease have a more insidious clinical pattern. The first metabol crisis may appear in late infancy or early childhood. The imagi findings also are less characteristic. Typically, brain atroph delayed myelination and pathological signal changes within t upper brainstem structures, the thalami, the globi pallidi and t centrum semiovale are observed. Diffusion-weighted imaging al shows signal abnormalities in these areas but they are often rath subtle (Figs 30.32A to E). From the imaging point of view, t intermittent form of maple syrup urine disease may, therefore, somewhat similar to Canavan disease in the early stage but t clinical context and the laboratory findings allow ea differentiation.

In treated MSUD cases, the conventional MRI and t diffusion-weighted imaging findings rarely return to norm Typically, variable but prominent residual abnormalities, includi diffuse brain atrophy, delayed myelination and structural lesio are noted. The pattern of the structural lesions is very similar those observed in the intermittent form of maple syrup uri disease. Changes are also present in the hypothalamic structur the dentate nuclei and the cerebellar or the cerebral hemispher white matter. Subtle residual diffusion weighted imagi abnormalities may also be noted. In successfully treated cas MR spectroscopy shows improvement but total normalization the branched chain amino acid peak complex is usually n achieved.

Classic Homocystinuria

Class homocystinuria is an autosomal recessive disorder caus by a defect in the enzyme crystathionine β synthetase resulti in elevations of homocystine and methionine. This results intimal irregularities that cause arteriosclerosis, arter

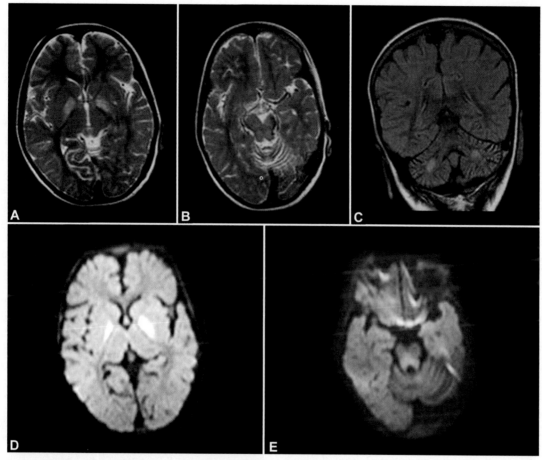

Figs 30.32A to E: Axial T2 W (A,B) and FLAIR coronal (C) MR images revealing symmetric areas of signal abnormality in the globus pallidi (A) dorsal brainstem (B) and the deep cerebellar white matter (C). Diffusion weighted MR images (D,E) revealing restricted pattern of diffusion in the globi pallidi and dorsal brainstem – Intermittent form of maple syrup urine disease

romboembolism and venous thrombosis in children and young adults.[109] The excess homocysteine generates superoxide and ydrogen peroxide, changes coagulation factor levels 'ncouraging clot formation), prevents small arteries from dilating nd causes proliferation of smooth muscle cells in arterial walls.

Clinical Features

he findings include dislocation of lens, osteoporosis, thinning nd lengthening of long bones. Lens dislocation (ectopia lentis) usually inferior which is the opposite of what is seen in Marfan yndrome. Untreated patients are at risk for seizures, psychiatric isorders, thromboembolic events including stroke myocardial ifarction and pulmonary emboli.

Imaging

naging studies reveal multiple cortical-subcortical and lacunar ifarctions both within the cerebral and the cerebellar emispheres. The disease may also present with a less specific, ffuse white matter involvement and the pattern is suggestive of etrograde' demyelination.

Nonketotic Hyperglycinemia

This is caused by a defect in glycine cleavage with resultant accumulation of glycine in the plasma, urine and CSF. Two clinical phenotypes are known: the more common neonatal type, which is characterized by practically absent glycine cleavage system activity and the late onset (infantile and juvenile) form, in which some residual glycine cleavage system activity is present. The neonatal form presents as lethargy and poor feeding after starting the protein feeds. The patients are hypotonic (glycine is an inhibitor neurotransmitter at the level of the lower motor neurons) and have frequent myoclonic seizures. This quickly progresses to persistent seizures, encephalopathy and coma. Apnea is common and persistent hiccups have been described. The prognosis for the neonatal form is poor. The late onset form has a milder and rather non-specific clinical presentation.

Imaging

The imaging hallmarks of non-ketotic hyperglycinemia are callosal abnormalities and delayed myelination.[110] The spectrum of morphological changes of the corpus callosum ranges from the rare true callosal dysgenesis to the more frequent callosal hypogenesis or hypoplasia but some degree of abnormality is always present. The delay in myelination is increasingly evident with the aging of the infant and is probably associated with global hypomyelination. Cortical gyral abnormalities have also been described. Acute hydrocephalus may contribute to the severe clinical picture. In the chronic stage of the disease, progressive atrophy of the brain develops.

MR spectroscopy is a useful adjunct to the MR work-up of patients with suspected non-ketotic hyperglycinemia since the concentration of glycine is particularly elevated in the brain. Glycine resonates at the 3.55 ppm level. Proton MR spectroscopy reveals a glycine peak at 3.55 ppm. In order to separate the glycine peak from that of myoinositol which has a similar chemical shift, the spectrum should be obtained with a long echo time. The myoinositol peak disappears on the long echo time.

5.10 Methylene-tetrahydrofolate Reductase Deficiency

5.10 methylene-tetrahydrofolate reductase deficiency is the best known of the defects of folate metabolism. This form has an autosomal recessive inheritance. The onset of the disease is variable, it is more frequent in infants but later onset cases, including an adult form, are also known. Neurologically, developmental delay is seen in conjunction with signs of spinal cord (combined degeneration of the cord) and peripheral nerve involvement.

MR imaging in 5.10 methylene tetrahydrofolate reductase deficiency may show rather prominent abnormalities in the brain. The cerebral white matter is diffusely abnormal, the lesions involve the corpus callosum, the external and extreme capsules, the laminae medullares and the anterior limbs of the internal capsules with sparing of the posterior limbs.[111] The corticospinal tracts within the centrum semiovale, the subcortical U-fibers in the occipital regions and the optic radiations are also spared. The basal ganglia and the thalami are normal but the globi pallidi show increased signal intensity on the T2 weighted images. Subtle signal changes may be present within the mesencephalon (hypersignal within the substantia nigra and the periaqueductal region) and the central tegmental tracts of the pons. The cerebellar white matter is not involved. Diffusion-weighted images show hypersignal within the white matter lesions, suggestive of vacuolating myelinopathy. The diffusion-weighted abnormalities (similar to the conventional MR imaging findings) may remain visible on follow-up studies even after a few years.

ORGANIC ACIDEMIAS

Many of the organic acidopathies fall into the group of devastating metabolic disease of the newborn, others have later and an often insidious onset. Typically, gray matter abnormalities dominate the imaging findings. White matter involvement may also be present which is usually less prominent. Occasionally, organic acidopathies present with a leukodystrophy like presentation but gray matter lesions are always conspicuous.[112]

Methylmalonic Acidemia

It is caused by a defect in methylmalonyl CoA mutase. Acidosis and hyperammonemia can be severe and a single attack can cause permanent cognitive disability. Seizures, spasticity, behavior problems and ataxia are common. Metabolic stroke with an acute decompensation can occur.

Imaging Findings during Metabolic Crisis

In methylmalonic aciduria, the most typical and often the sole abnormality is the symmetrical signal changes within the globi pallidi, which is associated with swelling[112] (Figs 30.33A to C). The caudate nuclei, the putamina and the thalami are spared. The cortex is normal. During the acute metabolic crisis, diffusion weighted images show hypersignal within the lesion areas. MR spectroscopy may show a small amount of lactate within the lesions. No disease specific metabolites are demonstrated.

Imaging Findings after Metabolic Crisis

The globus pallidus lesions undergo necrotic changes; they are markedly atrophic and continue to show hypersignal on the T2 weighted images. Sometimes, mild cerebellar atrophy may be present and subtle signal changes within the dentate nuclei suggest some damage too. In early onset cases, delayed myelination is frequently seen.

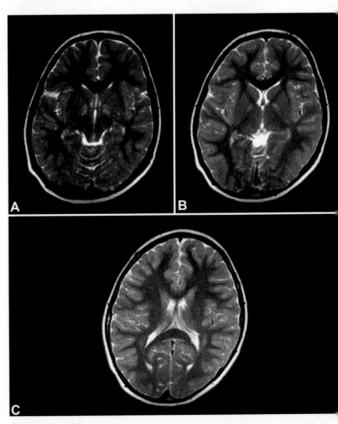

Figs 30.33A to C: Axial T2 W MR images showing symmetrical signal changes within the globi pallidi seen as a high signal (A,B). No other area of signal abnormality seen (C) – Methylmalonic acidemia

Differential diagnoses in bilateral globus pallidus disease without involvement of the other basal ganglia components include methylmalonic aciduria, kernicterus and carbon monoxide intoxication. In kernicterus, lesions of subthalamic nuclei are associated with the globus pallidus lesions. Carbon monoxide intoxication is usually encountered in suggestive clinical settings.

Management consists of vitamin $B_{1,2}$ supplementation and dietary protein restriction.

Propionic Acidemia

This is also a disorder of organic acid metabolism. It is a relatively common organic acidopathy. The deficiency enzyme is propionyl coenzyme A carboxylase. Clinical features include cognitive disability, cardiomyopathy, pancreatitis, osteoporosis and movement disorders

Imaging Findings

During metabolic crisis diffuse brain swelling is seen. Signal abnormalities within the basal ganglia and the dentate nuclei are seen on the T2-weighted images. Subtle signal changes may be present within the pulvinar of the thalami. The cerebral and cerebellar cortices are also affected. The involved gray matter structures are swollen at this stage. White matter structures also show signal changes, mainly subcortically, including the periinsular areas (external and extreme capsules). The corpus callosum, the internal capsule and corticospinal tracts are spared. Diffusion-weighted images usually show moderate signal increase within the involved gray matter structures and the subcortical white matter.

MR spectroscopy demonstrates lactate within the lesion areas consistent with impairment of the energy metabolism resulting in anaerobic glycolysis. No disease-specific metabolites are identified.

Methylmalonic Acidemia

Methylmalonic aciduria typically presents with basal ganglia disease but patchy white matter lesions may also be present within the cerebral hemispheres. The signal changes within the heads of the caudate nuclei and the putamina are patchy and inhomogeneous. This may help to raise the possibility of the disease and differentiate it from other organic acidopathies. A distinct clinical feature of the disease is the widespread cutaneous petechiae and ecchymoses indicative of vasculopathy.[113]

Methylglutaconic Aciduria

The disease has at least four clinical phenotypic presentations. Type 2 has an X-linked inheritance, the others are autosomal recessive. The typical imaging presentation in types 1 and 4 of this metabolic disorder is, as in many other organic acidopathies, also the symmetrical bilateral basal ganglia disease.

Imaging Finding

During the acute stage of the disease, the basal ganglia are swollen and exhibit high signal on the diffusion-weighted images suggestive of cytotoxic edema. Sometimes, only the globi pallidi,

the caudate nuclei and the anterior parts of the putamina are involved; posteriorly they are spared. With the progression of the disease, the putaminal abnormalities become complete. In some cases, ill defined, diffuse cerebral white matter signal changes are also present. During the metabolic crisis the cerebellar cortex and the dentate nuclei may also show signal abnormalities. Cerebellar atrophy is a very characteristic imaging finding. The vermis is usually more affected than the cerebellar hemispheres. **The association of cerebellar atrophy and basal ganglia disease is a suggestive imaging pattern of 3-methylglutaconic aciduria.**

On MR spectroscopy lactate is present within the lesion areas but no disease specific metabolite is identified.

3-Hydroxy-3-methylglutaryl (HMG)-Coenzyme a Lyase Deficiency

This is a relatively rare metabolic disorder of the L-leucine break down pathway. The disease may present with metabolic crises with hypoglycemia and ketoacidosis. MR imaging usually reveals non-specific abnormalities.

Since the disease usually starts in the early postnatal period or in early infancy, initially the gray matter abnormalities are easier to depict, since the white matter is not myelinated. Later, as the brain myelination progresses, the white matter changes, which correspond to demyelination become more apparent. The gray matter abnormalities involve the basal ganglia and the dentate nuclei. They are fairly subtle in most cases and do not seem to lead to necrosis if the disease is appropriately treated. The white matter abnormalities within the cerebral hemispheres are sometimes patchy, but usually confluent. The subcortical U-fibers are often spared. Diffusion-weighted imaging shows faint hyper signal within the involved white matter structures.

MR spectroscopy invariably demonstrates disease specific abnormalities with *two abnormal peaks at the 1.3 and 2.4 ppm levels.*

Glutaric Aciduria Type 1

Glutaric aciduria type 1 is usually an insidiously developing metabolic disease. The disorder may be diagnosed during a metabolic crisis, which is typically triggered by a febrile illness.

In the clinically mild phenotypes no parenchymal lesions may be seen. Patients with type 1 glutaric aciduria are usually macrocephalic. Another peculiar imaging finding is the bilateral enlargement of the sylvian fissures. They may correspond to arachnoidal cysts or disturbed and incomplete opercularization. They are usually bilateral but not necessarily symmetrical. Rarely, the abnormality is unilateral. These changes may be detected prenatally or in the early postnatal period by ultrasound. Macrocephaly and Sylvian fissure abnormalities are present in both the clinically benign and malignant phenotypes.

Prominent brain atrophy may also develop. Chronic subdural hematomas are relatively frequently seen in type 1 glutaric aciduria without any evidence of significant head trauma in the clinical history.

The presence of bilateral Sylvian fissure and temporal lobe CSF space enlargement and bilateral basal ganglia lesions in

Table 30.4: Disorders of amino acid metabolism[16]		
Disease	Imaging findings	Clinical findings
Maple syrup urine disease	Swelling and increase signal T2 WI: brainstem, GP, cerebellum, posterior limb of internal capsule	Neonate: coma Seizures Respiratory failure
Glutaric aciduria type I	Prominent extraaxial spaces, increase signal T2 WI: bilateral caudate, putamen; delay in myelination	Infancy /childhood Encephalopathy Macrocephaly
Phenylketonuria	Delay in myelination; increase signal T2 WI; periatrial WM	Normal at birth Developmental delay Varying severity
Nonketotic hyperglycinemia	Increase signal T2 WI: periventricular WM; delay in myelination	Early infancy Vomiting, seizures Apnea
Urea cycle defects	Neonates: brain swelling Acute stages: multifocal swollen areas cortex and subcortical WM Chronic stages: diffuse atrophy, delay in myelination	Infancy: lethargy, coma Childhood:episodic lethargy, confusion, ataxia, dysarthria, coma

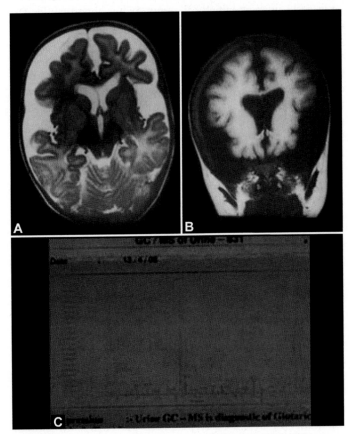

Figs 30.34A to C: Axial T2 W (A) and FLAIR coronal (B) MR images showing enlargement of bilateral sylvian fissures (A) with cysts in the temporal lobes (B) and signal abnormality in the bilateral putamen (A). Urine gas chromatography mass spectroscopy (C) revealing an abnormal glutaric acid peak – Glutaric aciduria type 1.

a macrocephalic child are almost pathognomonic of type 1 glutaric aciduria (Figs 30.34A to C). T2 prolongation is seen in the basal ganglia, most commonly the putamen, less commonly,

the caudate and rarely the globus pallidus and periventricular white matter.[114]

MR spectroscopy may show lactate within the basal ganglia during the acute stage of the disease. Although the possible role of glutamine glutamate complexes in the pathogenesis of basal ganglia disease has been raised (glutamine 'excitotoxicity' or glutamine 'suicide') increased glutamine glutamate levels have not been demonstrated within the basal ganglia by *in vivo* MR spectroscopy. Table 30.4 gives the differentiating features between various amino acid disorders.

METABOLIC DISORDERS PRIMARILY AFFECTING GRAY MATTER

Hallervorden-Spatz Disease

It is a rare metabolic disorder that is characterized clinically by progressive gait impairment, gradually increasing rigidity of all limbs, choreoathetoid movements, dysarthria and mental retardation. In the classic form onset of symptoms occurs before the age of 10 years while the atypical form has an older age of onset.

The striking pathologic finding in affected patients is rust brown pigmentation of the globus pallidus and zona reticulata of the substantia nigra. Iron is concentrated in these regions.

Imaging studies reflect the underlying pathology. Computed tomography scans show high or low density foci in the globus pallidi. Magnetic resonance shows a pronounced hypointensity in both the globus pallidus and substantia nigra on T2W imaging resulting from iron deposition.

Imaging reveals a characteristic "eye of the tiger sign" with marked pallidal hypointensity peripherally and hyperintensity centrally. The hyperintense signal represents pallidal destruction and gliosis.

Neuronal Ceroid Lipofuscinosis (NCL)

These are among the most common progressive encephalopathies of childhood. Eight types have been described and are grouped gether because of similar pathologic and clinical presentation. he first symptom is loss of vision followed by progressive :mentia, seizures and progressive impairment of speech and otor function. Definitive diagnosis is made by chromosomal alysis or by electron microscopic analysis of lymphocytes from eripheral blood which show characteristic curvilinear deposits.

naging Findings

here is variable cerebral and cerebellar atrophy associated with gh signal rims around ventricles and low signal intensity in the alami and globi pallidi on T2 weighted images. The T2 changes ppear to correlate with loss of myelin and gliosis of unknown igin. Thalamic atrophy develops later. MR spectroscopy shows complete loss of NAA peak, marked reduction of creatine and oline and elevation of myo-inositol and lactate in gray and white atter.[115] PET AND SPECT are useful in establishing the agnosis in NCL. Severe reduction of metabolism in the cortical d subcortical structures have been shown in 18 fluoro-oxyglucose PET studies.

ett Syndrome

ett syndrome is a progressive neurodevelopmental disorder aracterized by autistic like behavior, gait, ataxia, irregular spiration, seizures, dementia and microcephaly. On imaging, ere is a global reduction in gray and white matter volumes with e largest reductions in the prefrontal, posterior frontal, anterior mporal cortices and the caudate nucleus. Proton MRS shows creased NAA in older patients, more pronounced in gray matter an the white. The frontal and parietal lobes and insular cortex e the ones which are predominantly involved.

SORDERS OF METAL METABOLISM

ilson's Disease (Hepatolenticular egeneration)

ilson's disease results from an inborn error of copper meta-lism and is transmitted in an autosomal recessive manner. It characterized by a deficiency of ceruloplasmin, the serum insport protein for copper. As a result, copper is abnormally posited in various tissues with resultant toxicity to these organs. ver and brain are the most frequently involved with typical volvement of the lenticular nucleus.

linical Features

e peak age of presentation is between 8 and 16 years. Typical urologic signs include tremor, rigidity, dystonia, gait difficulty coordination and dysarthria. The Kayser-Fleischer ring, ring of een pigmentation in cornea, is virtually diagnostic of Wilson's sease.

naging

pical sites of cerebral involvement are deep gray matter. Gray atter involvement is usually bilaterally symmetric in the itamen, caudate, thalamus, globus pallidus, dentate nucleus, pons d mesencephalon and the claustra. *Involvement of the claustra a very characteristic finding and an important differential*

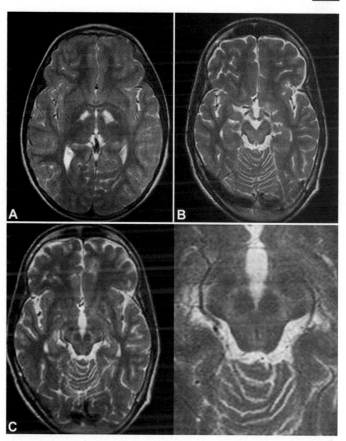

Figs 30.35A to C: Axial T2 W MR images showing symmetrical signal changes in the putamen seen as a high signal. High signal is also seen within the substantia nigra and tegmentum with sparing of the red nucleus and tectum (C) "face of giant panda sign" – Wilson's disease

diagnostic clue in Wilson's disease. The lesions are seen as hyperintensity on long TR images and reflect the pathologic changes of gliosis, edema and/or necrosis. *Mesencephalic involvement is characteristic, the so called "face of the giant panda sign"* (Figs 30.35A to C). This consists of high signal throughout the mesencephalon within the substantia nigra (mainly in the pars compacta) and the tegmentum of the mesencephalon in contrast with the normal or hypointense appearance of the red nuclei, the cerebral peduncles and the tectum. Some of these lesions appear to improve or reverse during treatment. In contrast to gray matter lesions, white matter lesions, if present are asymmetric, located in the subcortical regions and are commonest in the frontal lobes. The MR findings correlate well with neurologic findings. Lesion location is also useful. For example, dystonia correlates with putaminal lesions, dysarthria with both caudate and putaminal lesion and distractibility of gaze fixation with frontal lobe involvement. MR spectroscopy shows a decrease in all the metabolites.[116]

Menkes' Disease

Menkes' disease is related to a defect at the level of the membrane copper transport mechanism. One of the consequences of this is the impairment of the normal intestinal absorption of copper as a result of which a severe copper deficiency develops. On the other hand, transmembrane transport of copper is impaired, therefore, copper cannot be delivered to copper requiring enzymes, and hence copper is trapped and accumulated in connective tissues. Serum copper and ceruloplasmin levels are low. The most important manifestations of the disease are therefore connective tissue abnormalities and progressive degeneration of the central nervous system, the latter due to global failure of copper-requiring enzymes, in particular cytochrome C-oxidase.

The disease is of X-linked inheritance. The onset of the disease is neonatal but the patients are typically normal during the first 2 or 3 months of life. Then there is loss of milestones, convulsions, hypotonia followed by spasticity and eventually lethargy. Most affected children die during the first year of life. Menkes disease is often referred to as 'kinky hair' disease because of the peculiar appearance of the hair. Connective tissue abnormalities include bladder diverticula, inguinal hernia, loose skin, hyperflexible joints and vessel wall fragility.

At birth, the brain appears normal on MR imaging. During the course of the disease rapidly developing atrophy and prominent delay of the myelination become obvious. Shrinking of the brain can be so marked that spontaneous subdural fluid collections (hygroma, subdural hematoma) frequently develop. On the T1-weighted images the basal ganglia exhibit hypersignal, similar to what is seen in chronic hepatic encephalopathies, including Wilson disease. The cerebral vessels are usually tortuous and elongated; this can be seen on conventional images but is better appreciated on MR angiography.[117]

CONCLUSION

There are many different metabolic disorders, each of which has some distinctive features. MR imaging is highly sensitive in determining the presence and assessing the severity of underlying abnormalities in patients with metabolic disorders. Although the findings are often non-specific, systematic analysis of the finer details of disease involvement may permit a narrower differential diagnosis, which the clinician can then further refine with knowledge of patient history, clinical testing and metabolic analysis. MR imaging has a role in monitoring the natural progression of various metabolic disorders and response to therapy.

REFERENCES

1. Holland BA, Haas DK, Norman D, et al. MRI of normal brain maturation. Am J Neuroradiol 1986; 7:201-8.
2. Hasegawa M, Houdou S, Mito T, et al. Development of myelination in the human fetal and infant cerebrum: A myelin basic protein immunohistochemical study. Brain Dev 1992; 14:1.
3. Barkovich AJ, Kjos BO, Jackson DE, et al. Normal maturation of the neonatal and infant brain: MR Imaging at 1.5T. Radiology 1988; 166:173-80.
4. Johnson MA, Pennock JM, Bydder GM, et al. Clinical NMR images of the brain in children : Normal and neurologic disease. AJR 1983; 141:1005-18.

5. Dietrich RB. Maturation, myelination and dysmyelination. In Stark DD, Bradley WG (Eds): Magnetic Resonance Imaging (3rd ed) Mosby 1999.
6. Barkovich AJ, Jackson DE J. MRI assessment of normal and abnormal brain myelinization. MRI Decisions 1989; 19-25.
7. Dietrich RB, Bradley WG. Normal and abnormal white matter maturation. Seminars in Ultrasound, CT and MR 1988; 9:192-20.
8. Dietrich RB, Bradley WG, Zaragoza EJ, et al. MR evaluation of early myelination patterns in normal and developmentally delayed infants. Am J Neuroradiol 1988; 9:69-76.
9. Becker LE. Lysosomes peroxisomes and mitochondria: Function and disorder. Am J Neuroradiol 1992; 13:609-20.
10. Kendell BE. Disorders of lysosomes peroxisomes and mitochondria. Am J Neuroradiol 1992; 13:621-53.
11. Demaerel P, Faubert C, Wilms G, et al. MR findings in leukodystrophy. Neuroradiology 1991; 33:368-71.
12. Kim TS, Kim IO, Kim WS, et al. MR of childhood metachromatic leukodystrophy. Am J Neuroradiol 1997; 18:733-8.
13. Suzuki K, Armao D, Stone JA, Mukherji SK. Demyelinating diseases, leukodystrophies and other myelin disorders. Neuroimaging Clinics of North America 2001; 2:15-32.
14. Kolodny EH: Sulfatide lipidosis: Metachromatic leukodystrophy. In Scriver CR, Baedet AL, Syl W, et al (Eds): The Metabolic Basis of Inherited Diseases (6th ed) New York NY: McGraw Hill, 19.
15. Wolpert SM, Anderson ML, Kaye EM. Metabolic and degenerative disorders. In Wolpert SM, Barnes PD (Eds): MRI in Pediatric Neuroradiology. Mosby, 1992.
16. Nusbaum AO, Rapaleno, O Fung KM, Atlas SW. White matter diseases and inherited metabolic disorders. In Atlas SW (Ed) Magnetic Resonance Imaging of the Brain and Spine (4th ed) Lippincott Williams and Wilkins, 2009.
17. Waltz G, Harik SI, Haufman B. Adult metachromatic leukodystrophy. Arch Neurol 1987; 44:225.
18. Faerber EN, Melvin JJ, Smergel DM. MRI appearances of metachromatic leukodystrophy. Paediatr Radiol 1999; 29:669-.
19. Nowell MA, Grossman RI, Hackney DB, et al. MR imaging of white matter disease in children. Am J Neuroradiol 1988; 9:50.
20. Sener RN. Metachromatic leukodystrophy. Diffusion MR imaging findings. Am J Neuroradiol 2002; 22(3):461-76.
21. Patay Z. Diffusion weighted MR imaging in leukodystrophies. Eur Radiol 2005; 15(11):2284-2303.
22. Kruse B, Hanefeld F, Christen HJ, et al. Alterations of brain metabolites in metachromatic leukodystrophy as detected by localized proton magnetic resonance spectroscopy in vivo. J Neurol 1993; 241:68.
23. Suzuki Y, Suzuki K. Krabbe's globoid cell leukodystrophy. Deficiency of galactocerebrosidase in serum, leukocytes and fibroblast. Science 1971; 171:73-5.
24. Zlotogora J, Chakraborty S, Knowlton RG, et al. Krabbe disease locus mapped to chromosome 14 by genetic linkage. Am J H Genet 1990; 47:37-44.
25. Loes DJ, Peters C, Krivit W. Globoid cell leukodystrophy: Distinguishing early onset from late-onset disease using a brain MR imaging scoring method. Am J Neuroradiol 1999; 20:316-.
26. Demaerel P, Wilms G, Vendue P, et al. MR findings in globoid leukodystrophy. Neuroradiology 1990; 32:520.
27. Kolodny EH, Raghavan S, Krivit W. Late onset Krabbe disease (globoid cell leukodystrophy): Clinical and biochemical features of 15 cases. Dev Neurosci 1991; 13:232.

28. Lyon G, Hagberg B, Evard PH, et al. Symptomatology of late onset Krabbe's leukodystrophy: The European experience. Dev Neurosci 1991; 13:240.

29. Krivit W, Shapiro EG, Peters C, et al. Hematopoietic cell transplantation in globoid cell leukodystrophy. N Eng J Med 1998; 338:1119-26.

30. Barone R, Bruhl K, Stoeter P, et al. Clinical and neuroradiological findings in classic infantile and late onset globoid cell leukodystrophy (Krabbe's disease). Am J Med Genet 1996; 63:209-17.

31. Vanhanen SL, Raininko R, Santavilori P. Early differential diagnosis of infantile ceroid lipofuscinosis, Rett Syndrome and Krabbe's disease by CT and MR. Am J Neuroradiol 1994; 15:1443-53.

32. Choi S, Enzmann D. Infantile Krabbe disease : Complementary CT and MR findings. Am J Neuroradiol 1993; 14:1164-6.

33. Jones BV, Barron TF, Towfighi J. Optic nerve enlargement in Krabbe's disease. Am J Neuroradiol 1999; 20:1228-31.

34. Krabbe K. A new familial, infantile form of diffuse brain sclerosis. Brain 1916; 39:74-114.

35. Barker RH, Trautman JC, Younge BR, et al. Late juvenile onset Krabbe disease. Ophthalmology 1990; 97:1176-80.

36. Loes DJ, Hite S, Moser H, et al. Adrenoleukodystrophy: A scoring method for brain MR observations. Am J Neuroradiol 1994; 15:1761-5.

37. Vasconcellos E, Smith M. MRI nerve root enhancement in Krabbe disease. Pediatric Neurology 1998; 19:151-2.

38. Kim MJ, Provenzale JM, Law M. Magnetic resonance and diffusion tensor imaging in paediatric white matter diseases. Top Magn Reson Imaging 2006; 17(4):265-71.

39. Provenzale JM, Escolar M, Kurtzberg J. Quantitative analysis of diffusion tensor imaging data in serial assessment of Krabbe disease.Ann NY Acad Sci 2005; 1064:220-9.

40. Mc Graw P, et al. Krabbe disease treated with hematopoietic stem cell transplantation : serial assessment of anisotropy measurements –initial experience. Radiology 2005; 236:221-30.

41. Okada S, McCrea M, O'Brien JS. Sandhoff's disease (GM2 gangliosidosis Type 2): Clinical, chemical and enzyme studies in five patients. Pediat Res 1972; 6:606.

42. Boothman BR, Bamford JM, Parsons MR. Magnetic resonance imaging in Fabry's disease. J Neurol Neurosurg Psychiatry 1985; 51:1240-1.

43. Mirowitz SA, Sartor K, Prensky AJ, et al. Neuro-degenerative diseases of childhood: MR and CT evaluation. J Comput Assist Tomogr 1991; 15:210-22.

44. Murata R, Nakajma S, Tanaka A, et al. MR imaging of the brain in patients with mucopolysaccharidosis. Am J Neuroradiol 1989; 10:1165-70.

45. Johnson MA, Desai S, Hugh Jones K, et al. Magnetic resonance imaging of the brain in Hurler syndrome. Am J Neuroradiol 1984; 5:816-9.

46. Walts RWE, Spellacy E, Kendell BE, et al. Computed tomography studies on patients with mucopolysaccharidosis. Neuroradiology 1981; 21:9-23.

47. Moser HW. Adrenoleukodystrophy: Phenotype, genetics, pathogenesis and therapy. Brain 1997; 120:1485-1508.

48. Bezman L, Moser HW. The incidence of X-linked adrenoleukodystrophy and the relative frequency of its phenotypes. Am J Med Genet 1998; 76:415-9.

49. Griffin JW, Goren E, Schaumberg HH, et al. Adrenomyeloneuropathy: A probable variant of adrenoleukodystrophy. Neurology 1977; 27:1107-13.

50. Schaumburg HH, Powers JM, Raine CS, et al. Adrenoleukodystrophy: A clinical and pathological study of 17 cases. Arch Neurol 1975; 32:577-91.

51. Powers JM, Liu Y, Moser AB, et al. The inflammatory myelinopathy of adrenoleukodystrophy: Cells, effector molecules and pathogenetic implications. J Neuropathol Exp Neurol 1992; 51:630-43.

52. Jensen ME. MR imaging appearance of adrenoleukodystrophy with auditory, visual and motor pathway involvement. Radiographics 1990; 10:53.

53. Kumar AJ, Rosenbaum AE, Naidu S, et al. Adrenoleukodystrophy: Correlating MR imaging with CT. Radiology 1987; 165:497.

54. Ono J, Kodaka R, Imai K, et al. Evaluation of myelination by means of T2 value on magnetic resonance imaging. Brain Dev 1993; 15:433.

55. Melhem ER, Breiter SN, Ulug AM, et al. Improved tissue characterization in adrenoleukodystrophy using magnetization transfer imaging. Am J Roentgenol 1996; 166:689-95.

56. Melhem ER, Loes DJ, Georgiades CS, et al. X-linked adrenoleukodystrophy : The role of contrast enhanced MR imaging in predicting disease progression. Am J Neuroradiol 2000; 21:839-44.

57. Barkovich AJ, Ferriero DM, Bass N, et al. Involvement of the pontomedullary corticospinal tracts: A useful finding in the diagnosis of X-linked adrenoleukodystrophy. Am J Neuroradiol 1997; 18:95-100.

58. Castellote A, Vera J, Vazquez E, et al. MR in adrenoleukodystrophy: Atypical presentation as bilateral frontal demyelination. Am J Neuroradiol 1995; 16:814-5.

59. Tzika AA, Ball WAS, Vigneron DB, et al. Childhood adrenoleukodystrophy : Assessment with proton MR spectroscopy. Radiology 1993; 189:467-80.

60. Warren DJ, et al. Magnetic resonance spectroscopy changes following hematopoietic stem cell transplantation in children with cerebral adrenoleukodystrophy. Dev Med Child Neurol 2007; 49(2):135-9.

61. Wilken B, et al. Quantitative proton magnetic resonance spectroscopy of children with adrenoleukodystrophy before and after hematopoietic stem cell transplantation. Neuropediatrics 2003; 34:237-46.

62. Fatemi A, et al. Magnetization transfer MRI demonstrates spinal cord abnormalities in adrenomyeloneurophathy. Neurology 2005; 64(10):1739-45.

63. Barkovich AJ, Peck WW. MR of Zellweger's syndrome. Am J Neuroradiol 1997; 16:1163-70.

64. Cheon JE, Kim IO, Hwang YS, et al. Leukodystrophy in children: A pictorial review of MR Imaging features. Radiographics 2002; 22:461-76.

65. Hokezu Y, Kuriyama M, Kubota R. Cerebrotendinous xanthomatosis: Cranial CT and MRI studies in eight patients. Neuroradiology 1992; 34:308-12.

66. Matalon R, Michals K, Sebasta D, et al. Asparto-acyclase deficiency and N-acetylaspartic aciduria in patients with Canavan's disease. Am J Med Genet 1988; 29:463-71.

67. Grodd W, et al. In vivo assessment of N-acetylaspartate in brain in spongy degeneration (Canavan's disease) by proton spectroscopy. Lancet 1990; 336(8712):437-8.

68. Patel PJ, Kolawole TM, Mahdi AH, et al. Sonographic and computed tomographic findings in Canavan's disease. Br J Radiol 1986; 59:1226-8.

69. Brismar J, Brismar G, Gascon G, et al. Canavan disease: CT and MR imaging of Canavan disease. Am J Neuroradiol 1990; 11:805-10.

70. Mc Adam HP, Geyer CA, Done SL, et al: CT and MR imaging of Canavan disease. Am J Neuroradiol 1990; 11:397-9.

71. Srikanth SG, et al. Restricted diffusion in Canavan disease. Child Nerv Syst 2007; 23(4):465-8.

72. Lyon G, Fattal - Valevski A, Kolodny EH. Leukodystrophies: Clinical and genetic aspect. Top Magn Reson Imaging 2006; 17(4):219-42.

73. Brrett D, Becker LE. Alexander's disease: A disease of astrocytes. Brain 1985; 108:367-85.

74. Shah M, Ross JS: Infantile Alexander disease: MR appearance of a biopsy proven case. Am J Neuroradiol 1990; 11:1105-6.

75. Trommer BL, Naidich JP, Dal Canto MC, et al. Noninvasive CT diagnosis of infantile Alexander's disease: Pathologic correlation. J Comput Assist Tomogr 1983; 7:509-16.

76. Van der Knaap MS, Barth PG, Gabreels FJM, et al. A new leukoencephalopathy with Vanishing white matter. Neurology 1997; 48:845-55.

77. Sijens PE et al. [1]H chemical shift imaging, MRI and diffusion weighted imaging in vanishing white matter disease. Eur Radiol 2005; 15(11):2377-9.

78. Seitelberger F. Neuropathology and genetics of Pelizaeus-Merzbacher disease. Brain Pathol 1995; 5:267-73.

79. Silverstein AM, Hirsh DK, Trobe JD, et al. MR imaging of the brain in five members of a family with Pelizaeus-Merzbacher disease. Am J Neuroradiol 1990; 11:495-9.

80. Van der Knaap MS, Valk J: The reflection of histology in MR imaging of Pelizaeus-Merzbacher disease. Am J Neuroradiol 1989; 10:99-103.

81. Honkaniemi J, Kahari V, Latvala M, et al. Reversible posterior leukoencephalopathy after combination chemotherapy. Neuroradiology 2000; 42:895.

82. Kingsley PB, Shah JC, Woldenberg R. Identification of diffuse and focal brain lesions by clinical magnetic resonance spectroscopy. NMR Biomed 2006; 19(4):435-62.

83. Pavlakis SG, Philips PC, DiMauro S, et al. Mitochondrial myopathy, encephalopathy, lactic acidosis and stroke like episodes: A distinct clinical syndrome. Ann Neurol 1984; 16:481-8.

84. Barkovich AJ, Good WV, Koch TK, et al. Mitochondrial disorders: Analysis of their clinical and imaging characteristics. Am J Neuroradiol 1993; 14:1119-37.

85. Allard JC, Tilak S, Carter AP. CT and MR of MELAS syndrome. Am J Neuroradiol 1988; 9:1234-8.

86. Kim IO, Kim JH, Kim SUS, et al. Mitochondrial Myopathy encephalopathylactic acidosis and stroke like episodes (MELAS) syndrome: CT and MR findings in seven children. AJR 1996;166:641-5.

87. Rosen L, Phillips S, Enzmann D. Magnetic resonance imaging in MELAS syndrome. Neuroradiology 1990; 32:168-71.

88. Ducreux D, et al. MR diffusion tensor imaging, fiber tracking and single voxel spectroscopy findings in an unusual MELAS case. Am J Neuroradiol 2005; 26(7):1840-4.

89. Wray S, Provenzale J, Johns O, et al. MR of brain in mitochondri myopathy. Am J Neuroradiol 1995; 16:1167.

90. Fukuhara N, Tokiguchi S, Shirakawa K, et al. Myoclonus epileps associated with ragged red fibres (mitochondrial abnormalities Disease entity or a syndrome? J Neurol Sci 1980; 47:117-33.

91. Kearns TP, Sayre GP. Retinitis pigmentosa, external ophthal moplegia and complete heart block. Arch Ophthalmol 1958; 6 280-9.

92. Leutner C, Layer G, Zierz S, et al. Cerebral MR in ophthal-mopleg plus. Am J Neuroradiol 1994; 15:681-7.

93. Sandhu FS, Dillon WP. MR demonstration of leukoencephalopath associated with mitochondrial encephalomyopathy: Case report. A J Neuroradiol 1991; 12:375-79.

94. DiMauro S, Servidei S, Zeviam M, et al. Cytochrome C oxidas deficiency in Leigh syndrome. Ann Neurol 1987; 22:498-506.

95. Chi JG, Yoo HW, Chang KH, et al. Leigh subacute necrotizir encephalomyelopathy: Possible diagnosis by CT sca Neuroradiology 1981; 22:141-4.

96. Berkovic SF, Karpati G, Carpenter S, et al. Progressive dyston with bilateral putaminal hypodensities. Arch Neurol 1987; 44:118-7.

97. Koch TK, Yee MHC, Hutchinson HT, et al. Magnetic resonan imaging in subacute necrotizing encephalomyelopathy (Leig disease). Ann Neurol 1986; 19:605-7.

98. Medina L, Chi TL, DeVivo DC, et al. MR findings in patients wi subacute necrotizing encephalomyelopathy (Leigh syndrome Correlation with biochemical defect. Am J Neuroradiol 199 11:379-84.

99. Leigh D. Subacute necrotizing encephalomyelopathy in an infa J Neurol Neurosurg Psychiatry 1951; 14:216-21.

100. Atalar MH, et al. Magnetic resonance spectroscopy and diffusi weighted imaging findings in a child with Leigh disease. Pedia Int 2005; 47(5):601-3.

101. Chen YF., Huang YC, Liu HM, et al. MRI in a case of adult ons citrullinemia.Neuroradiology 2001; 43:845-7.

102. Connelly A, Cross JH, Gadian G, et al. Magnetic resonan spectroscopy shows increased brain glutamine in ornithi carbamoyl transferase deficiency. Pediatric Research 1993; 33:7 81.

103. Pearsen KD, Gean Marton AD, Levy HL, Davis K Phenylketonuria : MRI of the brain with clinical correlatio Radiology 1990; 177:437-40.

104. Phillips MD, Mc Graw P, Lowe MJ, Mathews VP, Hainline B Diffusion weighted imaging of white matter abnormalities in patie with phenylketonuria. Am J Neuroradiol 2001; 22:1583-6.

105. Pietz J, Kreis R, Schmidt H, et al. Phenylketonuria :findings at M imaging and localized in vivo H- I MR spectroscopy of the brain patients with early treatment. Raidology 1996; 201:413-20.

106. Brismar J, Aqueel A, Brusmar G, et al. Maple syrup urine disea Am J Neuroradiol 1990; 11:1219-28.

107. Fariello G, Dionisi – Vici C, Orazi C, et al. Cranial ultrasonograp in maple syrup urine disease. Am J Neuroradiol 1996; 17:311-5

108. Jan W, Zimmerman R, Wang Z, et al. MR diffusion imaging a MR spectroscopy of maple syrup urine disease during acu metabolic decompensation. Neuroradiology 2003; 45:393-9.

109. Rossi A, Cerone R, Biancheri R, et al. Early onset combin methylmalonic aciduria and homocystinuria. Neuroradiolog findings. Am J Neuroradiol 2001; 22:554-63

110. Press GA, Barshop BA, Haas RH, et al. Abnormalities of the brain in non ketotic hyperglycinemia: MR Manifestations. Am J Neuroradiol 1989; 10:315-21.

111. AI Tawari A, Ramadan P, Neubauer D, et al. An early onset form of methylene terahydrofolate reductase deficiency: A report of a family from Kuwait. Brain Dev 2002; 24:304-9.

112. Brismar J, Ozand P. CT and MR of the brain in the diagnosis of organic acidemias. Experiences from 107 patients. Brain Dev 1994; 16 (Suppl):104-24.

113. Ozand P, Rashed M, Millingtian D, et al. Ethylmalonic aciduria : an organic academia with CNS involvement and vasculopathy.Brain Dev 1994; 16 (supp):12-22.

114. Brismar J, Ozand P. CT and MR of the brain in glutaric academia type 1 : a review of 59 published cases and a report of 5 new patients. Am J Neuroradiol 1995; 16:675-83.

115. Brockmann K, et al. Localized proton magnetic resonance spectroscopy of cerebral metabolic disturbances in children with neuronal ceroid lipofuscinosis – Neuropediatrics 1996; 27:242-8.

116. Jayasunder R, Sahani A, Gaikwaid S, Singh S, Behari M. Proton MR spectroscopy of basal ganglia in Wilson disease : case report and review of literature. Mag Reson Imaging 2002; 20:131-5.

117. Jacobs DS, Smith AS, Finelli DA, et al. Menkes Kinky hair disease: characteristic MR angiographic findings. Am J Neuroradiol 1993; 14:1160-3.